THE CALORIEKING®
Calorie, Fat & Carbohydrate Counter

Contents

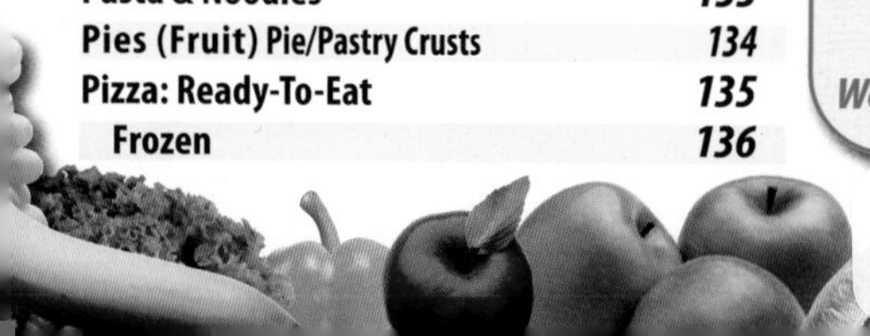

Weight Control Tips

Eat & Drink Sensibly

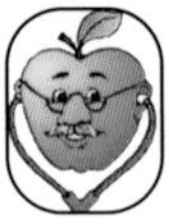

- Avoid fad diets. Eat 3 sensible portion-controlled meals daily.
- Limit fats, high-fat foods/snacks and sugar. Eat adequate fresh fruit & vegetables.
- Limit soft drinks, energy drinks, fruit juice and alcohol. Quench your thirst on water. (See Sample Meal Plan ~ Page 11)

Exercise Daily

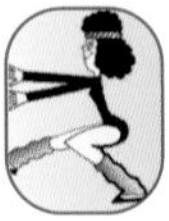

- Aim for at least 30 minutes daily – even in 5-10 minute lots. For motivation, find an exercise buddy, personal trainer or join a gym. *(Extra Notes ~ Page 12)*

Reshape Eating Behaviors

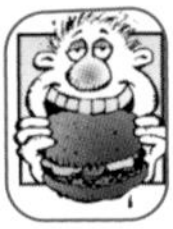

- Be aware of eating and shopping behaviors that lead to overeating.
- Also focus on social and emotional situations that may trigger compulsive eating. *(Extra Notes ~ Page 14)*

Keep a Food & Exercise Journal

- A journal helps you see exactly what you eat and drink, and how much you exercise. *(Extra Notes ~ Page 15)*

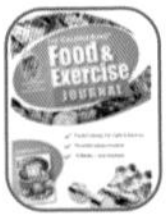

- An excellent motivator and proven weight loss aid. Keeps you honest!

Arrange Moral Support

- Gain the support of family and friends.
- Get extra professional help if required, from your doctor, dietitian, psychologist, exercise trainer, or slimming group.

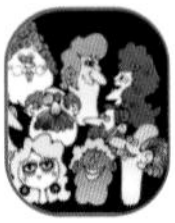

- Beware of family saboteurs who may discourage you from adopting a healthier diet and lifestyle!

DOCTOR CHECK-UP

Ask your doctor to check your blood pressure, blood sugar and blood cholesterol levels.

HEALTHY WEIGHTS
~ MEN & WOMEN ~
(Over 18 Years)

Based on weights with least risk of disease or death from heart disease, diabetes, stroke and cancer.

Based on Body Mass Index of 20-25

BMI calculated as: $\frac{\text{Weight (kg)}}{\text{Height (m)}^2}$

Height (No Shoes) Ft Ins		Healthy Weight Range (Pounds)
4'7"	~	86-108
4'8"	~	88-110
4'9"	~	92-114
4'10"	~	97-121
4'11"	~	99-123
5'0"	~	101-127
5'1"	~	105-132
5'2"	~	110-136
5'3"	~	112-140
5'4"	~	114-145
5'5"	~	119-149
5'6"	~	123-156
5'7"	~	127-158
5'8"	~	129-162
5'9"	~	134-167
5'10"	~	138-173
5'11"	~	143-178
6'0"	~	145-182
6'1"	~	149-187
6'2"	~	156-193
6'3"	~	158-198
6'4"	~	162-202
6'5"	~	170-211
6'6"	~	172-215
6'7"	~	175-220

Body Fat Distribution & Health

Moderate amounts of body fat do not compromise health. However, excess fat above the hips carries a far greater health risk than fat on or below the hips - better to be a 'pear-shape' than an 'apple-shape'.

Abdominal obesity greatly increases the risk of developing diabetes, heart disease, high blood fats, hypertension, stroke, sleep apnea, arthritis and some cancers. So-called 'cellulite' carries no extra health risk.

Waist Circumference directly reflects the increased health risk of abdominal obesity. Waist size associated with a high health risk:

Men ~ Over 40 inches **Women** ~ Over 35 inches

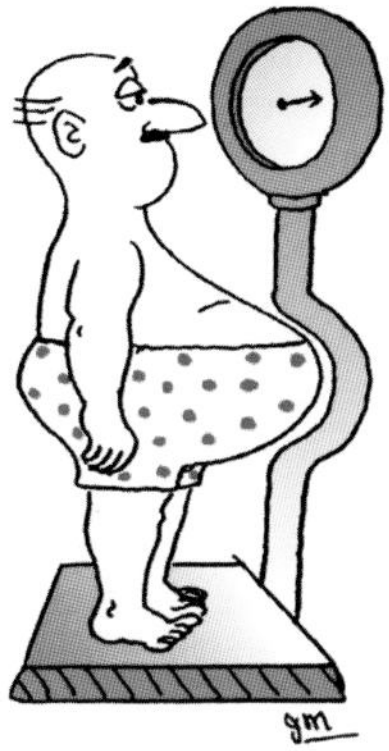

Abdominal obesity greatly increases the risk of ill-health and earlier death.

Body Mass Index (BMI)

BMI is a general (but not specific) indicator of body fatness. Although BMI alone is not diagnostic, the higher the BMI, the greater the health risk of developing diabetes, high blood pressure and heart disease. BMI does not apply to heavily muscled persons. BMI is used in a different way for children.

Check Your BMI: Find your height (no shoes) - look across the row to the weight nearest your own. Then track down to BMI.

Ht	WEIGHT (LBS) ~ ADULTS												
5'1"	100	106	111	116	122	127	132	137	143	148	153	158	185	211
5'2"	104	109	115	120	126	131	136	142	147	153	158	164	191	218
5'3"	107	113	118	124	130	135	141	146	152	158	163	169	197	225
5'4"	110	116	122	128	134	140	145	151	157	163	169	174	204	232
5'5"	114	120	126	132	138	144	150	156	162	168	174	180	210	240
5'6"	118	124	130	136	142	148	155	161	167	173	179	186	216	247
5'7"	121	127	134	140	146	153	159	166	172	178	185	191	223	255
5'8"	125	131	138	144	151	158	164	171	177	184	190	197	230	262
5'9"	128	135	142	149	155	162	169	176	182	189	196	206	236	270
5'10"	132	139	146	153	160	167	174	181	188	195	202	207	243	278
5'11"	136	143	150	157	165	172	179	186	193	200	208	215	250	286
6'0"	140	147	154	162	169	177	184	191	199	206	213	221	258	294
6'1"	144	151	159	166	174	182	189	197	204	212	219	227	265	302
6'2"	148	155	163	171	179	186	194	202	210	218	225	233	272	311
6'3"	152	160	168	176	184	192	200	208	216	224	232	240	279	319
6'4"	156	164	172	180	189	197	205	213	221	230	238	246	287	328
BMI	19	20	21	22	23	24	25	26	27	28	29	30	35	40

BMI Classification:

BMI Below 19
Underweight

BMI 19-24.9
Healthy Weight
(Low Health Risk)

BMI 25-29.9
Overweight
(Moderate Health Risk)

BMI 30-40
Obese (High Health Risk)

BMI Over 40
Morbid Obesity
(Very High Risk)

Interactive BMI Calculator
www.calorieking.com

Calories & Weight Loss

Calories in Food

Calories in food are derived from protein, fat and carbohydrate. Alcohol also provides calories. Vitamins, minerals and water provide no calories.

Calorie Values Per Gram

Fat/Oil	~ 9 Calories
Carbohydrate	~ 4 Calories
Protein	~ 4 Calories
Alcohol	~ 7 Calories

Note that fats have over double the calories of protein and carbohydrate. The higher the fat content of food, the higher the calories.

Sample Calculation

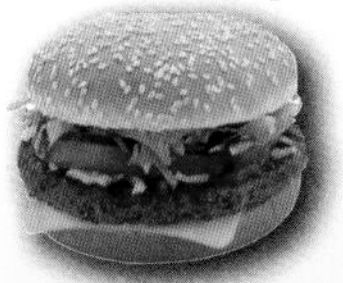

QUARTER POUNDER® WITH CHEESE has 510 calories derived from:

26g Fat (x 9 cals/gram)	= 234
40g Carbohyd.(x 4 cals/gram)	= 160
29g Protein (x 4 cals/gram)	= 116
Total Calories	= 510

Calorie Levels for Weight Loss

Start with a calorie-controlled diet that allows a moderate weight loss of ½ - 1 pound per week. Weight loss is usually much greater in the first few weeks due to extra fluid losses.

Note: It is better to increase exercise rather than lessen food calories too drastically.

Suggested Calories for Weight Loss

Women:	Non-active	1000 - 1200
	Active	1200 - 1500
Men:	Non-active	1200 - 1500
	Active	1500 - 1800
Teenagers:		1200 - 1800

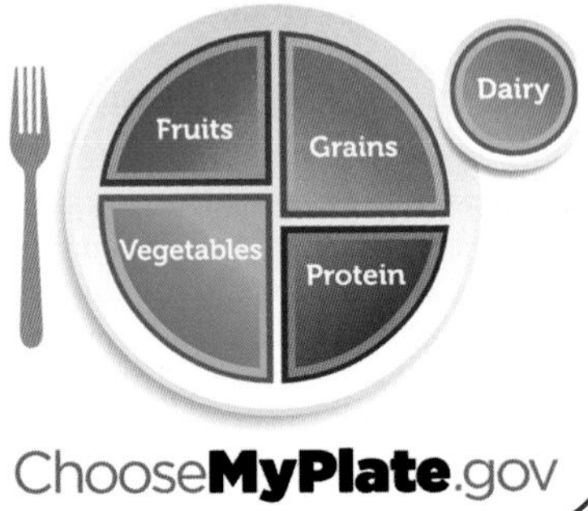

The MyPlate symbol represents the recommended proportion of foods from each food group. It focuses on the importance of making smart food choices in every food group, every day. Daily physical activity is also important. ***(More info: www.ChooseMyPlate.gov)***

Examples of Single Serving Sizes

Grains **(Eat 6 servings per day):**

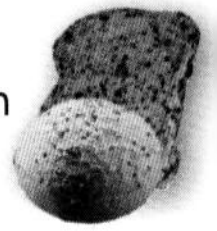

- 1 slice wholegrain bread (1 oz)
- ½ bun, small bagel or English muffin
- 4 small crackers or 1 tortilla
- 1 oz ready-to-eat wholegrain cereal
- ½ cup cooked cereal, rice or pasta

Vegetables **(Eat 3-5 servings per day):**

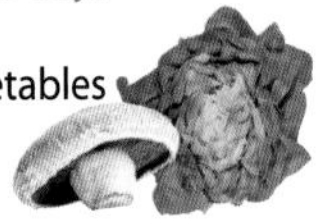

- 1 cup raw leafy vegetables
- 1½ cups raw chopped vegetables
- ½ cup cooked vegetables
- ½ - ¾ cup vegetable juice

Fruit **(Eat 3-5 servings per day):**

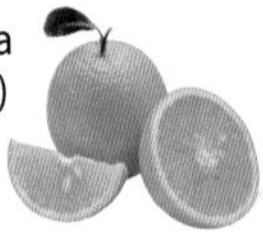

- 1 medium apple, orange, banana
- ½ cup canned fruit (in own juice)
- ¼ cup dried fruit
- ½ cup fruit juice (unsweetened)
- ¼ medium avocado

Protein **(2-3 servings per day):**

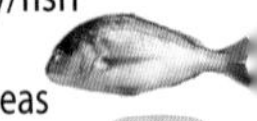

- 2-3 oz (cooked) lean meat/poultry/fish
- 2 eggs **or** 6 oz tofu **or** ¼ cup nuts
- 1 cup (cooked) dried beans **or** chickpeas

Dairy **(2-3 servings per day):**

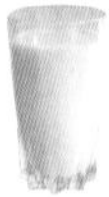

- 1 cup (8 fl.oz) milk/soy (enriched)/yogurt
- 1½ oz cheese or ½ cup cottage cheese

Portion Size Counts!

Food portion size is critical to controlling calorie intake for weight control.

Super-sized food servings have become more common when eating out and in the home. This can mean a day's worth of calories being consumed in one meal; or a snack being equivalent to a full meal.

It is easy to underestimate portion size of foods and drinks, and unwittingly consume excess calories – even if the fat content is low or even zero!

To more accurately estimate portion size of different foods, weigh and measure your food with food scales, measuring spoons and cups. Better control of calories will result.

For a visual idea of portion sizes, visit www.CalorieKing.com See examples (fries and cola) on this page.

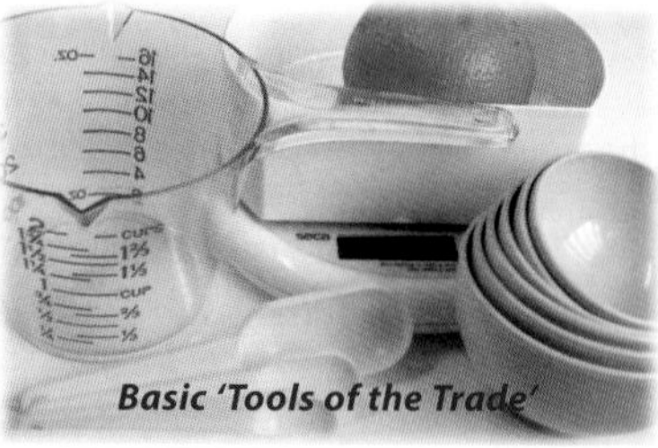

Basic 'Tools of the Trade'

CALORIEKING PORTION WATCH

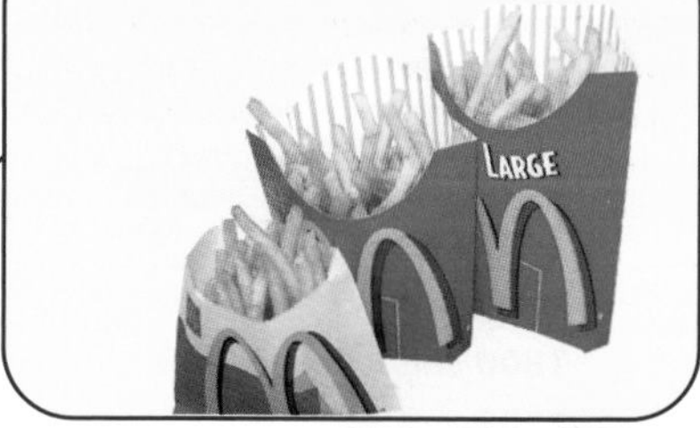

Fries	**Cal**	**Fat**	**Carb**
Small	230	11	29
Medium	380	19	48
Large	500	25	63

Allow for Extra Calories in Packaged Food

The actual weight of packaged foods is usually 5-10% more than the label net weight (the minimum legal weight) – and in some cases up to 50% more. However, manufacturers calculate the calories based on the net weight. For actual calories, weigh the product and calculate the extra calories.

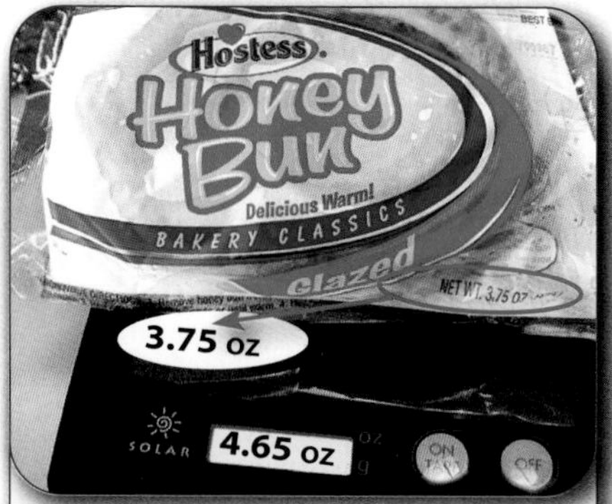

Actual weight of this bun is 24% more than the stated net weight.

CALORIEKING PORTION WATCH

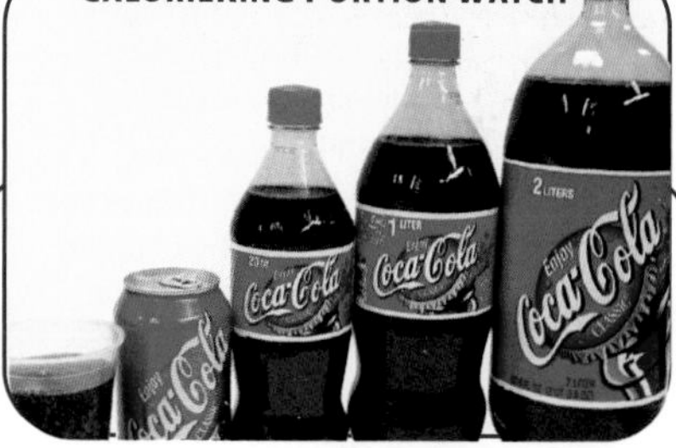

Cola	**Cal**	**Fat**	**Carb**
8 fl.oz Cup	100	0	25
12 fl.oz Can	150	0	37
20 fl.oz Bottle	250	0	63
1 Liter Bottle	400	0	100
2 Liter Bottle	800	0	200

Recommended Fat Intake

► Fat in the Diet

Fats in the diet are essential for good health. However, too much fat can contribute to obesity and a higher risk of heart disease, high blood pressure, diabetes, gallstone and certain cancers.

Dietary fat and oils have over double the calories of carbohydrates and protein. (Example: Changing from whole-milk to non-fat milk halves the calories.)

MAXIMUM DESIRABLE FAT INTAKE (DAILY)

Calories	Fat
1200 cals	30g fat
1500 cals	40g fat
1800 cals	50g fat
2000 cals	60g fat
2200 cals	70g fat
2500 cals	80g fat
3000 cals	110g fat

98% FAT-FREE NOT ALWAYS HEALTHY!

Don't be fooled by food product banners promoting "98% Fat Free".

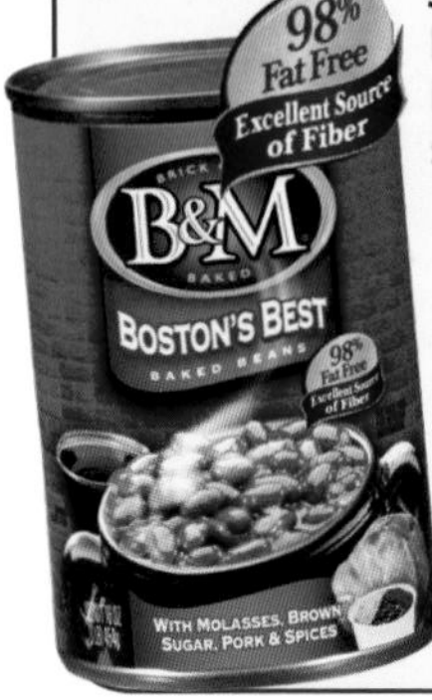

Such products may be hiding not-so-healthy ingredients such as sugar.

Baked beans are very healthy but this brand also hides 7 teaspoons of added sugar in an 8 oz serving (½ of 16 oz can).

(1 cup of soda has only 5 teaspoons of sugar)

► Beware low-fat foods

It is a mistake to think that eating low-fat or fat-free foods allows you to eat double the quantity. You can end up with even more calories than eating smaller amounts of regular-fat products.

Food products which are fat-free but high in calories include soda drinks, fruit juices, beer, alcoholic spirits, sugar and candy. Bread, rice and pasta also have negligible fat but need to be eaten in moderate amounts.

Ultimately, **it is food portion size as well as total calories that count** whether from fat, carbohydrate or protein. Remember, cows get fat on grass!

Reduced fat and fat-free foods are not necessarily low calorie. Portion size is still important.

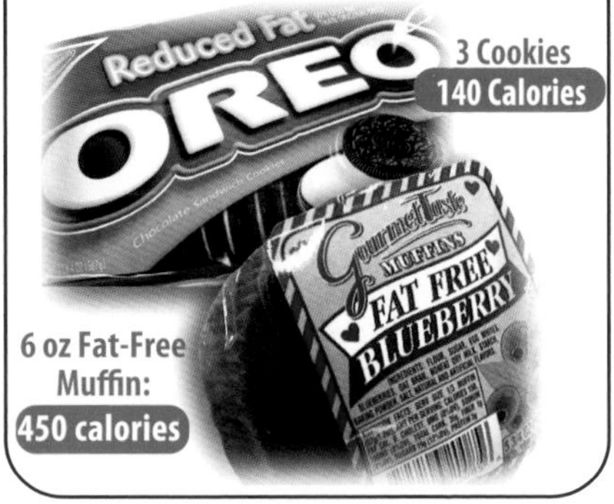

FOOD LABEL MEANINGS

FDA Nutrition Claim Definitions
(All are on a Per Serving Basis)

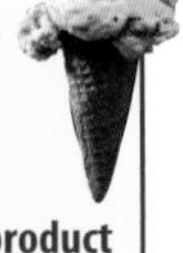

Low Calorie: **40 Calories or less**
Light or Lite: **One third fewer calories or, 50% or less fat than regular product**
Fat-Free: **Less than half a gram of fat**
Low-Fat: **3 grams or less of fat**
Reduced Fat: **25% less fat than regular product**
Fewer or Less Calories: **At least 25% fewer calories than regular product**

► Meats, Poultry, Fish

- **Choose lean cuts** of meat with little marbling. **Trim all visible fat** from meat and remove the skin from poultry. Removal of fat after cooking, is okay (to prevent dryness). Choose 'extra lean' ground beef.
- **Avoid high-fat meat products** such as salami, bacon, sausage and franks.
- **Broil or bake. Avoid frying in oil.** Allow casseroles to cool and skim off surface fat.
- **Avoid fried fish**, and fish in batter. **Choose** broiled or baked fish. Canned sardines and salmon have important omega-3 fats.

► Fats & Oils

- **Use minimal amounts** of all types of fat and oil. All are high in calories.
- **Choose** 'light' and 'reduced fat' spreads but still use sparingly.
- **Avoid frying.** Use minimal amounts of oil when stir-frying. Use no-stick sprays.

► Salad Dressings & Sauces

- **Avoid regular mayonnaise and oil dressings.** Choose 'light', 'reduced fat' or 'fat-free' brands.
- **Choose low-fat or fat-free sauces** (mainly tomato-based). Avoid 'pesto', 'alfredo', 'cheese' and 'creamy' sauces.

► Milk, Cheese

- **Choose low-fat or nonfat milks and yogurts.** Avoid full-cream milk, cream, Half & Half.
- **Cheese:** Choose fat-free, and low-fat cheese. Part-skim ricotta is still high in fat. Low-fat cottage cheese is a good choice. Cheese substitutes can still be high in fat.

► Snacks, Cookies, Candy

- **Avoid** high-fat snacks such as potato chips, corn/tortilla chips, cheese puffs, buttered popcorn and chocolate.

► Desserts/Sweets

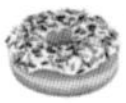
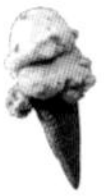

- **Avoid high-fat desserts**, such as cheesecake & ice cream.
- **Choose** fresh fruits, fresh fruit salad, canned fruit in water pack, low-fat ice cream. Use low-fat yogurt in place of cream.

► Fast-Foods & Take-Out

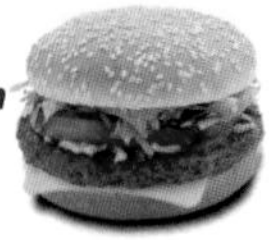

Check the Fast-Foods Section of this book for actual fat and calorie counts.

- **Avoid deep-fried foods such as** chicken, french fries and onion rings.
- **Pizzas:** Avoid sausage/pepperoni. Choose vegetarian topping and modest quantity of cheese. Eat a moderate serving. Eat extra salad and fresh fruit.
- **Hamburgers:** Choose medium size, lower fat burgers. Avoid bacon. Have a side salad (with fat-free dressing).
- **Delis:** Choose sandwiches/bread rolls, pitas with low-fat fillings and plain salad. Limit meat/cheese to small portions.
- **Coffees:** Avoid large sizes of latte and frappuccino. Request nonfat milk and no whipped cream. Avoid cookies and pastries.

Extra Information: www.CalorieKing.com

FRYING ADDS FAT!

The greater the surface area of potato exposed to fat or oil, the higher the fat content and calories.

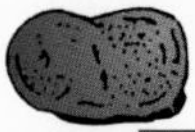

Whole Potato (3 oz)
0g Fat **65 Cals**

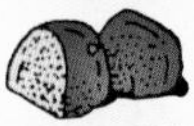

Roasted Potato (3 oz)
5g Fat **155 Cals**

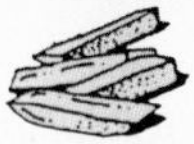

Fries (Large cut, 3 oz)
12g Fat **220 Cals**

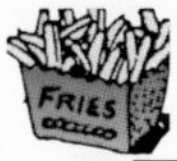

Fries (Small, 3 oz)
15g Fat **265 Cals**

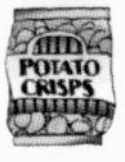

Potato Chips (3 oz)
30g Fat **450 Cals**

Carbohydrates ~ Friend or Foe?

Naturally-Friendly Carbs

- **Carbohydrate foods in their more natural forms** (not overly processed) are essential to good health. They are the main source of fuel for the body, and also provide important vitamins, minerals, antioxidants and fiber – all of which help protect against heart disease, diabetes, hypertension, constipation-related ailments and many other diseases.
- Carbohydrates even help the body produce serotonin, the 'feel good' brain chemical that helps control appetite and overeating. Too little serotonin can lead to mood swings and depression.

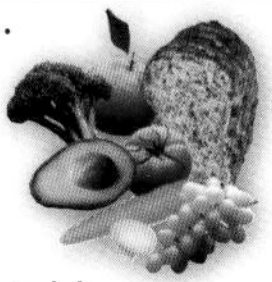

Carbohydrates are found in different forms in food as:

- Sugars in fruit, sugar cane, milk
- Starches in whole grains, legumes, nuts, seeds and vegetables
- Dietary fiber (See Fiber Guide ~ Page 264)

Glycemic Index & Diabetes ~ Page 21

Recommended Carbohydrate Intake

Calories (Daily)	Carbohydrate (Grams)	Percent Carbohydrate Calories
1200 cals	100-120g	35-40%
1500 cals	140-170g	40-45%
1800 cals	180-200g	40-45%
2000 cals	200-250g	40-50%
2500 cals	310-350g	50-55%
3000 cals	410-450g	55-65%

How Much Do We Need?

- As shown in the chart, well-balanced diets above 2000 calories contain 50-60% of total calories from carbohydrates.
- At lower calorie levels used for weight control (1200-1500 calories), carbohydrates account for as little as 40% of total calories. This is because protein calories have nutritional priority.
- Carbohydrates & Diabetes ~ *See Page 21*

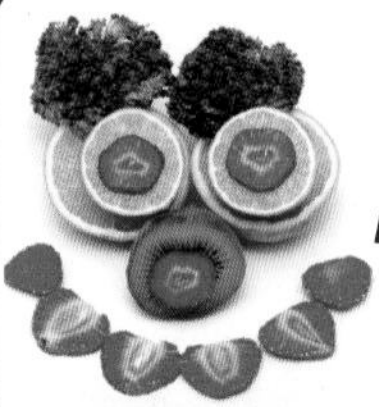

Carbohydrate foods (minimally processed) are essential to good health.

Be sure to eat adequate fruit and vegetables (5 - 7 servings) every day.

Low-Carbohydrate Diets

- Popular low-carbohydrate diets are extreme in their recommendations to initially cut carb intake to as little as 20 grams per day – the amount in 1 thick slice of bread, or 1 medium apple, or 1 small potato.

  This greatly increases the risk of nutritional deficiencies and compromises health, particularly if fat intake is excessive through fatty meats, high-fat dairy products, and fried foods.
- While overweight Americans do need to reduce carbohydrate intake, it should be done **sensibly as part of reducing portion size and total calories.**
- Simply eating 'low-carb' food products without regard to portion size, calories or fats, will do little to promote weight loss or good health.
- **Low-carb diets (and indeed any diet) only work if total calories are reduced.**
- Refined sugars should be one of the first targets in reducing carb intake.

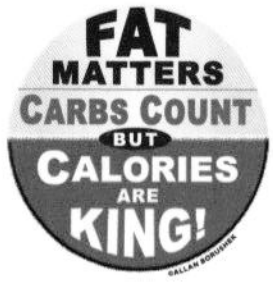

Extra Info ~ www.CalorieKing.com

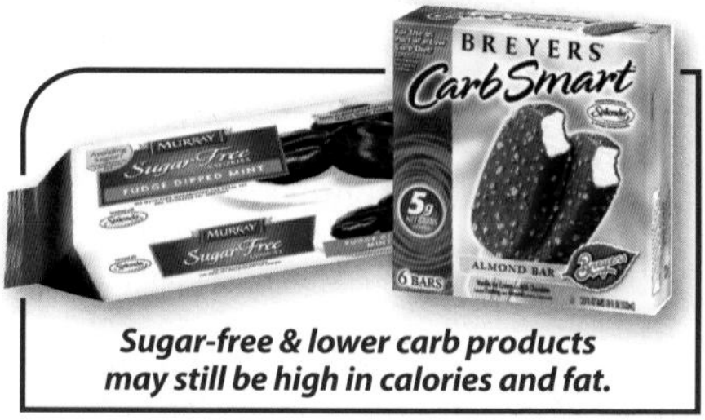

Sugar-free & lower carb products may still be high in calories and fat.

- **Excess Sugar:**
  Many overweight, inactive people consume over 500 calories of refined sugars per day, either self-added or as part of food products. This is equivalent to over 30 level teaspoons. For context, just one 12-ounce can of soda contains 10 teaspoons of added sugar.

  Maximum Sugar Recommended:
  Women ~ 6 teaspoons
  Men ~ 9 teaspoons

  Note: Naturally occurring sugars in fruits, vegetables and milk are fine when consumed in normal recommended amounts. These foods are also rich in other nutrients.

  Refined sugar is referred to as having **'empty calories'**. Sugar supplies calories but negligible nutrients and no fiber.

- **Most sugar in our diet is 'hidden'** in processed foods such as soft drinks, fruit drinks, candy, cookies, cake, jam, sauces, ice cream, desserts, canned foods, and processed breakfast cereals.

  For serious weight control, severely limit these foods and substitute healthier higher fiber wholefoods.

- **Be aware that sugar comes in different forms** such as sucrose, glucose, fructose, malt, high-fructose corn syrup, molasses, honey and maple syrup. Check the label.

- **Sugar alcohols** such as sorbitol, mannitol and maltitol are carb-based and have ½ - ¾ the calories of regular sugar. While not counted as sugar on food labels, they do add to the carb count. Excess amounts can cause bloating, gas and diarrhea.

- **Sugar-free sweeteners** make it easy to reduce sugar in drinks and recipes. However, use minimally since research suggests possible ill-effects of some artificial sweeteners on friendly gut microbes. This may increase the risk of glucose intolerance and an increase in appetite.

  Plant-based sweeteners like Stevia or monk fruit appear to be better choices.

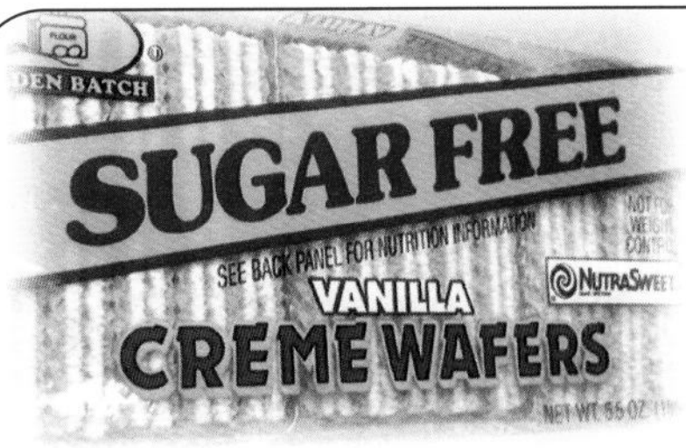

Sugar-free snacks and foods may be higher in fat and calories than the regular product.

Example ~ Creme Wafers (3):
Regular ~ 115 cals, 6g fat
Sugar-Free ~ 160 cals, 10g fat

SUGAR CONTENT OF SOME COMMON FOODS

	Teaspoons of Sugar
Coca Cola or *Pepsi,* 12 fl.oz	10
20 fl.oz size	17
Iced Tea, sweetened, 12 fl.oz	8
Energy Drink *(Red Bull),* 8.4 fl.oz	7
Chocolate Milk, 12 fl.oz	6
Baked Beans *(B&M),* 8 oz	5
Honey Smacks Cereal, 1 cup, 1 oz	4.5
Popcorn, caramel, 1 cup	3.5
Chocolate Bar, 1.5 oz	5
M&M's, 1.7 oz pkg	7
Muffin, large, 4 oz	6
Choc Chip Cookie, 1 oz	2
Donut, iced	6
Apple Pie, 1 piece	7
Jell-O, snack cup, 3.5 oz	4
Jam, 1 Tbsp, ¾ oz	2.5
Syrup, maple, 1 Tbsp	3

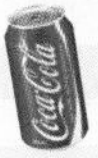

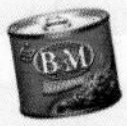

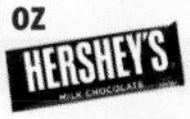

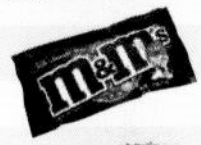

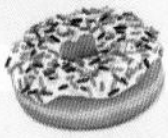
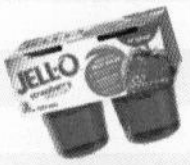

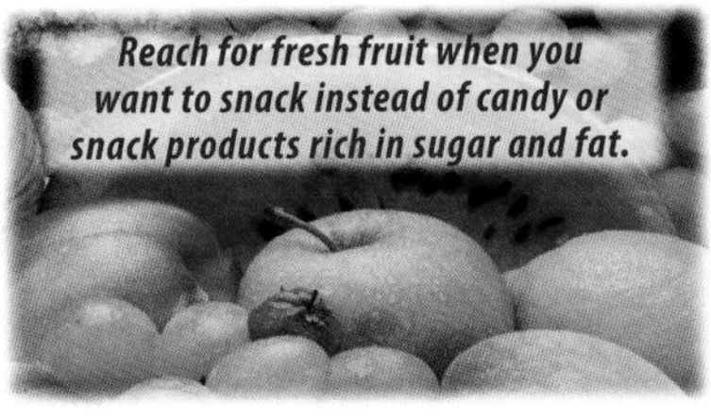

Tips for Overweight Kids & Parents

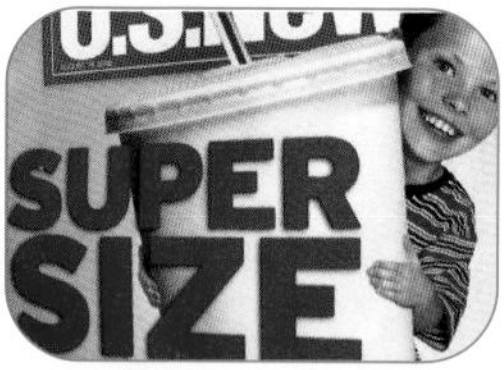

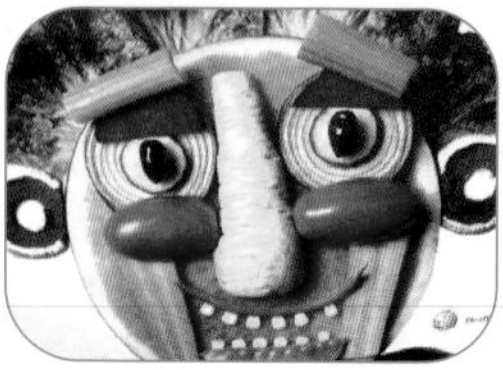

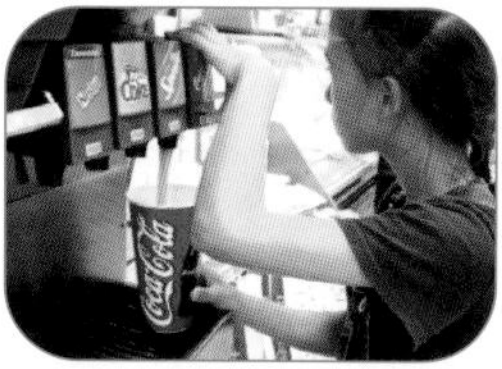

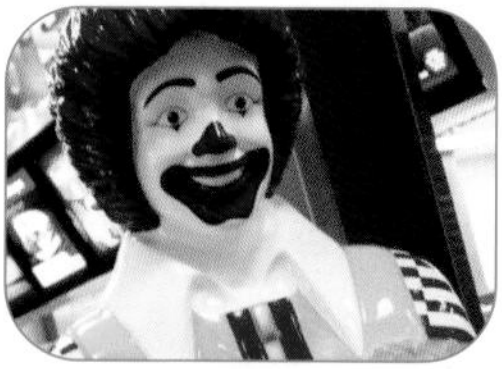

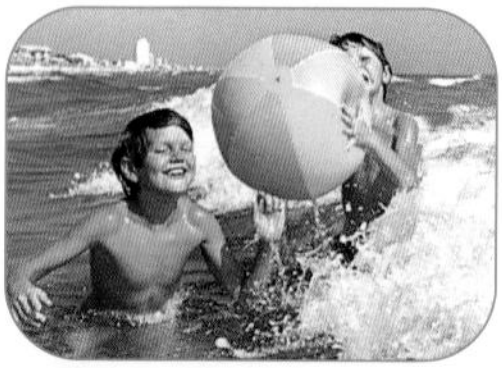

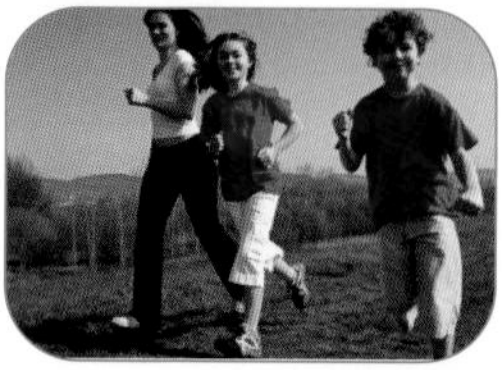

The XL Generation

Some 15% of American kids and adolescents are overweight; and childhood obesity has doubled over the last 20 years. Diabetes, high blood pressure and high cholesterol are major problem areas for overweight children and adolescents, as are depression, low self-esteem, sleep apnea and bone joint problems.

To address this problem, cooperation is required between kids, parents, schools and government. Weight control is a family and community affair.

Five Simple Tips To Get Started:

1 Watch Soda Intake

Limit soda and sugary drinks to one serving on the weekends. Soda should not be an everyday beverage – water should be. When at restaurants or using a soda fountain, choose small servings with ice or choose diet soda instead. Schools should provide water and restrict access to soda as should parents when eating out or in the home!

2 Cut back on Fast-Foods and Eating Out

Many more calories are consumed when you eat out. Healthy meals prepared at home are best for the whole family.

3 Say "No" to Super-Sizing

When meals are upsized, loads more calories are consumed. Choose sensible portion sizes when eating out and at home. Use smaller plates and choose smaller packages.

4 Limit Between-Meal Snacking

Watch out for high-fat and high-calorie snacks – they can have more calories than a meal! Keep your eye on portion sizes and limit salty snack foods and candy to parties and special occasions. Choose fresh fruit, vegetables, nuts and low-fat milk instead.

5 Get Moving ~ Watch Less TV

Kids need at least 60 minutes of physical activity every day. It's critical for their fitness, and greatly lessens the risk of obesity.

Encourage kids to be active out of school hours. Wearing a pedometer can be highly motivational for kids to move more – as can playing dance video games such as *Dance Dance Revolution. Dance Central* (XBox360) and *Wii Fit (Nintendo)* are also excellent fitness motivators.

Limit TV and non-active computer games to just one hour per day. Also limit the accompanying snacks! Include exercise in family activities.

Extra information and tips ~ www.CalorieKing.com

Sample Meal Plan ~ 1400 Calories

For Healthy, Overweight Persons ~ Not for Persons With Any Medical Condition
~ Please Check With Your Doctor & Dietitian ~

Breakfast (approx. 300 cal)

	1 Small Fruit or ½ oz Dried Fruit
Plus	Cereal: 1½ oz Dry (high fiber) or 1 cup cooked Oatmeal
Plus	½ oz Almonds/Seeds
Plus	Milk (from daily allowance) or Yogurt (low-fat)

Daily Milk Allowance (approx. 160 calories)
2 cups Non-Fat Milk or 1½ cups Low-fat (1%) Milk
or equivalent Soy Drink, Yogurt, Cheese, Tofu

Fat Allowance (140 calories; 15g Fat)
4 tsp Fat or 6-8 tsp Diet Margarine or 3 tsp Oil
or 1½ Tbsp Mayonnaise or ½ medium Avocado
or 1½ Tbsp Peanut Butter or 30g Nuts/Seeds

Lunch (approx. 440 calories)

	2 slices Wholegrain Bread (2 oz) or 4 Crispbreads/Crackers or 6" Pita
Plus	2 oz lean Meat, Chicken or Turkey or 3½ oz Tuna (in water) or 2½ oz Salmon or 1 oz Cheese or ½ cup (4 oz) Cottage Cheese or ½ cup (4 oz) Ricotta Cheese (low-fat) or ½ cup (4 oz) Fruit Yogurt (low-fat) or ½ cup (4 oz) Bean Salad
Plus	Large Salad
Plus	1 small Fruit or ½ oz Dried Fruit

Dinner (approx. 360 calories)

	Soup (fat-free)
Plus	3 oz lean Meat (cooked weight) or 4 oz Chicken Breast (no skin) or 3 oz Chicken Thigh/Leg (no skin) or 5 oz Fish (grilled, no fat) or ¾ cup (6 oz) Beans (Soy, Kidney, Pinto etc)/Lentils or Low-fat Entree (e.g. Lean Cuisine)
Plus	1 small Potato or ½ cup Rice/Pasta/Sweet Corn or 1 slice Wholegrain Bread
Plus	2-3 servings Vegetables/Salad

Breakfast ~ Choice 2

	1 Small Fruit
Plus	2 Eggs (no added fat) or 2 oz Cheese (low-fat) or 4 oz Cottage Cheese (low-fat) or 2 oz Lean/Canadian Bacon
Plus	1 Tomato
Plus	1 Slice Wholegrain Toast

Between Meals

Water, Coffee, Tea, Diet drinks, Fruit from main meals; Raw Vegetable Pieces, Milk from Daily Allowance

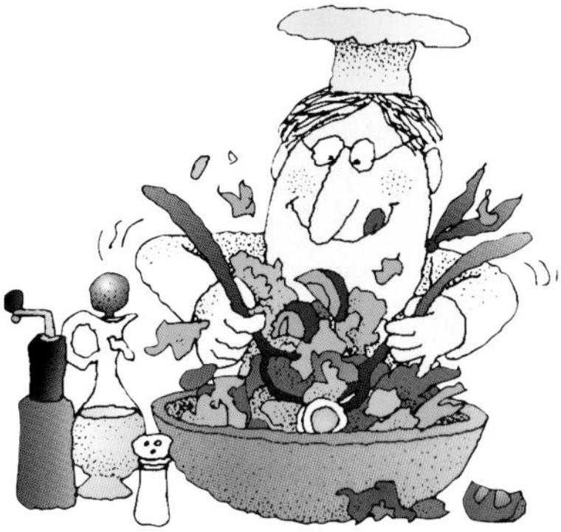

Exercise & Weight Control

- **Persons who exercise regularly lose more weight** and keep it off longer than non-exercisers. Blood glucose control also improves; as do beneficial gut microbes.
- **Exercise also improves general health and well-being.** Mood, confidence and self-esteem are also enhanced.
- **Exercise** is a good way to 'wake up' a sluggish metabolism and burn excess body fat.
- **Aerobic (huff and puff) exercise most days** is great for burning calories and for cardiovascular fitness. But, it is strength training that mainly builds the muscles that burn calories.
- **Strength training is the key to retaining or rebuilding muscles.** As we age, we lose some 6 pounds of muscle per decade. This results in a lower metabolism and fewer calories burnt.

  Muscles are the furnaces that burn calories. The more muscle you have, the more calories burnt – and as a bonus, the more food you can eat.
- **Regular strength training (2-3 times weekly)** can increase our metabolic rate for several days following exercise – with up to an extra 100 calories per day being burnt.

  While 2-3 pounds of muscle may be gained in the first 8-10 weeks, weight from exercised muscles is okay. It is excess fat (particularly abdominal fat) that is a potential health hazard.
- **Body reshaping** is enhanced by gaining muscle and losing fat - even if the scales don't show it.
- **Avoid injury** by beginning with walking, low impact aerobics, or weight-supported exercise (e.g. swimming, cycling). Avoid competitive sports. Allow 2-3 days of recovery between strength training sessions. Get professional advice.
- **How Much?** Start with 10-20 minutes per day and progress to 30-60 minutes per day. Also walk up stairs instead of using elevators. Take a brisk walk at lunch. Use an exercise bike, treadmill or stair machine while watching TV. Walk the dog.
- **How Often?** While aerobic fitness may require only 3-4 sessions weekly, **weight control is a daily event which requires daily exercise to burn calories.** Also add in strength training 2-3 times weekly.

Note: Persons on cholesterol-lowering statin drugs may experience muscle pains and weakness (as well as damage to muscle microfibrils). Supplementing with coenzyme Q10, magnesium, selenium, vitamins D and K2, may be beneficial. Check with your healthcare provider.

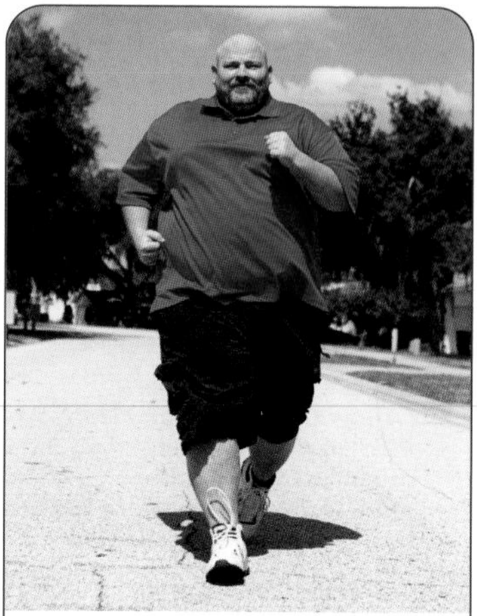

Brisk walking each day is a safe and effective way to burn calories and keep fit.
Try it – you'll like it!

Be sure to wear sun-protective clothing.

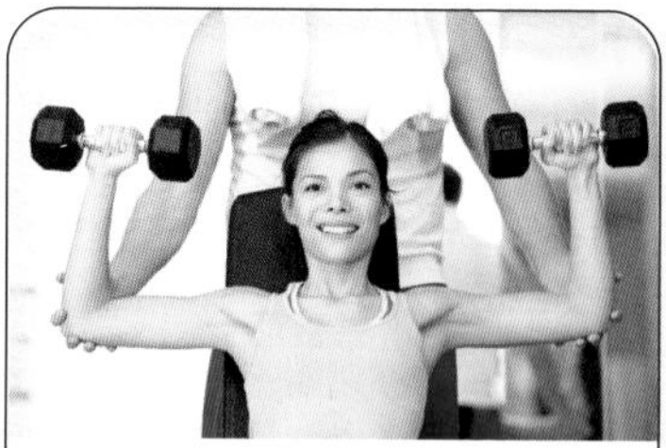

Strength training is the key to retain or rebuild muscles.

Exercized muscles burn extra calories even while you sleep.

For extra guidance and motivation, seek a qualified trainer or join a gym.

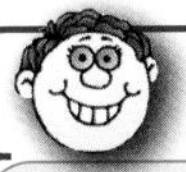

Calories Used in Exercise

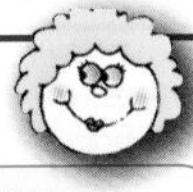

LIGHT

130 lbs ~ 3 Cals/Min

170 lbs ~ 4 Cals/Min

220 lbs ~ 5 Cals/Min

- Walking, slow
- Cycling, light
- Frisbee playing
- Gardening, light
- Golf, social
- Tennis, doubles
- Housework, cleaning
- Calisthenics, light
- Bowling
- Ping-pong, social
- Ice Skating, light
- Aquarobics, light
- Skate Boarding
- Line/Square Dancing
- Tai Chi, Yoga
- Volleyball

MODERATE

130 lbs ~ 5 Cals/Min

170 lbs ~ 6 Cals/Min

220 lbs ~ 7 Cals/Min

- Walking, brisk
- Cycling, moderate
- Swimming, crawl
- Weight-training, light
- Tennis, moderate
- Racquetball, beginners
- Aerobics, light
- Football, touch
- Basketball, Baseball
- Walking Downstairs
- Snow Skiing (downhill)
- Shovelling snow
- Dancing (ballroom)
- Rowing, moderate
- Volleyball, competitive

HEAVY

130 lbs ~ 8 Cals/Min

170 lbs ~ 10 Cals/Min

220 lbs ~ 12 Cals/Min

- Walking (power), Jogging
- Cycling (vigorous)
- Swimming, strenuous
- Weight-training, heavy
- Wrestling/Judo, advanced
- Racquetball, advanced
- Tae Bo, Kick Boxing
- Football, training
- Basketball (Pro)
- Climbing Stairs
- Skipping Rope
- Skiing (cross country)
- Aquarobics, advanced
- Dancing (strenuous), Zumba
- Rowing, vigorous
- Martial Arts

Note: Only those sports or activities that are sustained over a period of time (e.g running) qualify for heavy exercise. Stop-start sports such as tennis are considered 'moderate'.

WALKING PROGRAM

USE DISTANCE, STEPS OR TIME

Weeks	Distance	Steps (Pedometer)	Time
1-2	1 mile	2000	20 mins
3-5	1.5 miles	3000	28 mins
6-8	2 miles	3500	35 mins
9-10	2.5 miles	4500	45 mins
11+	3.5 miles	6000	60 mins

10,000 STEPS PER DAY

A pedometer can motivate you to be more active. It clips to your belt or waist band and registers each step.

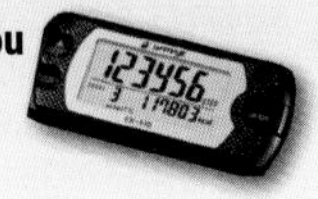

Alternatively, use a *Fitbit*, *Garmin* or *Striiv* activity tracker, or your smartphone inbuilt accelerometer.

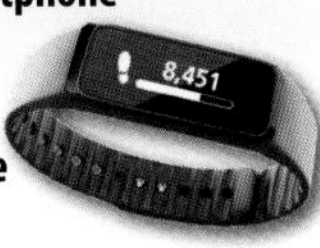

Aim for 8,000 - 10,000 steps per day, insead of an average of only 3,000 - 4,000 steps.

Reshaping Eating Behaviors

- Eating is a behavior that is largely controlled by people with whom we live or socialize, places in which we carry out our lives, and our emotions. Become aware of those situations that commonly lead to extra food being eaten.
- We may also be unaware of 'bad' eating habits that can lead to excess calorie intake; e.g. eating quickly, large mouthfuls, eating when tense or bored, finishing a large serving of food when not hungry.

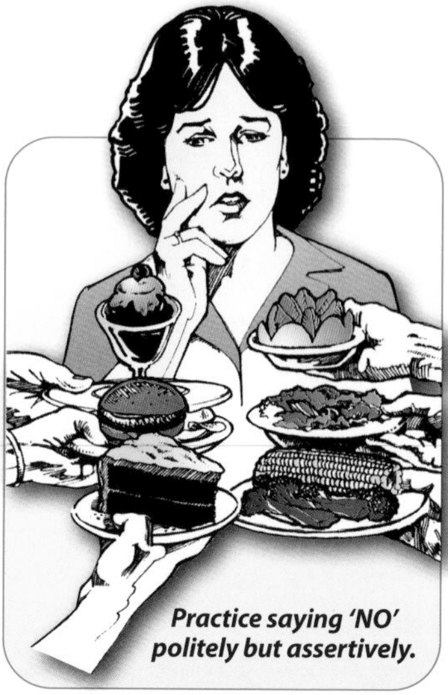

Practice saying 'NO' politely but assertively.

Tips to help uncover and correct those 'bad' or problem eating habits:

- **Don't eat while engaged in other activities;** for example, watching TV, reading. Eat only at the table, not at the fridge or while standing.
- **Don't eat quickly.** Chewing slowly allows time to register a feeling of fullness. Don't use fingers, only utensils. Cut food into smaller pieces. Don't load your fork until the previous mouthful is finished.
- **Don't purchase problem high calorie foods.** Shop from a set list to prevent impulse buying. Avoid shopping with children.
- **Buy snack foods** in the smallest package. The larger the serving size or package, the more you are likely to eat or drink.
- **Plan meals in advance. Stick to a set menu.**
- **Plan a strategy to avoid uncontrolled eating** and drinking at social events, or when your emotions urge you to binge.

  Rehearse repeatedly in your mind exactly what you will do in such situations. Remind yourself several times each day that you are in charge of your actions and that you can be strong-willed. Seek counseling or coaching on various strategies.
- **Distract yourself** when you feel the urge to snack impulsively. Engage in some activity that will distract you from thinking about food. Examples: go for a walk, brush your teeth, phone a friend.

  If you eat out of boredom, find some new hobby or interest that gets you out of the house. Even enrol in an adult education class.

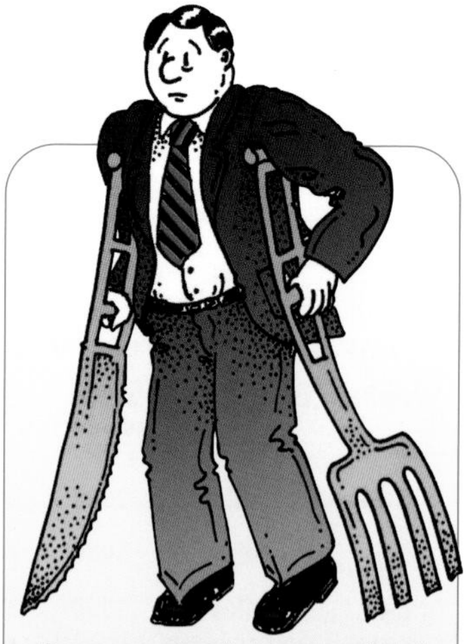

Do you use food as an emotional crutch? If so, professional counseling may be helpful.

The Value of a Food Journal

The food journal is the most powerful proven aid for dieters. Persons who keep a food and exercise journal not only lose more weight, they also keep it off. Here are some of the reasons:

- **Recording your eating and exercise habits** jolts you into realizing just what you do eat and drink each day; and also whether you exercise sufficiently.
- **Helps you identify problem foods** and drinks with excessive calories and fat.
- **Helps identify moods**, situations and events that lead to excessive eating of unwanted calories. You can then plan to overcome or avoid them.
- **Prevents 'calorie amnesia'**, the forgetfulness that leads to rebound weight gain after successful weight loss. Recording puts you back on the right track.
- **Helps you develop greater self-discipline.** You will think twice about overindulging if you have to record it - especially if someone checks your journal regularly. It certainly keeps you honest!
- **Motivates you** to carefully plan your meals and to exercise each day.
- **Serves as a check system** for your doctor, dietitian or counselor to assess your progress and make recommendations.

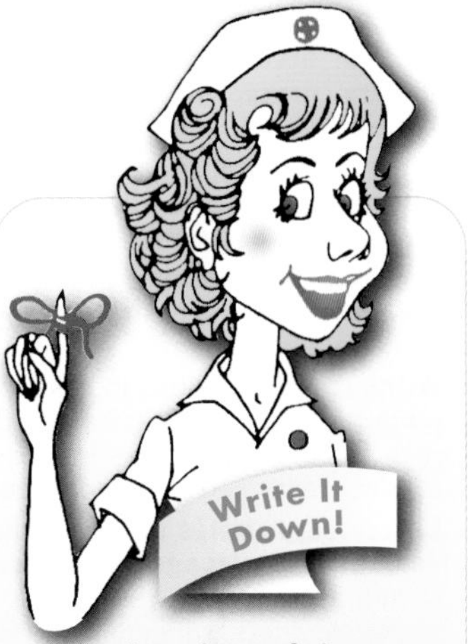

"Keeping a journal gives me feedback on exactly what I eat and drink each day.

It helps prevent 'calorie amnesia' and reminds me to exercise each day.

It's a 'must' for successful weight control!"

3 Easy Ways to Track Your Food & Exercise Calories!

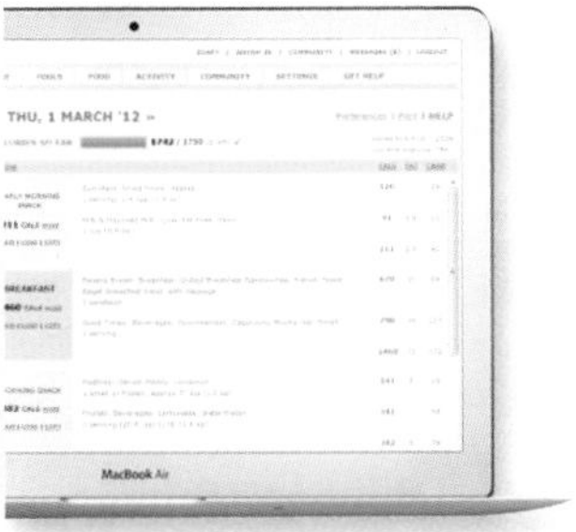

CalorieKing Online

Part of a comprehensive personalized program that includes tools, reports and a supportive community.

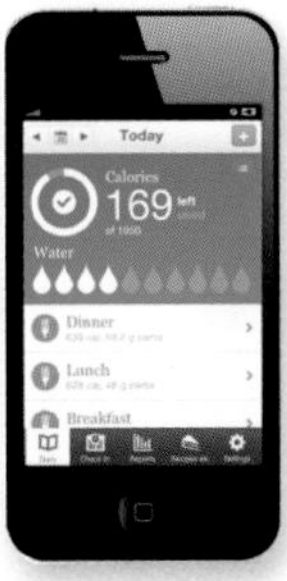

CalorieKing App

ControlMyWeight

Make smart food choices wherever you are! Easy to use.

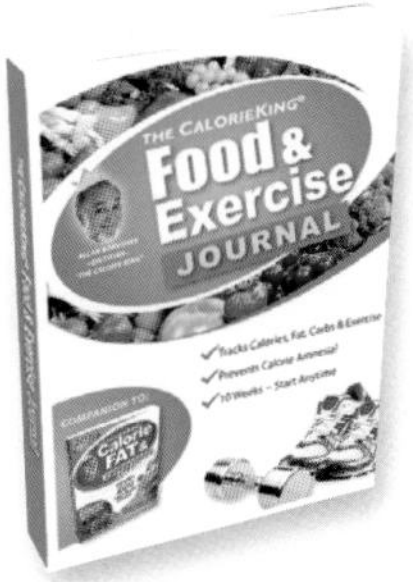

Book

A 10-week journal that fits in your pocket. Includes Weekly Summary page and Progress Checklist.

Extra Information ~ www.CalorieKing.com

Diabetes Guide

What is Diabetes?

Diabetes occurs when the body has difficulty processing glucose sugar in the blood.

- **After digestion**, sugar and starches are changed into **glucose** – the simplest form of sugar vital for body energy and growth.
- Insulin is the hormone which acts like a key that opens the door to body cells and allows glucose to enter.
- **Without enough insulin**, glucose builds up in the blood and passes into the urine. High blood glucose levels lead to frequent urination, extreme thirst, and tiredness.
- **Untreated diabetes increases the risk of damage to nerves and blood vessels.** This, in turn, increases the risk of heart disease, stroke, blindness, kidney damage, foot ulcers and gangrene (with amputation), impotence, Alzheimer's Disease and other problems.

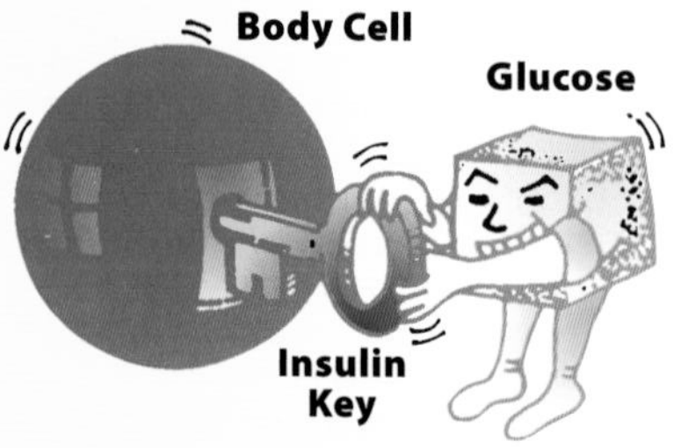

Insulin acts like a key. It opens the door to body cells and allows glucose to enter.

People with type 1 diabetes and some with type 2 have too few or no keys and require insulin injections.

Others (primarily type 2) make enough insulin but the body doesn't use it as well as it should – particularly if obese and inactive.

SYMPTOMS OF DIABETES

- Frequent urination
- Extreme thirst
- Unusual hunger
- Rapid weight loss
- Extreme fatigue
- Blurred vision
- Skin infections that are slow to heal
- Tingling/numbness in feet

Note: Diabetes can be present even with no symptoms.

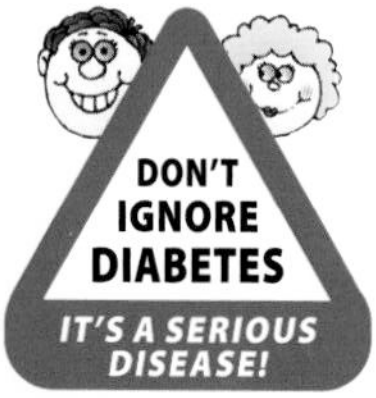

TYPE 2 DIABETES

- Occurs in 90% of diabetes cases
- Occurs mainly in adults - particularly in overweight and inactive persons
- Insulin is produced but body cells resist its action and glucose cannot enter cells
- Usually treated with meal planning and physical activity. Sometimes requires medication (pills or insulin)

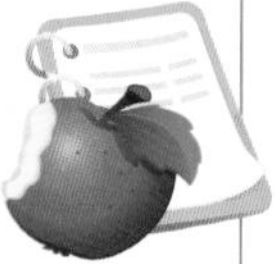

TYPE 1 DIABETES

- Occurs in 10% of diabetes cases
- Usually in children and young adults
- Pancreas produces little or no insulin. Daily insulin injections (or use of an insulin pump) are necessary, as well as:
  - matching pre-meal insulin to the amount of carbohydrate eaten
  - weight control and regular physical activity

GESTATIONAL DIABETES

- Occurs in some women during pregnancy. It usually disappears after the baby's birth but still leaves mothers (1 in 3) at high risk of type 2 diabetes within 5-10 years.
- Check your blood glucose **before** you become pregnant. High levels can harm the fetus, especially in the first 6 weeks.
- Requires weight control, a healthy lifestyle and regular medical checks.

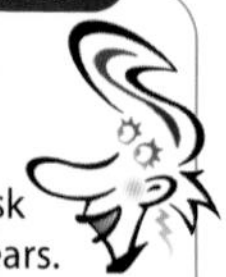

Are You At Risk for Diabetes?

Pre-Diabetes ~ An Early Warning!

Pre-diabetes means your blood glucose levels are higher than normal, but not high enough to be called diabetes.

If you have pre-diabetes, you have a higher risk for getting diabetes later on.

The good news is that you can start taking steps to prevent diabetes by making healthy lifestyle changes – such as losing weight if overweight, and being more physically active.

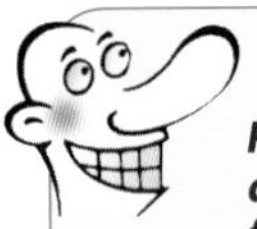

WHAT'S YOUR RISK?

Find out if you're at risk for diabetes by answering the following questions:

- ☐ I have been told I have pre-diabetes
- ☐ I have a family history of diabetes
- ☐ I am African American, Latino American, Asian American, Native American or a Pacific Islander
- ☐ I have had gestational diabetes (diabetes during pregnancy)
- ☐ I am over age 45
- ☐ I am overweight
- ☐ My waist is larger than: 35 inches (for a woman) or 40 inches (for a man)
- ☐ I get little or no physical activity
- ☐ My blood pressure is higher than 130 over 85
- ☐ My HDL (good cholesterol) is too low
- ☐ My triglycerides (blood fats) are too high

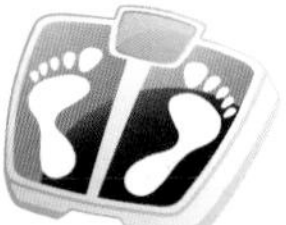

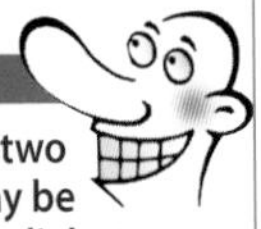

CHECK YOUR RESULT

- If you've put a check mark in two or more of the boxes, you may be more likely to develop type 2 diabetes.
- Talk with your healthcare provider to see if you should have a blood test for diabetes.

BLOOD GLUCOSE CLASSIFICATION OF DIABETES

Normal:	**Below 100 mg/dl***
Pre-Diabetes:	**100-125 mg/dl***
Diabetes:	**Over 125 mg/dl***

(*Fasting Blood Glucose)

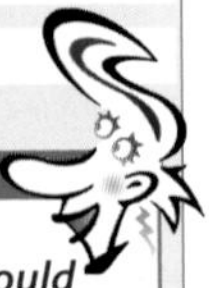

KNOW YOUR BGL

(Blood Glucose Level)

Everyone over the age of 45 should have a blood glucose test every three years.

Importance of Weight Control

- **Type 2 diabetes** is more common in people who are overweight.
- **Being overweight** means that your insulin doesn't work as well to control blood glucose levels.
- **Losing just 10 to 20 pounds** can help you better manage your diabetes and lower your risk for heart disease.

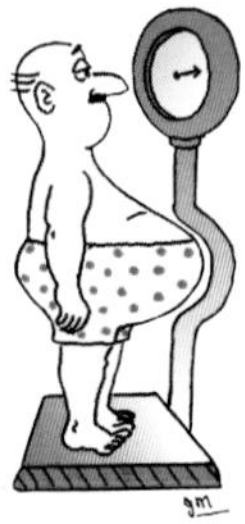

Keys to weight control include:

- Follow a healthy eating plan
- Control food portions.
- Be physically active every day. Track your daily activity.
- Keep food records ~ *See Page 15*
- Get the support of family and friends.
- **Work with a registered dietitian** who can help you reach a weight that's ideal for you.

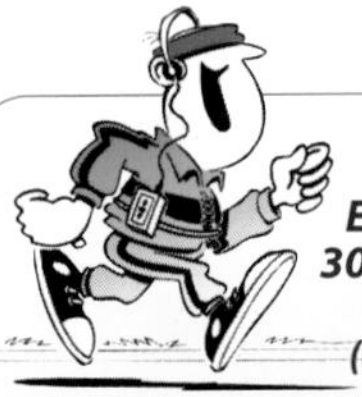

KEEP MOVING!

Every day, do at least 30 minutes of moderate intensity exercise. (even in 5-minute sets)

It's the key to improving insulin action. Add muscle strength training 3-4 times a week to double the benefits.

Managing Diabetes

Don't battle diabetes alone. Establish a partnership with your doctor, dietitian, certified diabetes educator, and pharmacist.

Extra Support:

- *American Association of Diabetes Educators*
- *American Diabetes Association*
- *BeyondType1.org* • *Joslin Diabetes Center*
- *Juvenile Diabetes Research Foundation*
- *National Diabetes Education Program*

Tips to keep blood glucose within safe limits:

- **Control your food intake.** Know what and when you will eat. Seek referral to a dietitian for expert advice.
- **Exercise daily.** It assists weight control and can improve sensitivity of body cells to insulin. Plan physical activity into your daily routine.
- **Take insulin or oral medication as prescribed.** If on insulin, know what action to take if hypoglycemia (low blood glucose) occurs. Also educate your family and friends.
- **Monitor your blood glucose** at home and work with a blood glucose meter or CGM system. It will help you become familiar with your blood glucose patterns, and the effects of food, activity and medication.
- **Continuous glucose monitoring (CGM) tracks** your glucose levels every few minutes by using a sensor (skin patch or insert) that measures glucose levels in the tissue just below the skin. This allows the user to see a graph of glucose levels – not just single measurements from fingerstick testing. Seeing trends and patterns can help to better manage diabetes. **This results in greater awareness of unnoticed highs and lows** (as illustrated below). CGM can also help to reduce A1C with less risk of hypoglycemia for people on insulin.

Blood glucose meter systems and insulin pumps can greatly improve control of diabetes

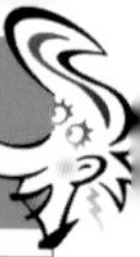

BLOOD GLUCOSE METERS (EXAMPLES)

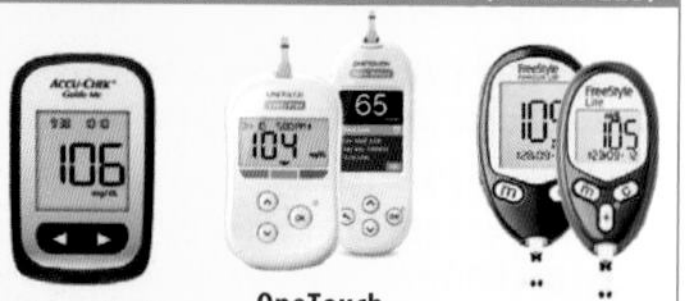

Accu-Chek | OneTouch Verio Models | FreeStyle

(CGM) CONTINUOUS GLUCOSE MONITORING SYSTEMS (EXAMPLES)

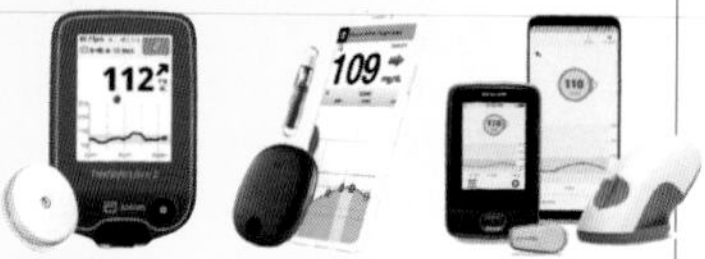

FreeStyle Libre 2 | Eversense System | Dexcom G6 System

INSULIN PUMPS & SYSTEMS (EXAMPLES)

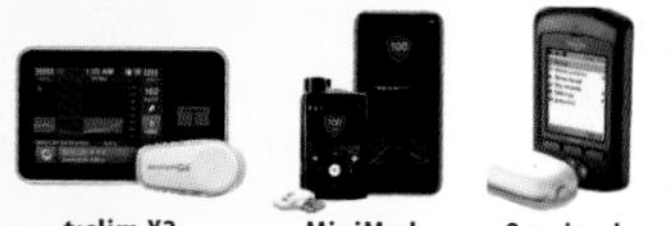

t:slim X2 Control-IQ | MiniMed 770G | Omnipod System

Hemoglobin A1C Target:

The hemoglobin A1C (A-one-C) test reflects your average blood glucose levels over the last 3 months. **Aim for 7-8%**

Benefits of Continuous Glucose Monitoring

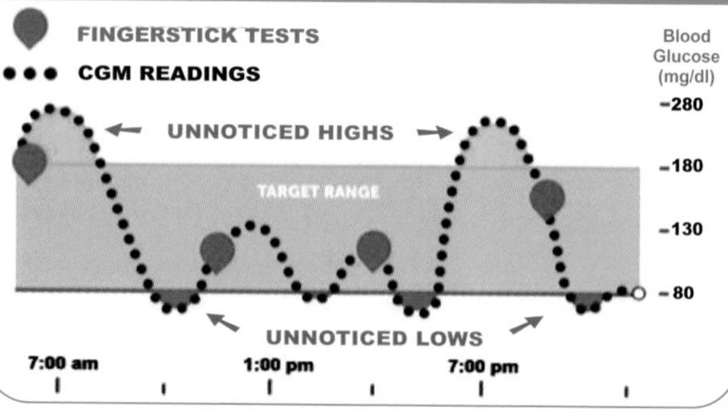

Target Blood Sugar Levels (ADA):

Before Meals:
Between 80 and 130 mg/dL

2 Hours After Meals:
Less than 180 mg/dL

Diabetes Guide ~ Meal Planning Tips

Guidelines for choosing a healthy diet apply equally to people with or without diabetes.

Eat a wide variety of whole foods that are minimally processed, moderate in fat, high in fiber and low in added sugars.

However, actual food quantities, as well as when you eat, will also influence control of blood glucose. Your dietitian will individualize a meal plan to suit your food preferences, lifestyle and medical status.

Eat a well-balanced diet with foods high in fiber and low in added sugars.

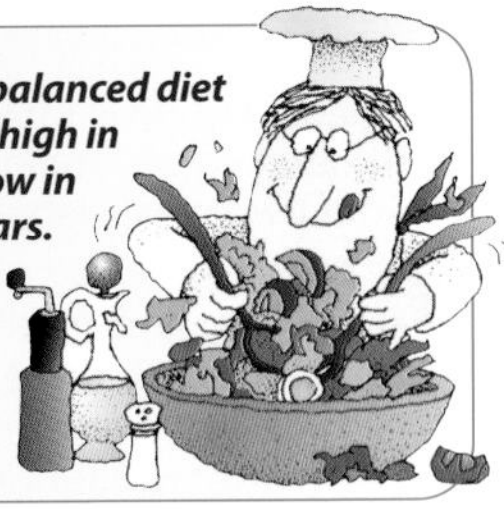

Healthy Diet Tips:

- **Maintain a healthy weight.** If overweight, even a modest weight loss plus daily physical activity can help manage blood glucose in type 2 diabetes.
- **Don't skip meals.** If you take insulin or an oral hypoglycemic agent, regular meals are important.

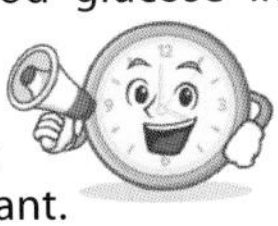

  If on insulin, eat meals at the same time each day. Eat a similar amount of food at each meal. Eating about the same amount of carbohydrate over the day will make best use of insulin and prevent wide variations in blood glucose levels.

- **Know which foods contain carbohydrate;** and learn how to check the *Nutrition Facts Label* on foods. Check the serving size, total fat and total carbohydrate – not just the sugar content. All carbohydrate breaks down to sugars after digestion.
- **Choose wholegrain breads, cereals and pasta.** Eat fresh fruits, vegetables and legumes. These foods contain more fiber and slow the release of glucose into your blood after a meal.

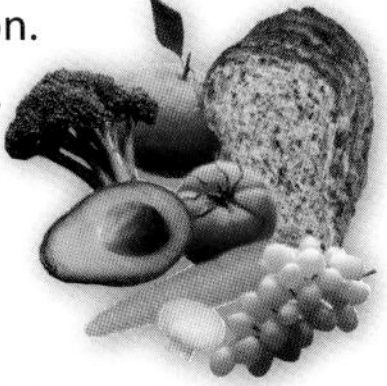

- **Limit sugars and foods high in added sugar** particularly if overweight. *(Extra Notes: Page 9)*
- **Choose foods with healthy fats** such as fatty fish, avocados, olives and nuts, flaxseeds, chia seeds, hemp seeds.Avoid excess use of seed oils. Ideally, use extra virgin olive oil. Avoid fried foods. Frying can oxidize seed oils that can harm our health.

A fiber-rich diet assists the growth of friendly gut microbes that can benefit our metabolism, weight and blood glucose levels – as well as hunger, mood and our immune system.
(Also see Fiber Guide ~ Page 264)

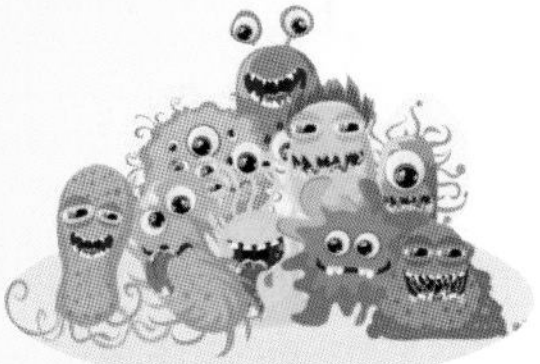

ALCOHOL TIPS

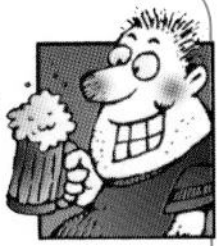

- **If you drink alcohol, have only moderate amounts:**
  Men ~ 1-2 drinks/day
  Women ~ 1 drink/day
  For some people, safe drinking will mean no alcoholic drinks at all.

(Also see Alcohol Guide ~ Page 23)

- **Drink along with your food –** especially if you use insulin or diabetes medication pills.
- **Do not omit any carb food** in exchange for an alcoholic drink. However, non-alcoholic beers (12 fl oz) count as one carb exchange.
- **Alcohol increases the risk of hypoglycemia** (low blood sugar) and drug interactions if you take insulin and certain types of diabetes pills.
- **Check with your doctor and dietitian.**

Diabetes Guide ~ The Plate Method

The Plate Method – An Easy Way to Eat Healthfully

The plate method is a helpful tool to guide your food choices until you see a dietitian for your own meal plan.

For a healthy meal:

- Fill half of your plate with non-starchy vegetables (broccoli, cabbage, green beans, salad greens, tomato).
- Fill a quarter of your plate with carbohydrate (wholegrain bread, pasta, potato, brown rice, corn, lentils, legumes).
- Fill the other quarter of your plate with 3-4 ounces of lean meat, poultry, or fish.
- Add a small piece of fruit or 8 ounces of skim/low-fat milk or yogurt.

How Much Carbohydrate Should You Eat?

A dietitian can best determine how much carbohydrate you need at each of your meals, based on your lifestyle, food preferences, and overall diabetes control.

Until you see a dietitian, aim to keep the amount of carbohydrate you eat the same at each of your meals.

Carb Choices Meal Plan
One Carb Choice = 15 Grams of Carb

The amount in: 1 slice Bread **or** ¾ cup Cereal (unsweetened) **or** 1 small Potato **or** 1 small Fruit

Breakfast
- Eat 2-3 carb choices (30-45 grams)
- Include a low-fat protein source such as egg whites or low-fat milk.

Lunch and Dinner
- Eat 3-4 carb choices (45-60 grams carb)
- Include fruit and non-starchy vegetables. Choose small portions of low-fat protein foods.

Snacks: If needed, eat 1-2 carb choices (15-30 grams carb).

Note: Above plan is for adults. Carbohydrate amounts will vary with physical activity level.

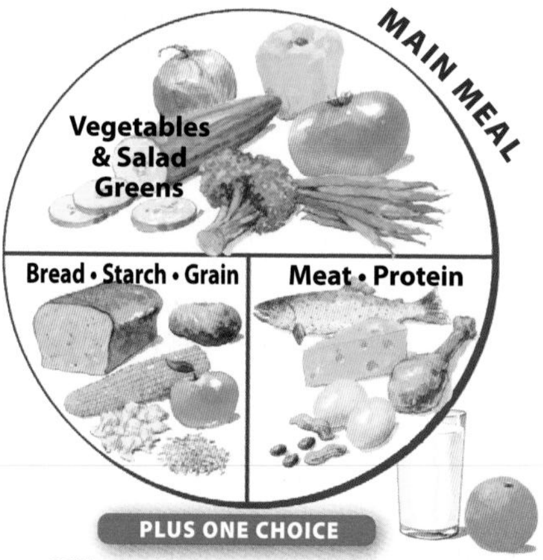

Milk, Fruit, Dessert or other Carb Food

HIDDEN SUGAR TRAPS
~ TEASPOONS OF SUGAR ~

Note: 1 Level Teaspoon Sugar = 4 grams

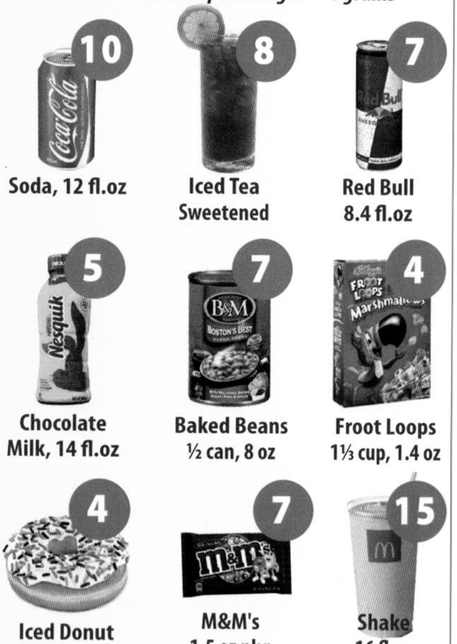

Item	Teaspoons of Sugar
Soda, 12 fl.oz	10
Iced Tea Sweetened	8
Red Bull 8.4 fl.oz	7
Chocolate Milk, 14 fl.oz	5
Baked Beans ½ can, 8 oz	7
Froot Loops 1⅓ cup, 1.4 oz	4
Iced Donut	4
M&M's 1.5 oz pkg	7
Shake 16 fl.oz	15

Carb Type Affects Blood Glucose

The various forms of carbohydrate affect blood glucose levels in different ways. It is difficult to predict the effect of particular foods, sugars, or meals, simply by their carbohydrate content.

Thus the same amount of carbohydrate from different foods may affect blood sugar levels very differently. **Many factors affect the rate of digestion and absorption such as:**

- the type of sugar, starch, and fiber
- the degree of processing and cooking (which increases digestion rate)
- the amount of protein and fat (which slow stomach emptying and digestion).

Glycemic Index (GI)

The GI is a method of ranking carbohydrate foods on a scale (0-100) according to how they affect blood glucose levels. (See next column).

The higher the GI value, the greater the food's ability to rapidly raise blood glucose levels; and the more insulin that is needed by the body (not desirable).

Eating low-GI foods may lead to better control of blood glucose and insulin levels (which in turn lowers the risk of damage to blood vessels and nerves). The slower digestion of low-GI foods may also help to delay hunger pangs and benefit weight control.

Cautionary Notes on GI

Choosing low-GI foods is not a license to eat unlimited amounts. Calorie restriction and portion control for weight control is of prime importance.

Also remember, **low-GI foods are carbohydrate foods** and must still be counted as part of any dietetic carbohydrate plan.

GI is not meant to be used by itself without regard to portion size, and other dietary recommendations for healthy eating. Foods are not good or bad on the basis of their GI.

While GI may be a helpful tool for some people with diabetes, what is most important is to control the total amount of carbohydrate that you eat.

LOWER-GLYCEMIC FOODS

Slower-Acting Carbohydrates

These foods are more slowly digested and absorbed. They help maintain more even blood glucose levels, as long as excessive amounts are not eaten. Use these foods regularly but still limit portion size for weight control.

Examples:

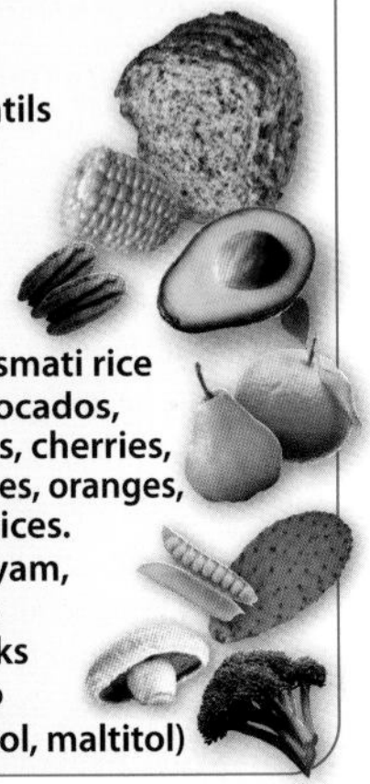

- **Dried beans, peas, lentils**
- **Nuts and seeds**
- **Wholegrain breads**
- **Bran cereals, oats**
- **Sweet corn, barley, quinoa buckwheat**
- **Wholegrain pasta, basmati rice**
- **Fresh fruit: apples, avocados, bananas (firm), berries, cherries, grapefruit, grapes, olives, oranges, pears, plums. Fresh juices.**
- **Vegetables: broccoli, yam, nopales, salad greens**
- **Milk, yogurt, soy drinks**
- **Dark chocolate, cacao**
- **Sugar alcohols (sorbitol, maltitol)**

HIGHER-GLYCEMIC FOODS

Quicker-Acting Carbohydrates

These foods more rapidly raise blood glucose levels. Eat only in moderation.

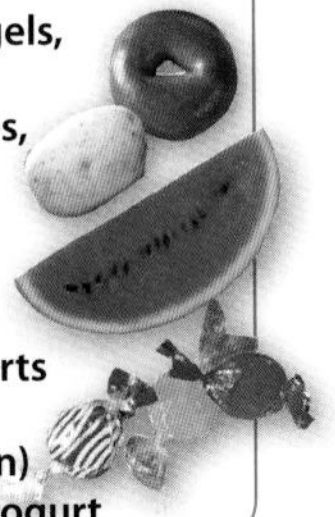

- **White bread, rice cakes, bagels, croissants, doughnuts**
- **Low-fiber cereals: Cornflakes, *Rice Krispies, Froot Loops***
- **White potatoes, white rice**
- **Watermelon, ripe bananas, cantaloupe, pineapple**
- **Soda, sugar-sweetened sports and energy drinks**
- **Sugar, candy, popcorn (plain)**
- **Ice cream (low-fat), frozen yogurt**

High-GI fruits and potatoes are still healthy choices when eaten in moderate amounts.

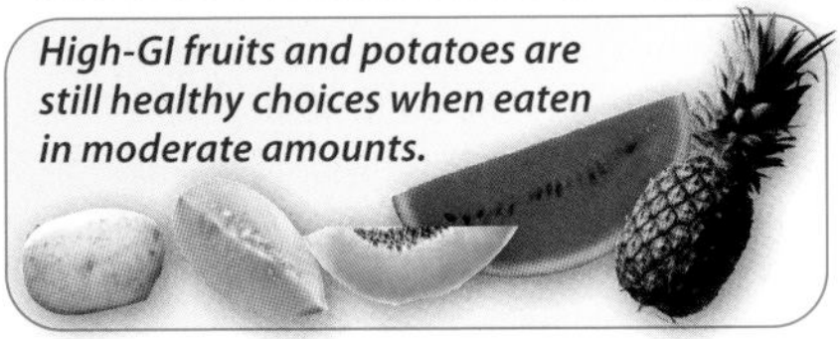

Notes ♦ Abbreviations ♦ Disclaimer

» **Calorie and fat values have been rounded off.**
Calories ~ to the nearest 5 or 10 calories.
Fat ~ to nearest half gram. **Note:** Trace amounts of fat (less than 0.3 grams) have been treated as zero.

» **Carbohydrate figures** in this book are for total carbohydrate, and not **Net Carbs** (which deducts fiber, polydextrose and sugar alcohols from total carbs).

» Because manufacturers' figures on labels are rounded off, figures in this book may differ slightly from the label. Serving sizes may also vary.

IMPORTANT DISCLAIMER

* The authors and publishers of this book are not physicians and are not licensed to give medical advice.This book is not a substitute for professional advice.Users should consult their medical professional before making any health, medical or other decisions based on the material contained herein.

* This book is a compilation of original material from other sources intended for educational purposes only. Because food manufacturers constantly change their products, only they are the authoritative source for food's most current nutritional information.

* Persons using the information herein for any medical purposes, such as matching insulin dosage to carbohydrate intake, should not rely solely on the accuracy of figures herein and should independently check food labels or contact the food manufacturer for the latest data.

Canadian Readers:

Please note that figures in this book are based on U.S. food products and restaurants. Equivalent Canadian foods may vary and should be checked independently.

* WARRANTY DISCLAIMER:

THE AUTHOR AND PUBLISHER DISCLAIM ANY LIABILITY ARISING DIRECTLY OR INDIRECTLY FROM THE USE OF THIS BOOK.THE INFORMATION HEREIN IS PROVIDED "AS IS" AND WITHOUT ANY WARRANTY EXPRESSED OR IMPLIED. ALL DIRECT, INDIRECT, SPECIAL, INCIDENTAL, CONSEQUENTIAL OR PUNITIVE DAMAGES ARISING FROM ANY USE OF THIS INFORMATION IS DISCLAIMED AND EXCLUDED.

This information is also provided subject to Family Health Publications' Terms and Conditions found at the website, www.calorieking.com/terms and incorporated herein.

C ~ Calories
F ~ Fat (grams)
Cb ~ Carbohydrate (grams)

Abbreviations

tsp = teaspoon
Tbsp or T = Tablespoon
oz = ounce(s)
c = cup
fl.oz = fluid ounce(s)
g = gram(s)
avg = average
pkg = package

Volume Measures

(All measures are level)
3 tsp = 1 Tbsp
2 Tbsp = 1 fl.oz
½ cup = 4 fl.oz
1 cup = 8 fl.oz
2 cups = 1 Pint
2 Pints = 1 Quart

Note: 8 oz weight is not the same as 8 fl oz volume (space occupied). Dense foods weigh more per set volume. Examples:
1 cup popcorn weighs ½ oz
1 cup milk weighs 8½ oz
1 cup pudding weighs 10 oz

Metric Conversion

½ oz = 14 grams
1 oz = 28.4 grams
2 oz = 57 grams
3½ oz = 100 grams
1 fl.oz = 30 mls
1 cup (8 fl.oz) = 240 mls
33 fl.oz = 1 liter (volume)

INFORMATION SOURCES

- U.S. Dept. of Agriculture
- U.S. Food Manufacturers
- Food Industry Boards & Councils
- Author extrapolations

FEEDBACK WELCOME!

Please contact the author with your queries and suggestions.
feedback@calorieking.com

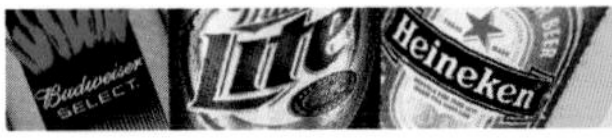

- **Health Hazards: Excessive alcohol intake** contributes to obesity, high blood pressure, stroke, heart and liver disease, some cancers, and even impotence. **Concentration and short-term memory** are reduced as well as athletic performance.

  Other alcohol hazards include: Fetal Alcohol Syndrome, stomach upsets, gut dysbiosis, menstrual and menopausal problems, depression, snoring, sleep problems, work absenteeism, impaired judgement, risky behaviors and social/family problems.
- **Alcohol contributes to obesity** through its high calories and by lessening the body's ability to burn fat. Fat storage is promoted, particularly in the belly – a health danger zone. Alcohol can also stimulate the appetite; and weaken the dieter's resolve!
- **Alcohol is potentially more harmful while dieting:** Blood sugar levels may drop with resultant fatigue and further impairment of concentration, reflexes and driving skills.

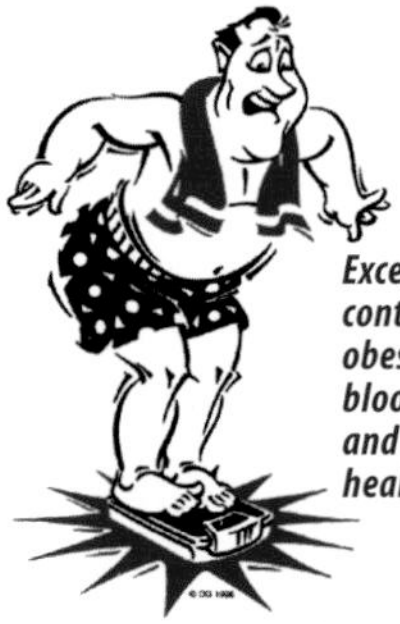

Excess alcohol contributes to obesity, high blood pressure and many other health problems

Lower Risk Alcohol Limits

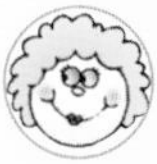

WOMEN:
No more than **1 drink** per day

MEN:
No more than **2 drinks** per day
(1 drink if over 65 y.o.)

(At least 2 days a week should be alcohol-free)

1 DRINK CONTAINS 14 GRAMS ALCOHOL →
- **12 fl.oz Regular Beer** (5% Alc.)
- **OR 14 fl.oz Light Beer** (4.2% Alc.)
- **OR 5 fl.oz Wine** (12% Alc.)
- **OR $1^1/_2$ fl.oz Spirits** (80 Proof)

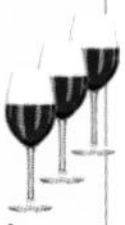

Note: You cannot save daily drinks for one occasion.
Binge drinking is particularly harmful:
4 drinks for males or 3 drinks for females (within 2 hours).

For some people, safe drinking means no alcohol at all. Even one drink may impair driving skills, particularly if tired. For women who drink frequently, breast cancer risk is increased by 9% for each drink after the first drink. In men, just 2 drinks a day doubles the risk of cancers of the mouth and throat.

It is advisable not to drink at all if you are:
- pregnant, trying to conceive or breastfeeding
- taking medication or have liver or heart disease (unless approved by your doctor or pharmacist)
- planning to drive, use machinery or play sports
- studying or needing to concentrate
- a child or adolescent

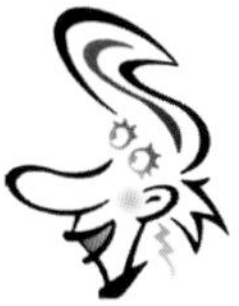

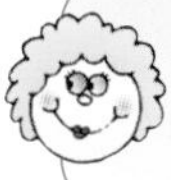

Women and adolescents are more prone to alcohol's ill-effects due to their lower body weight, smaller livers and lesser capacity to metabolize alcohol. As we age, our ability to handle alcohol decreases.

How To Calculate Alcohol Content

Percent alcohol on label refers to alcohol volume (ml alcohol/100ml).
Note: 100ml = 3½ fl.oz

To convert to grams (weight) of alcohol, multiply the alcohol volume by 0.8 – since 1 ml of alcohol weighs only 0.8 grams.

EXAMPLE:
12 fl.oz Can Beer
(5% alcohol)

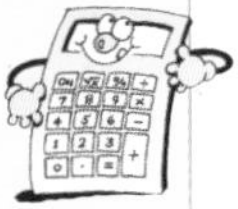

5% alc. volume
= 5% of 12 fl.oz = 0.6 fl.oz
= 18ml alcohol (Note: 1 fl.oz = 30ml)
Weight (18ml x 0.8) = 14.4g alcohol

Government Warnings!

(1) According to the Surgeon General, women should not drink alcoholic beverages during pregnancy because of the risk of birth defects.

(2) Consumption of alcoholic beverages impairs your ability to drive a car or operate machinery, and may cause health problems.

Extra Information

Alcohol & Diabetes ~ See Page 19
Alcohol & The Heart ~ See Page 18
Tips to Avoid Harmful Drinking ~ Page 19

Quick Guide

Alc ~ Alcohol (Grams)

Beer:

Cb ~ Carbohydrate

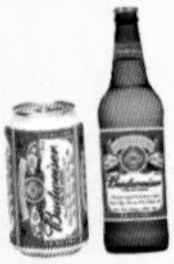

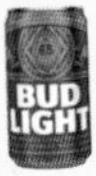

Beer Contains Zero Fat:	C	Alc	Cb
Regular Beer (5% Alc. Vol.):			
7 fl.oz Glass	80	8.5	4
12 fl.oz Bottle/Can/Glass	140	14	10
16 fl.oz/Pint	185	19	13
22 fl.oz Bottle	260	26	18
24 fl.oz Can	280	28	20
32 fl.oz/ ½ Yard	370	38	28
40 fl.oz Bottle	470	47	35
50 fl.oz Football	590	59	50
Light Beer (4.2% Alc. Vol.):			
7 fl.oz Glass	65	7	4
12 fl.oz Bottle/Can/Glass	110	12	7
16 fl.oz/Pint	145	16	9
22 fl.oz Bottle	200	22	13
24 fl.oz Can	220	24	14
Non-Alcoholic Brews: (Less than 0.5% alcohol by volume)			
Average all Brands, 12 fl.oz	70	1	14

Beer ~ Brands

Note: Figure shown are for the United States except for the states of Utah, Colorado, Kansas and Oklahoma who have certain restrictions limiting the alcohol content to not more than 4% by volume (3.2% by weight).

Percentage alcohol listed is by volume - not by weight.

Per 12 fl.oz Serving

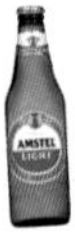

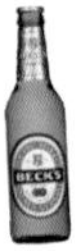

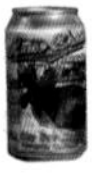

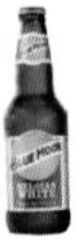

	C	Alc	Cb
Aguila (3.9%)	125	12	14
Amstel, Light (3.5%)	95	10	5
Anchor: Porter (5.6%)	210	16	23
Steam (4.9%)	160	14	14
Asahi: Kuronama (5.3%)	165	14	14
Select (4.7%)	140	13	11
Super Dry (4.9%)	150	14	11
Bass, Pale Ale (5.1%)	155	14	12
Beck's: Original (5%)	145	14	11
Premier Light (2.3%)	65	7	4
Sapphire (6%)	160	17	9
Big Sky: Original IPA (6.2%)	195	18	17
Moose Drool (5.3%)	175	15	16
Scape Goat (4.7%)	155	14	14
Trout Slayer Ale (4.7%)	145	14	12
Blatz: Original (4.6%)	145	13	13
Light (3.9%)	110	11	8
Blue Moon:			
Belgian White (5.4%)	170	15	14
Mango Wheat (5.4%)	175	15	16
Bohemia (4.73%)	140	14	12
Bud Ice (5.5%)	125	16	4

Brands (Cont)

Alc ~ Alcohol (Grams)

Per 12 fl.oz Serving

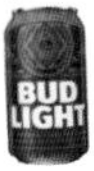

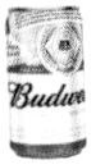

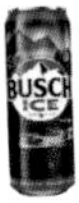

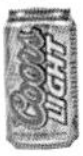

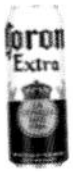

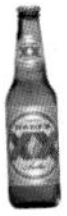

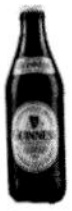

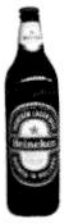

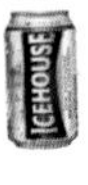

	C	Alc	Cb
Bud Light: Regular (4.2%)	110	12	7
Clamato Chelada: Orig. (4.2%)	150	12	16
Extra Lime; Mango (4.2%), av.	155	12	17
Lemonade (4.2%)	150	12	16
Lime (4%)	115	12	8
Orange (4.2%)	145	12	14
Platinum (6%)	140	17	5
Budweiser: Lager (5%)	145	14	11
Clamato Chelado (4.2%)	150	12	16
Discovery Reserve (5%)	155	14	13
Nitro Gold (5%)	170	14	15
Select (4.3%)	100	12	3
Select 55 (2.4%)	55	7	2
Zero (0%)	50	0	12
Busch: Original (4.3%)	115	12	7
Ice (5.9%)	135	17	4
Light (4.1%)	95	12	3
NA (0.4%)	60	1	13
Carlsberg, Pilsner (5%)	135	14	10
Carta Blanca (4.6%)	145	13	11
Cerveza, Aguila (4%)	125	11	11
Colorado Native, Amber (5.5%)	170	16	15
Colt 45, Malt Liquor (5.6%)	155	16	11
Coors: Banquet (5%)	145	14	12
Light (4.2%)	100	12	5
Non-Alcoholic	60	0	12
Corona: Extra (4.5%)	150	13	13
Light (4.1%)	100	12	5
Premier (4%)	90	11	11
Dos Equis XX: Ambar (4.7%)	145	14	12
Lager (4.5%)	140	13	11
Extra Gold (5%)	150	14	12
Fosters: Lager (5%)	145	14	11
Premium Ale (5.5%)	160	16	13
Genesee: Beer (4.5%)	145	13	13
Light (4%)	100	10	4
George Killian's, Irish Red (5.4%)	170	16	15
Goose Island, So-Lo (3%)	100	8	9
Grolsch, Premium (5%)	145	14	10
Guinness: Draught (4%)	125	12	10
Extra Stout (6%)	175	17	14
Blonde American (5%)	150	14	11
Nitro IPA (5.8%), 11.2oz	155	19	5
Hamm's: Original (4.7%)	145	13	12
Special Light (3.8%)	110	12	8
Heineken: Lager (5%)	140	14	10
Special Dark (5%)	165	14	15
Premium Light (3.5%)	100	10	7
0.0 (Alchohol-Free)	75	0	12
Hop Valley: Bubble Stash (6.2%)	195	17	16
Citrus Mistress (6.5%)	190	18	14
Hurricane: Malt Liquor (6%)	140	17	4
High Gravity (8.1%)	185	23	6
Icehouse, Original (5.5%)	150	16	10

Brands (Cont)

Alc ~ Alcohol (Grams) Cb ~ Carbohydrate

Beer Contains Zero Fat:
Per 12 fl.oz Serving

	C	Alc	Cb
Keystone: Ice (5.9%)	145	17	7
Light (4.1%)	100	12	5
King Cobra (6%)	135	17	4
Kirin: Ichiban (5%)	145	14	11
Light (3.2%)	95	9	8
Kokanee (5%)	145	14	11
Labatt: Blue (5%)	135	14	10
Blue Light (4%)	110	11	8
Laqunitas, Daytime (4%)	100	12	3
Landshark, Lager (4.6%)	150	13	13
Leinenkugel's: Original (4.7%)	150	13	15
Summer Shandy (4.2%)	135	12	13
Lone Star: Pale Lager (4.65%)	135	13	11
Light (3.85%)	110	11	8
Lowenbrau, Original (5%)	140	14	12
Magic Hat, #9 (5.1% alc)	165	15	15
Magnum, Malt Liquor (5.6%)	155	16	11
Michelob Ultra:			
Ultra Amber (4%)	100	11	5
Ultra Infusions, Lime (4%)	95	11	5
Ultra Light (4.2%)	95	12	3
Ultra Pure Gold (3.8%)	85	12	3
Mickey's, Malt Liquor (5.6%)	155	16	11
Miller:			
Genuine Draft/High Life (4.6%)	140	13	12
High Life Light (4.1%)	110	12	6
Lite (4.2%)	95	12	3
Miller64 (2.8%)	65	8	3
Milwaukee's Best:			
Ice (5.9%)	150	17	8
Light (4.1%)	95	12	4
Premium (4.8%)	145	14	12
Minnesota's Best, Original (4.9%)	140	14	10
Modelo, Especial (4.4%)	145	13	14
Molson Canadian: Ice (5.6%)	170	16	14
Lager (5%)	150	14	12
Canadian 67 (3%)	70	8	3
Moosehead, Lager (5%)	150	14	11
Natural: Ice (5.9%)	130	17	4
Light (4.2%)	95	12	3
Negra Modelo (5.4%)	175	15	16
Newcastle, Brown Ale (4.7%)	130	13	10
O'Douls: Amber (0.4%)	90	1	18
Original (0.4%)	65	1	13
Old Milwaukee: Lager (4.6%)	145	13	13
Light (3.8%)	110	11	8
Non-Alcoholic (0.4%)	60	1	12
Old Style: Lager (4.7%)	145	13	12
Light (4.2%)	115	12	7
Pabst: Blue Ribbon (4.8%)	145	13	12
Low Calorie (3.8%)	110	11	8
Pacifico, Clara (4.4%)	145	12	13

Per 12 fl.oz Serving Unless Indicated

	C	Alc	Cb
Palmier, (4.2%), 11.2 fl.oz	90	11	3
Peroni, Nastro Azzurro (5.1%)	150	14	12
Piels, Lager (4.3%)	125	12	9
Pilsner Urquell, Lager (4.4%)	155	12	16
Point: Amber Classic (4.7%)	160	13	14
Special Lager (4.7%)	150	13	12
Presidente (5%)	175	14	5
Redbridge, Lager (4%)	135	10	14
Red Dog, Lager (4.8%)	145	14	12
Red Hook: ESB (5.8%)	185	16	16
India Pale Ale (4.7%)	190	13	19
Red Stripe, Jamaican Lager (7%)	150	13	14
Redd's: Apple Ale (5%), 12 fl.oz	165	14	17
Wicked Hard Ale (8%), av. 10 fl.oz	230	19	25
Saint Archer: Blonde (4.8%)	150	14	13
Pale Ale (5.5%)	170	16	13
Samuel Adams:			
Boston Lager (4.9%)	175	14	17
Sam Adams, Light Lager (4%)	120	13	8
Sapporo, Prem. Lager (4.9%)	135	14	9
Schaefer: Lager (4.6%)	145	13	12
Light (3.9%)	110	11	8
Schell's: Deer (4.7%)	145	14	13
Light (3.5%)	100	10	7
Schlitz: Pale Lager (4.6%)	145	13	12
Light (3.8%)	110	11	8
Schmidt's: Pale Lager (4.6%)	145	13	13
Light (3.8%)	110	11	8
Sharps, *(Miller)*, N.A., 12 fl.oz	60	0	12
Sheaf, Stout (5.7%)	190	16	19
Shock Top: Belgian White (5.2%)	165	15	15
Lemon Shandy (4.2%)	145	12	15
Sierra Nevada: Bigfoot (9.6%)	330	28	32
Draft Pale Ale (5%)	155	14	13
Pale Ale (5.6%)	175	16	14
Sol: Lager (4.5%)	140	13	12
Chelada (3.5%)	160	10	20
Sparks, Lager (6%)	250	17	34
Steel Reserve:			
High Gravity Malt Liquor (8.1%)	220	23	15
Steel 6.0 (6%)	165	17	11
Stella Artois, (5%), 11.2 fl.oz	140	14	11
Stroh's: Classic (4.5%)	145	13	12
Light (4.1%)	120	12	7
Tecate: Pale Lager (4.6%)	140	13	11
Light (4%)	110	11	8
Third Shift, Amber Lager (5.3%)	185	15	18
Trader Jose: Premium, 11.2 fl.oz	145	14	14
Light (3.8%), 11.2 fl.oz	105	14	8
Victoria Lager (4%)	135	11	14
Wild Blue, Lager (8%)	240	23	20
Yuengling: Light (3.2%)	99	9	9
Traditional Lager (4.5%)	140	13	12
ZeigenBock, Amber (4.9%)	145	14	11

Updated Nutrition Data ~ www.CalorieKing.com
Persons with Diabetes ~ See Disclaimer (Page 22)

A Alcohol ~ Cider ◆ Wine

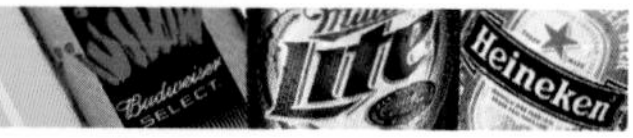

Alc ~ Alcohol (Grams) Cb ~ Carbohydrate

Ciders ~ Alcoholic/Hard

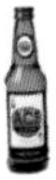
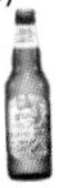
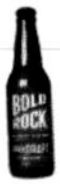
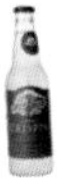
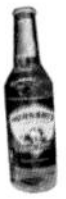
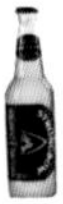
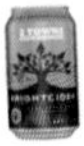
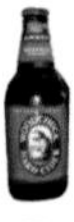
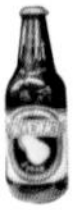

Per 12 fl.oz Unless Indicated	C	Alc	Cb
Ace: Apple (5%), 12 fl.oz	145	14	12
Berry (5%), 12 fl.oz	155	14	14
Joker (6.9%), 12 fl.oz	190	19	13
Perry (5%), 12 fl.oz	170	14	18
Pineapple (5%), 12 fl.oz	175	14	19
Angry Orchard: Crisp Apple (5%)	190	14	25
Easy Apple (4.2%), 12 fl.oz	150	12	19
Green Apple (5.5%), 12 fl.oz	210	14	31
Pear (5%), 12 fl.oz	160	14	17
Rosé (5.5%), 12 fl.oz	170	16	17
Bold Rock: Apple, (4.7%), 12 fl.oz	140	13	12
Carolina Draft (4.7%), 12 fl.oz	145	13	13
IPA (4.7%), 12 fl.oz	140	13	12
Pear (4.7%), 12 fl.oz	140	13	12
Premium Dry (6%), 12 fl.oz	140	17	6
Crispin: Original (5%), 12 fl.oz	160	14	15
Blackberry Pear (5%), 12 fl.oz	170	14	16
Brut (5.5%), 12 fl.oz	170	16	13
Honey Crisp (6.5%), 12 fl.oz	200	18	16
Pacific Pear (4.5%), 12 fl.oz	160	13	17
Rosé (5%), 12 fl.oz	160	14	13
The Saint (6.9%), 12 fl.oz	230	19	20
Hornsby's: Amber (5.5%)	180	16	19
Crisp (5.5%), 12 fl.oz	190	16	26
Johnny Appleseed, (5.5%)	210	16	26
Magners, (4.5%)	125	13	9
Michelob, Ultra Light Cider (4%)	120	10	10
Saint Archer, Hard Cider (6.1%)	170	17	11
Smith & Forge, Hard Apple (6%)	220	17	26
Stella Artois Cidre, (4.5%)	180	13	22
Strongbow: *Per 11.2 fl oz*			
Cherry Blossom, (4.5%), av.	155	12	25
Original Dry (5%), 12 fl.oz	145	14	10
Rosé Apple (5%)	140	13	11
2 Towns Ciderhouse:			
Brightcider Apple (6%), 12 fl.oz	145	17	7
Ginger Ninja (6%), 12 fl.oz	145	17	7
Made Marion (6%), 12 fl.oz	150	17	8
Outcider (5%), 12 fl.oz	155	14	14
Pacific Pineapple (5%), 12 fl.oz	150	14	12
Woodchuck: Amber (5%)	200	14	21
Granny Smith (5%), 12 fl.oz	160	14	11
Pear (4%), 12 fl.oz	150	12	18
Raspberry (4%), 12 fl.oz	170	12	22
Semi-Dry (5.5%), 12 fl.oz	160	14	13
Wyder's: Pear (4%), 12 fl.oz	140	11	22
Prickly Pineapple (5%), 12 fl.oz	180	14	22
Raspberry (4%), 12 fl.oz	120	11	17
Reposado (6.9%), 12 fl.oz	250	19	30

Quick Guide ~ Table Wines

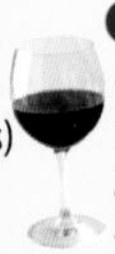
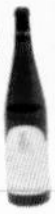

Average all Varieties (11.5% Alc.) *(Wine Contains Zero Fat)*	C	Alc	Cb
4 fl.oz, 1 small wine glass OR ½ large wine glass	100	11	3
6 fl.oz, (¾ large wine glass)	145	16	5
8 fl.oz, (1 large wine glass)	200	21	7
½ Carafe/Bottle, 12 fl.oz	300	32	10
1 Bottle, 750ml, 25.4 fl.oz	620	68	21
Red Wines: *Per 4 fl.oz*			
Burgundy/Cabernet/Merlot, av.	100	11	4
White Wines: *Per 4 fl.oz*			
Dry (Chenin; Fume Blanc; Chardonnay)	95	11	4
Sparkling, 4 fl.oz	95	11	4
Zinfandel Sweet, (Moselle/Sauterne), 4 fl.oz	85	11	2

Other Wines

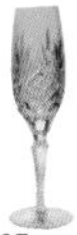

	C	Alc	Cb
Champagne: *Per 4 fl.oz*			
Average all types, 1 glass	85	11	2
with Orange Jce (3:1 orange)	75	8	4
with Orange Jce (1:1 orange)	65	5	7
Mulled Wine *(Gluhwein)*, 4 fl.oz	180	14	20
Non-Alcoholic Wine: *Less than 0.5% Alcohol*			
Ariel: White varieties, average, 4 fl.oz	35	0.5	8
Red varieties, average, 4 fl.oz	25	0.5	5
Flavored/Reduced Alcohol Wine:			
Average All Brands (6% alcohol): *(Arbor Mist, Wild Vines, Boone's Farm):*			
1 small wine glass, 4 fl.oz	80	6	10
1 large wine glass, 8 fl.oz	160	11	20
Skinnygirl, Red/White, (8.5%), 5 fl.oz	100	10	5
Sake *(Gekkeikan)*, (16%), 4 fl.oz	120	15	5
Sangria *(Skinnygirl)*, (4%), 5 fl.oz	130	5	23

Dessert Wines

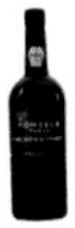

	C	Alc	Cb
Madeira (18%), 2 oz	85	9	5
Marsala (18%), 2 oz	110	9	11
Port, Muscatel (18%), 2 oz	85	9	5
Sherry (15%), 2 oz:			
Dry, 1 Sherry glass	90	7	7
Sweet/Cream, average	90	7	8
Vermouth *(Martini & Rossi)*:			
Extra Dry (18%), 2 oz	65	9	2
Martini Rosso (16%), 2 oz	90	8	8

Cooking Wines

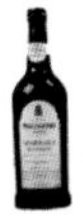

	C	Alc	Cb
Holland House:			
Marsala, (14%), 2 T., 1 fl.oz	45	4	4
Red/White, (10%): 2 T., 1 fl.oz	20	2	1
1 cup, 8 fl.oz	160	18	8
Sherry, (17%), 2 Tbsp, 1 fl.oz	45	5	2

Quick Guide

Alc ~ Alcohol (Grams)

Spirits/Liquors:
Includes Bourbon, Brandy, Gin, Rum, Scotch, Tequila, Vodka, Whiskey.
Note: All spirits with same alcohol proof have similar calories and zero fat.

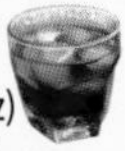

Average All Brands	C	Alc	Cb
80 Proof (40% Alcohol by Volume):			
1 fl.oz	65	9.5	0
1.5 fl.oz (1 shot)	100	14	0
3 fl.oz (Double shot)	195	28	0
½ Bottle, 350 ml (12 fl.oz)	770	113	0
1 Bottle, 700 ml (24 fl.oz)	1540	227	0
86 Proof (43% Alc), 1.5 fl.oz shot	105	15	0
100 Proof (50% Alc), 1.5 fl.oz	125	18	0
Shochu (Soju), av., (25% alc), 2 fl.oz	65	12	0

Flavored Spirits

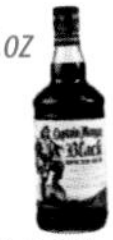

	C	Alc	Cb
Captain Morgan: *Per 1.5 fl.oz*			
Original (35%)	85	12	0.5
Black Spiced (47.3%)	115	14	1
Parrot Bay (21%), average	90	7.5	10
Silver Spiced (35%)	95	12	2
Malibu Rum, Orig,/Fruit (21%), 1.5 fl.oz	80	8	8
Southern Comfort (35%), 1.5 fl.oz	100	13	3

Hard Lemonade, Sodas, Seltzers & Tea

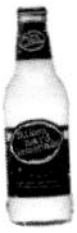

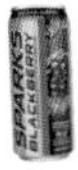

	C	Alc	Cb
Bud Light Seltzers, (5%), 12 fl.oz	100	14	2
Corona Seltzer, (4.5%), 12 fl.oz	90	12	0
Henry's Hard Soda:			
Grape (4.2%), 12 fl.oz	225	12	35
Lemon Lime/Orange (4.2%), 12 fl.oz	190	12	28
Labatt Blue Light Seltzer, (5%)	100	14	1
Margaritaville:			
Lime Margarita (8%), 12 fl.oz	310	23	30
Paradise Punch (8%), 12 fl.oz	340	23	46
Mike's Hard Lemonade:			
Black Cherry (5%), 11.2 fl.oz	220	13	33
Lite (5%), 11.2 fl.oz	150	13	15
Lemonade (5%), 11.2 fl.oz	220	13	33
Lite (5%), 11.2 fl.oz	100	13	4
Harder (8%), 16 fl.oz	395	31	44
Not Your Father's Root Beer, (5.9%), 12 fl.oz	195	17	20
Pabst Hard Coffee, (5%), 11 fl.oz	250	13	31
Platform Setzer, (5%), 11.2 fl.oz	110	13	4
Pura Still, (4.5%), 11.2 fl.oz	90	12	1
Redd's Wicked, (8%), av. 10 fl.oz	230	19	25
Social Club Seltzer, (7%), 12 fl.oz	150	20	2
Sparks, Original (6%), 16 fl.oz	335	23	45
Twisted Tea: Original (5%)	220	14	31
Half & Half (5%)	260	14	34
Zumbida Mango, (4.2%), 12 fl.oz	150	12	17

Coolers & Premix Cocktails

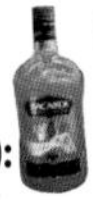

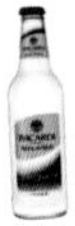

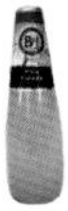

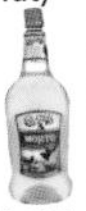

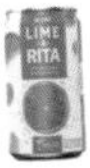

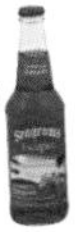

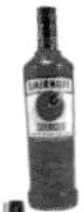

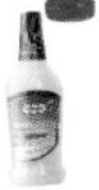

Ready-To-Drink: *Zero Fat Unless Indicated*	C	Alc	Cb
Bacardi: *Per 4 fl.oz*			
Party Drinks (Ready To Pour):			
Bahama Mama; Mai Tai (10%)	130	9	16
Mojito (15%)	160	14	16
Rum Island Ice Tea (12.5%)	150	12	16
Bacardi Silver: *Per 12 fl.oz*			
Lemonade/Sangria (6%), av.	270	17	41
Mojito/Raz/Strawberry (5%)	240	14	36
Bartles & Jaymes: *Per 11.2 fl.oz*			
Malt Based Coolers (3.2%):			
Exotic Berry	195	9	31
Fuzzy Navel	215	9	36
Margarita; Pina Colada, av.	245	9	44
Pomegranate Raspberry	205	9	35
Sangria	240	9	40
Strawberry Daiquiri	205	9	34
Cape Lime, Cocktails (4.5%), av. 12 fl.oz	120	13	9
Captain Morgan's, Parrot Bay (4.1%), all var. av., 11.2 fl.oz	210	10	35
Chi Chi's: Long Is. Iced Tea, 4 fl.oz	145	12	17
Mexican Mudslide, 4 fl.oz (8g fat)	240	2	42
Mojito, 4 fl.oz	160	11	21
Pina Colada, 4 fl.oz (6g fat)	240	4	42
White Russian, 4 fl.oz (7g fat)	245	2	43
Daily's, Frozen Pouches (5%), average all flavors, 10 fl.oz	285	12	47
Jack Daniels, Country Cocktails (4.8%), average all varieties, 10 fl.oz	200	9	30
Jose Cuervo:			
Margaritas: Classic Lime (10%), 6 fl.oz	210	14	29
Golden (12.7%), 4.7 fl.oz	170	14	19
Pabst, Hard Coffee (5%), 11 fl.oz	250	13	31
Ritas: Lime-A-Rita (8%), 8 fl.oz	220	15	29
Spritz (6%), av., 12 fl.oz	200	17	21
Seagram's:			
Escapes Coolers (3.2%):			
Bahama Mama, 11.2 fl.oz	200	9	36
Strawb. Daiquiri, 11.2 fl.oz	225	9	41
Skinnygirl:			
Vodka with flavors (30%), 1.5 fl.oz	75	11	0
Cocktails (10%), av., 3 fl.oz	70	8	4
Smirnoff:			
Ice (4.5%): Original, 11.2 fl.oz	220	13	33
Mango; Pineapple, av., 11.2 fl.oz	230	13	35
Sourced, Fruit Flavors, (4.5%), 11.2 fl.oz	160	12	20
Spiked Sparkling Seltzer, (4.5%), all flav., 12 fl.oz can	90	13	1
TGI Friday's:			
On The Rocks: *Per 6 fl.oz*			
Long Island Ice Tea (15%)	250	21	28
Margarita (7.5%)	185	11	29
Mudslide (10%)	365	14	31
Blenders (12.5%), Mudslide, 6 fl.oz	365	18	31

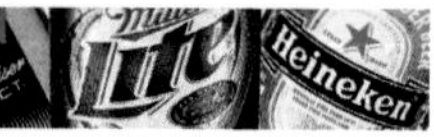

Coolers & Premix Cocktails (Cont)

Ready-To-Drink:	C	Alc	Cb
The Club Premix Cocktails: *Per 3.4 oz Serving (½ can)*			
Censored on Beach; Margarita (7.5%)	105	6	17
Gin/Vodka Martini (21%), av.	155	17	0.2
Ice Tea (15%)	145	12	17
Manhattan (17%)	115	13	5
Mudslide/Pina Colada (10%), av.	200	8	16
Screwdriver (7.5%)	95	6	14
Whiskey Sour (10%)	95	8	11

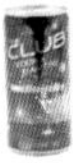

Shooters

Alc ~ Alcohol (Grams)

Alabama Slammer	110	14	2
Amaretto Sour	120	6	19
B52	145	14	11
Beam Me Up Scotty	145	13	13
Blue Tequila	160	18	6
Jager Bomb	205	8	30
Jager Bomb, w/ Sugar-Free Red Bull	155	8	18
Jell-O Shot: 3 oz, with 1.5 oz Vodka	180	14	19
with Diet Jell-O	110	14	0
Kamikaze	75	8	3
Kool-Aid	160	15	14
Orgasm	100	12	6
Peppermint Patty	195	8	11
Stinger	170	18	12
Surfer on Acid	90	7	11

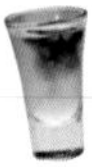

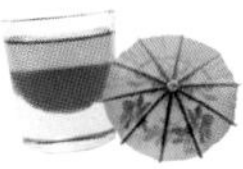

Cocktail Mixers ~ Non-Alcoholic

Bacardi: *Per 8 fl.oz, Prepared from 2 fl.oz Concentrate*			
Daiquiris; Rum Runner	120	0	32
Margarita	90	0	25
Mojito	110	0	30
Pina Colada	170	0	36
Baja Bob's: *Per 4 fl.oz*			
Cranberry Cosmo Martini	10	0	2
Pina Colada	30	0	4
Jose Cuervo:			
Margaritas: Av. all flav., 4 fl.oz	85	0	21
Light (Sugar Free), Lime, 4 fl.oz	5	0	1
Mr & Mrs T:			
Bloody Mary: Original, 5 oz	30	0	7
Bold & Spicy, 4 oz	35	0	7
Mai Tai	130	0	32
Margarita	100	0	26
Pina Colada	170	0	44
Strawberry Daiquiri	180	0	46
TGI Friday's:			
Mudslide, 2.3 fl.oz	110	0	23
Cosmo; Berrytini, 2 fl.oz	80	0	20
Strawb. Daiquiri; Marg., 4 fl.oz	190	0	46

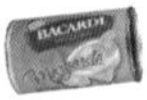

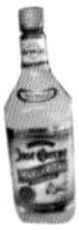

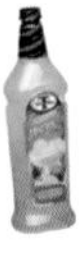

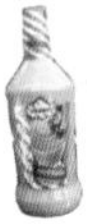

Cocktails

Alc ~ Alcohol (Grams)

Made to Standard Recipes (Standard Size):
(Main Reference: The New American Bartender's Guide)

Zero Fat Unless Indicated	C	Alc	Cb
Adios Mother F.	260	23	23
Bacardi & Coke (with 1.5 oz Bacardi)	160	14	17
Bellini, 4.5 fl.oz	95	11	7
Bloody Mary (with 1.5 oz Vodka)	125	10	7
Blushin' Russian (20g fat)	405	14	23
Bourbon & Soda (with 2 oz Bourbon)	130	19	0
Brandy Alexander (10g fat)	300	20	15
Chupa Naranjas (with 1.5 oz Tequila)	150	16	8
Cosmopolitan	215	24	12
Daiquiri (w/ 2 oz Rum), av. all types	140	19	4
Frozen Daiquiri (with 2 oz Rum):			
without fruit	155	19	6
with fruit (with 1.5 oz Rum)	145	14	11
Grasshopper	260	17	28
Harvey Wallbanger (2 oz)	200	19	17
Highball (1.5 oz Whiskey)	100	14	0
Irish Coffee (10g fat)	205	14	2
Kahlua Mudslide: with milk (3g fat)	145	11	12
with cream (12g fat)	230	11	10
Lemon Drop, 4 fl.oz	130	14	10
Long Island Iced Tea (with 3 oz Cola)	270	19	32
with 3 oz Diet Cola	235	19	22
Mai Tai (with 2 oz Rum)	290	24	33
Manhattan	130	17	5
Margarita	160	18	7
Martini: Dry, with 1.5 oz gin	100	14	0
Sour Apple, w/ 2 oz Vodka/1 oz Schnapps	250	31	10
Mint Julep (with 2½ oz Bourbon)	180	24	4
Mojito (with 2 oz rum)	170	19	9
Moscow Mule (with 1.5 oz Vodka)	180	14	20
Pina Colada (10g fat), 6 oz	250	15	18
Red Bull & Vodka (with 1.5 oz vodka)	210	14	28
with Sugar Free Red Bull	105	14	3
Rum & Coke (with 1.5 oz Rum)	160	14	17
Sake Bomb (1.5 oz Sake & 5 oz Beer)	105	12	7
Sangria: with 1 oz Fruit Juice, 5 oz	120	12	9
with 0.5 oz Brandy, 5.5 oz	150	17	9
Screwdriver	160	14	15
Sex On The Beach	235	19	25
Spritzer (with 3 oz Wine)	65	8	2
Tequila Sunrise	200	14	25
Tom Collins (with 2 oz Gin)	210	19	18
Vodka Soda (with 1.5 oz Vodka)	100	14	0
Vodka Tonic (with 1.5 oz Vodka)	165	14	18
Whiskey Sour (w/ 2 oz Whiskey)	155	19	7
White Russian (10g fat)	240	19	7
Non-Alcoholic:			
Cinderella	45	0	11
Shirley Temple (with 6 oz Ginger Ale)	140	0	34

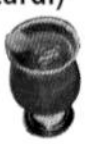

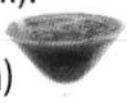

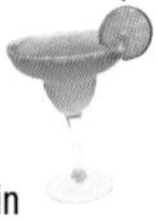

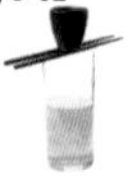

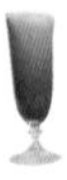

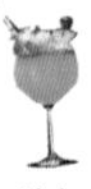

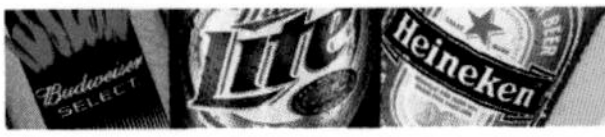

Liqueurs/Cordials

Per 1 fl.oz

	C	Alc	Cb
Advocaat (36 Proof; 2g fat)	85	4	9
Alizé: Cognac (80 Proof)	70	9	2
Gold/Red Passion (32 Proof)	105	4	11
Amaretto (56 Proof)	110	7	17
Baileys Irish Cream (34 Proof; 4g fat)	100	4	8
Benedictine (80 Proof)	90	9	5
Chambord (33 Proof)	105	4	11
Chartreuse (80 Proof)	100	9	9
Cherry Brandy (48 Proof)	80	6	9
Coffee Liqueur (53 Proof)	115	7	16
Cointreau (80 Proof)	95	9	7
Creme de Cacao (54 Proof)	100	6	15
Creme de Menthe (72 Proof)	125	9	14
Curacao (70 Proof)	95	8	6
Drambuie (80 Proof)	105	9	9
Frangelico (40 Proof)	65	5	12
Galliano (86 Proof)	100	10	8
Grand Marnier (80 Proof)	100	9	7
(40 Proof)	85	5	14
Kirsch (68 Proof)	80	8	6
Midori (42 Proof)	80	5	11
Ouzo (80 Proof)	105	9	11
Pernod (80 Proof)	75	9	11
Sambuca (84 Proof)	100	10	11
Schnapps (100 Proof)	115	12	9
Southern Comfort (70 Proof)	65	8	3
Tia Maria (40% Proof)	90	7	10

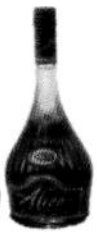

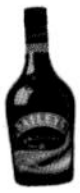

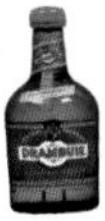

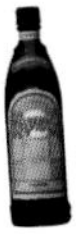
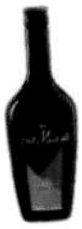

Liqueur Coffee & Hot Drinks

Per Standard Drink

	C	Alc	Cb
Liqueur Coffee: Av. all types	200	10	10
Irish, 1.5 oz Whiskey & 1 oz whip	205	9	4
Hot Toddy, with 1½ oz liquor, av. all	170	9	19
Mulled Wine *(Glühwein)*, 4 fl.oz, av	195	14	25

"The doctor told him to cut down to just one glass a day."

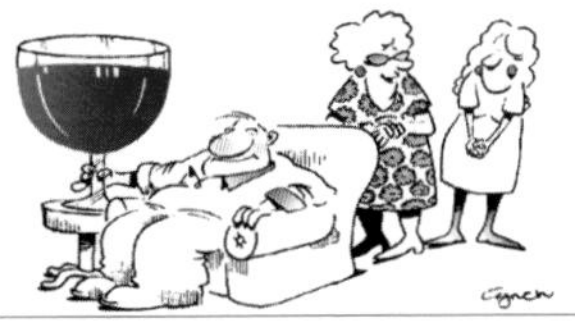

Updated Nutrition Data ~ www.CalorieKing.com
Persons with Diabetes ~ See Disclaimer (Page 22)

TEN TIPS TO AVOID HARMFUL DRINKING

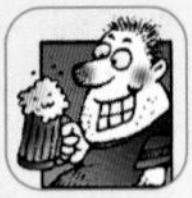

1. **Add up the alcohol** you typically drink each day and on social occasions. How does this compare with 'low risk' amounts? *(See page 23)*
2. **Compare the alcohol content** of different drinks and select the lowest. Request half shots of alcohol in cocktails and mixed drinks. Dilute them and keep topping off with non-alcoholic drinks.
3. **Go easy on 'Light' beers.** At 4% alcohol, on average, they are still high in alcohol compared to regular beer (5% alcohol).
4. **Try low alcohol or non-alcohol** alternatives such as fruit juices and mineral water. Take your own to parties.
5. **Before drinking alcohol,** quench your thirst with water and non-alcoholic drinks – particularly after vigorous exercise or sports.
6. **Slow the rate of drinking.** Chugging or drinking fast is the major cause of illness and death from alcohol poisoning.
7. **Avoid drinking in 'rounds'.**
8. **Have a non-alcoholic 'spacer'** between drinks (e.g. mineral water, orange juice).
9. **Don't drink on an empty stomach.** Food slows the rate of alcohol absorption.
10. **Keep track of the number of drinks** and know when to stop. Stick to a set limit.

Note: Alcohol can be very dangerous when taken with prescription or street drugs, or when you are very tired.

Extra Info: www.CalorieKing.com

Cocktail Mixers & Extracts

	C	Alc	Cb
Angostura Bitters, ¼ tsp	2	0	0.5
Grenadine, ½ tsp	6	0	2
Lime/Lemon Juice, 2 Tbsp, 1 oz	10	0	2
Maraschino Cherry, 1 small	8	0	2
Simple Syrup, 1 Tbsp, av.	50	0	14
Sweet & Sour Mix, 2 Tbsp, 1 oz	30	0	7
Tonic Water, 8 fl.oz	80	0	22
Flavor Extracts *(McCormick)*:			
Pure Lemon (83%), 1 tsp	0	3.5	0
Pure Vanilla (35%), 1tsp	0	1.5	0

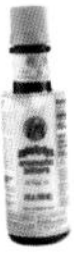
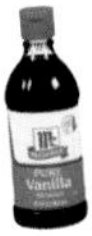

B Baking Ingredients

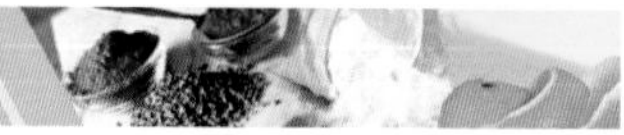

Baking Ingredients	C	F	Cb
Almond Flour, ¼ cup, 1 oz	160	10	10
Almond Paste,			
(Marzipan), 2 Tbsp	170	7	24
Apple Pie Filling,			
Sweetened, 9.4 oz	290	0	69
(Bean Water), ¼ c., 2 oz	10	0	2
Amaranth Flour *(Bob's Red Mill),*			
¼ cup, 1 oz	110	2	20
Baking Powder: Regular, 1 tsp	5	0	1
Cream of Tartar, 1 tsp	10	0	2
Baking Mix *(Bisquick)*:			
Original, ⅓ cup, 1.5 oz	160	5	26
Batter Mix (*Golden Dipt),*			
All Purpose, ¼ cup	100	0	20
Butter/Margarine, ½ cup, 4 oz	800	88	1
Stick *(Land O' Lakes)*, 0.5 oz	100	11	0
Cacao Butter, 2 Tbsp, 1 oz	240	28	0
Cacao Powder, raw: 1 Tbsp, 0.3 oz	35	2	3
¼ cup, 1 oz	150	9	11
Carob Flour, ½ cup	115	0.5	46
Cassava Flour, ½ cup, 70g	260	0	62
Chia Seed Protein Powder, 2 T., 0.5 oz	25	0	8
Chocolate Baking Bars: *Average all Brands*			
Sweet *(Baker's)*:			
1 oz portion	120	7	16
4 oz bar	470	28	64
Semi-sweet, 1 oz	140	9	16
White Baking, 1 oz	160	9	16
Unsweetened: 1 oz	140	14	8
Grated, 1 cup, 4.5 oz	660	69	39
Chocolate Baking Chips: *Average all Brands*			
Milk Choc./Semi Sweet, 1 oz	140	8	18
½ cup, 3 oz	420	24	54
1 cup, 6 oz	840	48	108
Dark, 1 Tbsp, 0.5 oz	70	5	3
Mini Kisses *(Hershey)*, 1 piece	5	0.5	1
Cocoa Powder, unsweetened:			
1 Tbsp, 0.2 oz	15	0.5	3
⅓ cup, 1 oz	60	4	17
Coconut, dried:			
Sweetened/Flaked: 1 oz	130	8	15
½ cup, 1.3 oz	195	12	22
Tsd *(Baker's)*, 1 oz	170	13	13
Unsweetened, 1 oz	190	18	7
Coconut Cream/Milk ~ *See Page 89*			
Coconut Flour, 2 Tbsp, 0.5 oz	60	2	8
Coconut Manna (*Nutiva)*, 1 Tbsp	100	9	3
Cornstarch, 1 Tbsp	30	0	7
Eggs: Large (1)	75	5	0
Jumbo (1)	90	6	0.5
Egg White: 1 Egg White	15	0	0
½ cup (4 egg whites), 4 oz	60	0	1

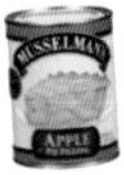
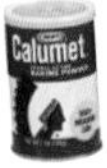

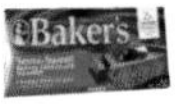

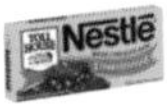

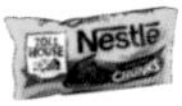

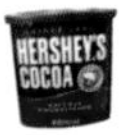

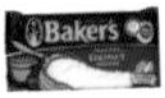

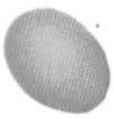

Flour:	C	F	Cb
Whole Wheat, 1 cup, 4.2 oz	400	2	84
White: 1 Tbsp, 0.3 oz	25	0	5.5
1 cup, 4.2 oz	400	1	88
Flavor Extracts: *Av. all Brands*			
Imitation, 1 tsp	10	0	2
Pure Extract, 1 tsp	10	0	0.5
Almond; Vanilla, 1 tsp	10	0	0.5
Fruit Pectin: Swtnd, ¼ tsp	5	0	1
Unsweetened, ¼ tsp	0	0	0
Gelatin, dry, unsweetened, 0.3 oz	20	0	0
Glaze *(Duncan Hines)*: Choc., 2 T.	150	7	21
Vanilla, 2 Tbsp	140	6	22
Hazelnut Meal/Flour, ¼ cup, 1 oz	160	12	8
Hemp Protein Powder, ¼ cup, 1.1 oz	120	3	10
Honey, ½ cup, 6 oz	515	0	145
Lemon/Orange Peel, ¼ cup	25	0	6
Lighter Bake *(Sunsweet)*:			
(Butter & Oil replacement)			
1 Tbsp, ½ oz	35	0	9
¼ Cup, 2.7 oz	140	0	36
Masa Harina *(Bob's Red Mill),*			
½ cup, 2 oz	220	2	47
Milk: Whole, 1 cup, 8 fl.oz	150	8	12
2%, 1 cup, 8 fl.oz	120	5	12
1%, 1 cup, 8 fl.oz	100	2.5	12
Fat-Free, 1 cup, 8 fl.oz	90	0.5	13
Oat Flour *(Bob's Red Mill)*, ⅓ cup, 1.5 oz	120	3	26
Pastry ~ *See Page 134*			
Pie Crusts ~ *See Page 134*			
Pie Fillings, Fruits ~ *See Page 134*			
Lemon Creme, ⅓ cup	130	1.5	28
Mincemeat, 3.5 oz	190	5	45
Pumpkin, 1 cup, 9.3 oz	270	1.5	60
Prune Puree, ¼ cup, 3 oz	220	0	55
Quinoa Flour, ¼ cup, 1 oz	110	1.5	18
Raisins, ½ cup, 2.8 oz	240	0.5	63
Rennin, 0.4 oz pkt	10	0	2
Rice Flour, ½ cup, 2.8 oz	290	1	63
Soy Milk ~ *See Pages 49-50*			
Soy Flour, *(Bob's Red Mill),*			
100% Whole Ground, ¼ cup, 1 oz	120	6	8
Sprinkles, all types, 1 tsp	20	1	3
Sugar: 1 Tbsp, 0.5 oz	55	0	14
1 oz	110	0	28
1 cup, 7 oz	775	0	195
16 oz (1 lb)	1760	0	454
Sweeteners & Sugar Substitutes ~ *See Page 156*			
Vinegar, average all types, 1 oz	5	0	1
Whey, sweet, dry, 1 oz	100	0.5	21
Yeast:			
Active, dry, 0.3 oz pkg	25	0.5	3
Bakers, compressed, 1 oz	30	0.5	5
Fleischmann's, 0.6 oz pkg	0	0	0

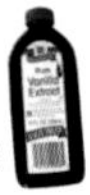
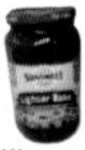
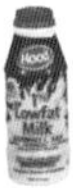
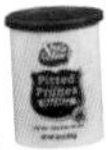
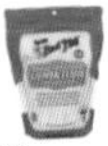
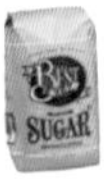

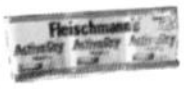

Note: Actual weight of bars is usually 5-10% more than label Net Weight. Weigh bar and allow extra calories.

Bars ~ Brands

Per Bar	C	F	Cb
AdvantEdge ~ *See EAS*			
Annie's Homegrown:			
Gluten Free, all varieties, 1 oz	110	3	20
Organic Chewy Granola Bars: *Per 0.9 oz Bar*			
Chocolate Chip	100	2.5	18
Oatmeal Raisin	90	1.5	19
PB Chocolate Chip	110	3.5	17
Organic Crispy, P'nut Butter, 0.9 oz	80	2	15
Protein, Choc. P'nut Butter, 1.2 oz	140	7	16
Atkins:			
Meal Bars: *Per 1.7 oz Unless Indicated*			
Birthday Cake	190	10	17
Blueberry Greek Yogurt	190	9	21
Choc. Almond Caramel	180	9	17
Chocolate Chip Granola	200	9	18
Chocolate Peanut Butter, 2 oz	240	15	23
Cookies 'n Crème, 1.76 oz	190	11	22
Peanut Fudge Granola	200	11	17
Vanilla Pecan Crisp	190	10	17
Note: Carb figures include 12-15g Fiber & Glycerin			
Snack Bars: *Per 1.55 oz Bar Unless Indicated*			
Caramel Chocolate Nut Roll	180	12	20
Caramel Chocolate Peanut Nougat	170	11	19
Caramel Double Chocolate Crunch	150	9	20
Choc. Chip Crisp, 1.23 oz	140	6	16
Cranberry Almond, 1.27 oz	140	6	16
Lemon Bar, 1.4 oz	150	7	15
Peanut Butter Fudge Crisp, 1.27 oz	140	8	13
Triple Chocolate, 1.4 oz	160	8	15
White Chocolate Macadamia, 1.4 oz	160	8	15
Note: Snack Bars Carb figures includes 14-16g Sugar Alcohol			
Protein Wafer Crisps, average	190	14	9
Balance:			
Original Bars:			
Average, 1.8 oz	205	7	21
Dark Chocolate var., av., 1.6 oz	180	7	22
Duo-licious: *Per 2 Pieces*			
Choc. Pepeprmint Patty, 1.4 oz	160	4	27
Dark Chocolate Turtle, 1.55 oz	190	8	24
Dulce De Leche & C'rml, 1.4 oz	150	5	24
Bounce: Caramel Sea Salt Ball, 1.4 oz	170	7	17
Peanut Chocolate Chip Ball, 1.4 oz	180	9	16

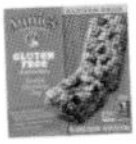
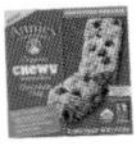
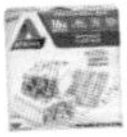
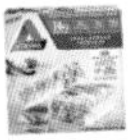
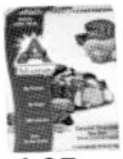
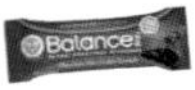

Per Bar	C	F	Cb
Cascadian Farms *(General Mills):*			
Chewy Granola:			
Dark Choc Chip, 1.2 oz	140	3.5	25
Harvest Berry, 1.2 oz	130	2	27
Crunchy Granola, av., 2 bars, 1.4 oz	190	7	27
Fruit Infused, av., 1.23 oz	140	3	25
Protein Granola Bars, av., 1.76 oz	250	15	20
Soft Baked Squares, av., 1.23 oz	150	5.5	23
Sweet & Salty, av. 1.2 oz	170	9	20
Clif:			
Original: Blueb. Crisp, 2.4 oz	250	5	44
Dark Choc. Mocha, 2.4 oz	250	5	44
Av. other flavors, 2.4 oz	255	7	42
Mini Bar, Chocolate Brownie, 1 oz	100	2	18
Bloks, av. all flavors, 3 pieces	100	0	24
Builder's, average, 2.4 oz	285	10	30
Fruit Smoothie, 1.76 oz	230	11	29
Kid Z-Bar, av., 1.27 oz	150	5	24
Nut Butter, av, 1.76 oz	230	11	27
Sweet & Salty, average, 2.4 oz	255	6.5	43
Whey, P'B & Chocolate, 2 oz	260	13	23
Corazonas:			
Heartbar Oatmeal Squares: *Per 1.8 oz Bar*			
Average all varieties	190	6	30
Detour:			
Lean Muscle:			
Cookie Dough Caramel Crisp, 3.2 oz	370	12	33
M&M's: Choc. Candy Crunch, 1.9 oz	210	2	27
PB Candy Crunch, 1.9 oz	250	3	25
P'nut Butter Choc. Crunch, 3.2 oz	420	18	33
Lower Sugar: *Average all flavors*			
Full Size, 3 oz	350	11	32
Snack Size, 1.5 oz	170	5	17
Protein Boost:			
Full size, 20g Protein, av., 2 oz	225	7	24
Snack size, 10g Protein, av., 1 oz	115	3	12
Smart:			
Coconut Almond, 1.3 oz	150	5	16
Cookie Dough, 1.3 oz	150	4	18
Fruit varieties, 1.3 oz	130	2.5	18
dotFIT:			
dotBAR:			
Double Choc. Brownie, 3.3 oz	370	13	38
Peanut Butter Crisp, 1.4oz	150	5	16
Vegan Chocolate Choc. Chip, 1.9 oz	260	9	24
Note: dotBARS Carb figures includes 7-21g Sugar Alcohol			
Extend Bar: Yogurt, av., 1.4 oz	150	5.5	23
Average Other Flavors	150	3	21
Note: Extend Bars Carb figure includes 3-8g Sugar Alcohol			

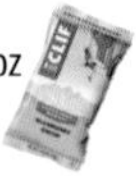
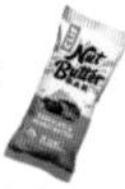
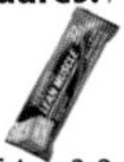
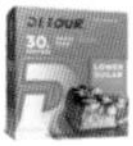
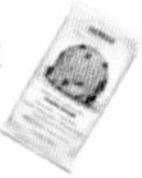
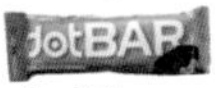

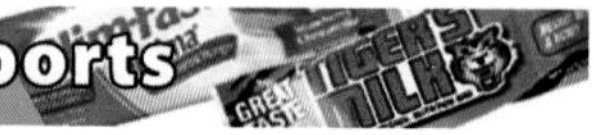

Bars ~ Brands (Cont)

Per Bar	C	F	Cb
Fiber One: *Per 0.8 oz Bar*			
Chewy: Choc.; Choc. Caramel & Pretzel	70	2	14
Chocolate Peanut Butter	70	2.5	13
Note: Carbohydrate figure includes 3g Sugar Alcohol			
General Mills: *Per 1.6 oz Bar*			
Milk 'n Cereal Bar, Honey Nut Cheerios 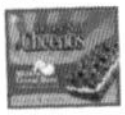	160	7	17
Glucerna: 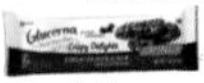			
Snack Bars,			
Peanut/Choc. Chip, av., 1.4 oz	155	5.5	20
Note: Carbohydrate figure includes 7g Sugar Alcohol			
Mini Snack Bar, average, 0.7 oz	80	3.5	11
Note: Carbohydrate figure includes 2g-4g Sugar Alcohol			
Great Value *(Walmart):*			
Cereal Bars, Fruit & Grain, 1.3 oz	130	3	24
Chewy Granola: 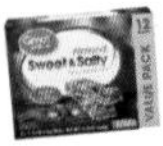			
Protein, average, 1.4 oz	190	12	14
Snack Size Variety Pack, average. 0.84 oz bar	100	2.5	19
Sweet & Salty, Almond, 1.23 oz	170	8	20
Crunchy Granola,			
Oats & Honey, 2 bars, 1.48 oz	190	7	29
Grenade:			
Carb Killa: Choc Chip Cookie Dough, 2 oz	220	9	24
Dark Chocolate Raspberry, 2 oz	220	10	21
Go Nuts Vegan Nut Bar, Spicy Chili, 1.4 oz 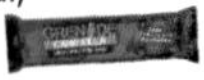	170	9	16
Peanut Butter, 2 oz	220	9	22
Health Valley,			
Multigrain, Cobbler Cereal Bars, all flavors, 3 oz	130	2	25
HMR, Benefit Bars, av. all, 1.4 oz	160	5	22
Init: *Per 1.4 oz Bar* 			
Dark Choc., average	180	10	23
Mixed Nut & Sweet Berries	180	9	24
Roasted Nuts & Honey Chipotle	190	13	18
Jenny Craig, all var., 1.2 oz	125	6	11
Kashi:			
Breakfast, Soft Baked, 1.26 oz	120	2.5	25
Go, Protein Bars, average, 1.76 oz	223	13	19
Granola Bars:			
Chewy, average all varieties, 1.3 oz	135	5	23
Chewy Nut Butter, av., 1.23 oz	150	7	21
Crunchy, all varieties, 2 bars, 1.4 oz 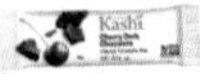	175	6	26
Layered, Dark Choc. Coconut	120	3.5	21
Kellogg's:			
Nutrigrain ~ *See page 33*			
Special K ~ *See page 34*			

Per Bar	C	F	Cb
Kind Bars: *Per 1.4 oz Bar*			
Almond & Apricot 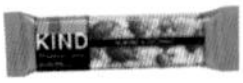	170	11	21
Almond & Coconut	180	12	21
Blueberry Vanilla Cashew	160	12	19
Cranberry Almonds with Macadamia	170	13	18
Dark Choc. Almond Coconut	180	12	21
Dark Chocolate Cherry Cashew	160	10	22
Honey Roasted Nuts & Sea Salt	180	15	15
Maple Glazed Pecan & Sea Salt	200	17	14
Milk Chocolate Almond 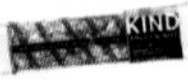	180	14	17
Peanut Butter Dark Choc	200	13	16
Raspberry Cashew Chia	170	11	21
Salted Caramel Dark Chocolate Nut	190	15	16
Breakfast Probiotics: *Per 2 Bars, 1.76 oz*			
Apple Cinn.; Or. Cranberry, av.	210	7	33
Peanut Buter Dark Chocolate	230	12	28
Kids, average all varieties,	95	3	16
Minis, Chewy, av all varieties, 0.8 oz	100	4	15
Kudos, av. all varieties, 0.9 oz	100	3	17
Kuli Kuli:			
Moringa Energy Bars: *Per 1.6 oz Bar*			
Black Cherry 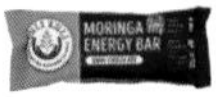	170	4	29
Dark Chocolate	210	11	22
Labrada:			
Lean Body Protein Bar: *Per 2.54 oz*			
Cookie Dough; Fudge Brownie	290	9	32
PB Chocolate Chip 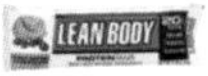	310	11	32
Larabar:			
Original Fruit & Nut, av.	205	10	26
Fruits & Greens, av. 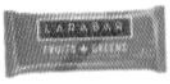	130	3	23
Protein, av., 1.83oz	220	8	25
Lindora Bars:			
Protein Bars: 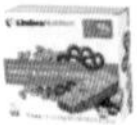			
Caramel Cocoa,1.6 oz	160	5	18
Chocolate Mint, 1.45 oz	150	4.5	21
Dark Chocolate S'mores, 1.6 oz	160	5	18
Oatmeal Cinnamon Raisin, 1.5 oz	150	4.5	19
Sweet & Salty Crunch. 1.4 oz	160	5	21
Zesty Lemon Crunch, 1.5 oz	160	7	16
Note: Carbohydrate figure includes 0.5g-4g Sugar Alcohol			
Luna Bars: 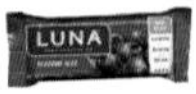			
Regular, av., 1.7 oz	185	7	20
Protein: Av. all varieties, 1.6 oz	175	5	21
Mini, Choc. Chip Cookie Dough, 1.1 oz	120	3.5	14
Mars, Protein Bar, 2 oz	200	4.5	22

Bars ~ Brands (Cont)

Per Bar	C	F	Cb
Medifast:			
Chewy, all varieties, 1.3 oz	110	3	15
Crunch, av. all varieties, 1.2 oz	105	3	13
Note: Crunch Bars Carb figure includes 2-3g Sugar Alcohol			
Maintenance, Cararmel Nut, 1.5 oz	160	5	20
Met-Rx:			
Big 100: *Per 3.52 oz*			
Crispy Apple Pie	400	10	48
Chocolate Toasted Almond	410	13	46
Peanut Butter Caramel Crunch	400	13	44
Peanut Butter Pretzel	410	12	47
Super Cookie Crunch	410	14	42
Protein Plus: Choc. Choc. Chunk, 3 oz	310	10	29
Choc. Roasted Peanut w/ Crml, 3oz	320	10	33
Peanut Butter Cup, 3 oz	300	10	34
Mojo Bars ~ *See Clif*			
Muscle Milk *(Cytosport):*			
15G Protein Bars: Cookies & Cream	180	5	23
Peanut Butter Cookie	190	6	22
20G Protein Bar, Choc P'nut Butter	250	9	27
Note: Protein Bars Carb figures include 6-14g Sugar Alcohol			
Nature's Path:			
Love Crunch, av., 1.1 oz	150	7	19
Nut Butter, av., 1.2 oz	170	10	17
Sunrise Chewy B'fast, av., 1.2 oz	140	4	25
Nature Valley:			
Chewy, XL Protein, average, 2 oz	290	19	21
Crunchy, 2 bars, average, 1.5 oz	190	8	29
Layered Granola Nut, average	190	11	20
Nut Crunch, Almond, 1.23 oz	190	14	14
Protein, all var., 1.4 oz	190	12	14
Sustained Energy, av., 1.7 oz	240	13	24
Sweet & Salty, average, 1.3 oz	160	7	22
Wafer, av., 1.3 oz	200	12	17
NuGo:			
Dark, average all varieties, 1.76 oz	200	6	25
Fiber d'Lish: Orange Cranb., 1.6 oz	150	3	31
Coc. Macaroon; P'nut Choc. Chip, 1.6 oz	160	6	28
Gluten Free, av. all varieties, 1.6 oz	180	4	27
Organic, all varieties, 1.6 oz	190	5	26
Slim: Espresso, 1.6 oz	170	5	20
Av.e other varieties	185	5	19

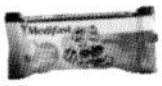
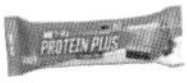

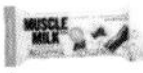

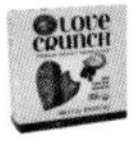

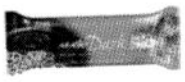
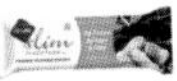

Per Bar	C	F	Cb
NuGo (Cont):			
Smarte Carb: Choc. Black Berry, 1.76 oz	150	3	22
Peanut Butter Crunch, 1.76 oz	160	5	19
Note: Carbohyrate figures include 12-14 g Sugar Alcohol			
Stronger: Peanut Cluster, 2.8 oz	330	14	36
Average other varieties, 2.8 oz	300	9	37
Nutri-Grain *(Kellogg's):*			
Kids, all varieties, 1.3 oz	140	3.5	27
Soft Baked B'fast Cereal Bars, all varieties, 1.3 oz	130	3.5	25
NutriSystem:			
Breakfast, Apple Streudel Bar	160	3	28
Lunch: Choc. P'nut Butter Bar	200	8	25
Double Chocolate Caramel	180	6	28
Snack, Dark Chocolate & Sea Salt Nut	190	14	16
Oh Yeah! (ISS):			
Original: *Per 3 oz Bar*			
Almond Fudge Brownie	350	13	27
Choc. Caramel Candies	340	13	32
Cookie Caramel Crunch	340	13	32
Peanut Butter & Caramel	380	19	30
Note: Carbohydrate figure includes 13g-14g Sugar Alcohol			
Good Grab, PB Crunch Bar	190	10	19
Note: Carbohydrate figure includes 4g Sugar Alcohol			
Optifast:			
800 Bars:			
Apple Cinnamon, 1.52 oz	160	4	18
Chocolate, 1.65 oz	160	4.5	18
Peanut Butter Chocolate, 1.52 oz	160	5	18
Note: 800 Bars Carb figures include 1-4g Sugar Alcohol			
PowerBar:			
Protein Plus, average, 1.4 oz	220	14	11
Note: Carbohydrate figures include 16-18g Sugar Alcohol			
Snack Bar, average	230	13	23
Power Crunch *(BNRG):*			
Orig. Protein Bar, av. all var., 1.4 oz	215	12	11
Power Crunch, Choklat, av., 1.5 oz	215	12	18
PR:			
Protein: Chocolate Mint, 2.1 oz	200	6	22
Chocolate Peanut, 1.8 oz	200	7	22
Oatmeal Raisin Granola, 1.8 oz	210	7	22
Premier Protein *(Premier Nutrition): 12G Protein*			
Chocolate Peanut Butter, 1.5 oz	180	10	17
Salted Caramel Cashew, 1.65 oz	190	10	19
Vanilla Almond Coconut, 1.65 oz	190	11	18

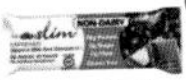
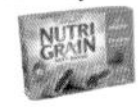

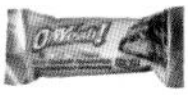

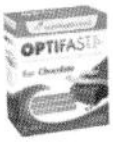

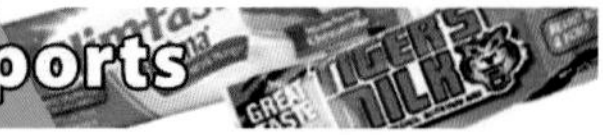

Note: Actual weight of bars is usually 5-10% more than label Net Weight. Weigh bar and allow extra calories.

Bars ~ Brands (Cont)

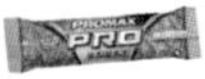

Per Bar	C	F	Cb
Promax:			
Original, av. all varieties, 2.6 oz	290	7.5	39
Lower Sugar, av. all varieties, 2.4 oz	215	7	32
Note: Lower Sugar Carbohydrate figures include 5-6g Sugar Alcohol			
Proti Bars *(Bariatrix)*:			
Almond Coconut, 1.76 oz	190	9	17
Chocolate/Vanilla Wafers (2), 1.4 oz	205	10	14
Note: Carbohydrate figures include 2g -5g Sugar Alcohol			
Salted Toffee Pretzel Bar, 1.75 oz	160	6	18
PureFit, Protein av. all varieties, 2 oz	225	7	25
Pure Protein:			
Hi Protein, av. all varieties, 1.76 oz	195	5	18
Note: Carbohydrate figures include 2-13g Sugar Alcohol			
Quaker:			
B'fast Flats: Banana Honey Nut (3)	170	7	28
Av. other varieties (3)	175	6.5	28
B'fast Squares: P'nut Butter, 2.1 oz	250	10	35
Other flavors, 2.1 oz	210	4.5	42
Granola Bars:			
Chewy: 25% Less Sugar, average, 0.8 oz	95	3	17
Big, average all varieties, 1.9 oz	175	6	30
Note: Big Bar Carbohydrate figure include 2g Sugar Alcohol			
Bites, average, 8 pieces	135	5	21
Dipps, average, 1.2 oz	140	6	22
Yogurt, Srawb., 1.2 oz	140	4.5	25
Quest Bar:			
Hero: Choc.Pnut Butter, 1.9 oz	200	12	18
Average other varieties, 2.1 oz	175	8	30
Note: Carbohydrate figure include 4g Sugar Alcohol			
Protein,, av., 2.1 oz	185	6	23
Note: Carbohydrate figures includs 1-6g Sugar Alcohol			
RX Bar:			
Protein: Average, 1.83 oz	215	9	24
Kids, average, 1.2 oz	135	5	16
Skratch Bars:			
Anytime Energy: *Per 1.76 oz Bar*			
Cherries & Pistachios; Savory Miso, av.	220	9	30
Choc. Chips & Almonds;PB & Strawb.	220	8	33
Slim-Fast:			
Bake Shop Bars, average all, 1.6 oz	180	6.5	17
Note: Carb includes 12g Sugar Alcohol + 5g Fibre			
Keto: Bars, av., 1.48 oz	190	14	15
Note: Carb includes 12g Sugar Alcohol + 9g Fibre			
Fat Bomb, P'But Butter, 1 cup	90	9	6
Snickers, Protein Bar, 1.8 oz	200	7	18
Solo, Gi, average all varieties 1.76 oz	195	7	26

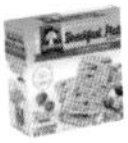

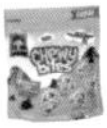

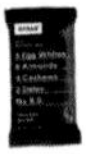

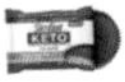

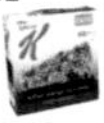

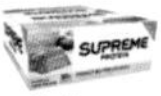

Per Bar	C	F	Cb
Special K:			
Chewy Nut Bars, av., 1.16 oz	165	8	18
Chewy Snack Bars, av. all varieties, 0.88 oz	100	2	19
Protein Snack, av. all var., 1.23 oz	155	7	17
Supreme Protein:			
High Protein:			
Caramel Nut Chocolate, 3.4 oz	390	15	36
PB Crunch, 3.38 oz	390	18	26
Note: Carbohydrate figures include 14-27g Sugar alcohol			
thinkThin: *Per Bar*			
High Protein, av. all flavors, 1.94 oz	235	9	25
Note: Carbohydrate figure includes 5-22g Sugar Alcohol			
Keto, Choc. Peanut Butter Pie, 1.4 oz	180	14	14
Note: Carbohydrate figure includes 4-5g Sugar Alcohol			
Protein + 150 Calorie, av., 1.4 oz	150	5	20
Vegan High Protein:			
Choc. Mint; Sea Salt Alm. Choc., 1.95 oz	230	8	28
PB Chocolate Chip, 1.76 oz	190	6	24
Note: Carbohydrate figure includes 9g Sugar Alcohol			
Tiger's Milk:			
Protein Rich, 1.2 oz	140	5	19
Peanut Butter Crunch, 1.2 oz	150	6	18
King Size, average all varieties, 2 oz	225	9	28
Trader Joe's:			
Hemp Seed Bar, 0.9 oz	120	7	11
Organic Granola Bar, Chocolate Chip, 0.85 oz	100	2.5	18
PB & J Bar, 1.2 oz	150	4	23
Simply Nutty Bars, av. , 1.4 oz	200	15	15
Vega:			
Protein Bars: 20G, 2.47 oz	290	10	26
Snack Bar, Choc. Caramel, 1.6 oz	190	8	20
Sports Bar, 2.47 oz	300	11	27
Wickedly Prime: *Per 1.4 oz Bar*			
Banana Nut	180	11	21
Cashews & Cranberry	170	9	24
Cherry Nut Crunch	190	14	15
Nuts & Sea Salt; Peanut Almond	200	16	14
Zone Perfect:			
High Protein Bars, average, 2 oz	235	9	22
Nutrition Bars:			
Chocolate Peanut Butter, 1.76 oz	220	8	24
Dark Choc. Almond, 1.58 oz	190	7	20
Salted Caramel Brownie, 1.58 oz	200	9	20

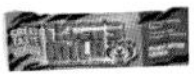

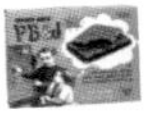

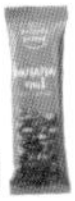

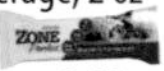

Cocoa & Hot Chocolate

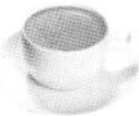

	C	F	Cb
Cocoa:			
Small (8 fl.oz):			
with Whole Milk	205	8.5	22
with Nonfat Milk	145	1	23
Tall (12 fl.oz): with Whole Milk	280	12	26
with Nonfat Milk	185	1	28
Hot Chocolate:			
Small (8 fl.oz): with Whole Milk	180	7	26
with Nonfat Milk	140	2	27
Tall (12 fl.oz): with Whole Milk	260	10	36
with Nonfat Milk	190	2	37
Cinnabon, Mochalatta Chill, 16 oz	420	17	63

Cocoa - Chocolate Mixes

Add extra cals/fat/carbohydrate for milk

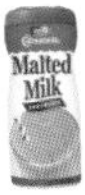

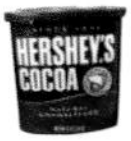

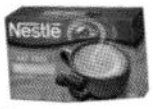

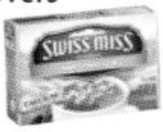

	C	F	Cb
Caffé D'Vita: *Per Singe Serve Envelope*			
Hot Cocoa, 1 oz	110	1.5	24
Hot Cocoa, Sugar Free	70	4.5	7
Carnation Breakfast Drinks ~ *See Page 38*			
Carnation: *Per 3 Tbsp*			
Malted Milk: Original	90	2	15
Chocolate	90	1	18
Ghirardelli:			
Premium Hot Cocoa:			
with Chocolate Chips, 1 oz	110	2	23
Double Chocolate, 2 Tbsp	90	1	20
Hershey's, Cocoa, Natural, unsweetened, 1 Tbsp, 0.2 oz	10	0.5	3
Land O Lakes:			
Arctic White Coccoa, 1.3 oz	160	6	26
Other varieties, 1.3 oz	140	3.5	26
Nestle: *Per Per Single Serve Envelope*			
Rich Milk Chocolate:			
Regular	80	2	15
Fat Free	25	0	4
with Mini Marshmallows	80	1.5	15
Nesquik Powder: *Per 2 Tbsp*			
Chocolate	50	0	12
No Added Sugar	40	0.5	8
Strawberry	45	0	12
Ovaltine, average all flav., 2 Tbsp	40	0	10
Swiss Miss: *Per Single Serve Envelope*			
Cafe Blends, Mocha	150	2.5	28
Classics: Marshmallow Lovers	190	2.5	39
Milk Chocolate	160	2.5	34
Indulgent Collection:			
Caramel Delight	160	2.5	34
Dark Chocolate Sensation	150	3.5	28
Sensibly Sweet,			
Milk Choc. Flavor, No Sugar Added	80	1.5	14
Simply Cocoa, Milk Chocolate	100	0	22

Updated Nutrition Data ~ www.CalorieKing.com
Persons with Diabetes ~ See Disclaimer (Page 22)

Instant Coffee

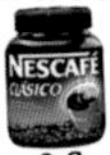

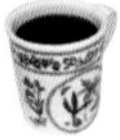

	C	F	Cb
Powder/Granules: *Regular or Decaffeinated,*			
1 level tsp	2	0	0.5
1 rounded tsp	4	0	1
Ground, 3 tsp	7	0	2
Brewed/Percolated, 1 cup, 8 fl.oz	4	0	1
Coffee with Milk/Cream/Creamers: *Per 8 oz Cup*			
Black:	4	0	1
with Whole Milk: Dash, 1 Tbsp	15	0.5	2
2 Tbsp, 1 fl.oz	25	1	2.5
with 2% Milk, 2 Tbsp	20	0.5	2.5
with 1% Milk, 2 Tbsp	20	0.5	2.5
with Fat Free Milk, 2 Tbsp	15	0	2.5
with Soy Milk: 1 Tbsp	10	0	1.5
2 Tbsp, 1 oz	15	0.5	2
with Half & Half: 2 Tbsp	50	3	3
1/4 cup, 2 fl.oz	90	6	4
with Cream (light coffee), 2 Tbsp	65	6	2
with Coffee Mate: Liquid, reg., 1 T.	20	1	3
Liquid Fat Free, 1 Tbsp	25	0	2
Powder, 1 heaping tsp	15	1	2
Sugar ~ Add Extra: 1 heaping tsp	25	0	6
Single portion, 1 package	25	0	6
Sweeteners, *(Equal/Splenda/Sweet N Low),* Powder, 1 package	0	0	0

Flavored Coffee Mixes

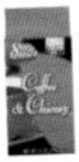

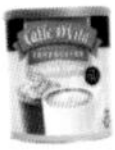

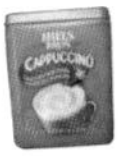

	C	F	Cb
Chicory:			
Instant Coffee, 1 tsp	5	0	1
Coffee Essence, 1 tsp	15	0	4
Caffé D'Vita:			
Cappuccino: Caramel, 3 tsp	60	2	10
English Toffee, 3 tsp	70	2.5	11
French Vanilla, 3 tsp	70	3	10
Mocha; Peppermint Mocha, av., 3 tsp	60	2.5	11
Iced, Caramel Latte, 3 tbsp	180	6	32
Sugar Free Cappuccino, Mocha, 2 tsp	40	2.5	4
General Foods International:			
Cappuccino: Hazelnut Belgian,1.3 oz	160	4	29
Suisse Mocha, 1.3 oz	150	5	28
White Chocolate Caramel, 1.3 oz	150	3	30
Hills Bros: *Per 3 Tbsp, 1 oz*			
Cappuccino: French Vanilla	110	3.5	19
Sugar Free	50	2	8
Double Mocha, Sugar Free	50	2	8
English Toffee	110	3	19
White Chocolate Caramel	120	4.5	19
Nescafe, Memento, 1 stick, average all varieties	100	2.5	19

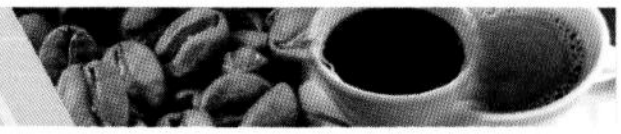

Coffee Shops/Restaurants

Per 8 fl.oz Cup (Unless Indicated)	C	F	Cb
Coffee, Regular/Percolated/Filtered	5	0	0
Americano Drip Coffee, 1 cup	7.5	0	1
Cafe Au Lait: 1 cup, 8 fl.oz	60	3.5	5
Nonfat Milk, 1 cup, 8 fl.oz	35	0	5
Caffe Latté:			
8 fl.oz cup: with Whole Milk	110	6	9
with 2% Milk	100	3.5	9
with Nonfat Milk	70	0	10
12 fl.oz: with Whole Milk	180	9	14
with Nonfat Milk	100	0	15
16 fl.oz: with Whole Milk	220	11	18
with Nonfat Milk	130	0	19
Cafe Mocha (Mochaccino): 8 fl.oz	150	6	20
12 fl.oz	230	9	31
16 fl.oz	290	12	41
Cappuccino:			
8 fl.oz cup: with Whole Milk	90	3.5	7
with 2% Milk	80	3	8
with Nonfat Milk	50	0	8
12 fl.oz: with Whole Milk	110	6	9
with 2% Milk	90	3.5	9
with Nonfat Milk	60	0	9
16 fl.oz: with Whole Milk	140	7	11
with 2% Milk	120	3.5	11
with Nonfat Milk	80	0	12
Mocha: *With Cream*			
8 fl.oz: with Whole Milk	200	11	22
with Nonfat Milk	160	6	22
12 fl.oz: Whole Milk	290	15	33
with Nonfat Milk	230	8	34
Iced Mocha: *Without Cream*			
12 fl.oz: with Whole Milk	170	6	26
with Nonfat Milk	130	2	27
Espresso: Single (Solo), 1 fl.oz	5	0	1
Double (Doppio), 2 fl.oz	10	0	2
Espresso con Panna,			
(w/ dollop wh. cream), solo, 1 fl.oz	30	2.5	2
Espresso Macchiato, solo, 1 fl.oz	5	0	1
Frappuccino: Tall, 12 fl.oz	180	2.5	37
Grande, 16 fl.oz	240	3	48
Frappuccino Mocha:			
(with Cream): Tall, 12 fl.oz	280	11	43
Grande, 16 fl.oz	380	15	57
Iced Latte, Similar to Caffe Latte			

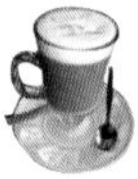

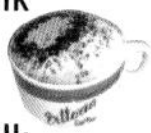

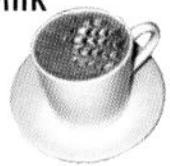

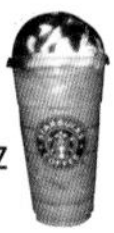

McCafe (McDonald's) ~ *See Fast Food, Page 216*
Starbucks ~ *See Fast-Foods Section, Page 243*

Coffee Substitute Mixes

	C	F	Cb
Roasted Cereal Beverages ~ *(No Caffeine)*			
Cafix, Instant Beverage, 1 tsp	5	0	1
Kaffree Roma, Instant Beverage, 1 tsp	10	0	2
Teeccino, Herbal Coffees, 1 tsp	10	0	2

Irish & Liqueur Coffees

	C	F	Cb
Irish Coffee, without sugar	175	10	0
Liqueur Coffee, with cream, all varieties, av., 1 fl.oz	100	5	7

Coffee Extras

	C	F	Cb
Chocolate (Cocoa) Topping, ½ tsp	5	0	1
Flavored Syrups: Regular, 2 Tbsp	80	0	20
Sugar-free, 2 Tbsp	0	0	0
Half & Half Cream: 2 Tbsp	40	3.5	1
Single serve pkg, ⅜ fl.oz	15	1.5	0.5
Light whipped cream, 2 Tbsp	15	1.5	1
Marshmallows, miniature (2)	5	0	1
Sugar:			
1 single portion package	20	0	5
1 level tsp	15	0	4
1 heaping tsp	25	0	6
Equal/Splenda/Sweet 'N Low	0	0	0

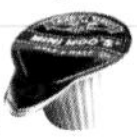

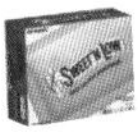

Coffee Shop ~ Cakes, Cookies

	C	F	Cb
Cookies:			
Biscotti, 1 oz	140	6.5	18
Chocolate Chip, 3 oz	350	15	54
Oatmeal Raisin, 3 oz	350	12	56
Peanut Butter, 3 oz	410	25	39
White Choc. Macadamia, 3.33 oz	420	20	55
Cakes/Pastries:			
Almond Croissant, 5 oz	620	35	67
Apple Danish, 5 oz	450	18	67
Banana Walnut, 4.5 oz	410	17	60
Brownie, 3 oz	390	24	42
Bundt, Chocolate, 4 oz	440	21	61
Carrot Cake, 4 oz	400	22	45
Chocolate Cake, 5 oz	530	28	65
Crumble Coffee Cake, 4.5 oz	500	25	65
Cupcake, 3 oz	330	16	43
Pound Cake, av., 3 oz	330	17	40
Cinnamon Roll, 6 oz	500	15	83
Donuts:			
Sugared, 1.8 oz	220	11	27
Glazed, 2 oz	250	12	34
Pretzel, large, 4 oz	290	5	52

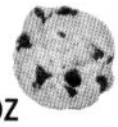

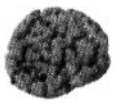

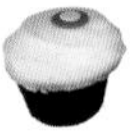

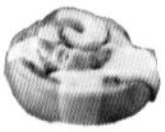

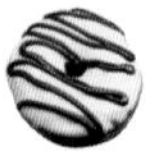

Starbucks Bakery Items ~ *See Page 244*

Ready To Drink Coffee

	C	F	Cb
Bottled & Chilled:			
Califia Farms: *With Almond Milk*			
Cold Brew Coffee: Cafe Latte, 12 fl.oz	**100**	4	15
Mocha, 12 fl.oz	**130**	4.5	21
Dunkin Donuts, Mocha, 13.7 fl.oz	**280**	9	44
International Delight:			
Iced, all flavors, 8 fl.oz	**120**	2.5	21
Light varieties, 8 fl.oz	**80**	2.5	13
Kahlua, Cappuccino Shake, 10.5 fl.oz	**130**	2	24
Starbucks:			
Cold Brew: *Per 11 fl.oz*			
Black, sweet	**50**	0	12
Black, unsweetened	**15**	0	2
Cocoa & Honey, with Cream	**150**	4	23
Vanilla & Fig, with Cream	**150**	4	24
Doubleshot Energy: *Per 15 fl.oz Can*			
Coffee Drink	**220**	3	35
Hazelnut Drink	**210**	3	34
Mocha/Vanilla Drink, av.	**210**	3	34
White Chocolate Drink	**210**	3	34
Doubleshot Espresso: *Per 6.5 fl.oz Can*			
Espresso/Salted Caramel & Cream	**140**	6	18
Espresso & Light Cream	**70**	4	5
Frappuccino Coffee Drink: *Per 9.5 fl.oz Bottle*			
Regular; Caramel; Vanilla, av.	**205**	3.5	37
AlmondMilk Mocha	**120**	3.5	21
Mocha	**190**	3.5	33
Light Mocha	**100**	3	12
Iced Espresso Classics (Chilled): *Per 12 fl.oz serving*			
Caffe Mocha	**200**	4	35
Caramel Macchiato; Van. Latte	**190**	4	32
Skinny, Caramel Macchiato, Van. Latte	**100**	0	15
Iced Latte: *Per 14 fl.oz Bottle*			
Regular, reduced fat milk	**220**	4.5	37
Vanilla, reduced fat milk	**220**	4.5	36
White Choc. Mocha, red. fat milk	**260**	4.5	44

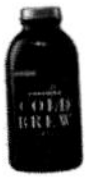
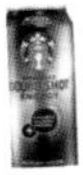
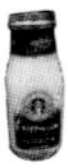

Starbucks Refreshers ~ *See Page 40*

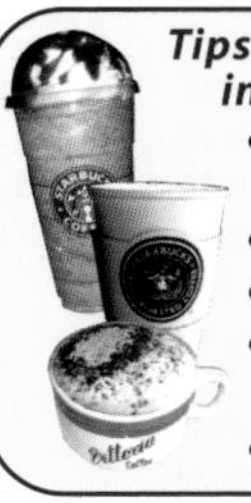

Tips to Reduce the Calories in Your Coffee Drinks:

- Request non-fat milk in place of whole or 2% milk
- Downsize to 8 fl.oz or 12 fl.oz
- Avoid cream on frappuccinos
- Replace sugar with *Equal, Splenda, Stevia* or *Sweet 'N Low*
- Avoid syrup add-ons

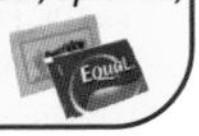

Caffeine Counter

Moderate caffeine intake is not harmful to healthy adults. However, frequent large amounts (over 350mg/day) may cause dependency ('caffeinism') and adversely affect health. **To be safe, limit caffeine to 200mg/day.** Avoid if pregnant, breastfeeding, a child under 8, have sleep problems, an overactive bladder or heart arrhythmia.

	Caffeine (mg)
Coffee: **Instant:** Weak, 1 level teaspoon	30
Medium, 1 rounded teaspoon	60
Strong, 1 heaping teaspoon	100
Decaffeinated, 1 rounded teaspoon	2
Bags (Folgers), 1 bag (6-8 fl.oz)	115
Ground, 1 Tbsp, 0.2 oz	60
Bottled (Ready-To-Drink), 9.5 fl.oz	70
Coffee Shop: Brewed, 8 fl.oz	110 -150
Cappuccino/Latte: 1 cup, 8 fl.oz	75
Tall, 12 fl.oz	110
Large, 16 fl.oz	150
Decappuccino, decaffeinated	5
Espresso: Regular/Single/Solo	75
Double/Doppio	150
Iced Coffee w/o Milk, 12 fl.oz	140
Latte, 1 cup, 8 fl.oz	75
Mocha, 1 cup, 8 fl.oz	90
Hot Chocolate, 8 fl.oz	15
Black Tea: Weak, 1 cup	20
Medium Strength, 1 cup	40
Strong, 1 cup	70
Decaffeinated Tea, 1 cup	0-5
Herbal Tea, 1 cup	0
Green Tea, 1 cup	20
Iced Tea, tall glass/can, 12 fl.oz	20-30
Soft Drinks: *Per 12 fl.oz Can*	
Coca-Cola; Pepsi (Regular/Diet)	35
Diet Coke; TAB; RC Cola (Regular)	45
Dr. Pepper; Sunkist Orange	40
Pepsi One; Mountain Dew; Mellow Yellow; Surge	55
Pepsi Max (Regular/Diet) Sun Drop (Reg/Diet)	70
7-Up, Fanta, Sprite, Fresca, Diet Rite Cola	0
Energy Drinks (with added caffeine):	
(AMP, Adrenaline Rush, Full Throttle Monster, No Fear, Red Bull, Rockstar)	
Average all brands: 8 fl.oz	80
16 fl.oz	160
NOS Energy, 16 fl.oz	260
Chocolate Bars: Milk Chocolate, 2 oz	20
Dark Chocolate, 2 oz	30
Choc Chip Cookies, 2 medium, 2 oz	6
Chocolate Syrup, 2 Tbsp, 1.4 oz	5
Guarana, *GNC*, 1 tablet	90
Medicinals: *Excedrin Extra*/Migraine, 1 tab.	65
Jet Alert/NoDoz, 1 tablet	200
Stay Awake (Walgreens), *Vivarin*, 1 tab.	200

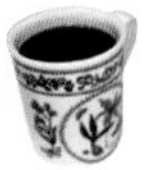
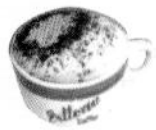
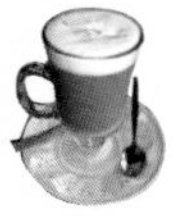
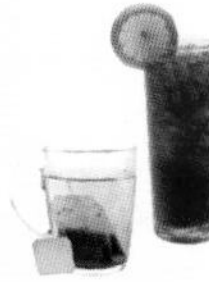
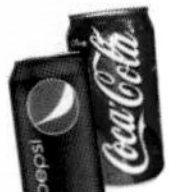
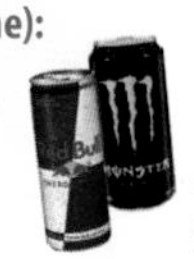
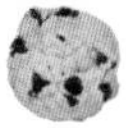
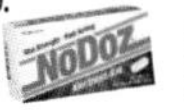

Energy/Protein Drinks	C	F	Cb
5-hour Energy, 2 fl.oz	4	0	1
A.B.B:			
Post Workout Pure-Pro:			
Pure Pro 50, all flavors, 14.5 fl.oz	260	4.5	7
Maxx Recovery, all flavors, 18 fl.oz	390	0.5	60
Pre Workout, Speed Stack Pumped, 22 fl.oz	30	0	8
AllSport Hydration:			
Regular, all flavors, 20 fl.oz	150	0	40
Zero, 20 fl.oz	0	0	0
AMP Energy: *Per 16 fl.oz Can*			
Original; Strawberry Limeade	220	0	58
Cherry Blast	120	0	31
Tropical Punch	100	0	26
Arbonne,			
Protein Shakes, av., 2 sc., 1.4 oz	165	3	13
Arizona:			
Green Tea Energy Shot, Extra Str., 2 fl.oz	5	0	1
Natural Energy, average, 8 fl.oz	70	0	19
Rx Energy, Herbal Tonic, 8 fl.oz	100	0	26
Atkins: *Per 11 fl.oz*			
Plus 30G Prot. Shakes, Choc./Van., av.	190	5	9
Shakes, average, 11 fl.oz	165	9	7
Bariatrix, Proti-Max, Ready to Drink			
Chocolate/Vanilla, av., 8.45 fl.oz	105	4	3
Bawls Guarana: *Per 10 fl.oz Bottle*			
Original; Cherry; Ginger	130	0	33
Orange; Root Beer, average	140	0	35
Beet It:			
Organic Beet Juice: 8.5 fl.oz	80	0	17
25.4 fl.oz Bottle	240	0	51
Shot, 2.4 fl.oz	95	0.2	20
BodyArmor, SuperDrinks, 16 fl.oz	120	0	28
Bolthouse: *Per 15.2 fl.oz*			
Bolts Energy, 2 fl.oz	25	0	6
Protein Keto, average all flavors	280	22	14
Protein Plus: Chocolate	390	6	55
Dutch Choc.; Banana;Van. Bean. av	345	6	46
Mango	375	1	62
Boost *(Nestle):*			
Original, all flavors, 8 fl.oz	240	4	41
High Protein, all flav, 8 fl.oz	240	6	28
Glucose Control, 8 fl.oz	190	7	16
Max 30g Protein, 11 fl.oz	160	2	7
Men, 8 fl.oz	220	6	24
Mobility, 8 fl.oz	180	4	16
Plus, all flavors, 8 fl.oz	360	14	45
Women, 8 fl.oz	180	7	14

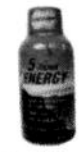
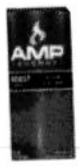
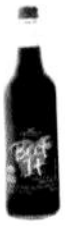
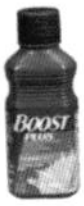
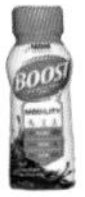

Carnation:	C	F	Cb
B'Fast Essentials, Powder:			
Original,av. all flav., 1.3 oz envelope	135	0	27
Light Start, av. , 0.7 oz	60	0.5	11
Probiotic, 1.3 oz envelope	140	1	27
Ready To Drink: Reg., all flav., 8 fl.oz	240	4	41
High Protein, average, 8 fl.oz	220	6	26
CeraSport:			
Powders: Endurance, Vanilla, 1 pkt	150	0	30
Plus Hydration, Strawb., 1 pkt	120	0	30
Ready To Drink, Citrus Drink, 8.5 fl.oz	40	0	10
Champion Performance:			
Heavyweight Gainer 900,			
av. all flavors, 4 scps, 5.4 oz	600	7	102
Metabolol II, 2 scoops, 2.3 oz	260	3	40
Pure Whey Plus, av., 1 scoop, 1.2 oz	130	2	5
UltraMet, 2.7 oz pkt	280	4	20
Clif: Hydration Mix, 0.4 oz pkt	40	0	10
Recovery Powder, Choc., 1.6 oz	160	0	31
Cocaine, Energy, 12fl.oz can	90	0	23
Core Power *(fairlife):*			
26g, av. all flavors, 11.5 fl.oz	240	3.5	27
Elite, 42g, av. all flav., 14 fl.oz	240	3.5	12
Curves, Protein Drink,			
Choc.; Vanilla, 2 scoops, 1 oz	120	1	12
Ensure: *Per Bottle*			
Original, all flavors, 8 fl.oz	220	6	33
Clear, all flavors, 10 fl.oz	180	0	37
Enlive, av. all flavors, 8 fl.oz	350	11	44
High Protein , all flav., 8 fl.oz	160	2	19
Plus, all flavors, 8 fl.oz	350	11	50
Enterex, Diabetic, all flavors, 8 fl.oz	220	8	25
Enu, Nutritional Shakes, av., 8.5 fl.oz	340	13	39
FRS, Energy Concentrate, 2 fl.oz	10	0	3
Fruit$_2$0 *(Veryfine)*: Classic 20 fl.oz	0	0	0
Sparkling, 20 fl.oz	0	0	1
Full Throttle: *Per 16 fl.oz*			
Energy, Citrus; Blue Agave	220	0	58
Gatorade G Series:			
Endurance: Powder, 1½ Tbsp	90	0	22
Thirst Quencher, 12 fl oz	90	0	22
Lower Sugar, 12 fl.oz	30	0	8
Protein: Chocolate Shake, 11.16 fl.oz	280	1	47
Super Shake, Chocolate, 11.16 fl.oz	190	1	12
Whey Protein Powder, ⅓ cup 1.1 oz	120	2	6
Sports Fuel Drink, 4 fl.oz	100	0	25
Glaceau:			
Smartwater, 8 fl.oz	0	0	0
Vitaminwater: Revive Punch, 20 fl.oz	120	0	32
Average other flavors, 20 fl.oz	100	0	27

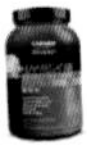
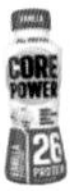
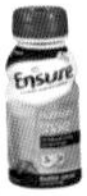
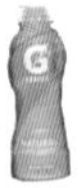

Glucerna:	C	F	Cb
Shakes, all flavors, 8 fl.oz	**180**	9	16
Advance Shakes, average., 8 fl.oz	**200**	7	27
Hunger Shakes, average, 8 fl.oz	**180**	8	15
GNC:			
Pro Performance:			
Amplified: Mass XXX,			
av. all flavors, 4 scoops	**745**	6	123
RTD, Wheybolic, all flavors, 14 fl.oz	**190**	1.5	6
Total Lean:			
Powders: All flavors, 1 pkt	**200**	3	18
Classics, Swiss Choc., 1 Heaping Scoop	**180**	2	31
RTD Shakes: 25, all flavors, 14 fl.oz	**170**	6	6
Burn, all flavors, 14.fl.oz	**170**	6	8
Guru:			
Org. Energy Drink: Regular, 8 oz can	**80**	0	21
Lite,12 oz can	**10**	0	3
Herbalife: Nutr. Shake, 1 scoop, 0.9 oz	**90**	1	13
Protein Drink Mix, 2 scoops, 1 oz	**110**	3	5
Hormel:			
Plus-2 Protein Shakes, all flav., 8 fl.oz	**480**	23	49
Vital Quisine 500, av. all flav., 8.5 fl.oz	**520**	21	60
Hype: *Per 8 fl.oz Can*			
Enlite	**25**	0	4
Energy: After Dark, Hype	**130**	0	30
MFP	**110**	0	25
Up, Ice Berry Max	**120**	0	28
Twisted, average all flavors	**110**	0	26
Jarrow:			
Optimal Plant Proteins, 2 scoops, 1.2 oz	**140**	3	8
Organic Plant Protein, Van., 1 oz	**120**	3	6
Rice Protein, Vanilla, Tbsp, 0.6 oz	**60**	0	3
Whey Protein: Unflavored, 0.8 oz sc.	**90**	2	1
Chocolate; Vanilla, 0..9 oz scoop	**100**	1.5	3
Knudsen: Recharge, average, 8 fl.oz	**75**	0	18
Simply Nutritious, av. all, 8 fl.oz	**115**	0	28
Kroger: *Per 8 fl.oz Bottle*			
Nutrutional Shake, all flavors	**190**	7	23
Nutrition Shake, Fortify Plus, av.,	**350**	11	50
La Brada:			
Lean Body, Meal Repl., 2.47 oz sc.	**285**	7	19
RTD, Lean Body, 17 fl.oz	**280**	9	9
Lindora:			
Powder: Berry Cream Smoothie	**100**	1	7
Creamy Chocolate; Vanilla	**90**	1	7
Ready To Drink Shakes, 8 fl oz	**110**	4.5	4

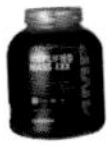

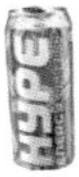

Liquid Ice:	C	F	Cb
Black, 8.3 fl.oz	**110**	0	26
Other Flavors, 8.3 fl oz	**120**	0	28
Met-Rx, 51 Shake,			
Chocolate, 15 fl.oz	**250**	2	6
Monster:			
Energy: 16 fl.oz can	**210**	0	54
Lo-Carb, 16 fl.oz	**25**	0	7
M-80, 16 fl.oz	**180**	0	46
Mixxd (with Juice), 16 fl.oz	**220**	0	54
Java Monster: All flav., 15 fl.oz	**190**	3	33
Light, Vanilla, 15 fl.oz	**95**	3	13
Shakes, 16 fl.oz can	**220**	4	20
MRM:			
Veggie Meal Replacement, 1.7 oz	**190**	5	14
Whey Protein, 1 scoop, 0.9 oz	**100**	1.5	4
Muscle Milk *(Cytosport):*			
Gainer, 4 scoops, 5.71 oz	**650**	9	109
Genuine Protein Powder:			
Real Chocolate; Vanilla, 2 sc., 2.47 oz	**310**	11	20
Other Flavors, 2 scoops, 2.47 oz	**280**	9	21
Non Dairy Ready To Drink:			
100 Calorie, Vanilla Creme, 11 fl.oz	**100**	1.5	5
Genuine, average all flavors, 11 fl.oz	**160**	4.5	6
Original, all flavors, 17 fl.oz	**320**	15	13
Pro Series, Go Bananas, 14 fl.oz	**200**	2.5	8
Yogurt Smoothies, 11 fl.oz	**180**	3	18
Muscle Tech:			
Mass-Tech Powder,			
Milk Choc., 5 scoops, 9 oz	**1000**	9	168
Nitro Tech Ripped Powder, 1.5 oz	**170**	4	4
Nature's Best:			
Isopure: 20G Protein, 16 fl.oz	**80**	0	0
Mass, all flavors, 20 fl.oz	**350**	0	53
Zero Carb, all flavors, 20 fl.oz	**160**	0	0
JavaPro Ready To Drink + Coffee,			
average all flavors, 8 fl.oz	**110**	2	3
Nestle Health Science,			
Diabetishield, Mixed Berry, 8 fl.oz	**150**	0	30
NOS, High Performance Energy,			
Grape, 16 fl.oz can	**210**	0	54
Av. other flavors, 16 fl.oz	**215**	0	53
Turbo, 16 fl.oz	**10**	0	3
Nutrament *(Nestle)*, 12 fl.oz can	**360**	10	52
Nutrilite *(Amway)*:			
BodyKey Meal Replacement Shakes,			
Powder, av. all flavors, 2 oz scoop	**230**	5	25

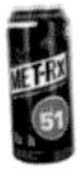

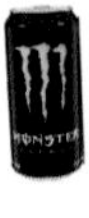

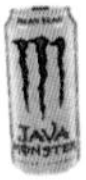

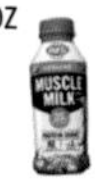

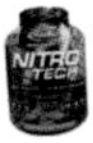

Updated Nutrition Data ~ www.CalorieKing.com
Persons with Diabetes ~ See Disclaimer (Page 22)

Energy/Protein Drinks (Cont)

Optifast: *(Nestle)*:	C	F	Cb
HP Shake Mix, 1 pkg	**200**	6	10
Ready To Drink Shakes, 8 fl.oz	**160**	3.5	18
Shake Mix, 1 pkg	**160**	3.5	18

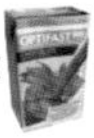

Optimum Nutrition: *Powder*	C	F	Cb
Gold Standard:			
100% Whey, av. all flavors, 1 oz scp	**120**	1	4
100% Plant, 1 scoop, 1.3 oz	**145**	2.5	6
Optisource *(Nestle)*,			
Very High Prot. Drink, Strawb., 8 fl.oz	**200**	6	12
OrGain:			
Organic Ready To Drink: 11 fl.oz	**250**	7	32
Van. Almond Milk Shake, Unsw., 8 fl.oz	**80**	3.5	4
Organic Plant Based Powders,			
Average all flavors, 2 scps, 1.62 oz	**150**	4	15
Powerade, av. all flavors, 12 fl.oz	**80**	0	21
PowerBar:			
Protein Plus 50G, Choc., 17 fl.oz	**315**	2	24
Power Gel Smoothie, av., 1.5 oz pkg	**110**	0	27
Premier Protein *(Premier Nutrition)*:			
Clear, Tropical Punch, 16.9 fl.oz	**60**	0	1
Shakes, average, 11 fl.oz bottle	**160**	3	5
Propel: Purified Water, 12 fl.oz	**0**	0	0
Vitamin Boost, all flavors, 20 fl.oz	**10**	0	2
Protein2O: Tropical Coconut, 16.9 fl.oz	**60**	0	1
Aveage other flavors, 16.9 fl oz	**55**	0	7
Pure Protein: *Per 11 fl.oz Bottle or Can*			
30 Gram Shakes, average	**140**	2	6
35 Gram Shakes: Banana	**150**	1	1
Average other flavors	**165**	1	3
Powder, Plant Based, Van. Bean, 1.3 oz	**140**	3.5	8
Red Bull:			
Energy Drink: Average, 8.4 fl.oz	**110**	0	29
12 fl.oz can	**160**	0	40
Sugar-Free, 8.4 fl.oz	**10**	0	3
Zero Calories, 8.4 fl.oz	**0**	0	0

Revival:	C	F	Cb
Soy Mix, unsweetened:			
Plain, 2 scoops, 0.95 oz	**105**	1	4
Average all flavors, 2 scoops	**115**	2.5	5
Rhino, Rush Drink, all flav., 2 fl.oz	**6**	0	2
Rip It, Energy Fuel, Citrus X, 16 fl.oz	**200**	0	52
Rockstar: *Per 16 fl.oz Can*			
Energy Drink: Original	**130**	0	32
Sugar Free	**0**	0	0
Rumble, Supershake, 12 fl.oz	**250**	8	26
Rush: *Per 8.4 fl.oz*			
Energy Drink: Regular	**120**	0	32
with Maca, 8 fl.oz	**130**	0	30

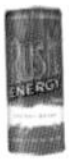

Skratch Labs:	C	F	Cb
Hydration Drink Mix: *Per Packet*			
Hyper, Passion Fruit, 0.9 oz	**80**	0	17
Sport Mix, average, 1 scoop, 0.78 oz	**80**	0	20
Wellness, Lemon & Limes, 0.6 oz	**70**	0	18
Sport Recov. Mix, average, 1.76 oz	**200**	3.5	35
Super Fuel, Lemon & Lime, 3.7 oz	**400**	0	100
Slim-Fast:			
Original: Protein Shakes, av., 11 fl.oz	**180**	5	24
Powder, average, 0.9 oz scoop	**110**	3.5	18
Advanced, High Protein, 11 fl.oz	**180**	9	7
Smoothie Mix, 1 scoop, 0.9 oz	**100**	3	7
Diabetic Wt. Loss, av., 1 sc., 26g	**100**	7	11
Keto Meal Shake, 2 sc, 38g	**180**	14	7
SoBe: *Per 20 fl.oz Can/Bottle*			
Citrus Energy Fruit Drink	**250**	0	64
Water, average all flavors	**0**	0	0
Solixir, Energy Drink, av. all, 12 fl.oz	**55**	0	13
Special K,			
Protein Shakes, av. all flav.	**185**	5	23

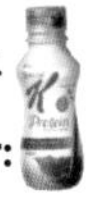

Spiru-Tein:	C	F	Cb
Energy Meal Shake Powder:			
Banana, 1.3 oz	**110**	0	15
Cappuccino, 1.1 oz	**100**	0	13
Gold: Chocolate, 1.3 oz	**90**	0	21
Strawberry,1.3 oz scoop	**125**	0	20
Note: Gold Products Contains 12 G Xylitol			
Sport, Vanilla, 2.25 oz scoop	**260**	7	27
Whey, Cookies & Cream, 1.2 oz sc.	**125**	2	15
Starbucks: Refreshers, av.,12 fl.oz	**90**	0	22
Doubleshot Energy ~ *See page 37*			
Steaz: Energy, all flav., 12 fl.oz	**140**	0	35
Zero Berry, 12 fl.oz	**0**	0	0
Shakeology:			
Beachbody Whey Prot. Powder,			
Chocolate, 1.45 oz	**160**	2.5	17
Twin Lab, MVP Fuel, all flav.,1 sc., 0.5 oz	**25**	0	6
Vega, Protein Shake, 11 fl.oz	**170**	5	14
Venom, av all flavors, 16 fl.oz	**235**	0	57
Vital: Organic Greens, 0,17 oz	**20**	0.2	2.3
Pea Protein, 0.9 oz	**90**	0.3	0.7
Weider:			
Mega Mass: 2000, 2 scoops, 3.5 oz	**400**	7	61
4000, 2 scoops, 3.5 oz	**400**	6	59
4000, Extreme Gainer, 7 sc., 11.8 oz	**1275**	19	247
XS *(Amway)*: Energy & Burn, 8 fl.oz	**10**	0	1
Energy, Summit 8.45 fl.oz	**10**	0	0
Zola: Energy Drinks, av., 12 fl.oz	**115**	0	27
Flavored Coconut Water, av., 8 fl.oz	**60**	0	15

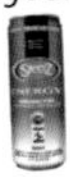

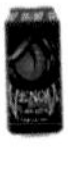

Quick Guide

Orange Juice

Average ~ Fresh	C	F	Cb
½ Cup, 4 fl.oz	55	0	13
Small Glass, 6 fl.oz	85	0	19
Regular Cup 8 fl.oz	110	0.5	26
Regular Glass, 12 fl.oz	160	0.5	39
10 fl.oz Bottle	140	0.5	32
11.5 fl.oz Can	160	0.5	37
16 fl.oz Bottle	225	1	52
20 fl.oz Bottle	280	1	64

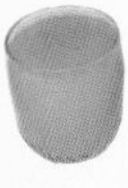

Juices ~ Generic

Average All Brands:	C	F	Cb
Aloe Vera Juice, unsweetened, 2 oz	10	0	0
Apple Juice: 8 fl.oz	120	0	29
10 fl.oz Bottle	145	0.5	36
16 fl.oz	235	0.5	58
Cactus Water, 1 Cup, 8 oz	25	0	6
Carrot Juice: Fresh, 6 fl.oz	35	0	8
Sweetened, 6 fl.oz	75	0	17
Coconut Water, 8 fl.oz	50	0.5	9
Cranberry Juice, Cocktail/Blend	140	0	34
Fruit Blends, average all, 8 fl.oz	110	0	27
Fruit Nectars, average all, 8 fl.oz	140	0	36
Grape Juice, 8 fl.oz	155	0	38
Grapefruit Juice, 8 fl.oz	95	0	22
Lemon/Lime Juice: 1 Tbsp	5	0	1
1 cup, 8 fl.oz	50	0.5	16
Concentrate, 1 tsp	0	0	0
Noni Juice:			
Tahitian, 2 Tbsp, 1 fl.oz	15	0	3
Tahiti Traders, 1 fl.oz	20	0	5
Papaya/Peach Nectar, av., 8 fl.oz	140	0	36
Passion Fruit Juice, Fresh:			
Purple, 1 cup, 8 fl.oz	125	0	34
Yellow, 1 cup, 8 fl.oz	80	1.5	14
Pear Nectar, 8 fl.oz	150	0	40
Pineapple Juice, 8 fl.oz	130	0	32
Pomegranate Juice, 8 fl.oz	160	0	40
Prune Juice, 8 fl.oz	180	0	45
Strawberry/Raspberry Juice, 8 fl.oz	100	0	23
Tangerine Juice, 8 fl.oz	105	0.5	25
Tomato Juice, 8 fl.oz	40	0	10
Vegetable Juice, 8 fl.oz	45	0	11
Wheat Grass Juice:			
1 fl.oz 'Shot'	10	0	1.5
2 fl.oz 'Shot'	20	0	3

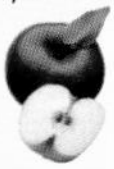
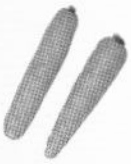
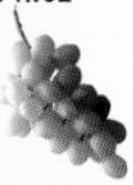
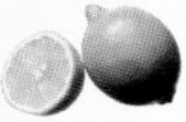
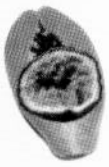
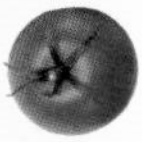
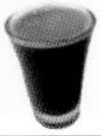

Updated Nutrition Data ~ www.CalorieKing.com
Persons with Diabetes ~ See Disclaimer (Page 22)

Quick Guide

Fruit Smoothies (Jamba Juice; Smoothie King)

Average All Brands	C	F	Cb
Fruit Only: 8 fl.oz	115	0.5	29
12 fl.oz	175	1	43
16 fl.oz	230	1	58
24 fl.oz	350	1	78
Fruit + Non-Fat Milk/Soy:			
12 fl.oz	135	0	29
16 fl.oz	155	0	37
24 fl.oz	265	1	59
Fruit + Non-Fat Frozen Yogurt/Sherbet:			
12 fl.oz	200	0.5	47
16 fl.oz	265	1	63
24 fl.oz	395	1.5	95

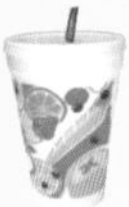

Juice ~ Brands

Per 8 fl.oz Unless Indicated

Apple & Eve:	C	F	Cb
100% Juice, No Sugar Added:			
Apple	110	0	26
Cranberry Blend/Raspberry	110	0	28
Cranberry Pomegranate	120	0	31
Strawb. Watermelon, 6.75 oz	90	0	24
Cool Waters, average, 6.75 fl.oz	15	0	4
Fruitables, av. all flav., 6.75 fl.oz	50	0	13
Organic Quenchers, all flav., 6.75 fl.oz	40	0	9
Bolthouse Farms: *Per 15.2 fl.oz Unless Indicated*			
B'fast Smoothie, Peach Parfait, 8 fl oz	190	2.5	34
Juice: 100% Carrot	130	0.5	29
100% Pomegranate, 8 fl.oz	150	0	38
Acai + 10 Superblend	240	0.5	60
Tropical + Carrot, 8 fl.oz	90	0.5	21
Fruit Smoothies: Amazing Mango	230	0	56
Berry Boost	250	0.5	61
Blue Goodness	290	0	72
C-Boost	210	0	52
Strawberry Banana	250	0.5	61
Tropical Goodness	220	1	51
Cactus Cooler, Orange Pineapple Blast,			
12 fl oz can	150	0	40

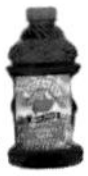
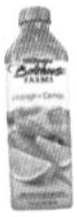
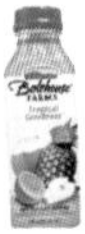

Juice Brands (Cont)

Per 8 fl.oz Unless Indicated

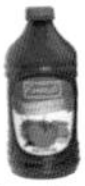

	C	F	Cb
Campbell's:			
Tomato Juice: 11.5 fl.oz can	70	0	14
8 fl.oz	50	0	10
Califia Farms: *Per 8 fl.oz Unless Indicated*			
Ginger Limeade	80	0	21
Meyer Lemonade	80	0	21
Orange Juice, 10. 5 fl.oz	140	0.5	32
Tangerine	110	0	25
Tart Cherry Lemonade	110	0	27

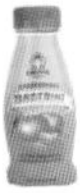

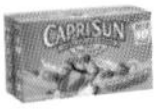

	C	F	Cb
Capri Sun: *Per 6 fl.oz*			
100% Juice, average,	85	0	21
Juice Drinks,			
(25% Less Sugar), all flavors	50	0	14
Refreshers, average, 6 fl.oz	45	0	11
Roarin' Waters, all flav., 6 fl.oz	30	0	8
Sport, average, 6 fl.oz	30	0	8
Sun Adventures, av., 6 fl.oz	50	0	13
Clamato: *Per 8 fl.oz*			
Original Tomato Cocktail	60	0	12
Picante	60	0	13
Coco Joy:			
Natural Coconut Water, 8.4 fl.oz	60	0	15
Sparkling Coconut Water, all, 11 fl.oz	80	2	20
Coco Libre, Flav. Coconut Water, 11 fl.oz	75	0	18
CocoZia, Coconut Water:			
100% Organic, 11.1 fl.oz pkg	70	0	16
Original, 8 fl.oz	40	0	10
Chocolate, 8 fl.oz	60	0.5	13

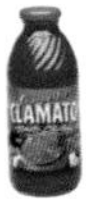

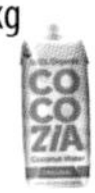

	C	F	Cb
Dole: *Per 8 fl.oz*			
Canned: 100% Juice, 6 fl.oz	100	0	25
Jaya Juice, av. all flavors, 8 fl.oz	145	0	36
Florida's Natural: *Per 8 fl.oz*			
Apple Juice	120	0	29
Lemonades, all flavors	110	0	28
Orange, No Pulp	110	0	26
Light Orange Juice	50	0	12
Ruby Red Grapefruit	90	0	22
Fuze: *Per 12 fl.oz*			
Blueberry Lemonade	80	0	21
Pineapple + Mango	80	0	21
Goya: *Per 9.6 fl.oz Can*			
Cocktail, Passion Fruit	130	0	34
Juice, Pineapple	110	0	27
Nectar: Mango	180	0	47
Peach	140	0	36
Pear & Passion Fruit	140	0	36
Soursop	130	0	35

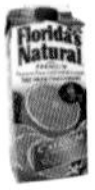

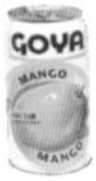

Per 8 fl.oz Unless Indicated

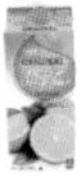

	C	F	Cb
Great Value *(Walmart):*			
100% Juice: *Per 8 fl.oz*			
Apple	110	0	28
Cranberry Blend	120	0	30
Grape	150	0	38
Orange	110	0	27
White Grape	140	0	38
Hansen's:			
Junior Juice,			
100% Juice, av. of flavors, 4.23 oz box	60	0	16
Natural, (64 fl.oz Bottles): *Per 8 fl.oz*			
Apple	120	0	28
Apple Strawberry	110	0	27
Cranberry Apple	110	0	27
Cranberry Grape	140	0	35
Grape	120	0	33
Orange Pineapple	110	0	27
White Grape	140	0	36

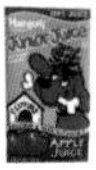

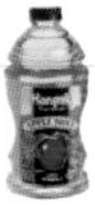

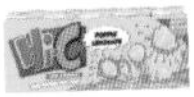

	C	F	Cb
Hawaii's Own, Frozen Concentrate, 100% Juice, average all flavors, 8 fl.oz prepared	105	0	27
Hi-C Juice Drinks: *Per 6.75 fl.oz Box*			
Flashin' Fruit Punch	90	0	25
Orange Lavaburst	90	0	25
Poppin' Lemonade	100	0	27
Hood: *Per 8 fl.oz*			
Lemonade	110	0	29
Orange	120	0	30
Jamba Juice ~ *See Fast-Foods Section*			
Juicy Juice *(Nestle):*			
Juicy Waters, 6.75 fl.oz	0	0	0
Organic Juice : *Per 8 fl.oz Unless Indicated*			
100%, Apple Juice; Fruit Punch	120	0	28
Fruitfuls, all flavors	70	0	16
6.75 fl.oz box	50	0	13
Plus Protein, all flavors, 6 fl.oz	90	0	17
Splashers, all f lavors, 1 pouch	40	0	9
Kerns:			
Nectars: *Per 11.5 fl.oz Can*			
Apricot	210	0	52
Guava; Strawberry, av.	180	0	45
Pear; Strawb. Banana, av.	195	0	46
Pineapple Coconut	230	6	43
L & A: *Per 8 fl.oz*			
All Cherry	180	0	45
All Cranberry	60	0	14
Papaya Delight	130	0	32
Pineapple Coconut	140	3	28

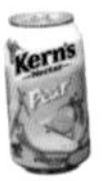

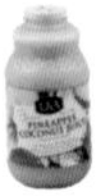

Juice Brands (Cont)

Per 8 fl.oz Unless Indicated	C	F	Cb
Lakewood Organic: *Per 8 fl.oz*			
Organic Blends:			
Black Cherry	130	0	32
Blueberry Blend	120	0	29
Pineapple Coconut	190	8	29
Pom Blue	120	0	29
Kale	80	0	19
Papaya	110	0	27
Tart Cherry	130	0	31
Veggie	80	0	17
Organic Pure: Beet	100	0	23
Blueberry	110	0	26
Carrot	90	0	20
Cranberry	80	0	19
Noni	5	0	1
Orange	120	0	28
Pineapple	130	0	31
Pink Grapefruit	110	0	26
Prune	180	0	43
Langers: *Per 8 fl.oz*			
100% Juice:			
Apple Juice	120	0	28
Red/White Grape Juice	160	0	40
Juice Cocktails (27% Juice):			
Blueberry Cranberry	135	0	34
Cranberry	140	0	35
Cranberry Grape	165	0	41
Cranberry Raspberry	140	0	35
20% Juice, all flavors	120	0	30
Martinellli's:			
Juice, 100% Apple, all varieties, 8 fl.oz	140	0	35
Sparkling: Apple Juice, 10 fl.oz	180	0	43
Apple Grape, 8 fl.oz	120	0	31
Apple-Pear, 8.4 fl.oz	130	0	31
Blush, 8 fl.oz	120	0	30
Cider, 8.4 fl.oz	150	0	37
Red Grape, 8.4 fl.oz	1270	0	42
White Grape, 8.4 fl.oz	170	0	42
Minute Maid:			
12 fl.oz Bottles: *Per Bottle*			
Apple Juice	170	0	41
Cranb. Apple Raspberry	180	0	48
Cranberry Grape	190	0	50
Pineapple Orange	180	0	43

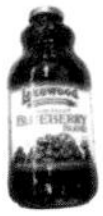
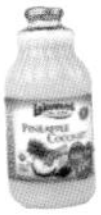
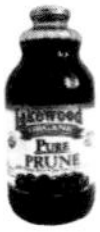
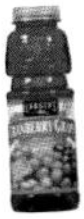
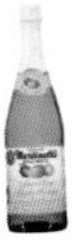
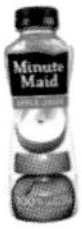

Per 8 fl.oz Unless Indicated	C	F	Cb
Minute Maid (Cont):			
Orange Juice,			
Original, 8 fl.oz	110	0	27
Just 15 Calories, Lemonade, 8 fl.oz	15	0	4
Kid's Juice Boxes, 100% Juice,			
Apple White Grape, 6.75 fl.oz	90	0	22
Light Juice, Cherry Limeade, 8 fl.oz	4	0	1
Soft Frozen Concentrate,			
Limeade, 8 fl.oz prepared	90	0	25
Mott's:			
100% Juice:			
Original Apple, 8 fl.oz	120	0	29
Apple Mango, 8 fl.oz	120	0	29
Apple White Grape, 6.75 fl.oz	130	0	31
Fruit Punch, 4.23 fl.oz	60	0	15
Juice Drink, Light Apple, 8 fl.oz	50	0	12
Mott's For Tots (47-54% Juice):			
40% Less Sugar: Fruit Punch, 8 fl.oz	70	0	16
Other flavors, 8 fl.oz	60	0	16
Sensibles, all flavors, 8 fl.oz	90	0	21
Naked Juice: *Per 15.2 fl.oz*			
100% Juice, No Sug. Added:			
O-J	210	0	51
Orange Mango	230	0	59
Pomegranate Blueberry	290	0	68
100% Juice Smoothie, No Sugar Added:			
Berry Blast	220	0.5	55
Mighty Mango	290	0	68
Orange Carrot	220	0	55
Pina Colada	310	3.5	66
Strawberry Banana	250	0	59
Half Naked 50% Less Sugar:			
Berry Almond	240	15	12
Lively Greens	150	0.5	32
Mango Orange	220	13	37
Watermelon with Passion Fruit	120	1	33
Machines: Blue	320	0	76
Power-C	220	0	55
Red	320	9	59
Vitamin D	230	0	55

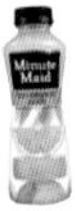
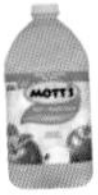
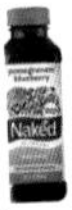
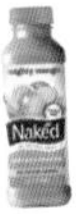
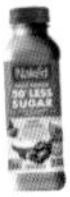
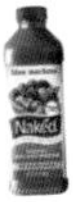

Juice Brands (Cont)

Per 8 fl.oz Unless Indicated	C	F	Cb
Nantucket Nectars:			
Juice: *Per 16 fl.oz*			
Orange Mango	220	0	59
Peach Orange	260	0	63
Pineapple Orange Banana	290	0	69
Pineapple Orange Guava	210	0	52
Pomegranate Cherry	230	0	57
Pomegranate Pear	230	0	57
Premium Orange Juice	220	0	51
Pressed Apple	240	0.5	59
Red Plum	220	0	55
Watermelon Strawberry	220	0	55
Juice Cocktail, Cranberry	240	0	59
Lemonade, Squeezed	180	0	47
Newman's Own: *Per 8 fl.oz*			
Lemonade, Regular; Pink	110	0	27
Limeade	140	0	34
Fruit Juice Cocktail:			
Grape	110	0	29
Orange Mango Tango	130	0	33
Northland: *Per 8 fl.oz*			
100% Juice:			
Blueberry Blackberry Acaí	110	0	27
Cranb. Blackberry/Raspberry, av.	110	0	27
Cranberry Cherry	120	0	30
Cranberry Grape	110	0	28
Cranberry Mango	120	0	29
Ocean Spray: *Per 8 fl.oz*			
Juice Cocktails:			
Cranberry	110	0	28
100% Juice Blends:			
Cranberry Concord Grape	130	0	36
Cranberry Mango	120	0	31
Cranberry Pineapple	110	0	31
Cranberry Raspberry	120	0	32
Juice Drinks:			
Cran-Apple	100	0	27
Cran-Grape	100	0	28
Cran-Tangerine	100	0	28
Diet Juice Drinks, all flavors	5	0	2
Growing Goodness, av., 6.75 fl.oz	45	0	12
Light Juice Drinks, av. all flavors	50	0	13
Sparkling, av. all flavors, 8.4 fl.oz	70	0	20

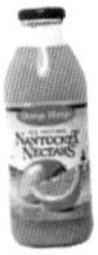
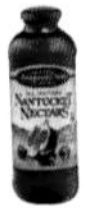
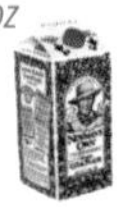
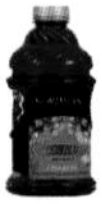
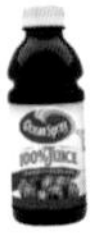
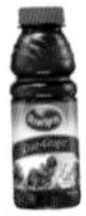

Per 8 fl.oz Unless Indicated	C	F	Cb
Orange Julius:			
Originals:			
Medium: Mango Pineapple	320	0.2	78
Orange	260	0.5	63
Strawberry	300	0.2	75
Large: Mango Pineapple	470	0.3	117
Orange	400	0.5	98
Strawberry	450	0.3	113
Smoothies ~ *See Fast-Foods Section*			
Orangina, 10 fl.oz bottle	130	0	32
Pom Wonderful,			
100% Juice (8 fl.oz Bottle),			
Pom Blueberry/Cherry/Pomegranate	155	0	38
R.W. Knudsen: *Per 8 fl.oz*			
Organic, 100% Juice: Apple	110	0	28
Acai Berry	110	0	26
Concord Grape	160	0	39
Cranberry Blueberry	110	0	27
Mango Nectar	120	0	29
Orange Carrot	110	0	27
Tomato	45	0	10
Natural, 100% Juice:			
Mango Peach	120	0	30
Papaya Nectar	130	0	32
Razzleberry	110	0	28
Rio Red Grapefruit	140	0	34
Just Juice:			
Just Blueberry	90	0	23
Just Black Cherry	190	0	45
Just Black Currant	110	0	24
Simply Nutritious:			
Lemon Ginger Echinacea	110	0	27
Average other flavors	115	0	28
Shots: Apple Cider Vinegar, 2.5 fl.oz	10	0	2
Beet , 2.5 fl.oz	25	0	5
Carrot, Black Pepper & Turmeric, 2.5 fl.oz	25	0	5
Pineapple Ginger, 2.5 fl.oz	30	0	9
Sparkling: Caramel Apple	110	0	28
Cranberry	110	0	27
Cherry; Pomegranate	130	0	32
Organic Pear	120	0	30

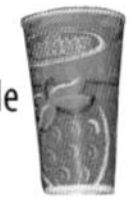
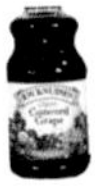
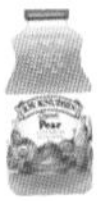
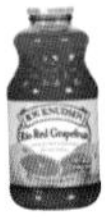
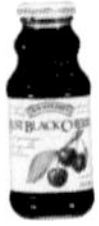
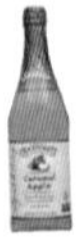

Juice Brands (Cont)

Per 8 fl.oz Unless Indicated	C	F	Cb
R.W. Knudsen (Cont):			
Organic Veggie Blends:			
Beet, Carrot Orange	90	0	22
Carrot Ginger Turmeric	70	0	16
Celery Apple Cucumber	50	0	11
Sweet Potato	100	0	24
Very Veggie; Low Sodium	50	0	10
Spicy	45	0	10
ReaLemon – ReaLime:			
Lemon/Lime Juice (from concentrate):			
1 teaspoon	0	0	0
2Tbsp, 1 fl.oz	10	0	2.5
Santa Cruz: *Per 8 fl.oz*			
Organic, 100% Juice:			
Apple; Apricot Mango, average	115	0	29
Concord/White Grape	160	0	39
Orange Mango; Red Tart Cherry	120	0	29
Pear Nectar	140	0	34
Lemonade:			
Regular; Peach	90	0	22
Blueberry; Raspberry; Strawberry, av.	90	0	23
Cherry	100	0	25
Peach	80	0	21
Simply Orange Juice Company:			
Lemonade; Limeade, average	120	0	31
Lemonade, with Raspberry	110	0	28
Mixed Berry; Tropical	100	0	26
Orange Juice,			
with or without pulp	110	0	26
Snap•E•Tom,			
Tomato & Chili Cocktail,			
11.5 fl.oz can	70	0	15
Snapple: *Per 16 fl.oz Bottle*			
Juice: Go Bananas.	230	0	55
Grapeade; Orangeade	190	0	46
Fruit Punch	200	0	48
Kiwi Strawberry	190	0	46
Mango Madness	190	0	45
Watermelon Lemonade	150	0	35
Diet, Cranberry Raspberry	20	0	5
Ssips, Juice Boxes,			
av. all flavors, 6 fl.oz box	80	0	21

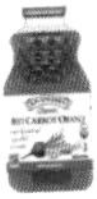
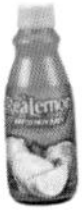
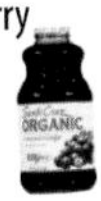
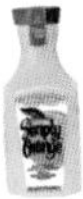
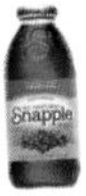
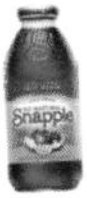

Per 8 fl.oz Unless Indicated	C	F	Cb
SunnyD: *Per 8 fl.oz*			
Blue Raspberry	60	0	15
Fruit Punch	60	0	16
Lemonade	60	0	15
Orange Mango/Strawberry	60	0	16
Orange Peach	60	0	17
Orange Pineapple	60	0	16
Orange Strawberry	60	0	16
Smooth Orange	50	0	14
Tangy Original	60	0	16
Sunsweet: *Per 8 fl.oz*			
Plum Smart: Original	160	0	36
Light	60	0	15
Prune Juice: Original	180	0	42
Light	100	0	26
Trader Joe's:			
All Natural Pasteurized, 32/64 fl.oz Bottle: *Per 8 fl.oz*			
100% Cranberry	70	0	16
Blueberry Pomegranate	140	0	34
Just Blueberry	100	0	24
Just Pomegranate	150	0	37
Mango PassionFruit	130	0	32
Omega Orange Carrot	110	0	26
Organic, 32/64 fl.oz Bottle: *Per 8 fl.oz*			
Apple Juice	120	0	30
Concord Grape Juice	160	0	39
Cranberry	70	0	18
Grapefruit Sunset	120	0	30
jalapeno Limeade	100	0	25
Mango Nectar	130	0	32
Pink Lemonade	130	0	32
Strawberry Lemonade	120	0	29
White Grape Juice	160	0	40
Cold Presssed, 12 fl.oz:			
Coconut Carrot	70	0	16
Spiced Fuji Apple Cider	200	0	48
Spiced Cider	130	0	31
Winter Wassail	100	0	26
Joe's Kids: *Per 6.75 oz Box*			
From Concentrate: Apple	90	0	23
Apple Grape	100	0	24
White Grape	120	0	30
10% Juice, Lemonade	90	0	22
Sparkling Juices, 25.4 fl.oz Bottle: *Per 8 fl.oz*			
Blueberry	120	0	30
Cranberry	140	0	35
Pomegranate	130	0	31

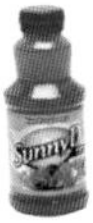
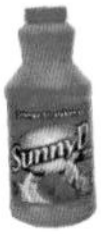
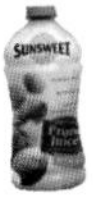
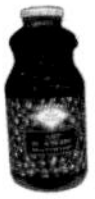
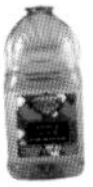
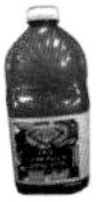
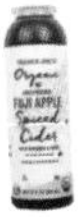
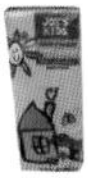

B Beverages ~ Fruit & Vegetable Juices

Juice Brands (Cont)

Per 8 fl.oz Unless Indicated	C	F	Cb
Tree Top:			
100% Juice, 64 fl.oz Bottle: *Per 8 fl.oz*			
Apple Berry/Grape, average	125	0	31
Mango Cherry	120	0	29
Orange Passionfruit ; P'apple Orange	120	0	30
5.5 fl.oz can, apple	80	0	19
6.75 fl.oz Box, Apple; Pear	100	0	24
Fruit & Water: Tropical, 6 fl.oz	45	0	11
All other Flavors, 6 fl.oz	50	0	12
Tropicana: *Per 8 fl.oz*			
Essentials Fiber,			
Strawberry Banana	140	0	35
Premium Drinks:			
Island Punch	90	0	21
Lemonade: Peach	110	0	27
Raspberry; Tangerine, average	100	0	25
Strawberry Peach	100	0	24
Pure Premium Orange Juice:			
Grovestand, Lots of Pulp	110	0	26
No Pulp	110	0	26
Trop 50: Pomegranate Blueberry	50	0	14
Orange Mango/Peach, av.	50	0	12
Tru Nopal:			
Cactus Water: 1 Cup, 8 fl.oz	25	0	6
16.9 fl.oz carton	50	0	12
Turkey Hill: *Per 12 fl.oz*			
All Natural Lemonade: Original	170	0	41
Blackberry; Watermelon	160	0	39
Pink	150	0	37
Watermelon	160	0	39
Fruit Punch	150	0	39
V8 Juices & Drinks *(Campbell's):*			
Original/Spicy 100% Vegetable Juice:			
5.5 fl.oz can	35	0	7
8 fl.oz cup	45	0	9
11.5 fl.oz can	70	0	14
12 fl.oz bottle	75	0	15
Blends: Peach Mango, 8 fl.oz	110	0	27
Healthy Greens; Carrot Mango, 8 fl.oz	60	0	14
Red Radiance, 8 fl.oz	70	0	17
Sparkling V8-Energy:			
Orange Pineapple, 11.5 fl.oz	140	5	20
Strawberry Kiwi, 11.5 fl.oz	50	0	12
Veryfine:			
100%: Apple, 8 fl.oz	120	0	29
Apple Strawb., Krazy Kiwi, 11.5 fl.oz	170	0	43
Orange, 8 fl.oz	120	0	30

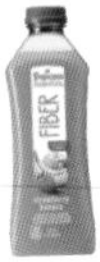

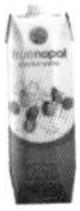

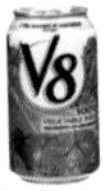

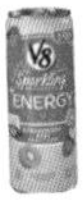

Per 8 fl.oz Unless Indicated	C	F	Cb
Vita Coco: *Per 8 fl.oz*			
Coconut Water: Regular	45	0	11
with Peach & Mango	90	3	16
with Pineapple	60	0	14
Walnut Acres: *Per 8 fl.oz*			
Organic: Apple	110	0	29
Apricot; Raspberry	130	0	32
Cherry	140	0	34
Concord Grape	120	0	31
Incredible Vegetable	50	0	12
Orange Carrot	110	0	27
Welch's: *Per 8 fl.oz Unless Indicated*			
100% Juice: Concord Grape	140	0	38
Red Sangria	140	0	34
White Grape	140	0	38
White Grape Peach	140	0	34
Juice Drink, Fruit Punch, 10 fl.oz	120	0	31
Refrigerated Cocktails: CherryBurst	100	0	23
Mango Twist	120	0	28
Peach Medley	100	0	25
Sparkling Juice Cocktail:			
Red/White Grape, av.	150	0	40
Rose; Mimosa, average	75	0	18
Zola:			
Acai: *Per 12 fl.oz Bottle*			
Original	185	3	38
with Blueberry/Pomegranate	180	3	38
Coconut Water, 17.5 oz Can:			
Original,	50	0	13
Chocolate, 8 fl.oz	50	0	12
Espresso, 8 fl.oz	60	0	13

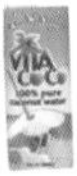

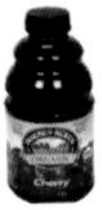

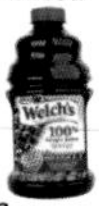

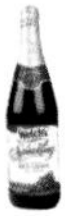

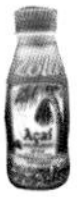

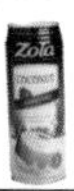

CalorieKing Portion Watch

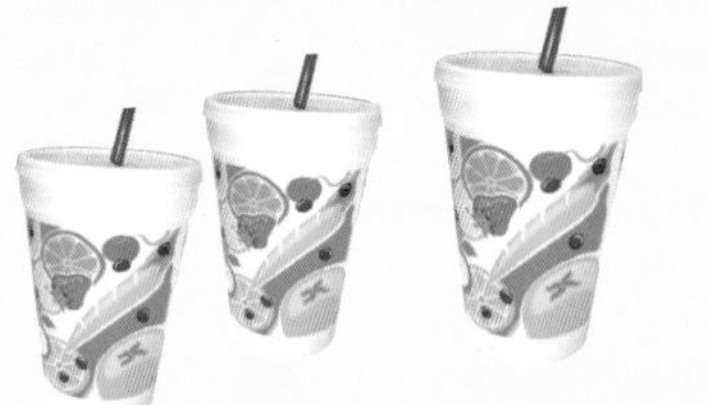

ORANGE JUICE	C	Cb
8 fl.oz	110	26
16 fl.oz	220	52
24 fl.oz	330	78
32 fl.oz	440	104

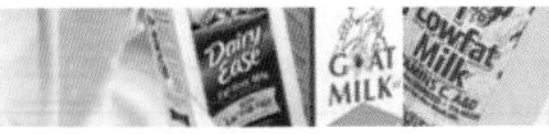

Quick Guide

	C	F	Cb
Cow's Milk ~ Average All Brands			
Whole (3.25% fat):			
2 Tbsp, 1 fl.oz	20	1	1.5
1 Cup, 8 fl.oz	150	8	12
1 Large Glass, 12 fl.oz	220	12	17
1 Pint, 16 fl.oz	295	16	22
1 Quart, 946 ml	590	32	44
Reduced-Fat (2% fat):			
2 Tbsp, 1 fl.oz	15	0.5	1.5
1 Cup, 8 fl.oz	120	5	12
1 Large Glass, 12 fl.oz	180	7.5	18
1 Pint, 16 fl.oz	245	10	23
1 Quart, 946 ml	490	20	46
Light/Low-Fat (1% fat):			
2 Tbsp, 1 fl.oz	13	0.3	1.5
1 Cup, 8 fl.oz	100	2.5	12
1 Large Glass, 12 fl.oz	150	4	18
1 Pint, 16 fl.oz	205	5	25
1 Quart, 946 ml	410	10	49
Fat Free/Skim (0% fat):			
2 Tbsp, 1 fl.oz	10	0	1.5
1 Cup, 8 fl.oz	90	0.5	13
1 Large Glass, 12 fl.oz	135	0.5	19
1 Pint, 16 fl.oz	180	1	26

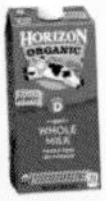
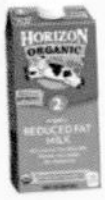
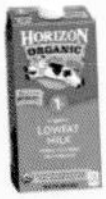
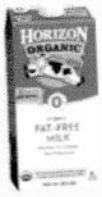

Half & Half ~ *See Page 89*

SWITCH & SAVE

Switch from whole milk to either 2%, 1% or 0% milk and save significant calories.

Per 8 oz Cup/Glass

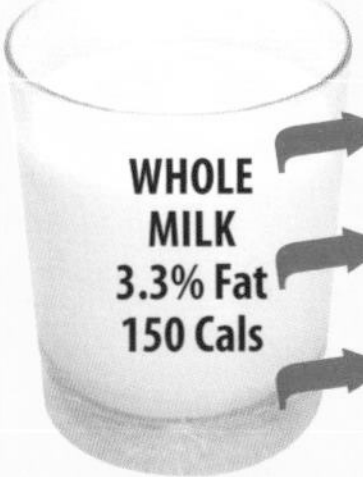

WHOLE MILK 3.3% Fat 150 Cals

2% MILK 120 Cals	SAVE 30 Cals
1% MILK 100 Cals	SAVE 50 Cals
0% FAT-FREE 90 Cals	SAVE 60 Cals

Switching to low-fat or fat-free milk also greatly reduces saturated fat.

Other Milks

	C	F	Cb
Buttermilk: *Average All Brands*			
Reduced-Fat (2%), 1 cup, 8 fl.oz	120	5	10
Low-Fat (1%), 1 cup, 8 fl.oz	100	2.5	12
Lactose Free:			
Lactaid 100: Whole	160	8	13
2% Reduced-Fat	130	5	12
1% Low-Fat	110	2.5	13
Fat Free; Calcium Enriched	90	0	13
Smart Balance,			
FF + Omega-3s & Vit. E	100	0	14
Lower Calorie/Carb Dairy Drinks: *Per 8 fl.oz Cup*			
Calorie Countdown (*Hood*):			
2% Reduced-Fat: Plain	70	4.5	3
Chocolate	80	4.5	6
Fat-Free	35	0	4

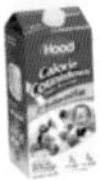

Goat/Sheep Milk, Kefir

	C	F	Cb
Goat's Milk (*Meyenberg*):			
Whole, 1 cup, 8 fl.oz	140	7	11
Low-Fat (1%), 8 fl.oz	100	2.5	11
Evaporated, reconst., 8 fl.oz	140	8	12
Kefir: *Per 8 fl.oz*			
Lifeway: Original, Plain	150	8	12
Greek, Plain, whole milk	210	14	12
Lowfat, average all flavors	140	1.5	20
Nancy's: Plain, low fat	140	3	17
Fruit flavors, average	205	2.5	38
Trader Joe's: Plain, 1%	110	2.5	8
Strawberry	160	2	21
Sheep's Milk, Whole, 1 cup	265	17	13

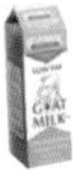
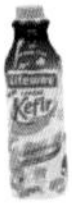
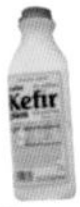

Canned & Dried Milk

	C	F	Cb
Condensed: Sweetened, 2 T., 1 fl.oz	130	3	22
Low Fat, 2 Tbsp	120	1.5	23
Fat-Free, 2 Tbsp	110	0	24
Evaporated: Whole, 2 Tbsp	40	3	3
Whole, 1/2 cup, 4 fl.oz	170	10	13
Carnation: Low Fat, 2 Tbsp, 1 oz	25	0.5	3
1/2 cup, 4 fl.oz	115	2.5	14
Fat-Free, 2 Tbsp, 1 oz	25	0	4
Dried: Whole, ¼ cup, 1 oz	160	9	12
Skim/Non-Fat, ⅓ cup	80	0	12
Made-up, 1 cup, 8 fl.oz	80	0	12
Buttermilk (sweet cream): 1 oz	110	2	14
Non-Fat, 1 Tbsp	25	0	3
Carnation, Malted, dry, 3 Tbsp, 0.7 oz	90	2	15
Horlick's, Malt Powder, dry, 1 oz	180	4	27

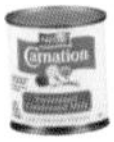
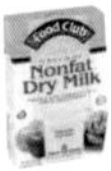

Soy/Non-Dairy Drinks ~ **See Page 49**

B Beverages ~ Flavored Milk

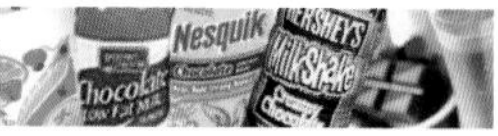

Quick Guide

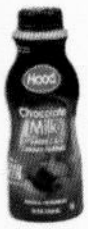
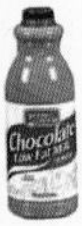

	C	F	Cb
Chocolate Milk:			
Average All Brands:			
Whole Milk, (3.3%):			
8 fl.oz cup	220	8	29
1 Pint, 16 fl.oz	440	16	58
Reduced-Fat, (2%):			
8 fl.oz cup	190	5	30
1 Pint, 16 fl.oz	380	10	60
Low-Fat, (1%):			
8 fl.oz cup	160	3	26
1 Pint, 16 fl.oz	315	5	52

Flavored Milk ~ Brands

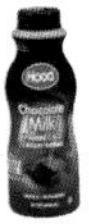
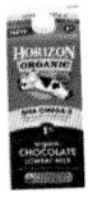
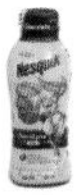
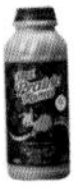
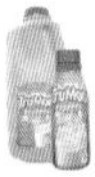

	C	F	Cb
Ready-To-Drink: *Per 8 fl.oz Unless Indicated*			
fairlife, Chocolate , reduced fat	140	4.5	13
Great Value *(Walmart),*			
Chocolate, low fat	140	2.5	29
Hood: Chocolate	220	8	30
Low-Fat (1%), Chocolate	160	2.5	28
Horizon Organic:			
HIgh Protein, Reduced Fat,			
Chocoalte	190	5	24
Low-Fat, with Omega 3,			
Choc./Vanilla, average	150	2.5	23
Kroger: *Per 8 fl.oz*			
1% Low Fat Chocolate Milk	170	3	29
Ultra Pasteurised	180	2.5	33
Simple Truth Organic:			
1% Chocolate	170	3	27
Whole Milk, Chocolate	210	8	27
Muscle Milk ~ *See Energy Protein Drinks*			
Nesquik: *Per 14 fl.oz*			
Low Fat, average all flavors	250	4	41
Prairie Farms: *Per 8 fl.oz*			
Chocolate: 2% Reduced Fat	180	5	26
Premium Whole Milk	220	8	29
Strawberry, 1% Low Fat	160	2.5	28
TruMoo: *Per 8 fl.oz*			
After Dark, Dark Choc Salted Caramel	230	8	30
Chocolate/Strawberry			
Whole	200	8	24
1% Low-Fat	130	2.5	19
High Protein 1% (25g),			
average all flavors, 14 fl.oz	360	4.5	55

Flavored Milk ~ Brands (Cont)

	C	F	Cb
Yoo-Hoo: Chocolate,15.5 fl.oz bottle	220	2	51
Chocolate Peanut Butter, 6.75 fl.oz	100	1	22
Strawberry, 6.5 fl.oz	90	0.5	22
Bottled Coffee Drinks ~ *See Page 37*			

Shakes

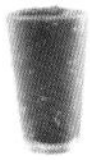
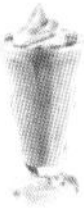

	C	F	Cb
Arby's: *Per Small Size*			
Chocolate; Jamocha	585	17	94
Burger King: *Per Medium 16 oz*			
Hand Spun Shakes: Chocolate	760	21	131
Strawberry	645	15	113
Vanilla	585	15	98
Other flavors ~ *See Fast Food Section*			
Denny's: *Per 16 oz*			
Cake Batter	1090	52	147
Chocolate	870	43	111
Oreo	1050	56	125
Strawberry	760	34	110
Vanilla	800	43	97
Hardees, all flavors, av., 14 oz	700	35	85
McDonalds, McCafe Shakes:			
Chocolate: 12 fl.oz	530	15	87
16 fl.oz	630	17	104
22 fl.oz	840	22	142
Strawberry/Vanilla, av.: 12 fl.oz	495	14	80
16 fl.oz	590	17	95
22 fl.oz	800	22	130
Other Restaurants ~ *See Fast-Foods Section*			

Smoothies

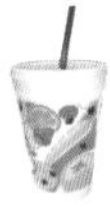

	C	F	Cb
Made Up Ready-To-Drink:			
8 fl. oz Milk/Soy + Fruit: *Per 12 fl.oz*			
Average all flavors:			
with Whole Milk	300	8	50
+ Ice Cream, 1 scoop	400	13	62
with Non-Fat Milk	240	0	50
Kroger/Ralph's Smoothies: *Per 8 fl.oz*			
Simple Truth: Mango	150	0	37
Strawberry Banana	130	0	32
Freshens; Jamba Juice; TCBY ~ *See Fast-Foods*			

Nut, Rice & Cereal Drinks

Per 8 fl.oz Cup Unless Indicated	C	F	Cb
Almond Breeze *(Blue Diamond):*			
Almond Milk: Original	60	2.5	8
Chocolate	100	2.5	21
Vanilla	80	2.5	14
Blended with Bananas	80	2	14
Red. Sugar: Original	45	2.5	6
Vanilla	60	2.5	8
Unsweetened: Chocolate	40	3	2
Original; Vanilla, average	30	2.5	1
Blends:			
Almond Cashew,			
Unsweetened, Plain; Vanilla	25	2	1
Almond Coconut: Original	60	3	7
Vanilla, unsweetened	40	3.5	1
Almond Dream ~ *See Dream*			
Amazake,			
Oh So Original, Rice Shake	150	0	31
Better Than Milk:			
Rice Vegan Powder Mix,			
Orig.; Van., 2 Tbsp, 0.7 oz	70	0	17
Cacique,			
Original Horchata, 12 fl.oz	230	5	46
Califia Farms: *Per 8 fl.oz Cup*			
Almond Milk: Original	60	4	6
Unsweetened	35	3	1
Vanilla	50	3	4
Barista Blend	70	4.5	7
Coconut: Chocolate	90	4.5	11
Toasted	45	4	1
Oatmilk, Barista Blend	130	7	14
Don Jose: *Per 8 fl.oz Cup*			
Horchata Rice Drink	140	4	25
Dream: *Per 8 fl.oz Cup*			
Almond Dream, unsweetened	50	3.5	3
Coconut Dream ~ *See page 50*			
Oat Dream: Original; Vanilla, av.	120	3.5	21
Unsweetened	70	3	8
Chocolate	170	3.5	32
Rice Dream: Classic Orig./Enriched	120	2.5	23
Enriched: Unsweetened	70	2.5	11
Vanilla	130	2.5	26
Horchata	160	2.5	33
Sprouted, unsweetened	70	2.5	11
Soy Dream ~ *See page 50*			

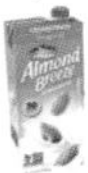
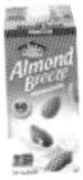
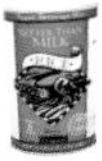
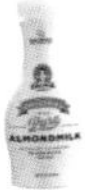
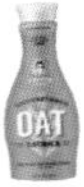

Note: Rice/Oat/Nut Drinks are very low in protein. Unless enriched with prtein (and calcium), they are not suitable for infants as a substitute for milk or calcium-enriched soy drinks.

Nut & Rice Drinks (Cont)

Per 8 fl.oz Cup Unless Indicated	C	F	Cb
Milkadamia: *Per 8 fl.oz Cup*			
Macadamia Milk: Original	70	5	7
Unsweetened, Orig./Vanilla	50	5	1
Latte da	70	4.5	8
Pacific Foods: *Per 8 fl.oz Cup*			
Cashew, Original	80	4.5	8
Hazelnut, Orig./Chocolate, av.	120	5	18
Hemp: Original	140	6	19
Unsweetened Orig./Vanilla	60	4.5	0
Chocolate	200	6	32
Vanilla	170	6	23
Organic Almond: Orig.; Vanilla, av.	65	3	10
Chocolate, single serve	110	3	19
Oat, Vanilla	130	2	25
Silk: *Per 8 fl.oz Cup*			
Organic Almond: Original	50	2	8
Unsweetened	30	2.5	1
Dark Chocolate	100	2	19
Vanilla, unsweetened	40	3	1
Cashew: Unsweetned Orig; Vanilla	25	2	1
Chocolate	90	2	19
Protein:			
Almond & Cashew: Original	130	8	3
Chocolate	150	5	18
Vanilla	140	7	8
Trader Joe's:			
Rice Drinks: *Per 8 fl.oz*			
Unsweetened: Original, Organic	120	2.5	23
Vanilla	130	2.5	26

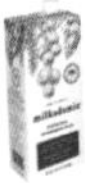
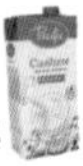
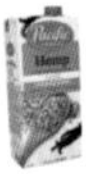
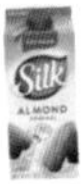

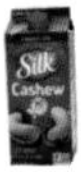

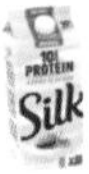

Soy Milk ~ Ready-To-Drink

	C	F	Cb
365 Organic *(Whole Foods): Per 8 fl.oz Cup*			
Original, unsweetened	70	3.5	3
Chocolate, unsweetened	40	3	1
8th Continent: *Per 8 fl.oz*			
Original	80	2.5	7
Vanilla	100	2.5	11
Edensoy: *Per 8 fl.oz Cup*			
Organic: Original	130	5	11
Unsweetened	120	6	4
Carob; Vanilla	150	3.5	23
Cocoa	200	4.5	32
Extra: Original	130	5	12
Vanilla	150	3	23
Great Value *(Walmart)*, Orig. Soy	100	4	9

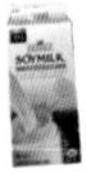
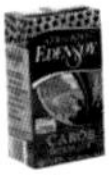

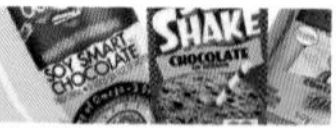

Soy Milk ~ Ready-To-Drink (Cont)

Per 8 fl.oz Unless Indicated	C	F	Cb
Odwalla: *Per 15.2 fl.oz Bottle*			
Soy & Dairy Protein Shakes:			
Chocolate	340	8	38
Strawberry	320	7	37
Vanilla	330	7	35
Pacific: *Per 8 fl.oz Cup*			
Soy, Organic, Orig., unswtnd	90	4	5
Ultra Soy, Original	140	5	13
Pearl *(Kikkoman): Per 8 fl.oz Cup*			
Organic: Original; Crmy Van.	130	4.5	13
Unsweetened	90	5	4
With Green Tea	140	4.5	18
Chocolate; Coffee, av.	135	3	21
Silk *(Whitewave): Per 8 fl.oz Cup*			
Organic: Original; Vanilla, av.	105	4	10
Chocolate	150	5	19
Very Vanilla	130	3.5	18
Light, Original	60	2	5
Unsweetened: Original	80	4	3
Vanilla	80	4	4
Slim-Fast ~ *See Page 40*			
Soy Dream *(Dream): Per 8 fl.oz Cup*			
Enriched: Original	100	4	8
Vanilla	120	4	14
Soylent:			
Ready To Drink Bottles: *Per 14 fl.oz*			
Original	400	24	37
Banana; Cacao; Strawberry	400	21	37
Creamy Chocolate; Vanilla	400	24	36
Mint Chocolate	400	24	36
Cafe, Chai; Mocha; Vanilla, average	400	22	36
Stacked, Chocolate, 11.15 fl.oz	180	10	12
Soy Slender *(Westsoy): Per 8 fl.oz Cup*			
Soy Milk,			
Cappuccino; Vanilla; Chocolate	70	3	4
Trader Joe's: *Per 8 fl.oz*			
Soy Milk: Original	110	2	13
Chocolate	130	2.5	23
Vanilla	100	2	16
Organic: Original	130	3.5	18
Chocolate	120	3	17
Vanilla	130	3	19

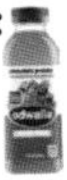
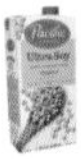
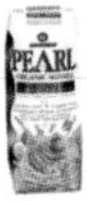
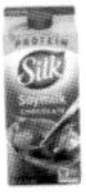
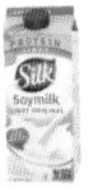
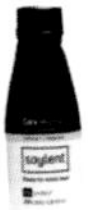
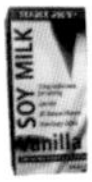
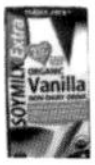

Soy Milk ~ Ready-To-Drink (Cont)

Per 8 fl.oz Unless Indicated	C	F	Cb
WestSoy:			
Soy Milk: Chocolate Peppermint Stick	180	3.5	30
Organic: Original	130	3.5	18
Unsweetened: Plain	100	5	4
Vanilla	100	4.5	5
Organic Plus, Plain/Vanilla	110	4.5	11
Low-Fat: Plain	90	2	15
Vanilla	120	2	23
Non-Fat: Plain	70	0	10
Vanilla	80	0	12

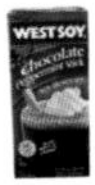
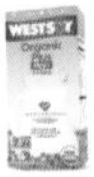

Soy Powder Mix

1 oz (¼ cup) mix makes 8 fl.oz Cup	C	F	Cb
Soy Protein Isolate, dry, 1 oz	95	1	2
Better Than Milk:			
Original, 2 Tbsp	90	1.5	18
Vanilla, 2 Tbsp	90	1.5	18
Now:			
Soy Protein Isolate:			
Plain, ⅓ cup, 0.8 fl.oz	90	0.5	0
Chocolate, 1 scoop, 1.6 oz	160	1.5	9
Vanilla, 1 scoop, 1.6 oz	180	2.5	13
Soylent:			
Meal Replacement Powders:			
Original, ⅔ cup, 3.2 oz	400	20	41
Cacao, 2 rounded scoops, 3.2 oz	400	20	41
Cafe Mocha, ⅔cup, 3.2 oz	400	20	41
Whole Foods:			
Chocolate, with Spirulina, 1 oz	100	1	10
Vanilla, with Spirulina, 1 oz	100	0	11

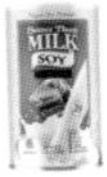
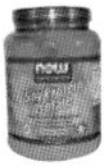

Coconut Milk Drinks

	C	F	Cb
Califia Farms: *Per 8 fl.oz Cup*			
Blend, Coconut Almond, Chocolate	90	4.5	11
Go Coconuts, Coconut Water Blend	45	4	2
Coconut Dream *(Dream): Per 8 fl.oz Cup*			
Enriched: Original	80	5	7
Unsweetened	60	5	1
Vanilla	90	5	9
Great Value *(Walmart),*			
Original Unsweetened	50	5	1
Pacific, Organic, Original Unsweetened	45	4	1
Silk: Original	70	4.5	6
Unsweetened	40	4	1
So Delicious: *Per 8 fl.oz cup*			
Organic, Unswtn'd Shelf Stable	45	4	2
Trader Joes: *Per 8 fl.oz cup*			
Unsweetened	60	5	1
Vanilla	90	5	9

(Enriched with calcium + vitamins D & B12)

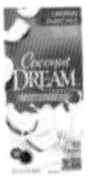
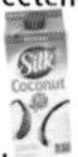
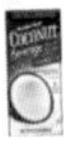

Quick Guide

	C	F	Cb
Cola:			
Drinks: *Average all Brands*			
8 fl.oz Cup/Can	100	0	26
12 fl.oz Can	150	0	39
16 fl.oz Bottle	200	0	52
20 fl.oz Bottle	250	0	65
24 fl.oz (Pepsi)	300	0	84
1-Liter Bottle (34 fl.oz)	400	0	100
2-Liter Bottle (68 fl.oz)	800	0	200
Other Soda Drinks: *Per 12 fl.oz, average all brands*			
Club Soda	0	0	0
Cream Soda	190	0	48
Ginger Ale	125	0	31
Lemonade, Regular/Pink	180	0	45
Orange	180	0	45
Root Beer	150	0	39
Tonic Water	125	0	32
Mineral Water: Plain	0	0	0
Sweetened/flavored	150	0	37
with Fruit Juice	120	0	30
Soda Water/Seltzer: Plain/Diet	0	0	0
Sweetened/flavored	155	0	39
with Fruit Juice	160	0	40

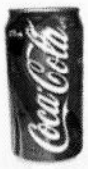

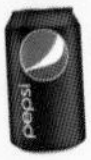

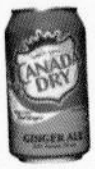

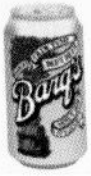

Fountain, Movie Theater & Take-Out

	C	F	Cb
Average All Flavors			
Small Cup, 12 fl.oz: No Ice	160	0	40
with ⅓ Ice	120	0	30
Regular, 16 fl.oz: No Ice	215	0	53
with ⅓ Ice	160	0	40
Medium, 22 fl.oz: No Ice	295	0	73
with ⅓ Ice	220	0	55
Large, 32 fl.oz: No Ice	430	0	105
with ⅓ Ice	320	0	80

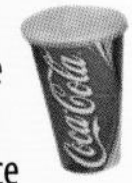

Note: ⅓ Cup of Ice = ¼ Cup Liquid

Soft Drink ~ Brands

Per 12 fl.oz Unless Indicated	C	F	Cb
A&W: Root Beer, 20 fl.oz	290	0	78
Cream Soda, 20 fl.oz	170	0	46
Albertson's:			
Signature Select: Cola	160	0	44
Diet Cola	0	0	0
Barq's: Root Beer	160	0	44
Creme Soda: Fr. Vanilla	160	0	45
Red	170	0	45
Big Red, Red Soda, 20 fl.oz	250	0	63
Blue Sky, Root Beer	130	0	32

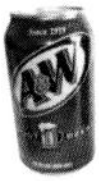

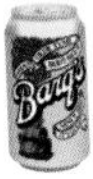

Soft Drink Brands (Cont)

Per 12 fl.oz Unless Indicated	C	F	Cb
Bubble Up,			
Lemon-Lime Soda	140	0	42
Cactus Cooler	150	0	40
Canada Dry:			
Club Soda; Diet Ginger Ale	0	0	0
Ginger Ale; Tonic Water, av.	140	0	36
Cheerwine	150	0	42
Coca-Cola:			
Classic; Orange/Cherry Vanilla	140	0	39
Vanilla	150	0	42
Diet Coke; Zero	0	0	0
Energy: Regular	140	0	39
Cherry	140	0	39
Zero Sugar	0	0	0
Life	140	0	39
Crush: *Per 20 fl.oz*			
Cherry; Strawberry	290	0	77
Grape; Orange	270	0	72
Peach; Pineapple, average	315	0	84
Dad's: Cream Soda, 12 fl.oz	200	0	51
Root Beer, 12 fl.oz	180	0	45
Diet Rite, Pure Zero	0	0	0
Dr Pepper: *Per 12 fl.oz Can*			
Regular	150	0	40
Cherry	160	0	43
Ten	10	0	3
Fanta: Orange	160	0	44
Zero, all flavors	0	0	0
Fresca, all flavors	0	0	0
Great Value *(Walmart)*, Cream Soda	180	0	49
GuS, Cola; Root Beer, av.	95	0	24
Hansen's: *Per 12 fl.oz*			
Natural Cane Sugar:			
Original Cola; Root Beer	160	0	41
Pomegranate	140	0	35
Diet, all flavors	0	0	0
Hawaiian Punch, all flavors	60	0	15
Henry Weinhard's: Root Beer	170	0	43
Orange/Vanilla Cream, av.	180	0	44
Hires, Root Beer	170	0	45
IBC: Cream Soda; Black Cherry	175	0	44
Root Beer; Cherry Limeade, av.	165	0	40
Icee: Cola; Orange; Lemon Lime, 6 fl.oz	80	0	20
Average other flavors	80	0	21
Jarritos, av. all flavors, 8 fl.oz	110	0	28
Jelly Belly, all flavors	180	0	42
Jolt, Cola, 16 fl.oz	190	0	50

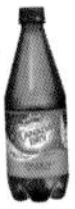
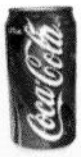

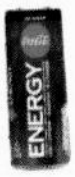

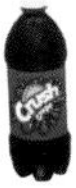

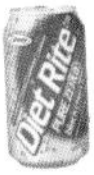

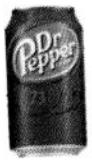

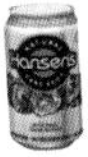

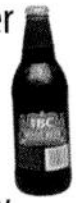

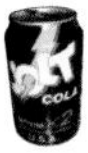

Updated Nutrition Data ~ www.CalorieKing.com
Persons with Diabetes ~ See Disclaimer (Page 22)

Soft Drink Brands (Cont)

Per 12 fl.oz Unless Indicated	C	F	Cb
Jones Soda:			
Regular, all flavors, 12 fl.oz	160	0	36
Stripped, all flavors, 12 fl.oz	30	0	8
Zilch, sugar free, 12 fl.oz	0	0	0
Kool Aid, Bursts, av., 6.75 fl.oz	20	0	5
Mello Yello: Regular, 12 fl.oz can	170	0	47
Cherry; Peach, 20 fl.oz	290	0	78
Mountain Dew: All flavors, can	170	0	46
Diet, 20 fl.oz	10	0	0.5
Dewshine, 12 fl.oz can	160	0	42
Kickstart, all flavors, 16 fl.oz	80	0	20
Mug, Root Beer	160	0	43
Natural Brew: Draft Root Beer	170	0	43
Outrageous Ginger Ale	180	0	44
Vanilla Cream Soda	160	0	39
Nehi, Peach	190	0	51
Pepsi: *Per 12 fl.oz*			
Regular; Mango Flavor	150	0	41
Black Currant; Citrus Flavor	150	0	39
Zero	0	0	0
7.5 Fl.oz, Regular	100	0	26
Perrier, Carbonated Water	0	0	0
Pibb: Xtra	140	0	38
Zero	0	0	0
RC Cola: Regular, 12.fl.oz	160	0	43
Cherry, 12.fl.oz	160	0	45
Reed's: Ginger Beer, all varieties	145	0	35
Ginger Ale	140	0	35
7•UP: Lemon Lime; Cherry	140	0	39
Diet flavors	0	0	0
Safeway ***(Albertson's):*** *Per 12 fl.oz Can*			
Refreshe: Cherry Cola	160	0	44
Dr Dynamite	140	0	38
Grape	200	0	53
Root Beer	170	0	47
Signature Select, Ginger Ale, 12 fl.oz	140	0	37
Schweppes: Ginger Ale	120	0	33
Tonic Water	130	0	33
Shasta: Cream Soda	190	0	47
Cola	130	0	33
Club Soda; Diet, all flavors	0	0	0
Dr. Shasta	150	0	38
Ginger Ale; Orange	130	0	33
Lemon Lime	120	0	29
Tiki Punch	150	0	39
Average other flavors	170	0	41
Sierra Mist, Lemon Lime	120	0	30
Sprite: Original, 12 fl.oz	140	0	37
Zero, all flavors	0	0	0

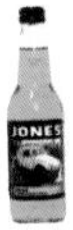

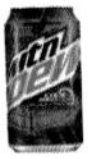
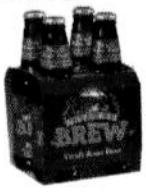
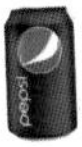
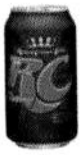
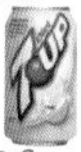
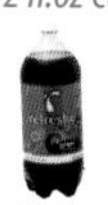
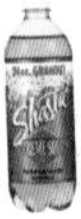
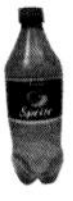

Per 12 fl.oz Unless Indicated	C	F	Cb
Squirt, Ruby Red	170	0	45
Stewarts: Cherries 'n Cream	190	0	46
Grape; Orange 'n Cream	180	0	45
Root Beer	150	0	38
Average Other Flavors	180	0	44
Sun Drop: Citrus Soda, 20 fl.oz	290	0	76
Diet Citrus Soda	10	0	1
Sunkist: Orange; Grape, av., 12 fl.oz	165	0	45
Pineapple, 12 fl.oz	190	0	51
Surge, Original 16 fl.oz	230	0	62
Tab, Original	0	0	0
Tampico: *Per 8 fl.oz*			
Lemonade, with Lime	50	0	14
Punch: Blue Raspberry	60	0	14
Pineapple Coconut	70	0	17
Average other flavors	55	0	14
Thomas Kemper: *Per 12 fl.oz*			
Black Cherry	170	0	44
Ginger Ale; Vanilla Cream	150	0	36
Root Beer	160	0	41
Trader Joe's:			
Sparkling:			
French Berry Lemonade:			
1 cup, 8 fl.oz	130	0	31
1 bottle, 33.8 fl.oz	520	0	124
Lime Ade: 1 cup, 8 fl.oz	110	0	28
1 bottle, 33.8 fl.oz	440	0	108
Pink Lemonade: 1 cup, 8 fl.oz	130	0	31
1 Bottle, 33.8 fl.oz	520	0	124
Vernors, Ginger Soda, 20 fl.oz	240	0	65
Virgil's, Root Beer	160	0	42
Walgreens: *Per 12fl.oz*			
Nice: Cherry Cola	170	0	45
Diet Cola	0	0	0
Root Beer	160	0	45
Zevia, all flavors,	0	0	0

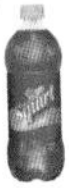
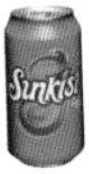

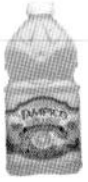
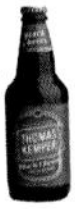
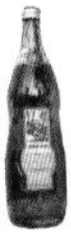
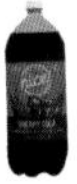

Powdered Soft Drink Mixes

Per 8 fl.oz Prepared, Unless Indicated	C	F	Cb
Country Time: *Per 12 fl.oz*			
Lemonade; Pink Lemonade	100	0	26
Strawberry Lemonade	130	0	33
Crystal Light ***(Kraft):***			
Fruit Drinks, all flav., 1/2 tsp	5	0	0
On The Go, 1 pkt, 3 grams	10	0	3
Flavor Aid, 1/8 package	0	0	0
Kool-Aid, sweetened, 0.6 oz	60	0	16
Tang, Regular, 1 cap, 0.9 oz	90	0	22

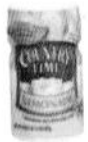
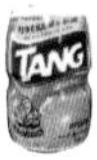

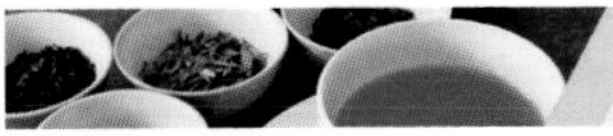

Quick Guide

	C	F	Cb
Teas			
Regular: Bag, Loose or Instant			
Brewed, 1 cup, 8 fl.oz (Add extra for sugar/milk)	2	0	0.5
Herbal, av. all flav., 1 cup	2	0	0.5
Bubble Milk Tea, w/ Pearls, 8 fl.oz	175	0	41
Chai Tea Latte Mix, 1 oz	110	1	24
Kombucha Tea, *Average all Brands:*			
Low Sugar, 1 cup, 8 fl.oz	30	0	7
Higher Sugar, 1 cup, 8 fl.oz	50	0	12
Iced Tea			
Average All Brands			
Sweetened: 8 fl.oz cup	90	0	22
12 fl.oz glass/can	140	0	35
16 fl.oz bottle	180	0	45
20 fl.oz bottle	225	0	55
Unsweetened, 8 fl.oz	0	0	0

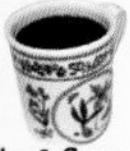

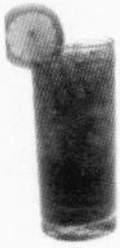

Iced Tea Mixes

Per 8 fl.oz Made-Up Unless Indicated

	C	F	Cb
4C Iced Tea: *Per 12 fl.oz*			
Average all flavors, 0.9 oz	100	0	25
Light, all flavors, 1 Tbsp	25	0	6
Crystal Light, sugar free	5	0	0
Lipton:			
Sweetened: Lemon	70	0	18
Mango; Peach	80	0	19
Unsweetened	0	0	0
Diet, all varieties	5	0	0.5

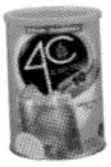

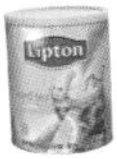

Bottled & Canned Teas

	C	F	Cb
Arizona: *Per 8 fl.oz*			
Brewed Tea, Southern Style, Sweet	130	0	33
Green Tea, with Ginseng & Honey	70	0	18
Half & Half, Mango	50	0	14
Iced Tea, Lemon Flavor	100	0	25
White Tea, Blueberry	70	0	19
Fuze: *Per 12 fl.oz*			
Lemon + Sweet Black Tea	80	0	22
Strawberry + Peach Green Tea	80	0	21
Watermelon + Lime Green Tea	80	0	21
Gold Peak, Lemon, 18.5 fl.oz	180	0	45
Health-Ade: *Per 8 fl.oz*			
Original Kombucha	30	0	7
Blood Orange Carrot Ginger	35	0	7
Ginger Lemonade	35	0	7
Pink Lady Apple; Bubbly Rose	40	0	9

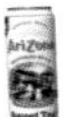

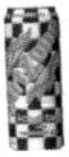

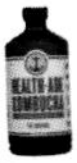

Updated Nutrition Data ~ www.CalorieKing.com
Persons with Diabetes ~ See Disclaimer (Page 22)

Bottled & Canned Teas (Cont)

	C	F	Cb
Honest Tea:			
Honey Green Tea, 16.9 fl.oz	70	0	19
Mango White Tea, 16 fl.oz	70	0	19
Peach Oolong, 16.9 fl.oz	70	0	19
Lipton:			
Green Tea, Citrus Flav. & Juice, 20 fl.oz	100	0	25
Half & Half	90	0	24
Flavored Iced Tea:			
Lemon Flavor, 12 fl.oz	70	0	19
Mango Flavor, 20 fl.oz	120	0	30
Peach Flavor, 12 fl.oz	70	0	18
Pear & Peach, 20 fl.oz	100	0	26
Tropical, 16.9 fl.oz	90	0	22
Sweet Tea, Black, 12 fl.oz	70	0	17
Nestea:			
Classics, all flavors, 8 fl.oz	50	0	13
Flash Brewed, all flavors, 17.6 fl.oz	100	0	25
POM:			
Antioxidant Super Tea: *Per 12 fl.oz*			
Pomegranate:			
Honey Green Tea	130	0	35
Lemonade Tea	140	0	35
Peach Passion White Tea	130	0	32
Sweet Tea	120	0	30
Snapple: *Per 16 fl.oz*			
Green Tea	120	0	31
Diet Green Tea	0	0	0
Half & Half	210	0	51
Lemon Tea; Raspberry Tea	150	0	37
Diet Lemon/Raspberry Tea	5	0	0
Straight Up Tea: *Per 18.5 fl.oz Bottle*			
Sorta Sweet	90	0	22
Sweet	180	0	45
SoBe, Elixir, Green Tea, 20 fl.oz	200	0	52
Ssips, Lemon Iced Tea, 8 fl.oz	100	0	24
Steaz, Iced Green Tea, lightly sweetened, av., 16 fl.oz	80	0	20
Tampico, Iced Tea, Peach, Lemon, 8 fl.oz	40	0	10
Tazo, Giant Peach, 13.8 fl.oz	150	0	37
TeaZazz, NaturalZ, all flav., 12.8 fl.oz	70	0	20
Trader Joe's:			
Org. Tea & Lemonade, 8 fl.oz	100	0	25
Hibiscus Tea & Lemonade, 16 fl.oz	40	0	9
Turkey Hill: Iced Tea, 12 fl.oz	120	0	31
Orange Tea, 12 fl.oz	150	0	38
Peach Tea, 12 fl.oz	140	0	34
365 Organic *(Whole Foods)*:			
Unsweetened: Black Tea	0	0	0
Green Tea	0	0	0

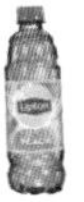

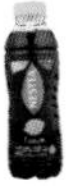

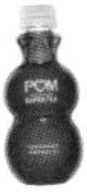

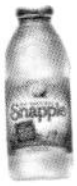

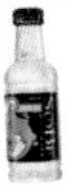

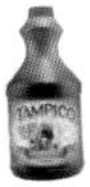

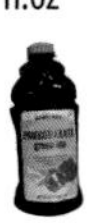

B Bread & Bread Products

Note: Most breads have similar calories on a weight basis. However, volume may vary.

For example, 1 oz of bread may equal 1 slice regular bread or 2 slices of a lighter bread. It is best to weigh bread used and calculate using: 1 oz bread = 70 calories, 14g carb.

Quick Guide

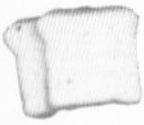

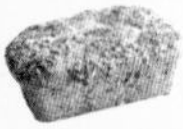

Bread	C	F	Cb
White or Wheat: *Average Per Slice*			
Thin or Light, 0.75 oz	50	0.5	9
Sandwich slice, 1 oz	70	1	14
Thick or Large, 1.5 oz	105	1.5	18
Thick, 2 oz	140	2	23
Extra Thick, 3 oz	210	3	35
Whole Loaf: 16 oz	1120	15	185
24 oz Loaf	1680	24	280
Multi Grain/Whole Grain: *Per Slice*			
Sandwich Slice, 1 oz	75	1.5	12
Thick Slice, 2 oz	150	2.5	25
Toast: *Based on same counts as White/Wheat as above*			
1 Slice (1 oz fresh):			
with 1 tsp butter/margarine	105	5	12
with 1 tsp "light" butter/marg.	90	3.5	12
with 2 tsp butter/margarine	140	9	12
with 2 tsp "light" butter/marg.	110	6	12

Breads

Per Slice Unless Indicated

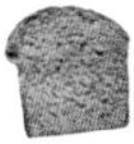

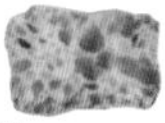

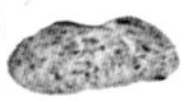

	C	F	Cb
12-Grain, 1.5 oz	110	1.5	22
Bran style/Dark, 1 oz	70	1	14
Buttermilk, average, 1.5 oz	110	1	22
Challah, 0.75 oz	85	1.5	17
Chapati, 1 oz	110	3	18
Ciabatta, 2 oz	130	1	26
Cornbread, average, 3 oz	220	6	37
Cracked Wheat Sourdough, 1.5 oz	130	0.5	27
Croissants ~ *See Page 134*			
Crustless Bread, regular, slice, 0.75 oz	40	0.5	8.5
Crusts Only, regular slice, 0.25 oz	30	0	7
English Toasting, 2 oz	140	1.5	27
Flax & Grain, 1.5 oz	120	3	19
Foccacia: Plain, 2 oz serve	150	2.5	28
Cheese & Garlic; Pesto, 2 oz serve	160	6	21
Tomato & Olive, 2 oz serve	150	5	21

Breads (Cont)

Per Slice Unless Indicated

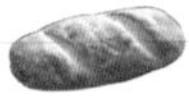

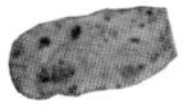

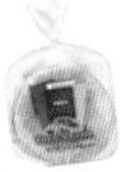

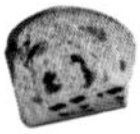

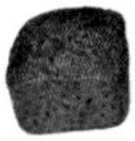

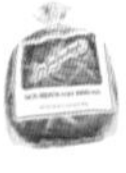

	C	F	Cb
French Stick/Baguette, 1 oz	70	1	15
French Toast: Slice, 1.5oz	140	2	26
Aunt Jemima, Sticks, av., 2 oz	110	2	18
Garlic Bread/Toast:			
Small slice + 1 tsp spread, 0.75 oz	80	5	7
Medium slice + 2 tsp spread, 1.5 oz	160	10	14
Thick slice + 3 tsp spread, 1.8 oz	220	14	20
Pepperidge Farm, Texas, 1 sl., 1.4 oz	150	8	15
Hawaiian Sweet Bread, 1.5 oz	110	2	19
Hemp Bread, 1.2 oz	95	2	12
Italian Bread, 2 oz	140	1	28
Lower Carb, (higher protein/fiber), average all brands, 1 oz	60	1.5	9
MultiGrain, 1.5 oz	100	2	21
Naan Flatbread, 2 oz	160	3.5	29
Nut/Health Nut, 1.35 oz	90	1.5	18
Oatmeal/Oatbran Bread, 1.5 oz	90	0.5	19
Pita, average all types:			
Small (4" diam), 1 oz	90	0	18
Large (6½" diam), 2 oz	140	1.5	27
Extra Large (9" diam), 4 oz	300	1.5	60
Popovers, (1), without butter	130	2	18
Pumpernickel:			
Cocktail/Party size	30	0.5	6
Large slice, 1.35 oz	80	0	15
Raisin Bread, 1 oz	80	1	15
Rye: 1 thin slice, av., 1 oz	80	1	14
1 thick slice, 2 oz	150	2	25
Cocktail size, 0.4 oz	25	0.5	4
Sandwich Pockets, 2 oz	140	1.5	27
Sourdough: Regular, 1.5oz	120	1	25
French Style, 1 oz	75	0	14
Spelt, 1.6 oz	130	1	26
Sprouted 7-Grain, 1.5 oz	110	0.5	18
Squaw, 1.1 oz	85	0.5	13
Tacos/Tortillas ~ *See Page 172*			
Turkish/Middle Eastern, 1 oz	80	1.5	16
Wheat-Free Breads: Spelt, 1.6 oz	130	1	26
Rice, with Fruit Juice, 1.5 oz	110	2	21
Healthseed Rye, 1.6 oz	90	1	20
Millet, 1.5 oz	100	1	20

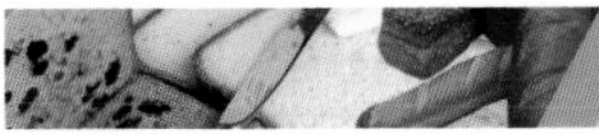

Bread ~ Brands

Per Slice Unless Indicated

	C	F	Cb
Bimbo: 100% Whole Wheat, 1 slice	60	1	12
Pan Integral Grande Wheat, 1 slices	75	1	14
Soft Wheat, 1 slice	65	1	12
Ener-G, Gluten-Free:			
Classic White, Regular, 1 sl., 1.4 oz	110	6	15
Multigrain: Regular, 1 slice, 1.4 oz	100	5	15
Light, 1 slice, 0.8 oz	60	3	9
Rice: Brown Loaf, regular, 1 sl., 1.2 oz	100	3	16
White Rice, 1 slice, 1.34 oz	100	3.5	17
Home Pride:			
Butter Top, Wheat/White, 1 sl., 0.9 oz	70	1	13
Nature's Harvest: *Per 2 Slices*			
100% Whole Wheat	120	1.5	26
Honey 7 Grain	160	2.5	28
Light Multigrain, 0.7 oz	80	1	18
Nature's Own: *Per Slice*			
100% Whole Wheat, 0.9 oz	60	0.5	11
Butterbread, 0.9 oz	60	1	12
Honey Wheat, 0.9 oz	70	0.5	13
Oroweat: *Per Slice*			
100% Whole Wheat, 1.3 oz	100	1	19
Country Sourdough, 1.35 oz	100	1.5	18
Health Nut, 1.34 oz	100	1.5	18
Honey Wheat Berry, 1.2 oz	90	1	17
Oatnut, 1.3 oz	110	2	19
Organic 22 Grains & Seeds,			
Regular, 1.7 oz	140	3	23
Sweet Hawaiian, 1.34 oz	110	2	20
Pepperidge Farm: *Per Slice*			
100% Whole Wheat, 1.7 oz	120	2	23
15 Grain, 1.7 oz	130	2.5	22
Family, White Sandwich, 1 oz	75	1.5	13
Honey White Bread, 1.6 oz	130	1	24
Italian, w/ Sesame Seeds, 1.1 oz	90	1.5	17
Oatmeal, 1.7 oz	130	2	25
Swirl, Brown Sugar Cinn., 1.34 oz	110	2	21
Roman Meal: 100% Whole Grain, 1 sl	80	1	16
Honey Split Top, 2 slices, 2 oz	130	1.5	25
Sara Lee: *Per Slice*			
100% Whole Wheat, 0.9 oz	60	1	12
Artesano: Brioche, 1 sl., 1.34 oz	110	1.5	21
Golden Wheat, 1 slice	100	1.5	19
Honey Wheat, 0.9 oz	70	1	13
Trader Joe's: Gourmet White, 1.5 oz	120	3.5	19
Sprouted Wheat Cranberry, 1.2 oz	90	1	16
Wonder: 100% Wh. Wheat, 1 sl., 0.9 oz	60	0.5	11
Classic White, 1 slice, 1oz	70	1	14
Whole Grain White, 1 slice, 1 oz	60	1	12

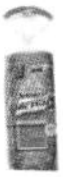
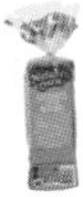
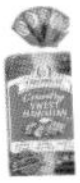

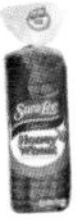

Persons with Diabetes ~ See Disclaimer (Page 22)

Biscuits, Bread Rolls & Buns

	C	F	Cb
Biscuits: *Average, 2½" diameter*			
Plain/Butter Milk:			
Prepared from Recipe	210	10	27
Refrig. Dough, Baked	95	4	13
Brown 'n Serve, av., 1 oz	70	1	13
Refrigerated Dough:			
Pillsbury, Buttermilk Biscuit, (3), 2.25 oz	150	2	30
Buns:			
Frankfurter/Hot Dog: 1.25 oz	110	1.5	21
1.5 oz	130	2	25
Hamburger: Regular, 1.5 oz	110	1.5	22
Large, 3 oz	210	3	40
Hoagie/Submarine, Plain, 2.3 oz	200	1	38
Rolls:			
Ciabatta Roll, 3.5 oz	230	4	41
Crescent Roll, Original, 1 oz	100	6	11
Dinner:			
1 small, 1 oz	90	1.5	17
1 medium (3" diam),1.5 oz	110	1	23
French: 1 medium 1.3 oz	110	1.5	22
1 large, 3 oz	230	2.5	42
Kaiser:			
Small, 2 oz	200	2.5	35
Large, 3.5 oz	350	4	61
Plain, 6", average all, 2.5 oz	200	1	38
Sourdough, 1.3 oz	110	1	21
Wheat Rolls: Small, 1.2 oz	100	1	17
Medium, 1.8 oz	130	1.5	23
Large, 3.5 oz	260	3	46

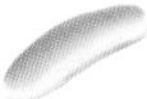

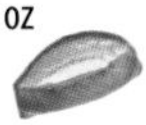
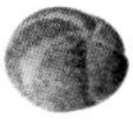
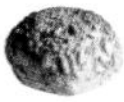

Breadsticks, Croutons

	C	F	Cb
Breadsticks:			
Salt Sticks, plain, 1 oz	110	1	20
Fresh baked (1), 2 oz	180	2.5	34
Stella D'oro: Original (1)	45	1	7
Sesame (1)	50	2	7
Croutons: Seasoned, 2 Tbsp, 0.3 oz	35	1.5	4
Pepp. Farm, Zesty Italian, 6 croutons	30	1	5

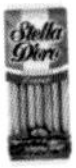

Bread Products

	C	F	Cb
Bread Crumbs, dry:			
Plain or seasoned: 1 oz	110	1.5	20
1 cup, 3.5 oz	385	5	70
Corn Flake Crumbs, 1 oz	120	0	29
Graham Cracker Crumbs *(Keebler)*,1 oz	110	2.5	20
Bread Dough, average:			
Frozen, 1 slice, 2 oz	140	2	26
Refrigerated: French, 1" sl.	60	1	13
Wheat; White, 1" slice	80	2	14
Coating Mixes, av., 2 Tbsp., 1 oz	100	0.5	20
Stuffing: Dry mix, average all,1 oz	110	1	10
Prepared, ½ cup, 4 oz	180	9	22

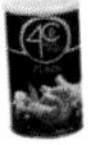

Quick Guide

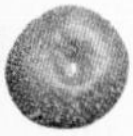

	C	F	Cb
Bagels			
Average All Brands			
Plain/Onion:			
1 mini/bagelette, 1 oz	**65**	0.5	13
1 small bagel, 2 oz	**145**	1	29
1 medium bagel, 3 oz	**220**	1.5	43
1 large bagel, 4 oz	**290**	2	57
Bagel Chips, 1 oz	**130**	4.5	19
Pizza Bagel Bites (Bagel Bites), average all varieties., 4 pieces, 3 oz	**190**	5.5	27
Bagel Crisps *(New York Style),* average all varieties, 6 crisps, 1 oz	**130**	5	17
Bagel Thins *(Thomas'),* 1, 1.5 oz	**110**	1	25

Bagel ~ Brands

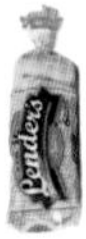
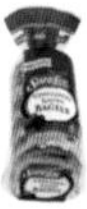

	C	F	Cb
Per Bagel			
Bubba's: Plain	**220**	1.5	45
Blueberry	**230**	2	49
Cinnamon Raisin	**230**	1.5	48
Costco Bakery: Plain	**330**	1.5	70
Cinnamon Raisin	**340**	1.5	73
Whole Grain	**300**	5	56
Lender's, Fresh, NY Style:			
Plain, 3.3 oz	**240**	2	46
Blueberry, 3.3 oz	**240**	2	46
Cinnamon, 3.3 oz	**240**	2	46
French Toast, 2.86 oz	**220**	1.5	45
Whole Wheat, 3.3 oz	**240**	2	46
Panera Bread: Plain	**280**	1	57
Cinnamon Swirl & Raisin, 3.8 fl.oz	**310**	1.5	65
Everything, 4 oz	**290**	1.5	58
Whole Grain, 4.3 oz	**330**	2.5	66
Sara Lee: Plain, 3.4 oz	**260**	1	52
Blueberry, 3.4 oz	**260**	1	54
Cinnamon Raisin, 3.7 oz	**260**	0.5	54
Everything, 3.4 oz	**270**	3	50
Onion, 3.4 oz	**260**	1	53
Western, The Alternatives, av., 2 oz	**120**	0.5	29

Bagel Spreads

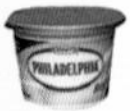
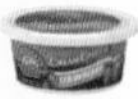

	C	F	Cb
Cream Cheese:			
Plain: 2 Tbsp, 1 oz	**100**	9	1
2 oz mini-tub	**200**	18	2
Reduced Fat: 2 Tbsp, 1 oz	**60**	5	2
2 oz mini-tub	**120**	10	4
Flavors: Lox, 1 oz	**90**	8	2
Honey Nut, 1 oz	**80**	7	4
Strawberry, 1 oz	**90**	7	5
Sundried Tomato, 1 oz	**80**	7	2
Vegetable, 1 oz	**90**	8	2

English Muffins

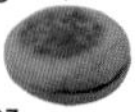

	C	F	Cb
Average All Brands			
Plain/Whole Wheat: Regular, 2 oz	**135**	1.5	26
Heavier, 2.5 oz	**155**	2	31
Super Size, 3.2 oz	**190**	2	38
Raisin-Cinnamon, 2.2 oz	**150**	1	30

Note: Actual weight of packaged muffins can be 10-15% heavier than stated net weight.

Rice Cakes

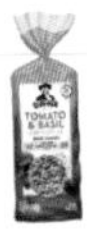

	C	F	Cb
Hain, Mini, White Cheddar (10), 1.2 oz	**70**	2.5	11
Lundberg:			
Minis, av. all flavors, 13 pieces	**130**	5	20
Thin Stackers, All flavors, (4)	**110**	1	24
Quaker: Apple Cinn., (1)	**50**	0	11
Butter Popcorn, (1)	**35**	0	7
Chocolate, (1)	**60**	1	12
Tomato & Basil, (1)	**50**	2	8
White Cheddar, (1)	**45**	1	8

Tortillas & Shells

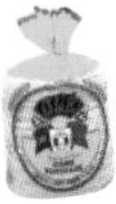
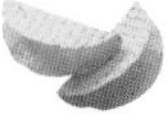
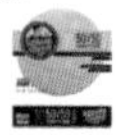
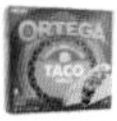

	C	F	Cb
Tortillas: *Per Tortilla*			
Corn Flour, White/Yellow: 6", 1 oz	**55**	1	11
7", 1.2 oz	**75**	1	14
Wheat Flour:			
6", 1.2 oz	**100**	3	16
8", 1.4 oz	**130**	4	20
10", 2.3 oz	**200**	6	31
Shells: *Per Shell, without Fillings*			
Corn Taco Shells: Mini, 3", 0.2 oz	**25**	1	3
Medium, 5", 0.5 oz	**60**	2.5	8
Large, 6½", 0.7 oz	**100**	4.5	13
Salad Shell, 10"	**310**	17	34
Tostada Shells, fried:			
White Corn, 5½" diam., 0.4 oz	**55**	2.5	8
Yellow Corn, 5½" diam., 0.5 oz	**80**	3.5	11
Sopes, 1 shell, 4" 2 oz	**110**	1.5	23
La Tortilla Factory:			
Non GMO: Hand Made Style, White Corn & Wheat, 1.45 oz	**90**	1	15
Gluten Free, Casava Flour, 1.4 oz	**190**	3	20
Low Carb, Quinoa & Flax, 1.45 oz	**60**	2	15
Whole Wheat Protein, 1.76 oz	**120**	3.5	12
Traditional, Flour, Burrito Size, 2 oz	**170**	4.5	24
Mission Foods:			
Corn, Yellow, Super Soft:			
Low Fat, 2 Tortillas, 1.65 oz	**100**	1.5	20
Flour, Large Burrito Size (1), 2.47 oz	**210**	4	37
Ortego:			
Cauli/Corn: Taco Shell (1)	**65**	3	9
Tortillas (1)	**120**	2	22

Quick Guide

Cooked Cereals		F	Cb
Barley, pearled, cooked, 1 cup	195	0.5	44
Buckwheat Groats, roasted:			
Dry, 1/2 cup, 3 oz	285	2	61
Cooked, 1 cup, 6 oz	155	1	34
Bulgur: Dry, 1/2 cup, 2.5 oz	240	1	53
Cooked, 1 cup, 6.5 oz	150	0.5	34
Corn/Hominy Grits:			
Dry: Regular, 1/4 cup, 1.4 oz	140	0.5	32
Instant: 0.8 fl.oz packet	75	0	18
w/ Imitation Bacon Bits, 1 oz	100	0.5	22
Cooked, 3/4 cup, 6.5 oz	110	0.5	23
Cream of Rice, cooked, 3/4 cup, 6.5 oz	95	0	21
Cream of Wheat:			
Cooked: Regular, 3/4 cup, 6.5 oz	95	0.5	20
Instant, 3/4 cup, 6.5 oz	105	0.5	21
Quick, 3/4 cup, 6.5 oz	100	0.5	22
Farina, cooked, 3/4 cup, 6 oz	95	0.5	19
Millet, dry, 1/2 cup, 1.8 oz	190	2	36
Oat Bran: Raw, 1/3 cup, 1 oz	70	2	19
Cooked, 1/2 cup, 3.8 fl.oz	45	1	13
Oatmeal:			
Dry: Regular, 1/3 cup, 1 oz	100	1.5	18
Instant: Regular, average, 1 oz	105	1.5	18
Flavored, average, 1.5 oz	165	2	34
Cooked: Regular, 3/4 cup, 6 oz	125	2.5	21
1 cup, 8 fl.oz	165	3.5	28
Whole Wheat, cooked, 3/4 cup, 6.5 oz	115	0.5	25

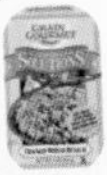
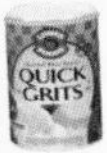

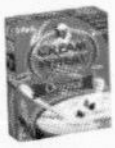
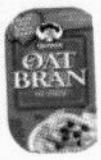

Brans, Wheat Germ, Add-Ons

Bee Pollen Granules, 1 Tbsp, 0.3 oz	25	1	2
Bran:			
Oat Bran: Raw, 1 Tbsp, 0.2 oz	20	0.5	3
1/3 cup, 1 oz	100	2	17
Rice Bran: Raw, 1 Tbsp, 0.2 oz	15	1	2.5
¼ cup, 1 oz	95	6	15
Fruit: Dried, average, 1 oz	70	0	18
Banana, 1/2 medium	55	0	14
Prunes in Syrup (5), 3 oz	90	0	23
Honey, 1 Tbsp, 0.75 oz	65	0	17
Lecithin Granules, 1 Tbsp, 0.4 oz	55	4	0.5
Nuts, Almonds (6), 0.3 oz	40	4	1.5
Psyllium Husks, 1 Tbsp, 0.2 oz	10	0	4
Wheat, unprocessed, 1 Tbsp	5	0	2
Wheat Germ: Raw, 1 Tbsp, 0.3 oz	25	0.5	4
1/4 cup, 1 oz	105	3	15

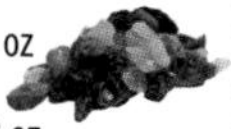

Updated Nutrition Data ~ www.CalorieKing.com
Persons with Diabetes ~ See Disclaimer (Page 22)

Hot/Cooked Cereals ~ Brands

Per Serving, Dry Mix only	C	F	Cb
Albers,			
Quick Grits, 1/4 cup, 1.4 oz	140	0.5	31
B&G:			
Cream of Wheat Instant:			
Original, 1 oz	100	0	20
Maple Brown Sugar, 1.3 oz	130	0	29
Bob's Red Mill:			
Brown Rice Farina, ¼ cup	150	1	32
Extra Thick Rolled Oats,			
½ cup, 1.7 oz	190	3.5	33
Dr. McDougall's:			
Stay Full,			
Organic Maple Hot Oatmeal, no sugar	250	3.5	46
Great Value *(Walmart):*			
Instant Oatmeal:			
Cinnamon Swirl, 1.6 oz	160	2	34
Original, 1 oz packet	100	2	19
McCann's:			
Instant Irish Oatmeal:			
Apples & Cinn., 1.3 oz	130	1	28
Maple & Brown Sugar, 1.5 oz	160	1.5	34
Malt-O-Meal: Orig.; Creamy, 3 tbsp	130	0	27
Maple Brown Sugar, 1/4 cup	170	0	38
Natures Path:			
Oatmeal: Flax Plus, 1.76 oz	210	0	38
Apple Cinnamon, 1.76 oz	210	2.5	40
Maple Nut, 1.7 oz	210	4	38
NutriSystem,			
Oatmeal, Maple Brown Sugar, 1 pkg	150	1.5	29
Quaker:			
Gluten Free, Instant, Orig., 1.23 oz pkt	130	2.5	24
Instant Grits, Butter, 1.45 oz	150	1.5	32
Quick Grits, Original, 1/4 cup, 1.3 oz	130	0.5	29
Instant Oatmeal:			
Maple & Brown Sug., 1.5 oz	160	2	33
Peaches & Cream, 1 oz	110	2	23
Old Fash'nd/Quick Oats, 1/2 c., 1.4 oz	150	3	27
Wegmans: *Per Packet*			
Instant Oatmeal: Original, 1 oz	110	2	19
Raisin & Spice, 1.5 oz pkt	160	2	32

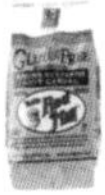
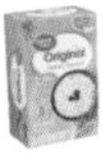
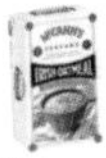
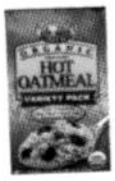

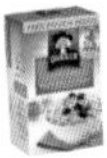

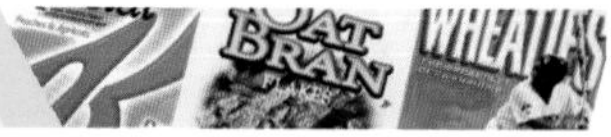

Quick Guide

Cold Cereals

Average All Brands

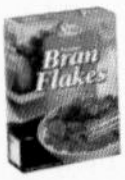
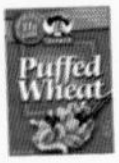

	C	F	Cb
Bran Flakes, 3/4 cup, 1 oz	**95**	0.5	24
Corn Flakes, 1 cup, 1 oz	**100**	0	22
Frosted Flakes, 3/4 cup, 1 oz	**110**	0	27
Granola, 100% Nat., 1/2 cup, 1.7 oz	**205**	6	35
Oat Bran Cereal, 1/2 cup, 1.5 oz	**145**	3	25
Puffed Rice, 1 cup. 0.5 oz	**55**	0	13
Puffed Wheat, 1 cup, 0.5 oz	**45**	0	10
Raisin Bran, 1/2 cup, 1 oz	**90**	0.5	22
Rice Crisps, 1 cup, 1 oz	**105**	0.5	24
Shredded Wheat, 1 biscuit, 1 oz	**85**	0.5	20
Wheat Flakes, 3/4 cup, 1 oz	**105**	1	24

Breakfast/Cereal Bars ~ *See Page 31*

Ready-To-Eat Cereal ~ Brands

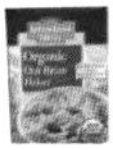
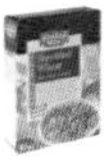
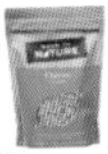
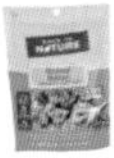
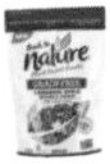

	C	F	Cb
Arrowhead Mills:			
Organic:b Bulgar Wheat, 1.5 oz	**150**	0.5	34
Flakes: Amaranth, 1.2 oz	**140**	2	26
Maple Buckwheat, 1.5 oz	**170**	1	35
Oat Bran, 1.2 oz	**140**	2.5	24
Spelt, 1 oz	**120**	1	24
Sprouted Corn, 1.3oz	**110**	1	25
Organic Puffed: Corn, 0.5 oz	**60**	1	12
Kamut, 0.5 oz	**50**	0	11
Millet, 0.5 oz	**60**	0.5	11
Rice, 0.5 oz	**60**	0	14
Wheat, 0.5 oz	**60**	0	12
Rise & Shine, 1.45 oz	**150**	1	32
Sprouted, Corn Flakes, 1.3 oz	**110**	1	25
Back to Nature: *Per 1/2 Cup*			
Granola: Apple Blueberry, 1.76 oz	**200**	3	39
Chocolate Delight, 1.76 oz	**210**	5	37
Classic, 1.76 oz	**200**	2.5	40
Cranberry Pecan, 1.65 oz	**190**	5	36
Dark Chocolate Coconut, 1.76 oz	**230**	11	32
Granola Clusters:			
Almond Chia, 1.8 oz	**200**	5	33
Banana & Walnut, 1.8 oz	**210**	5	36
Peanut Butter, 1.8 oz	**220**	9	27
Granola Crunch:			
Cinnamon Apple, 1 oz	**170**	13	8
Cocoa, 1 oz	**170**	12	7
Vanilla Almond, 1 oz	**160**	12	8

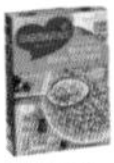
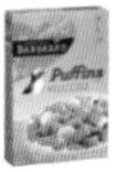
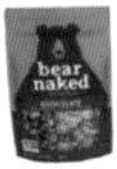
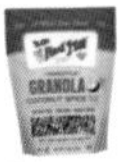
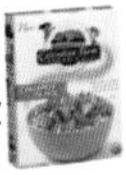
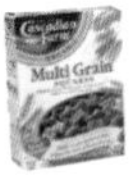
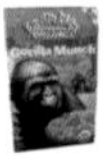

	C	F	Cb
Barbara's Bakery:			
Classics, Organic & Sweetened:			
Brown Rice Crisps, 1.4 oz	**160**	1	35
Corn Flakes, 1.4 oz	**150**	0	34
Honest O's, Orig., 1.4 oz	**150**	2	30
Morning Oat Crunch, Original, 2 oz	**210**	2.5	45
Puffins:			
Original; Cinnamon, 1.4 oz	**130**	1	32
Honey Rice, 1 oz	**150**	1	34
Multigrain, 1.4 oz	**130**	0.5	33
PB/PB & Choc., av.,1.3 oz	**150**	2	30
Snackimals, all var., 1 1/4 cup, 1.4 oz	**145**	0.5	35
Shredded Wheat, 2 biscuits, 1.8 oz	**170**	1	41
Spoonfuls, Multigrain, 1.4 oz	**140**	1.5	31
Squarefuls, Multigrain, 1.95 oz	**200**	1	48
Bear Naked:			
Granola: Chocolate, 1.83 oz	**210**	7	36
Fruit & Nut, 2 oz	**270**	12	39
Maple Pecan, 2 oz	**260**	9	43
Original Cinnamon, 2 oz	**260**	12	31
Peanut Butter, 2.2 oz	**290**	13	42
V'nilla Almond, 2 oz	**210**	5	40
Bob's Red Mill:			
Granola:			
Coconut Spice; Maple Sea Salt, 1 oz	**150**	7	17
Lemon Blueberry, 1 oz	**140**	6	19
Muesli: Old Country Style, 1/4 c.,1.23 oz	**140**	3	23
Paleo Style, 1/4 cup, 0.85 oz	**140**	10	9
Cascadian Farm:			
Buzz Crunch, 21.9 oz	**210**	2.5	44
Cinnamon Crunch, 1.3 oz	**140**	3	29
Graham Crunch, 1.3 oz	**150**	3	30
Granola: Ancient Grains, 2 oz	**250**	6	42
Coconut Cashew, 2.2 oz	**330**	19	37
Dark Chocolate Almond, 2.2 oz	**260**	8	45
French Vanilla Almond, 2 oz	**240**	7	42
Lemon Blueberry, 2 oz	**240**	7	38
Honey Nut O's, 1.5 oz	**160**	1.5	35
Multi Grain Squares, 1 cup, 2 oz	**260**	1.5	54
Raisin Bran, 2.2 oz	**210**	1.5	50
EnviroKidz: *Per 1 oz*			
Amazon Frosted Flakes, 1.4 oz	**160**	0	36
Gorilla Munch, 1.4 oz	**150**	1	35
Leapin' Lemurs, 1.4 oz	**160**	2	33
Panda Puffs, 1.4 oz	**170**	4.5	31

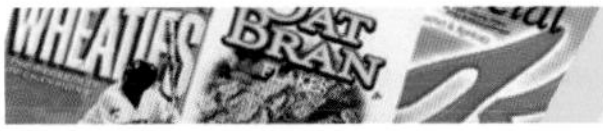

Ready-To-Eat Cereal (Cont)

Ezekiel 4.9:	C	F	Cb
Sprouted Whole Grain Cereal:			
Original, ½ cup, 2 oz	190	3	35
Almond, ½ cup, 2 oz	200	3	34
Cinnamon Raisin, 2 oz	190	1	38
Sprouted Flakes: Almond, ¾ c., 1.94 oz	200	2.5	40
Flax & Chia, ¾ cup, 1.94 oz	200	1.5	41
Original, ¾ cup, 1.94 oz	210	21	42

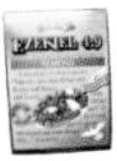

General Mills:	C	F	Cb
Cheerios: *Per Cup Unless Indicated*			
Original, 1 ½ cups1.4 oz	140	2.5	29
Apple Cinnamon, 1.3 oz	150	2.5	30
Banana Nut, ¾ cup, 1 oz	110	1.5	22
Chocolate, 1.3 oz	140	2	28
Cinnamon, 1.3 oz	140	3	29
Frosted, 1.3 oz	140	1.5	29
Fruity, 1.3 oz	140	2	29
Multi Grain, 1 ⅓ cups, 1.4oz	150	1.5	32
Very Berry, 1.3 oz	140	2	29
Chex: Choc., 1.5 oz	180	3.5	36
Cinnamon, 1.4 oz	170	4	33
Corn, 1 oz	120	0.5	26
Honey Nut, 1 ¼ cups, 1.4 oz	150	1	33
Rice,1 ⅓ cups, 1.4 oz	160	1	35
Vanilla, 1.4 oz	170	3.5	33
Wheat, 2 oz	210	1	51
Crunch: Blueberry, 1 oz	120	3	22
Cinnamon Toast, 1.1 oz	130	3	25
Fiber One: Original, ⅔ cup, 1.4 oz	90	1	34
Honey Clusters, 1.8 oz	170	1.5	43
Strawberry & Vanilla Clusters, 2 oz	190	3	45
French Toast Crunch, 1.3 oz	150	1.5	32
Kix: Original, 1 ¼ cups1 oz	120	1	27
Berry Berry; Honey, av., 1 ¼ cups, 1.2 oz	120	1.5	27
Lucky Charms:			
Original, 3/4 cup, 1 oz	110	1.5	23
Honey Clovers, 1.25 oz	140	1	31
Monster: Berry varieties, 1 cup 1.2 oz	130	1.5	28
Count Chocula, 3/4 cup, 1 oz	100	1.5	23
Total, Whole Grain,¾ cup1 oz	110	0.5	25
Wheaties, 1.4 oz	130	0.5	30

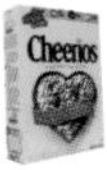

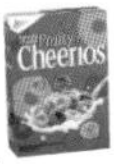

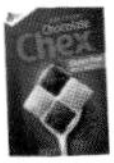

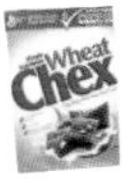

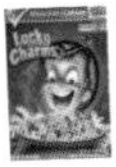

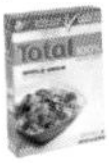

Great Value *(Walmart):*	C	F	Cb
Apple Blasts, 1 ⅓ cups, 1.4 oz	150	1	34
Awake, Fruit & Yogurt, 1 cup, 1.94 oz	210	1.5	46
Cinnamon Crunch, 1 cup, 1.4 oz	180	5	32
Corn Flakes, 1 ⅓ cups	160	0	35
Crunchy Nuggets, ½ cup, 2 oz	200	1	47
Extra Raisin Raisin Bran, 1 cup, 2.1 oz	200	1	48
Frosted Shredded Wheat (21), 2 oz	210	1	50
Fruit Spins, 1 ½ cups, 1.4 oz	170	1.5	36
O's Oat, 1 ½ cups1 oz	150	2.5	30

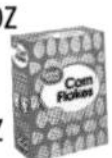

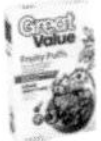

Kashi:	C	F	Cb
7 Whole Grain: Flakes, 1 ¼ cups, 1.8 oz	210	1	51
Whole Grain Puffs, 1½ cups, 1.4 oz	150	1.5	32
Go: Original, 1¼ cups, 2 oz	180	2	40
Cinnamon Crisp, 1 cup, 2.1 oz	230	5	39
Crunch: Original, 3/4 cup, 2 oz	190	3	38
Chocolate, 3/4 cup, 1.83 oz	210	7	32
Coconut Almond, ¾ cup, 1.85 oz	210	8	32
Honey Almond Flax, ¾ cup, 1.86 oz	200	5	35
Peanut Butter, ¾ c., 1.87 oz	220	9	31
Toasted Berry Crisp, ¾ cup, 1.87 oz	200	4.5	36
Organic:			
Honey Toasted Oat, 1 cup, 1.45 oz	150	2.5	34
Indigo Morning, 1 cup, 1.4 oz	140	1.5	32
Sprouted Grains, 1⅓ cups, 2 oz	210	1.5	48
Strawberry Fieldfs, 1 cup, 1.8 oz	200	1	47
Whole Wheat Biscuit:			
Autumn Fruit, 32 biuscuits	200	1	47
Cinnamon Crunch, 31 biscuits	200	1	48
Island Vanilla, 29 biscuits	200	1	47

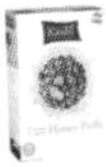

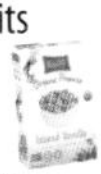

Kellogg's:	C	F	Cb
All-Bran: Original, ½ cup, 1 oz	80	1	23
Bran Buds, 1/3 cup, 1 oz	80	1	24
Compl. Wheat Flakes, 1.3 oz	90	1	30
Apple Jacks, 1 cup, 1 oz	110	1	25
Choco Krispis, 1.4 oz	160	0.5	37
Corn Flakes,			
Original, 1 ½ cups, 1.4 oz	150	0	36
Cracklin' Oat Bran, 3/4 cup, 2 oz	230	8	41
Crispix, Original, 1 ⅓ cups, 1.4 oz	150	0	34

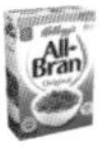

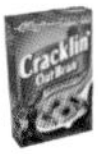

continued next page...

B Breakfast Cereals

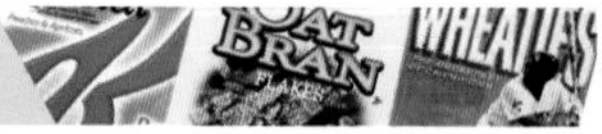

Ready-To-Eat Cereal (Cont)

Kellogg's (Cont):	C	F	Cb
Despicable Me 3 Minion, 1 c., 1.2 oz	120	1	27
Froot Loops: Original, 1 ⅓ cups, 1.4 oz	150	1.5	34
Marshmallow, 1 ⅓ cups, 1.4 oz	150	1	35
Frosted Flakes: *Per 1 oz*			
Chocolate, 1 cup, 1.4 oz	150	1	33
Cinnamon, 1 cup, 1.4 oz	140	0	34
Honey Nut, 1 cup, 1.4 oz	140	0	33
Original Flakes, 1 cup, 1.4 oz	140	0	34
w/ Marshmallows, 1 ¼ cups, 1.4 oz	150	0	36
Happy Inside, all flavors, 1.94 oz	210	4	44
Honey Smacks, 1 cup, 1.3 oz	130	0.5	32
Krave, Double Choc., 1 cup,1.45 oz	170	5	31
Krispies:			
Original, 1 ½ cups, 1.4 oz	150	0	36
Cocoa, 1 cup, 1.4 oz	160	1	35
Frosted, 1 cup, 1.38 oz	150	0	35
Mini-Wheats, Frosted:			
Original (25), 2 oz	210	1.5	51
Blueberry (25), 2 oz	210	1	51
Strawberry (25), 2 oz	210	1	51
Little Bites, Orig., 1 c., 2 oz	190	1	47
Mini Wheats, unfrosted:			
Bite Size (30), 1.8 oz	190	1	45
Mueslix, 1 cup, 2.36 oz	250	3.5	50
Raisin Bran: Reg., 1 c., 2 oz	190	1	47
Crunch, 1 cup, 1.94 oz	190	1	46
Smart Start,			
Orig. Antioxidants, 1¼ cups, 2.25 oz	240	1	56
Special K: Orig., 1¼ cups, 1.4 oz	150	0.5	29
Apple Cinnamon Crunch, 1.5 oz	160	1.5	35
Banana, 1 cup, 1.4 oz	160	2.5	35
Chocolate Strawberry, 1 cup, 1.5 oz	160	2	35
Chocolatey Delight, 1 cup, 1.48 oz	170	3	34
Fruit & Yogurt, 1 cup, 1.48 oz	160	1	36
Red Berries, 1¼ cups, 1.4 oz	140	0.5	34
Vanilla & Almond, 1.4 oz	150	1.5	33
Kind:			
Clusters: *Per ⅓ Cup*			
Almond & Coconut Nut,1 oz	140	10	11
Almond Cashew Sunflower, 1 oz	140	13	10
Dark Choc. Nuts & Sea Salt, 1 oz	140	11	11
Peanut Butter Dark Choc. Nut, 1 oz	150	12	10

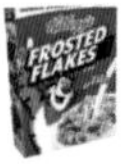

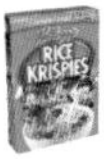

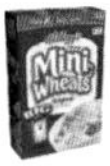

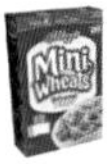

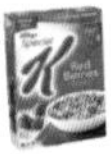

Malt-O-Meal:	C	F	Cb
Apple Zings, 1 ⅓ cups, 1.4 oz	140	1	34
Cocoa Dyno-Bites, 1.4 oz	170	1.5	37
Coco Roos, 1 ¼ cups, 1.45 oz	170	2	38
Frosted Flakes, 1 ¼ cups, 1.4 oz	160	0	37
Fruity Dyno-Bites, 1 cup, 1.27 oz	140	1	32
Frosted Mini Spooners, 21 biscuits	210	1	50
Golden Puffs, 1 cup, 1.35 oz	150	0.5	34
Honey Nut Scooters, 1.4 oz	160	2	33
Marshmallow Mateys, 1.4 oz	160	1.5	35
Peanut Butter Cups, 1.4 oz	170	4.5	31
Raisin Bran, 1 ¼ cups, 2.1 oz	190	1	48
Nature's Path:			
Flax Plus: *Per 1 Cup*			
Maple Pecan Crunch, 2.1 oz	240	8	41
Multibran Flakes, 1.4 oz	150	2	31
Granola: Coconut Chia, ¾ c., 1.94 oz	270	11	36
Honey Almond, ⅓ cup, 1 oz	140	4.5	21
Maple Almond, Grain Free, ⅓ cup, 1 oz	170	14	8
Heritage Flakes, 1.4 oz	160	1.5	31
Love Crunch Granola: *Per ¼ Cup Unless Indicated*			
Apple Chia Crumble, 1 oz	140	4	22
Espresso Vanilla Cream, 1 oz	130	4.5	21
Salted Caramel Pretzel, 1 oz	140	5	21
Sunrise: *Per ⅔ Cup*			
Crunchy Honey, 1 oz	120	1	26
Crunchy Maple, 1 oz	110	1	25
Superflakes,			
Qi'a Cocoa Coconut, 1.94 oz	240	7	39
New England Natural Bakers:			
Organic Granola:			
Berry Coconut, unswtnd, 2 oz	290	13	37
Blueberry Harvest, ⅔ cup, 2 oz	270	7	41
Chocolate Peanut, ⅔ cup, 2 oz	270	9	42
Cranberry Almond, ⅔ cup, 2 oz	240	9	36
Granny Smith Apple ⅔ cup, 2 oz	260	7	41
Salted Caramel Apple, ⅔ cup, 2 oz	260	7	43
Strawberry, ½ cup, 2 oz	290	16	34
Toasted Coconut, ⅔ cup, 2 oz	270	10	42
NutriSystem,			
NutriFlakes, 1 pkt	90	1	22

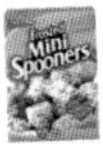

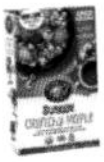
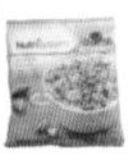

Ready-To-Eat Cereal ~ Brands (Cont)

Post:

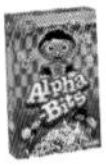

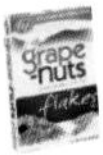

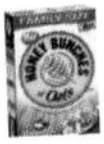

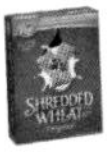

	C	F	Cb
Alpha Bits, 1 cup, 1.3 oz	140	1.5	29
Bran Flakes, 1 cup, 1.3 oz	110	1	29
CoCo Wheats, 1.1 oz	110	0	24
Golden Crisp, 1 cup, 1.34 oz	150	0.5	34
Grape-Nuts: Original, 2 oz	200	1	47
Flakes, 3/4 cup, 1.45 oz	150	1.5	34
Great Grains:			
Banana Nut Crunch, 1 cup, 2 oz	230	4.5	45
Cranb. Alm. Crunch, 1 cup,1.9 oz	210	3	44
Crunchy Pecan, 3/4 cup, 1.8 oz	210	5	39
Honey Bunches of Oats:			
Frosted; Honey Roasted, 1.4 oz	160	2	34
Honey Roasted Granola, 1.92 oz	230	7	40
Pecan & Maple Brown Sugar, 1 oz	160	3.5	33
With Almonds, 1.42 oz	170	3	34
W/ Cinnamon Bunches, 1.4 oz	160	2	34
Malt O Meal ~ *see Page 60*			
Nutter Butter, 1¼ cups, 1.4 oz	180	5	31
Oreo O's, 1⅓ cups, 1.4 oz	160	2	34
Pebbles, Marshmallow, 1.4 oz	160	1	36
Raisin Bran, 1¼ cups, 2 oz	190	1	48
Shredded Wheat, Spoon Size:			
Original, 1⅓ cups, 2 oz	210	1.5	49
Wheat & Bran, 2 oz	210	1.5	49
Shredded Wheat, Frosted,			
Choc. Strawb., 21 bisc., 2 oz	210	1	49

Quaker:

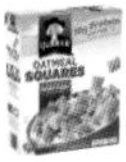

	C	F	Cb
Life, all types, 1 cup, 1.4 oz	160	2	33
Oatmeal Squares,			
all varieties,1 cup., 1.58 oz	210	3	44
Multigrain Flakes, av., ¾ cup, 2.1 oz	240	3.5	49
Real Medleys:			
Granola, Summer Berry, ⅔ c., 1.83 oz	210	5	39
Multigrain, Cherry Alm. Pecan, ¾ c., 1.9 oz	240	7	41
Supergrains, all flavors, ½ c., 1.83 oz	220	8	37
Simply Granola:			
Apple Cranberry Almond, 2.2 oz	260	7	49
Oats, Honey, Raisins & Alm., 2.4 oz	270	7	51

Sweet Home Farm:

	C	F	Cb
Granola: Blueberry, w/ Flax, 1.94 oz	240	8	40
Cinnamon with Raisins, 1.94 oz	200	3	43
French Vanilla with Almond, 1.94 oz	250	8	41
Honey Nut with Almonds, 1.87 oz	240	10	36
Maple Pecan with Syrup, 2 oz	260	9	42
Pumpkin Flax, 1.94 oz	240	9	37

Trader Joe's:

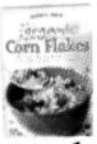

	C	F	Cb
Bran Flakes, 1¼ cups cup, 1.4 oz	170	1	37
Cinnamon Squares, ¾ cup, 1.1 oz	130	2.5	24
Cocoa Crunch, 1 cup, 1.4 oz	150	1	33
Cornflakes, 1 cup, 1 oz	110	0	26
Frosted Flakes, 3/4 c., 1 oz	110	0	24
High Fiber Cereal: Reg., 2/3 cup, 1 oz	80	0.5	23
Fruit & Nut, Multigrain, 2/3 cup, 1 oz	90	1.5	25
Granola: Ancient Grains & Nuts, 1.8 oz	220	10	29
Low Fat, av., 3/4 cup, 2 oz	210	3	44
Org., Apple/Mango, av., 2/3 cup, 2 oz	240	8	37
Joe's O's, 1 cup, 1 oz	110	2	20
Just The Clusters, av., 2/3 cup, 2 oz	240	9	36
O's, av. all flavours, 3/4 - 1 cup, 1 oz	120	2	24
Oatmeal (Instant): *Per 1.4 oz Pkt*			
Ancient Grains	160	6	24
Mango; Maple & Brown Sugar, av.	160	2	32
Unsweetened	160	3.5	27
Oatmeal Complete: Plain, 1.4 oz pkt	170	3	29
Maple Brown Sugar, 1.4 oz pkt	210	3	38
Raisin Bran: Regular, 1 cup, 1 oz	170	1	44
Clusters, 1 cup, 2 oz	190	3	41
w/ Pomegr. Blue. Flakes/Clusters, 1 c.	210	2	44
Shredded Wheat, 1 cup, 1.7 oz	180	1	38
Toasted Oatmeal Flakes, 3/4 c.,1 oz	110	1	23

Udi's:

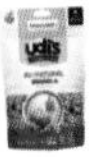

	C	F	Cb
Simple Gluten Free:			
Original; Cranb., av., 2 oz	270	11	42
Almond Butter, ½ cup, 2 oz	280	12	36
Au Naturel Honey; Vanilla, av., 2 oz	275	10	39

Uncle Sam:

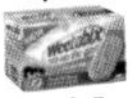

	C	F	Cb
Original, Wheat Berry, 3/4 cup, 2 oz	220	6	43
Skinner's Raisin Bran, 1 cup, 2 oz	200	1	48
Weetabix, 3 bisc., 1.84 oz	180	1	43

Wegmans:

	C	F	Cb
Chocolaty Rice Crisps, 1 cup,1.5 oz	170	1.5	37
Crunchy Raisin Bran, 1 cup, 1.8 oz	230	0	50
Granola:			
Oats & Honey, with Alm., ⅔ cup, 2.3 oz	270	8	46
Vanilla & Almonds, ⅓ cup, 1.1 oz	130	4	21
Shredded Wheat,			
Frosted Bite Size, 21 biscuits	210	1	50
Toasted Grains, 1 cup	150	0	29

Whole Foods 365:

	C	F	Cb
Organic: Bran Flakes, ¾ up, 1.1 oz	100	0	24
Blueberry Almond Granola, 2 oz	240	9	38
Brown Rice Crisps, 1.1 oz	110	1	25
Fruit & Nut Granola, ½ cup, 1.9 oz	250	10	36
Honey Almond Flax, ¾ cup, 1.87 oz	210	5	35
Honey Flakes & Oat Clusters, 1.1 oz	120	1	25
Morning O's, Honey & Nut, 1.4 oz	150	2	32

Ready-to-Eat

Per Piece/Slice

	C	F	Cb
Angel Food, Plain: without oil, 2 oz	145	0	33
with oil, 2 oz	145	1	27
with Cream Frosting	255	7	45
Almond Croissant, 5 oz	620	35	67
Apple Danish, 5 oz	450	18	67
Apple Pie ~ *See Pies/Tarts Page 134*			
Baklava, 1½" square, 1.75 oz	200	10	27
Banana Cake, with Butter Cream, 2 oz	230	9	37
Banana Walnut Cake, 3 oz	270	11	40
Bear Claw, 4.5 oz	540	24	71
Black Forest, 3 oz	345	11	59
Brownie: Small, 2" Square, 1 oz	130	8	14
Large, 3 oz	390	24	42
Bundt Cakes, average all types:			
3 oz slice	300	13	42
Mini-Bundt, 5 oz	500	22	70
Cannoli's: Mini, 1 oz	85	3	11
Regular, 2.5 oz	215	8	28
Carrot Cake: Plain, 3 oz	300	16	37
with Cream Cheese Frosting	400	22	48
Cheesecake:			
Small serving, 3 oz	240	13	26
Large serving, 5 oz	400	21	44
with Low-Fat Cheese/Fruit, 3 oz	170	4	28
Denny's, NY Style, 5oz	510	34	43
Chocolate Cake:			
with Chocolate Frosting, 4 oz	415	18	62
without Frosting, 1/12 of 9", 3.5 oz	340	14	51
Chocolate Croissant, 4.25 oz	470	26	54
Chocolate Eclair, w/ custard, 3.5 oz	260	16	24
Chocolate Fudge Cake, 3 oz	270	12	40
Chocolate Meringue, 2.5 oz	320	13	48
Churros, 1 stick, 1.5 oz	165	8	21
Cinnamon Crumb Cake, 2.5 oz	260	9	40
Cinnamon Rolls: Small, 2 oz	220	8	34
Regular, 4 oz	440	16	68
Large, 6 oz	660	24	102
Brands ~ *See Page 67*			
Coffee Cake, 2 oz	180	6	30
Concha: Small, 2 oz	240	9	33
Large (5" diameter), 5.5 oz	615	23	85
Cream Puff, custard filled, 4.6 oz	335	20	30
Cream Horn, 3 oz	210	5	36
Crumble Coffee Cake, 4.5 oz	500	25	65
Danish Pastries:			
Small, 2.5 oz	250	14	25
Large, 5 oz	500	28	50
Donuts ~ *See Page 66*			
Eclair, Chocolate, custard filled, 3.5 oz	260	16	24
Fig Bars, average	160	3	31

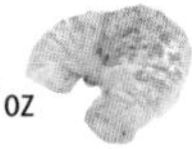
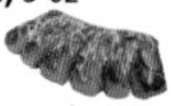
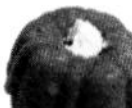
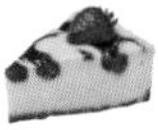
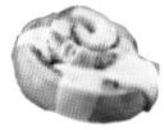
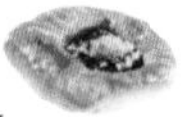

Ready-to-Eat (Cont)

Per Piece/Slice

	C	F	Cb
Fruit Cake, Dark/Light, 2 oz	185	5	34
Fudge Nut Brownie, 3.5 oz	380	18	54
Gingerbread, from mix, 3" square	210	4	41
Honey Bun, 2.7 oz	310	15	39
Jelly Roll, 1/12 roll, 1.8 oz	150	2	32
Key Lime Pie, 4.3 oz	400	25	41
Kringles: Almond; Pecan, average	205	12	24
Blueberry: Cherry; Raspberry, av.	165	8	24
Lady Finger, 3 oz	310	4.5	59
Lemon Cake, 4 oz	440	24	49
Lemon Poppy Seed Creme, 1.6 oz	180	9	23
Marble Cake, 4 oz	430	23	50
Mississippi Mud Pie, 4 oz	480	22	67
Mud Cake, 4.5 oz	380	20	44
Muffins ~ *See Page 67*			
Palmier Cookie, large, 4.5 oz	490	25	62
Pineapple Upside Down Cake,			
2.5 oz	230	9	36
Peach Melba, 3.5 oz	300	8	52
Pecan Sticky Roll, 6.5 oz	690	22	91
Pecan Twirls, 1.3 oz	170	7	26
Pies & Tarts ~ *See Page 134*			
Pound Cakes: Iced Lemon, 3.5 oz	360	17	50
Marble, 3.75 oz	350	13	53
Raspberry Rugulah,			
1.2 oz	110	9	7
Scone, fruit, 2 oz	200	9	30
Sponge Cake: Plain, 2.5 oz	220	10	33
with Chocolate Frosting	290	12	45
with Cream & Strawberry Jam	390	12	69
Starbucks Cakes ~ *Page 244*			
Strawberry Cream Cake, 4.7 oz	400	27	33
Strudel Bites, 0.75 oz	60	2.5	9
Strudel, fruit, av., 4.5 oz	300	17	32
Swiss Rolls, 1 oz	135	6	19
Tiramisu, 4.5 oz	440	22	34
Turnovers, fruit, average, 3 oz	290	15	35

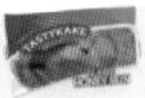

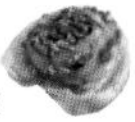
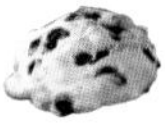
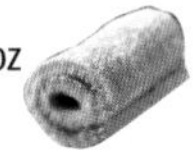

Cupcakes

Average all Varieties

	C	F	Cb
Regular:			
Cake only, 1.5 oz	140	5.5	20
Cake + Icing, 2.5 oz	260	13	34
Large, (Muffin Size):			
Cake only, 2.5 oz	235	9	34
Cake + Icing, 5 oz	520	27	67
Mini, (2-Bite):			
Cake only, 0.4 oz	40	1.5	5.5
Cake + Icing, 1 oz	110	5.5	13
Icing Only: Per 1 oz	115	7	13
Thick/Tall amount, 2.5 oz	290	17	32

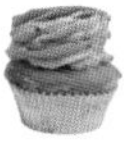
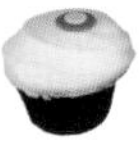
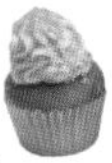

Cakes ~ Brands

	C	F	Cb
Albertson's Bakery:			
Ring Cakes: *Per 1/10 Cake*			
Angel Food	135	0	27
Cake Slices: *Per Slice Unless Indicated*			
Banana Nut Loaf	330	17	39
Creme Cake (2), 3.2 oz	300	12	43
Cinn. Streusel (2), 3.2 oz	350	18	43
Bimbo Bakery:			
Conchas, Vanilla, 2.12 oz	230	9	32
Pound Cakes: *Per Slice*			
Panque/Chocolate, 2.2 oz	240	10	35
Panqecitos, 3.5 oz	410	18	54
Bon Appetit Bakery:			
Banana Bread, 4 oz	440	25	49
Cream Cheese Cake, 4 oz slice	430	24	49
Danish: Apple (1), 5 oz	210	11	25
Bear Claw (1), 5 oz	240	13	27
Cheese & Berries (1), 5 oz	250	14	26
Vienna Cream (1), 5 oz	240	14	27
Slices: Cheesecake, 4 oz	430	24	49
Lemon Cake, 4 oz	430	24	49
Marble Cake, 4 oz	430	24	50
Walnut Brownie, 3.5 oz	380	18	54
Cheesecake Factory ~ *See Fast-Foods Section*			
Entenmann's: *Per Slice*			
Crumb Cakes: Butter French, 2.3 oz	280	14	36
Cheese-Filled Coffee, 2 oz	200	9	27
NY Style, 1/9 cake, 2 oz	230	10	34
Danish: Cheese, 1/8, 1.86 oz	210	10	27
Pecan Twist, 1/6, 2 oz	260	16	27
Raspberry Twist, 1/8, 1.86 oz	220	11	29
Iced Cakes:			
Chocolate Fudge, 1/6, 3.17 oz	330	13	53
Lemon, 1/6, 3 oz	370	19	48
Marshmallow Devil's Food, 3.17 oz	370	17	52
Loaf Cakes: Banana Bread, 2.2 oz	200	7	32
Blueberry Crumb, 1.76 oz	200	9	28
Chocolate, 1.9 oz	190	8	29
Choc. Chip Crumb, 1.7 oz	190	9	27
Lemon, 1.9 oz	210	10	28
Glenny's:			
100 Calorie:			
Blondie, Choc. Chip, 1.5 oz	100	4	15
Brownies: Chocolate Chip, 1.5 oz	100	4	12
Peanut Butter, 1.5 oz	100	4	15

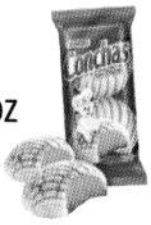
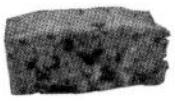
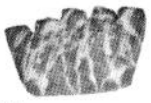
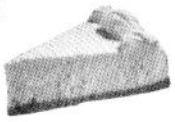
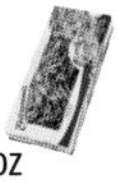
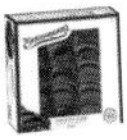
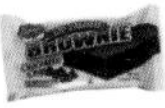

Muffins/Sweet Rolls ~ See Page 67

	C	F	Cb
Great American Cookies:			
Original Cookie Cakes: *Per Slice*			
By the Slice, 4.4 oz	530	25	75
14" Heart Shaped, 3 oz	350	16	51
with M&M, 3 oz	360	17	52
Great Value *(Walmart):*			
Angel Food, 2 oz slice	110	0	27
Cheese Crumb Cake, (1), 2 oz	230	10	32
Chocolate Cup Cake, (1), 2 oz	200	6	35
Chocolate 3 Layer Cake, 2.36 oz	260	13	35
Pink Snowballs (1), 2 oz	210	5	38
Pound Cake, 2 oz sl.	240	13	29
Hostess:			
Cup Cakes, Choc.; Orange, av., 1.6 oz	165	6	30
Ding Dongs, (2), average, 2.53 oz	325	15	43
Ho Hos, (3), 3 oz	380	20	52
Snoball (1), all flavors, 1.76 oz	160	5	29
SuzyQ's, (1), 2.6 oz	290	13	38
Twinkies:			
Classic (2), 2.7 oz	280	9	47
Chocolate (2), 2.7 oz	260	8	45
Fudge Covered (1), 1.9 oz	230	10	34
Pumpkin Spice (2), 2.7 oz	260	8	44
Zingers, Vanilla (2), 2.53 oz	290	10	49
Donettes ~ *Page 66*			
Little Debbie:			
Cinnamon Streusel Cake, (1),1.6 oz	180	7	26
Cocoa Cremes, (1), 1.4 oz	170	8	24
Cookies & Creme Cake, (2)	320	15	43
Devil Cremes, (1), 1.66 oz	200	9	29
Pumpkin Spice Roll, (1), 2.2 oz	260	11	40
Strawberry Shortcake Rolls, (1), 2.1 oz	240	8	40
Swiss Rolls, (1), 2.1 oz	270	12	39
Zebra Cake, (1), 2.6 oz	320	14	48
Ne-Mo's:			
Brookie, (1), 3 oz	320	14	48
Bundt: Chocolate, 4 oz	380	14	62
Orange Dreamswirl, 4 oz	410	16	64
Cake Breads: Banana; Carrot, 4 oz	420	21	53
Cream Cheese Coffee Cake, 4 oz	430	19	60
Peanut Butter & Jelly, 4 oz	400	16	57
Sweet Potato,, 4 oz	420	20	55
Wild Blueberry, 4 oz	410	19	58
Zesty Lemon, 4 oz	410	18	56
Cake Slices: All Butter, 4 oz	400	17	56
Marble, 2 oz	210	11	27
Cake Squares: Carrot, 3.6 oz	360	19	44
Banana; Chocolate, av, 3 oz	285	11	43
Danish: Cheese, 4 oz slice	430	19	58
Cinnamon, with Icing, 4 oz slice	440	20	60

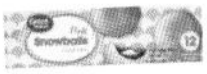
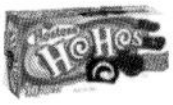

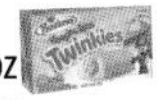

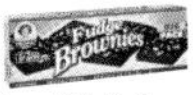

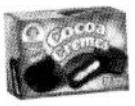

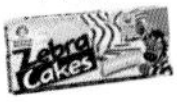

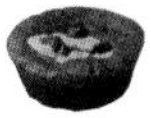
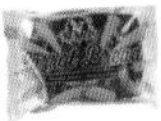

Cakes ~ Brands (Cont)

	C	F	Cb
Pepperidge Farm:			
Layer Cakes (Frozen): *Per ⅛ Cake, 2.43 oz*			
Chocolate Fudge	240	13	32
Chocolate Fudge Stripe	250	13	32
Coconut 	250	12	34
Creamy Red Velvet	240	13	30
German Chocolate	240	12	31
Lemon; Tangy Key Lime; Vanilla	240	12	34
Turnovers (Frozen):			
Apple; Cherry; Raspberry (1), av.	245	13	30
Peach (1)	270	13	34
Pop-Tarts *(Kellogg's):*			
Brown Sugar Cinnamon, (2)	400	13	68
Chocolate Fudge, (2) 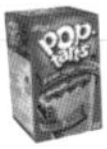	400	10	74
Cherry, (2)	370	9	70
Fruit, Unfrosted, average (2)	380	10	69
Bites, Strawberry, 1.4 oz pouch	150	3	30
Prairie City:			
Brownie, Big n' Fudgy, 3.5 oz pkg	440	23	58
Cinnamon Roll, Bigger Big, 6 oz	630	34	76
Danish: Ooey Gooey Cheese (1)	470	24	57
Raspberry (1)	420	17	64
Turnovers: Apple & Maple Strudel (1)	500	23	67
Blueberry Cheese (1)	430	20	56
Cherry/Strawberry Cheese (1)	500	23	67
Safeway Select,			
Molten Chocolate Lava Cake (1)	390	23	43
Sara Lee:			
Butter Streusel Coffee Cake,			
⅙ Cake, 1.9 oz	200	9	26
Cheesecakes:			
Classic: Cheesecake, 4.27 oz	330	17	37
Cherry, 4.76 oz 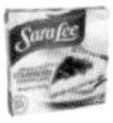	360	12	55
Strawberry, 4.76 oz	330	12	50
French Style: Classic, 4.7 oz	410	26	38
Strawberry, 4.34 oz	310	18	35
NY Style, 4.73 oz 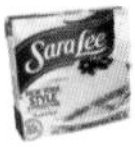	460	27	47
Pecan Coffee Cake,			
⅙ Cake, 1.9 oz	190	9	25
Pound Cakes: *Per ¼ Cake*			
All Butter, 2.68 oz	340	21	34
Blueberry, 2.57 oz 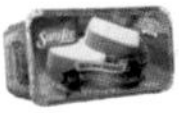	210	7	36
Lemon, 2.68 oz	240	8	39
2 Slices: Original, 2.8 oz	250	8	41
Double Chocolate, 3 oz	280	10	45
Special K, Pastry Crisps,			
all varieties, 1 pouch, 0.9 oz	100	2	20

	C	F	Cb
Tastykake:			
Creme Filled Cupcakes:			
Chocolate (2), 2.4 oz 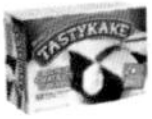	270	10	42
Koffee Cake (2), 2.1 oz	240	9	38
Swirly Choc. (1), 2 oz	200	6	35
Kandy Kake: Choc. (2), 1.3 oz	180	9	24
Peanut Butter (2), 1.3 oz	190	10	20
Krimpets: Butterscotch (2), 2 oz	220	6	39
Creme Filled (2), 2.4 oz 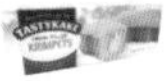	280	11	44
Jelly (2), 2 oz	190	3.5	37
Lemon Flavored (2), 2 oz	220	6	40
Toaster Strudel *(Pillsbury): Per 1.9 oz*			
Boston Cream Pie 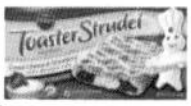	180	7	26
Cream Cheese,			
average all varieties	190	9	25
Fruit flavors, all var. 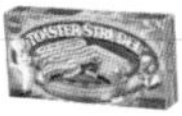	180	7	27
Trader Joe's:			
Bakery Fresh:			
Apricot Almond Tart, 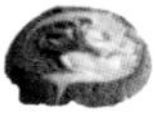			
4 oz slice	450	24	56
Cheesecake Brownie Bites (1)	110	7	9
Chocolate Ganache Cake, 3 oz slice	390	22	44
Flourless Chocolate Cake,			
1 slice, 2 oz	260	17	23
I Dream of Chocolate, 2.68 oz slice	250	13	31
Lemon Cake, 3.3oz slice	350	19	43
Mini Carrot Cake, 5 oz 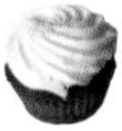	450	19	68
Whoopie Pie (1), 2.5 oz	350	14	54
Bread Cake:			
Banana Bonanza, 2.6 oz slice	250	9	39
Pumpkin Nut, 2.6 oz slice	270	10	43
Walnut Streusel Coffee, 2 oz slice	180	8	25
Zucchini Carrot, 2 oz slice	200	7	32
Loaf Cake:			
Cranberry Pumpkin, 2 oz slice	140	2	30
Pumpkin Nut, 2.6 oz slice	270	10	43
Frozen:			
Apple Raspberry Turnover, 3.2 oz	280	14	34
Chocolate Dilemma Cheesecake:			
Plain, 3.5 oz	320	19	30
Choc. Chip; Triple Choc, av., 3.5 oz	345	20	35
Tuxedo, 3.5 oz	320	17	34
Choc Lava Cake, 4 oz 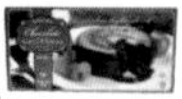	360	23	40
Karat Cake, 3 oz slice	320	19	37
N.Y. Style Cheesecake, 4.5 oz slice	400	28	32
Tiramisu Torte, 3.2 oz slice	230	12	24
Tarts: 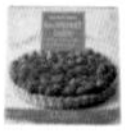			
Pear, 3.5 oz slice	250	9	39
Raspberry, 5 oz slice	290	10	51
Wild Blueberry, 3.5 oz slice	260	6	52

Cakes ~ Mixes

	C	F	Cb
Arrowhead Mills: *Dry Mix Only*			
All Purpose Mix, 1.4 oz	130	1	28
Betty Crocker: *Dry Mix Only*			
Brownie Mix:			
Dark Chocolate, 1 oz	110	1	24
Fudge, 0.9 oz	100	1	22
Milk Chocolate, 1 oz	110	1	25
Salted Caramel, 1.15 oz	120	1.5	26
Supreme:			
Chocolate Chunk, 1.1 oz	130	2	26
Fudge, 1.2 oz	120	1.5	26
Triple Chunk, 1.1 oz	130	2.5	26
Walnut, 1.1 oz	120	2.5	23
Cake Mix: Gingerbread, 1.8 oz	220	6	38
Pound Cake, 2 oz	220	2.5	47
Fat Free Cake Mix: Angel Food, 1.34 oz	140	0	32
Pineapple Upside Down Cake, 3.6 oz	140	0	32
Super Moist Delights Cake Mix: *Per 1.5 oz Dry Mix*			
Butter Recipe Yellow	160	1.5	36
Butter Pecan	160	1.5	36
Carrot; Devil's Food	160	1.5	35
Cherry Chip	160	1.5	36
French Vanilla	160	1	36
German Chocolate	160	1.5	35
Lemon	160	1.5	36
Red Velvet	160	1.5	35
Strawberry	160	1.5	36
Triple Chocolate Fudge	160	2	34
Dessert Bars: *Dry Mix Only*			
Coconut White Chip Oat Bar, 1.1 oz	150	6	22
Reese's PB & Chocolate, 1.1 oz	130	1.5	27
Duncan Hines: *Dry Mix Only*			
Brownie Mix: Chewy Fudge, 0.9 oz	110	1.5	22
Decadent, Choc. Peanut Butter, 1 oz	130	3.5	24
Perfectly Moist Cake Mix:			
Classic: Butter Golden, 1.5 oz	170	3	35
Dark Choc. Fudge, 1.5 oz	170	4	33
White, 1.5 oz	170	4	34
Signature Cake Mix:			
French Vanilla, 1.5 oz	180	4	34
German Chocolate, 1.5 oz	180	4	34
Orange, 1.5 oz	180	4	34
Triple Chocolate, 1.5 oz	170	3.5	34

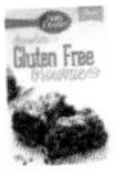

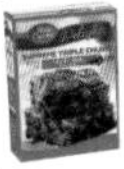
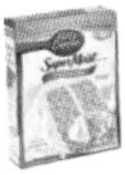
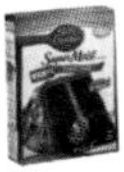
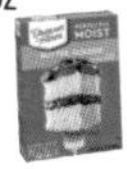

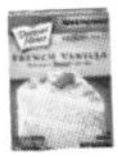

	C	F	Cb
Jell-O: *Dry Mix Only*			
No Bake: Classic Cheesecake, 1.83 oz	210	5	41
Double Choc. Cheesecake, 1.5 oz	180	5	33
Strawberry Cheesecake, 2.2 oz	210	4	42
Krusteaz: *Dry Mix Only*			
Bars: Meyer Lemon, 1.1 oz	130	3	26
Pumpkin Pie, 1 oz	110	1	24
Raspberry, 1.2 oz	100	0.5	22
Cakes: Lemon Pound Cake, with Glaze, 1.87 oz	180	1	41
Pumpkin Spice Cake Bread, 1.23 oz	140	1.5	30
Gluten Free Cakes: Choc., 1.24 oz	130	1	29
Yellow Cake, 1.5 oz	170	1	37
Pillsbury: *Per 1 oz Dry Mix Only*			
Classic Brownie Mix: Choc Fudge	110	0.5	25
Classic Fudge	120	1	28
Dark Chocolate	110	1	25
Milk Chocolate	110	0.5	25
Funfetti Brownie Mix: Blondie, 1.1 oz	120	2	26
Chocolate Fudge, 1 oz	110	1	24
Premium Brownie Mix:			
Caramel Swirl, 1.2 oz	120	1	28
Cheesecake Swirl, 1 oz	110	1.5	25
Chocolate Chunk, 1 oz	120	2.5	24
Chocolate Walnut, 1.1 oz	130	3	25
Toffee Flavored Brownie Bark, 1 oz	110	1	25
Moist Supreme Cake Mix:			
Devils Food, 1.5 oz	160	2	35
White/Yellow, 1.5 oz	160	1.5	35
Traditional Cake Mix, Vanilla Flavored, 1.5 oz	160	1.5	35

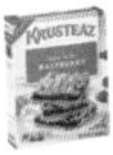

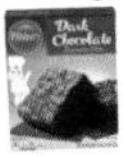

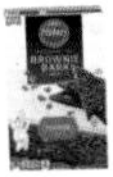
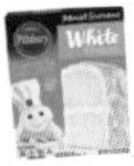

Cake Frostings

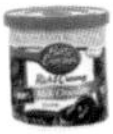

	C	F	Cb
Betty Crocker: *Per 2 Tbsp*			
Rich & Creamy: Coconut Pecan, 1.23 oz	140	8	18
Av. other flavors, 1.23 oz	135	5	23
Whipped, av. all flavors., 0.9 oz	100	4.5	15
Cool Whip, Original, 2 Tbsp, 0.3 oz	25	1.5	3
Duncan Hines: *Per 2 Tbsp*			
Creamy, average all flavors, 1.23 oz	140	6	23
Whipped, av. all flavors, 0.9 oz	100	5	15
Pillsbury: *Per 2 Tbsp*			
Creamy Supreme:			
Choc Fudge; Milk Choc., 1.2 oz	130	6	21
Strawb.; Vanilla; White,1.2 oz	140	5	22
Funfetti, av. all flavors, 1.2 oz	140	5	23
Sugar Free, average, 1.1 oz	100	6	16

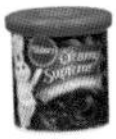

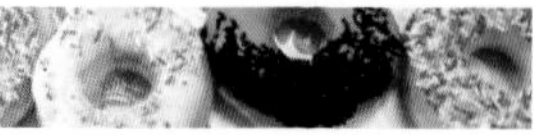

Quick Guide

Donuts	C	F	Cb
Average All Brands			
Cake: Plain, 1.8 oz	205	12	23
Chocolate Iced, 2 oz	255	14	29
Sugared, 0.8 oz	205	10	29
Non-Cake, Glazed, 2 oz	225	11	29
Croissant-Donuts			
(Includes Cronuts/Frissants)			
Average all Brands			
Cream-filled, 3.5 oz	430	26	45
Custard-filled, 3.5 oz	360	19	45

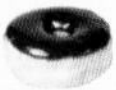
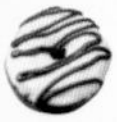
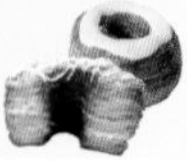

Extra Listings ~ *See CalorieKing.com*

(Cronut is a trademark of Dominique Ansel Bakery, New York)

Donuts ~ Brands

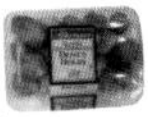
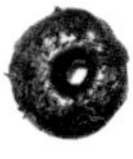
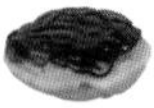
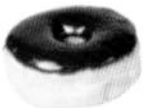
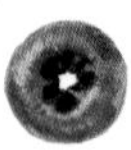
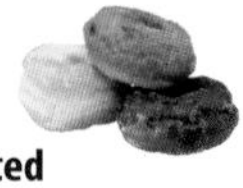

	C	F	Cb
Albertson's:			
Donut Holes:			
Glazed Old Fashioned (4)	240	12	31
Powdered Sugar (4)	210	12	24
Gem Donuts: Plain Cake (3)	190	12	20
Cinnamon Sugar (3)	240	15	23
Glazed (1)	140	6	21
Bon Appetit:			
Mini Donuts:			
Chocolate (4)	270	16	29
Crumb (4)	240	12	32
Powdered (4)	250	12	34
Dunkin':			
Apple Crumb	290	11	44
Apple N' Spice	230	10	31
Barvarian Kreme	240	11	31
Boston Kreme	270	11	39
Chocolate Frosted Cake	260	11	34
Chocolate Headlight	310	14	41
Coconut	410	21	50
Glazed Chocolate	240	11	33
Jelly Filled	250	10	36
Lemon	230	10	31
Powdered	330	20	34
Strawberry Frosted	260	11	35
Sugared	210	11	24
Vanilla Creme	300	15	37

Extra Listings ~ *See Fast Food Section*

Donuts ~ Brands (Cont)

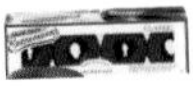
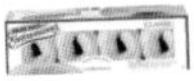
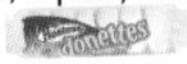
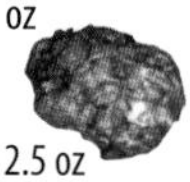
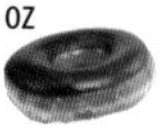
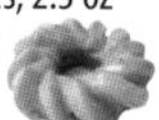
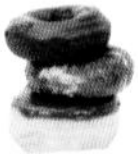
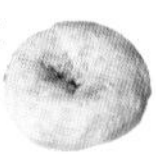
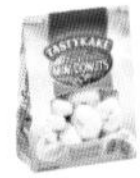

	C	F	Cb
Entenmann's:			
8 Pack: *Per Donut*			
Apple Cider, 2 oz	240	11	34
Crumb Topped, 1.94 oz	240	11	33
Frosted: Devil's Food, 2.1 oz	290	17	33
Rich Frosted, 2 oz	290	18	30
12 Count' Softees Variety Pack: *Per Donut*			
Glazed, 1.4 oz	180	11	19
Plain, 1.4 oz	180	11	19
Cinnamon; Powdered, 1.5 oz	210	12	24
Pop'ems Donut Holes: Glazed (4)	240	13	28
Party Sprinkled Devil's Food (4)	230	12	31
Rich Frosted (4)	330	26	24
Hostess:			
Mini Donettes: Crumb, 6-pack, 4 oz	430	18	63
Frosted, 6-pack, 3 oz	360	22	38
Powdered, 6-pack, 3 oz	340	17	43
Krispy Kreme:			
Apple Fritter, 3.5 oz	350	19	42
Chocolate: Iced Cake, 2.5 oz	280	13	37
Iced Custard Filled, 3 oz	300	15	37
Iced Glazed Cruller, 2.5 oz	260	10	40
Iced Glazed, 2.2	240	11	33
Iced Kreme Filled, 3 oz	350	19	41
Iced Glazed w/ Sprinkles, 2.3 oz	250	11	36
Cinnamon Twist, 1.9oz	210	11	26
Glazed Cruller, 1.9 oz	210	10	29
Glazed Doughnut Holes:			
Original (5)	220	11	25
Blueberry (4)	190	7	28
Cake (4)	190	8	28
Chocolate Cake (4)	180	7	27
Glazed Kreme Filled, 3 oz	340	19	40
Maple Iced Glazed, 2.2 oz	240	11	34
New York Cheesecake, 3.3 oz	310	17	35
Original Glazed, 1.7 oz	190	11	22
Powdered Cake, 2.3 oz	240	11	29
Traditional Cake, 2 oz	230	12	26
Little Debbie,			
Donut Sticks, 1.9 oz	270	16	29
Tastykake: *10 oz Bags*			
Mini: Black & White (4), 2 oz	220	10	33
Blueberry (4), 2 oz	260	14	31
Cinnamon (4), 1.9 oz	230	10	31
Lemon (4), 2 oz	260	14	30
Orange (4), 2 oz	260	14	31
Salted Caramel Flavored (4), 2 oz	260	10	39

Quick Guide

	C	F	Cb
Muffins: Ready-To-Eat			
Average All Brands			
Small, 1 oz	90	3.5	14
Medium, 2 oz	185	6.5	28
Large, 3 oz	275	10	42
Extra Large, 4 oz	365	13	57
Giant, 6 oz	550	20	84
Super Size, 8 oz	730	27	112

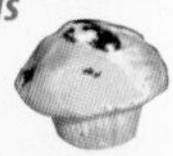
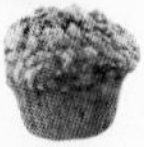

Muffins Ready-To-Eat ~ Brands

	C	F	Cb
Albertsons: *Each*			
Banana Nut	450	23	54
Blueberry	420	21	53
Entenmann's,			
Blueberry; Corn (2), average, 3.5 oz	380	18	50
Garden Lites: *Per 2 oz Muffin*			
Banana Choc. Chip	120	3	22
Blueberry Oat	110	2	21
Double Chocolate	110	2	21
Great Value *(Walmart):*			
Banana Nut Filled, (4), 4 oz	410	19	56
Blueberry Filled, (1), 4 oz	430	17	65
Chocolate Filled, (1), 4 oz	430	19	62
Little Debbie:			
Mini Muffins: Blueberry (1), 1.9 oz	170	6	28
Chocolate Chip (1), 1.9 oz	190	8	27
My Favorite Muffin: *Per Large*			
Banana Nut	650	38	71
Blueberry	590	28	78
Boston Cream Pie	740	33	105
Chocolate Chip	790	39	100
Lemon Poppyseed	670	32	90
Otis Spunkmeyer:			
Banana, 2 oz	220	10	30
Banana Minis (3), 2.2 oz	260	12	35
Blueberry, 2 oz	210	9	29
Starbucks ~ *See Fast-Foods Section*			
Trader Joe's: *Per Muffin*			
Apple Cranberry, 4.8 oz	220	5	38
Banana Chocolate Chip, 4 oz	400	18	57
Carrot, 4 oz	320	11	52
Triple Berry, 4 oz	310	11	49
Vitalicious:			
VitaTops: Banana Choc. Chip, 2 oz	130	2	25
Deep Chocolate, 2 ozimage	100	2	26
Wild Blueberry, 2 oz	120	1.5	27
Weight Watchers,			
Blueberry, 1.9 oz	150	1.5	35

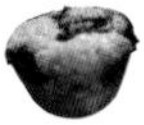
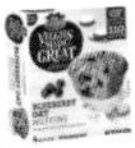
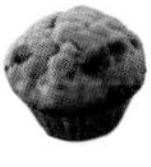
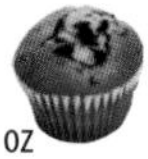
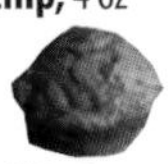
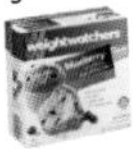

Muffin Mixes

	C	F	Cb
Dry Mix Only			
Betty Crocker: *Makes 2 Muffins*			
Boxed: Banana Nut, 2 oz	230	4.5	44
Cinnamon Streusel, 2.3 oz	270	6	51
Wild Blueberry, 2.8 oz	230	2.5	49
Pouch Mix:			
Banana Nut, 2.1 oz	240	5	45
Blueberry, 2.1 oz	250	5	46
Chocolate Chip, 2.1 oz	250	6	46
Krusteaz: *Dry Mix Only*			
Almond Poppy Seed, 1.4 oz	150	1.5	35
Choc Chunk, 1.5 oz	180	3.5	35
Cranb. Orange, 1.23 oz	140	0	33
Trader Joe's, Triple Berry	150	2	28

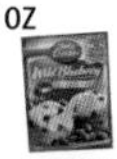
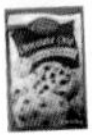
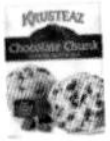

Sweet Rolls & Buns

Note: It is best to weigh for accuracy as actual weight can be 10-50% higher than label weight.

	C	F	Cb
Per Sweet Roll or Bun Unless Indicated			
Bimbo, Crispy Wheels, 4 pcs, 2.33 oz	360	22	41
Bon Appetit, Super Cinn. Roll, 5 oz	480	16	72
Cinnabon: Classic	880	37	127
Caramel Pecanbon	1080	51	146
Cloverhill Bakery,			
Big Texas Cinnamon Roll, 4 oz	430	18	62
Entenmann's, Iced Honey Bun, 4 oz	450	19	62
Little Debbie:			
Honey Bun: 1.5 oz	230	13	26
Individual, 3 oz Bun	360	20	41
Pecan Spinwheels: Single, 1 oz	110	3.5	18
2 Pack, 2.1 oz	210	7	32
O&H Danish: *Per 1.95 oz*			
Kringles: Apple: Wisconsin, av.	185	9	26
Almond; Turtle, average	215	13	27
Cinn. Roll; Cream Cheese, average	220	14	25
Pillsbury:			
Sweet Rolls, Refrigerated: *Per Roll Unless Indicated*			
Orig; Cinnamon, w/ Crm Cheese Icing	140	4.5	24
Cinn., Flaky w/ Butter Cream Icing	160	7	23
Orange, with Orange Icing	160	5	26
Grands, Refrigerated: *Per Roll*			
Cinnabon: Cinnamon Roll, with Cream Cheese Icing	300	7	54
w/ Extra Rich Butter Icing, 3.5 oz	300	7	56
Flaky Supreme Cinnamon Roll, with Icing, 3.5 oz	360	16	50
7-Eleven: Iced Honey Bun, 6 oz	820	58	68
Glazed Honey Bun, 5 oz	620	35	70

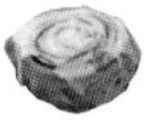
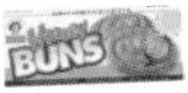

Updated Nutrition Data ~ www.CalorieKing.com
Persons with Diabetes ~ See Disclaimer (Page 22)

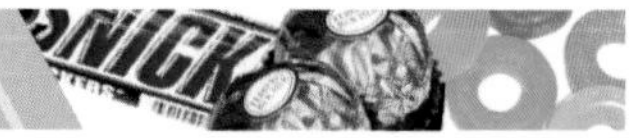

Quick Guide

Item	C	F	Cb
Chocolate:			
Average All Brands			
Milk Chocolate, regular:			
Plain/Nuts/Fruit, average, 1 oz	150	9	17
1.5oz Bar	230	13	25
2 oz Bar	305	17	34
4 oz Block	610	34	68
8 oz Block	1220	68	136
1 Pound, 16 oz	2440	136	272
Dark/White Chocolate: 1 oz	155	9	17
Hershey's, Sugar Free, 5 pieces	110	13	24
Milk Chocolate-Coated:			
Almonds, 5-6, 1 oz	150	10	15
Cherry Cordial Centers, 2 pcs, 1 oz	145	6	21
Clusters, Nut, 3 pieces, 1.2 oz	210	14	20
Coffee Beans, 1.4 oz	220	13	22
Macadamias, 10 pieces, 1.4 oz	220	16	21
Mints, 1 medium, 0.5 oz	55	1	11
Nougat & Caramel, 1 oz	150	9	15
Peanuts, 12 medium, 1 oz	145	10	14
Raisins, 28 medium, 1 oz	110	4	19
Baking Chocolate:			
Baker's: Bittersweet, 1 oz	140	12	14
Semi-sweet, 1 oz	140	9	16
Nestle, Chips: Dark, 1 Tbsp. 0.5 oz	70	5	3
Semi-Sweet, 1 Tbsp. 0.5oz	70	4	9
Unsweetened, 1 oz	140	14	8
Carob, Plain, 1 oz	155	9	16

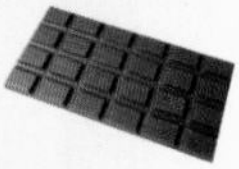

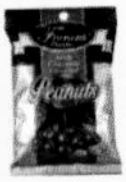

Candy ~ Brands & Generic

Per Piece/Serving	C	F	Cb
3 Musketeers: Orig., 1 bar, 1.9 oz	240	7	42
2 To Go, 1.7 oz Bar	200	6	36
Fun Size, 3 bars, 1.6 oz	190	6	34
Minis, 7 pieces, 1.4 oz	170	5	32
100 Grand: 1.5 oz bar	190	8	30
Snack Size (1), 0.8 oz	95	4	15
Super Size, 2.8 oz	360	14	58
Abba Zabba, 2 oz bar	250	5	48
After Dinner Mints, 1 small	25	1.5	3
After Eight Mint, each	35	1.5	4
Airhead, 1 bar, 0.5 oz	60	1	14
Almond Joy: 2 bars, 1.6 oz	220	13	26
King Size, 4 bars, 3.2 oz	440	26	53
Snack Size, 2pieces, 1.2 oz	160	9	20
Miniatures, 2 pieces, 1 oz	130	7	15

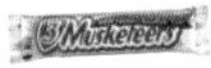

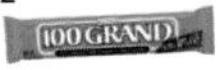

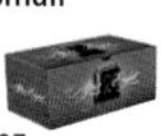

Per Piece/Serving	C	F	Cb
Almond Roca, 3 pieces, 1.3 oz	200	15	17
Almonds: Sugar-coated (15), 1.4 oz	190	7	27
Jordan, 15 pieces, 1.4 oz	180	8	28
Almond Clusters:			
True North, 5 pieces, 1 oz	170	12	9
Trader Joe's, 2 pieces, 1.2 oz	190	14	13
Almond Pecan Crunch:			
True North, 5 pieces, 1.2 oz	150	11	10
Altoids: Original, 3 mints	10	0	2
Artic, 3 mints	5	0	2
Andes, Thins (8), av. all var., 1.4 oz	205	13	22
Anthon Berg:			
Creamy Mint (4), 1.4 oz	180	6	31
Marzipan with Plum, in Madeira	120	6	14
Atomic Fireball, 1 piece, 0.3 oz	35	0	9
Baby Ruth: King Size, 3.5 oz bar	500	24	66
2 oz bar	280	14	39
Fun size, 2 bars	170	8	24
Minis, 4 bars	210	11	28
Baci *(Perugina),*			
1 piece, 0.5 oz	75	6	7
Bark Thins, Snacking Chocolate,			
Dark Choc. Mint/Pretzel, av., 1 oz	140	6	20
Baskin-Robbins: Sugar Candy, 3 pcs	60	1	12
Sugar Free, 4 pieces, average, 0.6 oz	40	1	16
Note: Carb figure includes 16g sugar alcohol			
Big Hunk, 2 oz Bar	230	3	47
Bit-O-Honey:			
1.7 oz bar	180	3.5	39
Chews, 6 pcs, 1.4 oz	150	3	32
Blow Pops, each, 0.6 oz	60	0	17
Bon Bons, 3 pieces	65	0	15
Boston Baked Beans, (11)	70	2	11
Brach's: Almond Supremes (10)	200	14	20
Bridge Mix (15)	190	10	26
Double Dippers (15)	210	14	22
Gummi Bears (14)	130	0	30
Lemon Drops, Sugar Free, 4 pieces	35	0	17
Note: Carb figures include 17g Sugar Alcohol			
Mandarin/Orange Slices (3), 1.6 oz	150	0	37
Maple Nut Goodies (8)	190	9	27
Milk Maid Crmls (4)	150	4	25
Peanut Cluster (3)	210	15	20
Breath Savers, (1),all var.	5	0	2
Bubble Gum ~ *See Page 75*			
Bulls Eyes, 3 pieces, 1.2 oz	130	3	23
Buncha Crunch: 1.4 oz	180	9	25
Movie Box, 3.2 oz	450	20	65
Burnt Peanuts, 1.4 oz	170	6	29

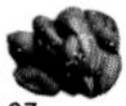

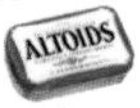

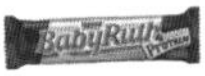

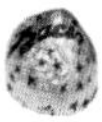

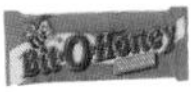

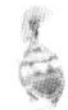

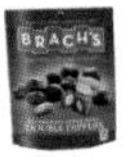

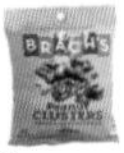

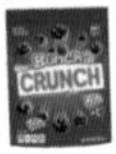

Candy ~ Brands & Generic (Cont)

Per Piece/Serving	C	F	Cb
Butterfinger:			
Bars: 1.9 oz bar	250	10	36
Fun Size Bars (2), 1.3 oz	170	7	25
Minis, 1.1 oz	140	6	20
Bites, 6 pieces, 1.1 oz	140	6	20
Crisp Bar, 1 pkg, 2 oz	300	17	35
Dessert Toppers, 2 Tbsp, 1.3 oz	180	7	25
Butter Mints, 7 pieces, 0.5 oz	50	0	12
Butterscotch: 3 pieces	60	0	15
Discs (*Walgreens*), 3 pieces, 0.6 oz	70	0	17
Cadbury: Caramello Bar, 1.6 oz	220	10	29
Caramel Egg, 1.2 oz	170	8	22
Dairy Milk Bar, 7 pcs, 1.4 oz	200	11	23
Mini Eggs (Candy), 12 pcs, 1.4 oz	190	8	28
Candy Apple, medium, 6.5 oz	280	0	60
Candy Cane, medium, 5", 0.5 oz	40	0	14
Candy Corn, 20 pieces, 1.4 oz	150	0	38
Candy Jar Mix (*Jewel*), 3 pcs, 0.6 oz	60	0	14
Candy Necklace (*Smarties*), (1), 0.8 oz	90	0.5	20
Caramels: Each, 0.4 oz	40	1	8
Chocolate, each, 0.3 oz	25	0.3	6
Creams (3), 1.3 oz	130	3	23
Caramel Popcorn, 2/3 cup	150	6	23
Cella's,			
Milk Choc. Cherries, 3 pieces, 1.5 oz	160	6	27
Certs, Breath Mints, 1 piece	5	0	2
Charleston Chew:			
Chocolate Bar (1), 1.4 oz	160	4.5	30
Mini Bars, 13 pieces	190	6	34
Charms: Blow Pop	60	0	17
Flat Pop, 0.5 oz	50	0	14
Chew-ets, Peanut Chews,			
Original (4), 1.6 oz	230	12	29
Chewz, 1 roll, 1 oz	120	1	28
Chick O Stick, 2 oz	240	9	42
Chunky Bar (*Nestlé*),			
King Size, 2.5 oz	340	19	44
Chupa Chups, 1 Pop	50	0	12
Cinn. Buttons (*Walgreens*), 3 pieces	60	0	16

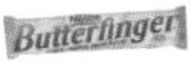

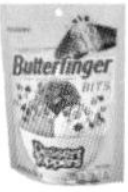

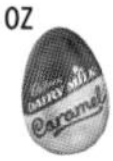

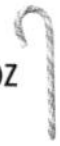

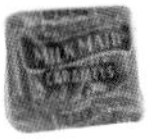

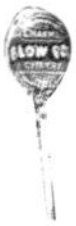

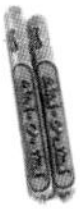

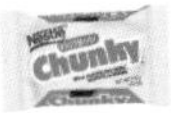

Per Piece/Serving	C	F	Cb
Cinnamon Disks (*Walmart*), 3 pieces	70	0	18
Circus Peanuts (*Spangler*),			
6 pieces, 1.3 oz	165	0	41
CocoaVia, Orig., 0.8 oz	100	6	12
Coconut Stacks, (8)	320	16	46
Coffee Go, Candy, (4)	60	1	12
Conversation Hearts (*Necco*):			
Small (40), 1.4 oz	160	0	39
1 large	10	0	3
Cookie Dough Bites, 1.4 oz	200	10	27
Cote d'Or: Dark 86% Coca, 4 pcs	270	22	14
Dark, 70%, Orange, 3.5 oz	575	46	34
Dark, Raspberry, 3.5 oz	580	46	34
Milk, Intense, 3.5 oz	575	40	45
Cotton Candy, 1 oz	110	0	28
Cough Drops ~ *See Page 75*			
Cracker Jack, 1/2 cup, 1 oz	120	2	23
Creme Savers:			
3 pieces, 0.5 oz	60	1	11
Sugar-Free, 3 pieces	30	1	8
Crisped Rice, Choc Chip, 1 bar, 1 oz	115	4	20
Crows, 11 pieces, 1.4 oz	130	0	33
Crunch Bar ~ *See Nestle*			
Dots, 11 dots, 1.4 oz	130	0	33
Double Dip Stick, 1 stick	15	0.5	3
Dove:			
Milk Choc: Singles Bar, 1.4 oz	220	13	24
Large Tablet Bar, 9 pcs, 1.5 oz	230	13	25
Choc. Cov. Almonds, 13 pcs, 1.4 oz	220	15	19
Promises: Milk Choc., 1 pce, 0.3 oz	45	2.5	5
w/ Caramel, 1 piece, 0.3 oz	40	2	5
w/ Peanut Butter, 1 pce, 0.3 oz	45	3	4
Swirls, all var., 9 pieces 1.5 oz	230	14	25
Dark Choc: Singles Bar, 1.3 oz	220	13	24
Large Tablet Bar, 9 pcs, 1.5 oz	220	14	25
Choc. Cov. Almds, 13 pcs, 1.4 oz	210	15	19
Promises, Almond, 1 piece, 0.3 oz	40	3	4
Swirls, Raspberry, 9 pcs, 1.4 oz	220	14	24
Sugar Free, all flav., 5 pcs, 1.4 oz	195	15	21
Dum Dum Pops (*Spangler*), 1 pop	25	0	7
Drops (*Hershey's*):			
Cookies 'n' Creme, 14 pieces, 1.5 oz	210	11	26
Milk Chocolate, 15 pieces, 1.4 oz	200	12	25

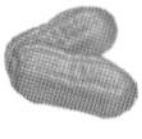

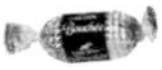

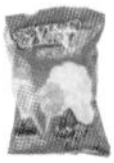

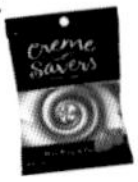

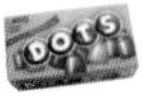

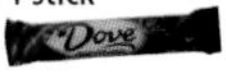

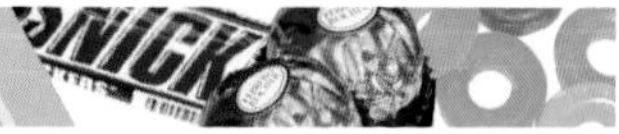

Candy ~ Brands & Generic (Cont)

Per Piece/Serving	C	F	Cb
English Toffee, 1 piece, 0.4 oz	70	4	6
5th Avenue: 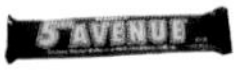			
Bars: 2 oz	260	12	38
King Size, 3.5 oz	440	20	64
Fannie May: 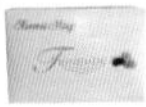			
Mint Meltaway, (1)	240	16	24
Pixie (1), 1.5 oz	210	13	23
Trinidad (1), 1.5 oz	200	12	23
Fast Break (Reese's):			
Bars: 1.8 oz bar 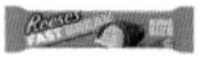	230	11	32
King Size, 3.5 oz	460	22	63
Ferrero Rocher: 			
Pieces:1 piece	75	5	5
3 pieces, 1.3 oz	220	16	16
Rondnoir, 3 pieces, 1 oz 	180	13	14
Fifty 50 Snack Bars: 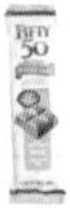			
Milk Chocolate: 5 pieces, 1 oz	135	11	14
Almond, 5 pieces, 1 oz	135	12	14
Crunch Bar, 7 pcs, 1 oz	140	12	16
Dark Chocolate, 5 pieces, 1 oz	120	11	15
Note: Carb figures include 9-12g Sugar Alcohol			
Fluffy Stuff *(Charms),* 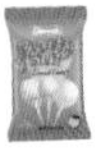			
Cotton Candy, 1.4 oz	150	0	40
Fondant: Choc-coated, 1.2 oz	125	3	27
Mint, 1 oz	105	0	25
Fran's: Gold Bar, Macadamia (1) 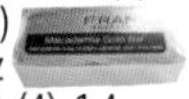	250	14	27
GoldBite, Almond (1)	120	7	13
Fruit Drops, (1), 1/4 oz	20	0	4
Fruit Gems *(Sunkist)*, (4), 1.4 oz	130	0	33
Fruit Leathers, average, 0.5 oz	50	0.5	12
Fruit Pastilles *(Rowntree)*, 1 roll	185	0	45
Fruit Roll-Ups *(Betty Crocker/Sunkist)*,			
1 roll, 0.5 oz 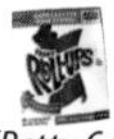	50	1	12
Fruit Runts *(Walgreens)*,			
12 pieces	60	0	14
Fruit Flavored Shapes *(Betty Crocker)*,			
all varieties, 0.8 oz 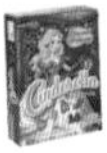	80	0	19
Fudge:			
Chocolate; Mint, 1 oz	130	8	14
P'nut Butter & Choc., 1 oz	130	8	13
Brevin's: Cashew, 1 oz 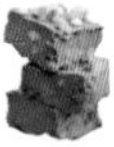	195	9	28
Triple Decker, 1 oz	165	7	25
Ghirardelli:			
3 oz Bars: Dark Choc., 4 squares	220	17	23
Filled, P'nut Butter, 4 squares	250	17	22
Intense Dark Bars, 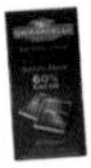			
Ev'ng Dream, 3 pcs	190	15	20
Squares: Dark Choc. (4)	210	16	23
Milk & Caramel (3)	220	12	27

Per Piece/Serving	C	F	Cb
Godiva: 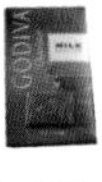			
Bars: Milk/Dark, av., 1.5 oz	230	14	26
Extra Dark: 75%, 1.5 oz	230	17	18
85%, 1.4 oz	260	21	14
Chocoiste: Dk Choc. Cherries (12)	190	7	30
Milk Chocolate Cashews (14)	230	15	19
Hearts: Dark Ganache (4) 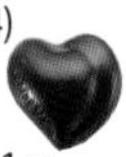	200	12	23
Milk Praline (4)	220	13	23
Go Lightly:			
Assorted Toffee, 5 pieces, 1 oz	85	2	24
Fruit Chews, 5 pieces, 1 oz	95	2	26
Hard Candy, Assorted (4), 0.5 oz	45	0	15
Note: Carb figures include 15-25g sugar alcohol			
Goobers Peanuts, 1 package, 1.4 oz	200	13	21
Good & Plenty *(Hershey's)*, (33), 1.8 oz	180	0	46
GooGoo Clusters, 1 piece, 1.8 oz	240	12	30
Gum ~ *See Page 75*			
Gum Drops: 1 small, 0.1 oz 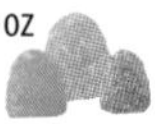	15	0	3
5 pieces, 0.5 oz	75	0	15
Gummi *(Shur Fine):* 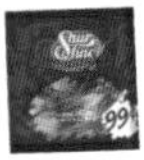			
Bears (15), 1.4 oz	130	0	29
Chewy Sweet Tarts (4)	160	0	36
Worms (9), 1.5 oz	140	0	31
Guylian:			
Bars: Dark Chocolate (3), 1 oz	150	12	11
Milk Choc. w/ Hazelnuts (3),1 oz	170	11	15
No Sugar Added Bars:			
Milk Chocolate, 3 squares	150	11	16
54% Cocoa, Dark Choc., 3 sqrs.	140	11	16
Seashells: 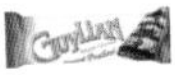			
Bar, 1.4 oz	210	13	21
Boxed, Originals (1), 0.4 oz	60	4	6
Truffles, (1), 0.4 oz	70	5.5	5
Heath: Original (1), 1.4 oz	210	13	24
King Size, 2.8 oz 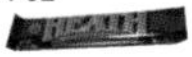	410	22	49
Miniatures, 4 pieces, 1 oz	150	9	17
Hershey's:			
Cookie Layer Crunch, 2, 1.4 oz	190	11	24
Cookies 'n' Creme: 1.55 oz Bar	230	12	28
Snack Size, 2 pieces, 0.95 oz	130	7	17
Milk Chocolate: 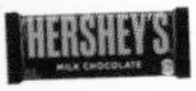			
Bars: 1.55 oz	220	13	26
with Almonds, 1 bar, 1.45 oz	210	14	20
Golden Almond			
Kisses, 7 pieces, av., 1.2 oz	160	9	19
Nuggets: Milk Choc., 3 pieces	150	9	19
with Almonds, 3 pcs, 1 oz	150	10	15
Special Dark Choc., 1.45 oz bar	200	13	24

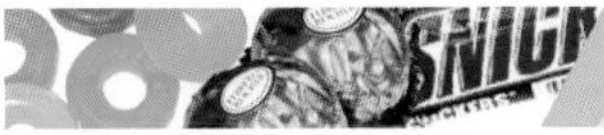

Candy ~ Brands & Generic (Cont)

Per Piece/Serving	C	F	Cb
Hershey's, (Cont):			
Candy-Coated Eggs, 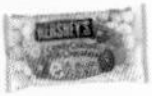			
Milk Chocolate, (5)	140	9	17
Pot of Gold Chocolate Asstd:			
Milk Choc: Carmel, 4 pieces, 1.4 oz	190	10	26
Av. other var., 4 pieces, 1.4 oz	210	12	24
Honeycomb: Plain, 1 oz	115	0	27
Choc-coated, 2 pieces	180	7	31
Hot Tamales, 20 pieces, 1.4 oz	150	0	36
Hugs ~ *See Kisses*			
Jawbreakers *(Sathers)*, (15), 0.6 oz	60	0	16
Jells *(Joyva)*, Raspb., 3 pieces, 1.6 oz	160	0	38
Jelly Beans, average all brands:			
Small Size (Jelly Belly): 1 bean	5	0	1
12 beans, 0.5 oz	50	0	13
Regular Size: 1 bean 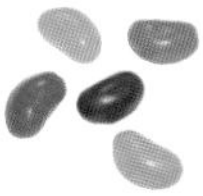	10	0	2
10 beans, 1 oz	105	0	26
Large Size: 1 bean	15	0	38
10 beans, 1.5 oz	150	0	38
Sugar Free, av. all brands, (25), 1 oz	60	0	26
Note: Carb figure include 26g sugar alcohol			
Jelly Belly: 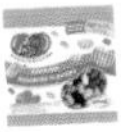			
25 beans, 1 oz	105	0	26
Sugar Free, 25 beans, 1 oz	60	0	26
Note: Carb figure include 26g sugar alcohol			
Chocolate Dips, all flavors:			
1 bean 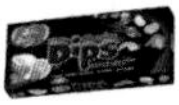	4	0	1
10 beans	40	1	8
2.8 oz bag	300	8	62
Jolly Rancher: 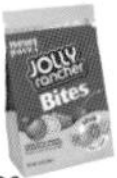			
Bites: Filled, 11 pieces	140	0	32
Sours, 16 pieces	130	0	34
Crunch 'N Chew, 1 oz pkg	160	0.5	40
Filled Fruity Bites, 22 pieces	140	1	31
Gummies, 9 pieces 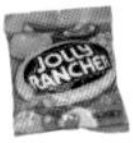	120	0	28
Hard Candy, 3 pieces	70	0	17
Jelly Beans/Sours, 1.4 oz	140	0	36
Lollipops (1), 0.55 oz	60	0	15
Triple Pop, 1 pop	80	0	19
Jujubes, all varieties (52), 1.4 oz	110	0	28
Juju Bears, 5 pieces	130	0	34
Juju Mix (Sathers), 11 pieces, 1.5 oz	150	0	36
Jujyfruits, 16 pieces, 1.4 oz	120	0	32
Junior Caramels: 13 pieces, 1.5 oz	190	6	33
Mini, 2 boxes, 1 oz	130	4	23
Junior Mints, 5 pieces 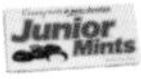	55	1	11

Per Piece/Serving	C	F	Cb
Justin's:			
Peanut Butter Cups: Dark Choc (1)	230	15	20
Milk Choc, (1)	230	15	20
Kinder Joy, 1 egg, 0.7 oz 	110	6	12
Kisses *(Hershey's):*			
Candy Cane Mint, (6)	140	8	18
Dark Chocolate, Mint Truffles (7)	160	10	19
Milk Chocolate: 1 Kiss 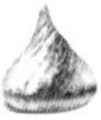	20	1	3
7 Kisses	160	9	19
With Almonds (7)	160	10	16
Filled with: Cherry Cordial (6)	120	5	19
Vanilla Creme (9)	210	13	24
Hot Cocoa (7) 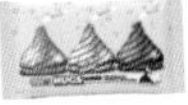	160	10	19
Hugs (9)	210	12	24
Kit Kat *(Hershey's):*			
Dark Chocolate: 1.5 oz pkg	200	12	27
Mint & Dark Chocolate, 1.5 oz pkg	210	12	27
Milk Chocolate: 4 pce bar, 1.5 oz	210	11	28
Miniatures (4), 1.2 oz 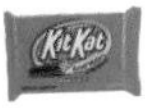	170	9	22
Snack Size (3), 1.5 oz	210	11	27
Apple Pie, 1.5 oz pkg	220	12	27
Halloween: 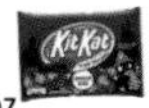			
1.5 oz package	210	11	28
White Choc., 1.48 oz	220	11	27
White Chocolate, Snack (3), 1.5 oz	220	11	27
Lemon Drops: (4), 0.6 oz	60	0	16
Walgreens, Sugar Free (3), 0.6 oz	50	0	17
Lemonhead, (26), 1.4 oz 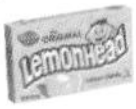	140	0	36
Lance, Peanut Bar, 2.2 oz	340	19	29
Licorice:			
Average all varieties, 1oz	100	0	25
Chews *(Panda)*, (1) 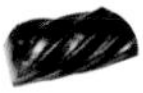	10	0	3
Tid Bits (1)	10	0	2
Twists: Black/Red, av., 1 pc	35	0	8
Sugar Free, 1 piece	15	0	2.5
American Licorice Co.:			
Natural Vines: Black (9), 1.4 oz	140	1	33
Strawberry (9), 1.4 oz	150	1	34
Red Vines (4), 1.4 oz	140	0	34
Sip-n-Chew, 1 oz package 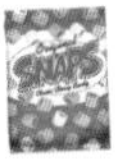	100	1	23
Snaps (31), 1.4 oz	140	0.5	33
Sour Punch (6), 1.4 oz	150	0.5	34
Super Ropes (1), 2 oz	200	0	46
Lifesavers: Large size, 1 candy	15	0	3
Regular: All flavors, 1 candy	10	0	3
1 Roll (14 candies), 1.2 oz	140	0	35
Creme Savers, 3 pcs, 0.5 oz 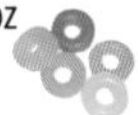	60	1	11
Fruit Splosion (10), 1.4 oz	130	0	31
Pep-o-mint: (3), 0.2 oz	20	0	5
Sugar-Free (4), 0.5 oz	35	0	14
Note: Carb figure includes 14g sugar alcohol			

Candy ~ Brands & Generic (Cont)

Per Piece/Serving	C	F	Cb
Lik-m-aid *(Nestle)*, Fun Dip, 1 package	50	0	13
Lindt:			
Dark Choc. Truffles, w filling, (7)	240	18	18
Lindor Truffles (1), average	75	6	5
Swiss Milk Chocolate Bars:			
70% Cocoa, 4 pieces	220	17	13
Classic, with Hazelnuts, 10 pieces	230	16	20
Raspberry filled, 7 pieces	200	10	25
Lollipops: Mini, 0.3 oz	25	0	6
Small, 0.5 oz	50	0	12
Medium, 1 oz	100	0	25
Giant (4" diam), 7 oz	790	0	198
M & M's:			
Dark Chocolate/Mint, 1.5 oz pkg	210	10	29
Milk Chocolate: 28 pieces, 1 oz	145	6.5	21
1.5 oz package	210	9	30
Minis, 1 tube, 1 oz	150	6	21
Almond, 1.5 oz	220	12	25
Coffee Nut, 1.1 oz	160	8	19
Crispy, 1.5 oz	200	7	31
Fudge Brownie, 11 pieces, 1 oz	140	6	20
Halloween, Popcorn Candy, 1 oz	130	5	21
Peanut 12 pieces, 1 oz	140	7	17
Peanut Butter, 1.62 oz pkg	240	13	26
Pretzel, 1.3 oz package	150	5	24
Red, Whie & Blue, 1 oz	140	5	20
White Chocolate, 1.5 oz pkg	210	11	29
Mamba Sours,			
Fruit Chews, 6 pieces, 1 oz	100	1	22
Marshmallow Egg, 1 egg, 1 oz	120	3	22
Mary Jane *(Necco)*, 5 pieces, 1.4 oz	160	3.5	32
Marshmallows: Firm/Soft, 1 oz	90	0	23
Regular size, 4 pieces, 1 oz	100	0	24
Mini-Marshmallow, 2/3 cup, 1 oz	95	0	24
Joyva, Choc-coated Twists	95	2	10
Fluff, 2 Tbsp, 0.6 oz	60	0	15
Kraft: Creme, 0.5 oz	45	0	11
Funmallows, 2/3 cup, 1 oz	100	0	24
Jet-Puffed, 5 pieces, 1 oz	100	0	24
Mini, 1 oz	90	0	23
Marzipan, 2 Tbsp, 1.4 oz	160	4	29
Mauna Loa, Mountains, 4 pcs	230	17	21
Mexican Hats, (7), 1.4 oz	120	0	30
Mentos: Regular	10	0	3
Sugar Free	5	0	2
Mike & Ike:			
Original: 2.1 oz package	220	0	55
23 pieces, 1.4 oz	140	0	36
Milk Duds, 1 box, 1.8 oz	230	8	38

Per Piece/Serving	C	F	Cb
Milky Way *(Mars)*:			
Bars: Single, 2 oz	240	9	37
Fun Size, 2 bars, 1.2 oz	160	6	24
To Go, 1.8 oz	230	9	36
Minis, 5 pieces, 1.5 oz	190	7	30
Midnight Bars: 1.8 oz	230	8	36
Minis, 5 pieces, 1.4 oz	190	7	30
Simply Caramel, 1.9 oz	250	11	37
Mints: *Average All Brands*			
1 mint , medium	7	0	1
1 large mint	15	0	3
Mon Cheri *(Ferrero)*, 4 pieces, 2 oz	260	18	20
Mounds: 1.75 oz bar	240	13	28
King Size, 4 pces, 3.5 oz	480	26	56
Snack Size, 1 piece, 0.6 oz	80	4.5	10
Mr Goodbar: 1.8 oz bar	250	17	26
King Size, 2.6 oz bar	380	26	38
Munch Bar, 1.4 oz	220	15	18
Necco, Candy Wafers (40), 2 oz	220	0	56
Nestle: Original,1.6 oz bar	220	11	30
Fun Size, 3 bars, 1.4 oz	180	9	26
Miniatures, 4 bars, 1.4 oz	200	10	27
Buncha Crunch, 1/3 cup, 1.2 oz	180	9	25
Crunch Crisp, 1.8 oz	240	13	32
Newman's Own:			
Milk Choc.: Caramel Cups (3)	160	8	21
Peanut Butter Cups (3)	180	12	17
Dark Choc.: Caramel Cups (3)	160	9	20
Peanut Butter Cups (3)	180	13	16
Nips, all varieties, 2 pieces, 0.5 oz	60	2	11
Nougat: 3 pieces, 1.5 oz	170	1	39
Chocolate Covered, 1 oz	125	4	22
Nutrageous Bar *(Reese's)*, 1.8 oz	260	16	28
Oh Henry!: Fun Size, 0.9 oz	120	5	16
1.8 oz bar	230	11	33
Orange Slices:			
Jewel, 3 pieces, 1.5 oz	140	0	35
Walgreens, 4 pieces, 1.6 oz	160	0	39
Oreo Choc. Candy Bars *(Milka)*:			
Regular, 1.44 oz bar	230	14	24
Big Crunch, 3.5 oz	550	35	57
Cookies & Creme, 1.44 oz bar	230	14	25
Fun Size, 2 pieces	170	10	18
Mint, 1.44 oz bar	230	13	24
Pastel Mints *(Walgreens)*, 20 pieces	60	0	14
PayDay Bar: 1.8 oz bar	240	13	27
King Size, 3.5 oz bar	440	24	50
Snack Size, 0.7 oz	90	5	10
Avalanche, 1.8 oz bar	250	13	29
Peanut Bar *(Planter's)*, 1.6 oz	240	14	21
Peanut Butter Cups ~ *See Reese's; Newman's Own*			
Peanut Brittle: 1 piece, 1.5 oz	190	5	32
Sugar Free (*Russell Stover*), 4 pieces, 1.3 oz	140	10	24

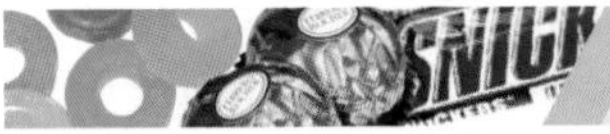

Candy ~ Brands & Generic (Cont)

Per Piece/Serving	C	F	Cb
Peanuts, choc-covered, 14 pieces	230	14	23
Pearson's, Mint Patties, (5), 1.3 oz	150	2.5	31
Peppermints: 7 small, 0.5 oz	60	0	15
Brach's, Star Brites (3)	60	0	16
Pez, 1 roll	35	0	9
Planters,			
Double Peanut Bar, 1.6 oz	240	14	21
Pop Rocks, 0.4 oz package	35	0	9
Pot of Gold *(Hershey's):*			
Assortment: Caramel, 4 pieces	190	10	25
Nut, 4 pieces	210	13	23
Pretzels: Choc-covered, Mini (6)	200	9	25
White Chocolate Bites (23), 1.4 oz	200	9	25
Pretzel Flipz *(Nestlé),* 8 pcs, 1 oz	130	5	20
Raisinets:			
Milk Choc: 1.58 oz pkg	190	8	32
Movie Pack, 3.5 oz	380	16	64
Dark Chocolate, 1/4 cup, 1.6 oz	180	8	32
Reese's:			
Peanut Butter Cups:			
Dark Chocolate, (2), 1.5 oz	210	14	23
Milk Choc:			
1.5 oz Pkg	210	12	24
Big Cup, King Size, 2.8 oz pkg	400	22	46
King Size (2), 1.4 oz	200	12	22
Minis, 2 packages, 1.23 oz	180	11	20
Snack Size (1), 0.8 oz	110	6	12
Crunchy, 1.4 oz pkg	220	13	22
Outrageous Stuffed,			
Snack Size (1), 0.7 oz	100	4.5	13
Pieces: 3 pieces, 0.9 oz	130	7	16
2 pkgs, 1.4 oz	210	12	25
Thins (3), 1.25 oz	170	10	20
White Cups, 1.5 oz pkg	220	13	23
Rice Krispies Treats *(Kellogg's),*			
1 bar, average all varieties, 0.8 oz	95	2.5	17
Riesen, Choc. Chew, 4 pcs, 1.3 oz	170	6	28
Rocky Road, Milk/Dark, 1.8 oz bar	240	11	34
Roca Thins, 3 pieces, av. all var.	210	14	24
Rolo:			
Regular, all var., 1.7 oz roll	220	10	33
Mini Chews, Caramel in milk choc. (11)	190	9	26
Root Beer Barrels, (3), 0.6 oz	60	0	17

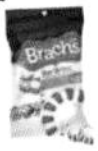

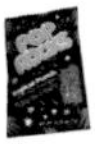

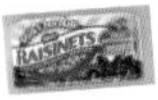

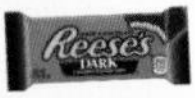

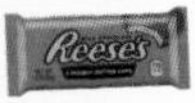

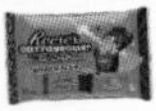

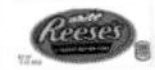

Per Piece/Serving	C	F	Cb
Russell Stover Candy:			
Boxed Chocolates Choc. Coated:			
Assorted (2), 1.2 oz	150	7	22
Cherry Cordials (3), 0.4 oz	150	5	25
Dairy Crm Caramels (2), 1.2 oz	160	7	22
Elegant Collection (3), 1.6 oz	210	10	25
French Choc. Mints (4), 1.4 oz	220	13	22
Nut, Chewy & Crisp Centers (2)	160	8	21
Sugar Free: Ass'td Hard Candies (3)	210	16	24
Bags: Caramel (3), 1.3 oz	180	8	25
Coconut (3), 1.5 oz	160	10	28
Mint Patty (3), 1.5 oz	180	12	26
Peanut Butter Cups (2), 1.2 oz	160	12	17
Pecan Delight (2), 1.2 oz	160	12	19
Note: Carbohydrate figures include sugar alcohol			
Salt Water Taffy *(Brach's),* (5)	170	2.5	36
Seashells *(Guylian),* (4), 1.6 oz	260	17	24
See's Candies:			
Almond Royal (5)	190	13	18
Butterscotch Chews (5)	210	12	27
Krispy's: Caffe Latte (5)	180	8	27
Mint (5)	170	8	27
Little Pops:			
Butterscotch (4), 0.5 oz	60	2	12
Av. other flavors (4)	55	3	10
Lollypops, average, 0.7 oz	90	3	17
Milk Molasses Chips (6), 1.4 oz	180	8	27
Milk Peppermints, 2 pieces, 1.3 oz	150	4	28
Peanut Brittle Bar, 1 oz	150	10	15
Peanut Butter Patties (2), 1.2 oz	170	10	16
Peppermint Twists, (3)	60	0	15
Toffee-ettes, 3 pieces	270	21	18
Sugar Free: Dark Bar, 1.5 oz	180	16	24
Dark Walnut Clusters (4), 1.5 oz	230	21	17
Peanut Brittle, 1.5 oz	170	14	17
Note: Carbohydrate figures include 12-18 g sugar alcohol			
Skinny Cow:			
Dreamy Clusters, all var., 1 pouch	120	6	20
Heavenly Crips, all varieties, 1 bar	110	6	14
Skittles:			
Original, 2 oz	230	2.5	52
Sour, 1.8 oz	200	2	44
Tropical; Wild Berry, 2.2 oz	250	2.5	56
Fun Size, 1 bag, 0.5 oz	60	1	14
Tear & Share, 4 oz bag	420	4.5	93
Skor, Toffee Bar (1), 1.4 oz	200	12	25
Smarties: Candy Rolls (1), 0.3 oz	25	0	6
Giant, 1 roll, 1 oz	100	0	25

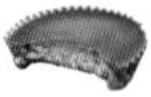

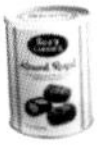

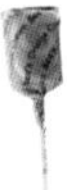

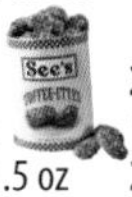

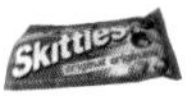

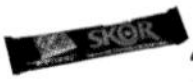

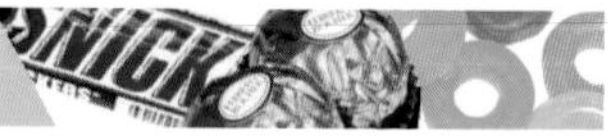

Candy ~ Brands & Generic (Cont)

Per Piece/Serving

	C	F	Cb
Snickers:			
Milk Chocolate Bar:			
Original, 1.9 oz bar 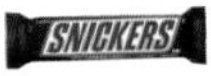	**250**	12	33
Fun Size, 2 bars, 1.2 oz	**160**	7	22
Minis, 3 pieces, 0.9 oz	**130**	6	17
Almond Bar, 1.8 oz 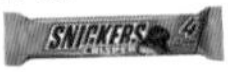	**230**	10	33
Crisper (2)	**190**	9	26
Crunchy Peanut Butter (2)	**250**	14	29
Hazelnut, 1 bar 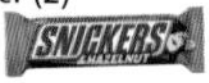	**240**	11	31
Sno Caps, ¼ cup, 1.4 oz	**180**	8	30
Soft 'N Chewy, Butter Toffee, 1 piece	**30**	0.5	5
Sorbee, Crystal Light Hard Candy (4)	**25**	0	13
Note: Carb figure includes Isomalt which has fewer calories than sugar.			
Sour Patch: Kids, average, 2 oz	**210**	0	52
Extreme, 1.8 oz	**190**	0	47
Spearmint Leaves: 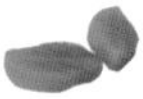			
Jewel, 5 pieces, 1.4 oz	**140**	0	35
Walgreens, 4 pieces, 1.6 oz	**160**	0	39
Spree Candies: Original, 15 pieces	**50**	0	13
Chewy, 8 pieces	**60**	0	13
Starburst: 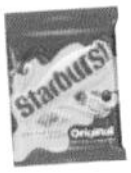			
Candy Canes, 0.5 oz	**70**	0	18
Fruit Chews: Original (1)	**20**	0.5	4
8 pieces, 1.4 oz	**160**	3.5	33
Gummibursts, 9 pieces, 1.4 oz	**130**	0	31
Jellybeans, 1.5 oz	**150**	0	37
Starlight Mints, 3 pieces, 0.5 oz	**60**	0	15
Suckers *(Walgreens),* 1 piece, 0.4 oz	**45**	0	11
Sugar Babies, Original, 1.4 oz	**160**	1.5	37
Sugar Coated Peanuts, 1 oz	**120**	8	10
Sunbursts Sunflowers *(Kimmie)*:			
ChocoRocks Milk, 3.5 oz	**525**	25	67
Habanero Corn, 3.5 oz	**500**	23	70
Sunburst Mix, Milk, 3.5 oz	**500**	28	55
Swedish Fish, 7 pieces, 1.5 oz	**150**	0	38
SweeTARTS: 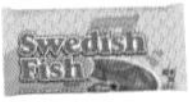			
Orig., 8 pieces, 0.5 oz	**50**	0	13
Mini Chewy, 23 pieces, 0.5 oz	**50**	0.5	12
Symphony *(Hershey's)*: 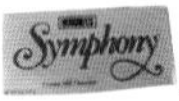			
Milk Choc: 1.5 oz bar	**220**	14	23
Large Block: 5 pieces, 1.4 oz	**200**	12	22
w/ Almond & Toffee, 5 pcs, 1.3 oz	**200**	13	21

Per Piece/Serving

	C	F	Cb
Taffy, Fruit Chews, 1 piece	**20**	0.5	4
Take 5 *(Hershey's)*: 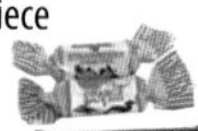			
Bars: Original, 1.5oz	**200**	11	25
King Size, 2.3 oz 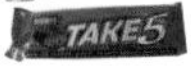	**300**	16	37
Snack Size, 2 pcs, 1 oz	**150**	8	19
3 Musketeers: 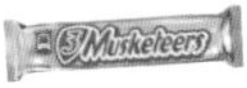			
Original, 1.9 oz	**240**	7	42
2 To Go, 1 bar, 1.6 oz	**200**	6	35
Fun Size, 3 bars, 1.6 oz 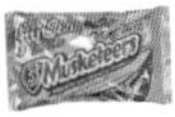	**190**	6	34
Minis, 7 pieces, 1.4 oz	**170**	5	32
Tang-a-Roos, 1 roll	**25**	0	6
Terry's:			
Chocolate Orange (5), 1.5 oz	**230**	12	27
Dark Chocolate Orange (5), 1.5 oz	**240**	13	28
Tic Tac, all flavors, 1 piece	**2**	0	0
Toblerone: 1.23 oz bar	**190**	10	22
Pieces, 5.3 oz pkg, 5 pieces, 1.5 oz	**230**	13	27
Fruit & Nut, ⅓ bar, 1.2 oz	**170**	8	21
Dark/White Chocolate, ⅓ bar 1.2 oz	**180**	10	20
Toffees, Regular, 1 oz	**160**	9	18
Tootsie Pops, (1), 0.6 oz	**60**	0	15
Tootsie Roll: 2.25 oz roll 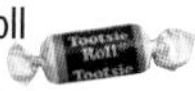	**220**	5	45
Midgees, 1.4 oz	**140**	3	28
Truffles: Reg., 1 piece, 0.4 oz	**60**	4	6
Large *(Godiva),* 0.8 oz	**110**	6.5	12
Extra Large *(J.Schmidt),* 1.5 oz	**220**	13	24
Turtles: Original, 1 piece, 0.6 oz	**85**	5	10
Sugar Free, 1 piece, 0.4 oz	**50**	3.5	7
Twists, Licorice; Strawb., sugar free, 7 pieces, 1.4 oz	**90**	0	25
Twix: 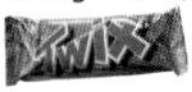			
Caramel: 2 cookies, 1.8 oz	**250**	12	34
Fun Size, 1 cookie, 0.6 oz	**80**	4	11
4 To Go, 1 cookie, 0.8 oz	**110**	5	15
Minis, 3 pieces, 1 oz	**150**	7	20
Milk Chocolate, Bites, 5 pcs, 1 oz	**140**	7	18
White Chocolate, 2 cookies, 1.6 oz	**110**	12	29
Twizzlers:			
Cherry Bites, (13), 1.4 oz	**110**	0.5	25
Cherry Twists, 3 pieces, 1.2 oz	**120**	0.5	27
Pull 'n' Peel, Cherry, 1 piece, 1.2 oz	**110**	0.5	26
Twists, Strawberry, 1 twist	**25**	0	6
Watermelon Soft Bites, 11 pieces	**150**	1.5	33
U-No Bar, 1.5 oz	**250**	17	22
Weight Watchers *(Whitman's)*:			
Caramel Medallions, (3)	**160**	9	24
Coconut, (3)	**150**	9	23
English Toffee Squares, (3)	**150**	9	21
Mint Patties, (3) 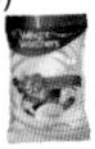	**150**	9	23
Peanut Butter Cups, (4)	**180**	8	31
Pecan Crowns, (3)	**160**	10	24

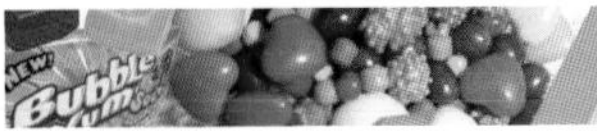

Candy ~ Brands & Generic (Cont)

Per Piece/Serving

	C	F	Cb
Werther's:			
Hard Candy: Original (3), 0.5 oz	70	1.5	14
Sugar-Free Original (5)	40	1.5	15
Note: Carb figure includes 14g sugar alcohol			
Soft, Chocolate Caramel (4), 1.4 oz	190	8	28
Whatchamacallit: 1.5 oz Bar	230	12	28
King Size Bar, 2.5 oz	370	20	45
Whitman's:			
Boxed Chocolates: Sampler (4)	220	12	27
12 oz Box, 3 pieces, 1.2 oz	170	9	21
Reserve, 7 oz Box, 2 pieces, 1.2 oz	160	9	21
Sugar Free, 10 oz Box, 3 pcs, 1.5 oz	190	13	25
Whoppers, av. all varieties, 18 pcs	190	7	31
Wonka:			
Bar, 2.5 oz	360	19	49
Exceptional Bars, average, 4 pieces	200	13	23
Gobstopper, 9 pieces, 0.5 oz	60	0	14
Laffy Taffy: Ropes, all var., 0.8 oz	80	1.5	18
Stretchy & Tangy, all var., 1.5 oz	150	3.5	29
Nerds, Giant, Chewy, 1.8 oz package	180	0	42
Yogurt Candy, Coated Raisins, 1.4 oz	180	8	28
York: Mints, (3)	10	0	3
Peppermint Pattie, reg, 1.4 oz	140	2.5	31
Pieces (50)	170	8	28
Zagnut, 1.75 oz bar	220	9	35
Zero Bar: 1.8 oz bar	230	8	37
King Size, 3.5 oz	400	14	68

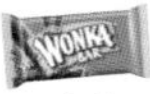
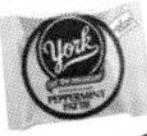
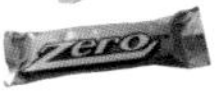

Gum

Per Piece

	C	F	Cb
Bazooka	15	0	4
Beechies	6	0	2
Big League Chews	10	0	2
Bubble Yum: Original	25	0	6
Sugarless	10	0	3
Candilicious	30	0	2
Carefree, Sugarless/Regular	5	0	2
Chiclet	5	0	1
Dentyne	5	0	0.5
Double Bubble Ball	20	0	5
Estee, Bubble/Regular	5	0	2
Extra *(Wrigley's)*, Sugar-Free	5	0	2
Freshen-Up	10	0	3
Hubba Bubba: Regular	25	0	6
Sugar-free, average	14	0	0.5
Ice Breakers	5	0	2
Jolt Gum	5	0	2
Super Bubble	15	0	4
Trident, Orig.; White	5	0	1
Wrigley's, all flavors	10	0	2

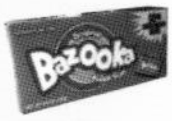
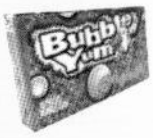
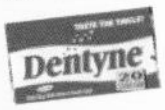
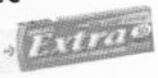
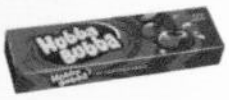
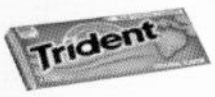

Updated Nutrition Data ~ www.CalorieKing.com
Persons with Diabetes ~ See Disclaimer (Page 22)

Carob Candy

Per Piece/Serving

	C	F	Cb
Carob, Plain/Natural, 1 oz	155	9	15
Carob Coated: Raisins, 1 oz	130	8	15
Almonds/Peanuts, 1 oz	150	10	14
Caramels, 1 oz	110	4	18
Dates, 1 oz	125	5	20
Malt Balls, 1 oz	135	8	15
Soybeans	145	9	16
Trail/Party Mix, 1 oz	150	9	15

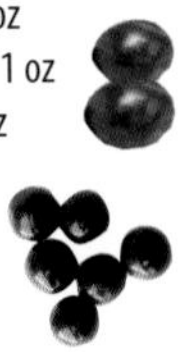

Cough Drops

Per Drop/Piece

	C	F	Cb
Beech Nut, 1 drop	10	0	2
CVS, Honey Lemon Cough Drops	15	0	4
Diabetic Tussin	0	0	0
Halls, Defense Vitamin C:			
Regular	15	0	4
Sugar Free	5	0	3
Fruit Breezers	15	0	4
Menthol Drops: Regular	15	0	4
Sugar Free	5	0	4
Plus	20	0	5
Listerine *(Amer. Chicle)*, Lozenge	10	0	2
Luden's, Throat Drops: Reg., all var.	10	0	2
Sugar Free	0	0	0
Pine Bros, Cough Drops	10	0	2
Ricola:			
Cough Drops:			
Natural Herbs	10	0	3
Sugar-Free Lemon Mint	0	0	1
Rolaids, Sodium Free	5	0	1
Sathers, Peppermint Lozenges	15	0	3
Sucrets *(Beecham)*, Lozenges	10	0	2.5
Wintergreen, Lozenges	15	0	3

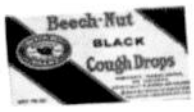
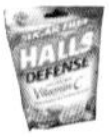
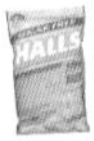
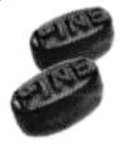
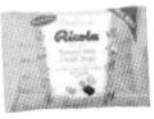
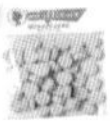

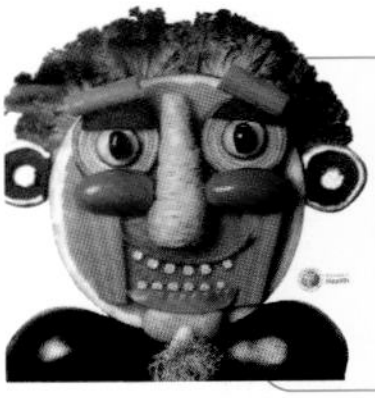

Eat at least 5 servings of fruit and vegetables every day . . . and Enjoy Better Health!

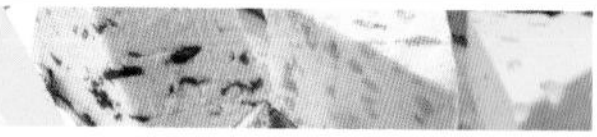

Quick Guide

Firm/Hard Cheeses

American, Cheddar, Jack, Swiss:
Average All Brands

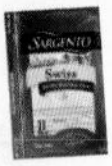
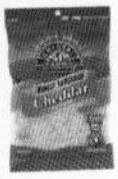

	C	F	Cb
Regular Cheese:			
Thin Deli slice, 0.8 oz	80	6	0.5
1 oz slice/piece	110	9	0.5
8 oz package	880	72	3
Cubes: 1" cube, 0.6 oz	70	5.5	0.5
1¼" cube, 1 oz	115	9	0.5
Diced, 1 cup, 4.5 oz	510	41	3
Melted, ¼ cup, 2 oz	245	20	1
Shredded: ¼ cup, 1 oz	110	9	0.5
1 cup, 4 oz	440	36	2

Cheese & Cheese Products

Per 1 oz Unless Indicated

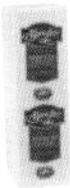
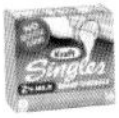
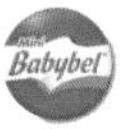
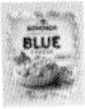
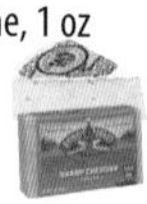

	C	F	Cb
Almond, *(Lisanatti)*, Chunks/Shreds, av.	70	4	3
American:			
Regular: 1 slice, 1 oz	105	9	0.5
Borden, Singles, 0.67 oz slice	70	4.5	2
Kraft, Singles, 0.67 oz slice	50	3.5	2
Land O'Lakes, Yellow, 0.67 oz slice	70	6	1
Reduced Fat:			
Alpine Lace, Yellow/White, 1 oz	90	6	2
Kraft, 2% Milk, 0.67 oz	45	2.5	2
Land O Lakes, White, 2% Milk, 1 oz	90	6	2
Babybel *(Laughing Cow)*, Mini:			
Original (1), 0.75 oz	70	6	0
Light (1), 0.75 oz	50	3	0
Gouda (1), 0.75 oz	70	6	0
White Cheddar (1), 0.75 oz	70	6	6
Blue/Bleu: Average all Brands			
Crumbled, ¼ cup, 1 oz	100	8	0
Castello, Blue Danish, 1 oz	110	10	0
Light, 0.8 oz	35	1.5	2
Brie: Average, 1 oz	95	8	0
Alouette, Original Creme, 1 oz	100	9	1
Camembert, 1 oz	85	7	0
Caraway, 1 oz	105	8	1
Cheddar:			
Regular: Medium/Sharp, av., 1 oz	110	9	1
Shredded, ¼ cup, 1 oz	110	9	1
Cracker Barrell: Extra Sharp, 1 oz	110	10	0
Vermont Sharp White, 1 oz	110	10	0

Cheese & Cheese Products (Cont)

Per 1 oz Unless Indicated

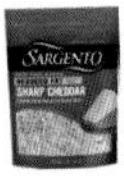
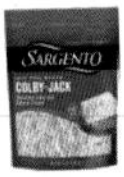
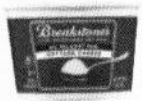
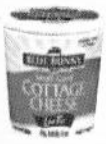

	C	F	Cb
Cheddar (Cont):			
Reduced Fat, 2% Milk, *Kraft,* Shredded, 1 oz	90	6	2
Curds, Cheddar Cheese,			
Cheese Curds ~ *See Cottage Cheese*			
Cheese Logs *(Kaukauna)*, average	100	7	4
Cheez Whiz ~ *See Dips*			
Cheshire, 1 oz	110	9	1.5
Colby, Regular, 1 oz	110	8	0
Colby-Jack:			
Big Slice, 0.8 oz	90	7	0
Cottage Cheese (Curds): *Average All Brands*			
Creamed (4% milk fat):			
2 Tbsp, 1 oz	30	1	1.5
½ cup, 4 oz	110	5	4
with fruit, ½ cup, 4 oz	115	4	5
Reduced-Fat (2%): 2 Tbsp, 1 oz	25	0.5	1
½ cup, 4 oz	100	3	4
Low-Fat (1%): 2 Tbsp, 1 oz	20	0.5	1
½ cup, 4 oz	80	1	3
Fat-Free/Non-Fat: 2 T., 1 oz	20	0	1
½ cup, 4 oz	80	0	5

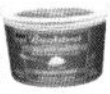
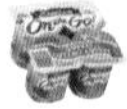
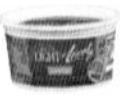
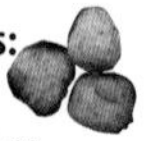

	C	F	Cb
Cottage Cheese (Curds): *Brands*			
Friendship:			
1% Low-Fat with Pineapple, 5 oz	120	1.5	12
Nonfat with Pineapple, ½ cup, 4 oz	110	0	18
Pot Style, 2%, ½ cup, 4 oz	100	2.5	4
Hood, Low Fat, 4 oz	90	1.5	5
Knudsen/Breakstone's:			
Free, Non-Fat, ½ cup, 4.25 oz	80	0	8
2% Milk Fat, ½ cup, 4 oz	90	2.5	6
On the Go!, Low-Fat, 4 oz carton	90	2.5	7
Lactaid, 4% Lowfat, ½ cup, 4 oz	110	5	5
Light n' Lively:			
Fat-Free, ½ cup, 4.4 oz	80	0	8
Low-Fat, ½ cup, 4.4 oz	80	1.5	6
Breaded & Fried Curds:			
A&W, 5 oz	570	40	27
Culver's, Wisconsin, 5.3 oz	510	25	51

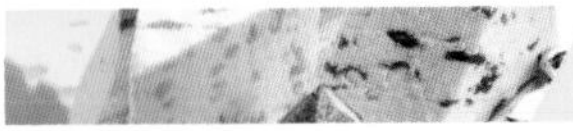

Cheese & Cheese Products (Cont)

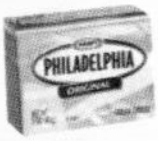

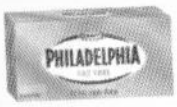

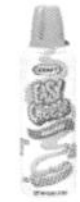

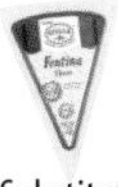

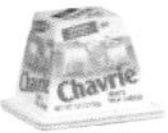

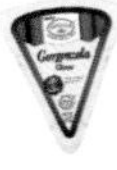

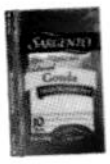

Per 1 oz Unless Indicated	C	F	Cb
Cream Cheese: *Average All Brands*			
Regular/Soft:			
2 Tbsp, 1 oz	95	10	1
3 oz package	290	29	3.5
8 oz package	780	78	9
Light, Plain, 1 oz	60	4.5	2.5
Fat-Free, Plain, 1 oz	30	0	2
Better Than Cream Cheese (Tofutti),			
all varieties, 1 oz	85	5	9
Easy Cheese *(Kraft),*			
American, 2 Tbsp, 1.2 oz	80	6	2
Edam, 1 oz	100	8	0.5
Farmer, Low-Fat, 1 oz	40	2.5	0
Feta: Regular, 1 oz	75	6	1
Crumbled, ½ cup, 2.5 oz	190	15	3
Athenos, Reduced-Fat,			
1 oz	50	3	1
Fontina, 2 Tbsp, 1 oz	110	9	0.5
Galaxy, Go Vegan Cheese Substitute:			
Grated Parmesan Flavor, 2 tsp, 0.2 oz	20	1	3
Slices: Cheddar, 1 slice, 0.6 oz	40	3	0.5
Mozzarella, 1 slice, 0.6 oz	40	2.5	0.5
Goat's Milk Cheese:			
Chevre: Original, 2 Tbsp	80	7	0
Semi-Soft, 1 oz	100	8.5	1
Hard, 1 oz	130	10	0.5
Chavrie, Logs:			
Original, 2 Tbsp, 1 oz	80	7	0
Honey, 1 oz	80	5	6
Sundried Tomato & Garlic, 1 oz	80	6	2
Gjetost, fresh, 1 oz	130	8	12
Myzithra, grated, 1 oz	80	4	2
Gorgonzola, 1 oz	100	8	0.5
Galbani, Dolcelatte, 1 oz	95	8	1
Gouda, 1 oz slice	100	8	0.5
Gruyere, 1 oz	115	9	1
Havarti *(Sargento),* 0.7 oz	80	6	0
Jarlsberg: Average, 1 oz	100	8	0
Reduced Fat, shredded, 1 oz	70	3.5	0
Labneh, (Lebanese Cream Chse), 1.8 oz	70	4	4

Cheese & Cheese Products (Cont)

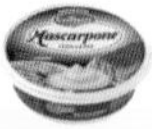

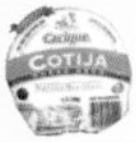

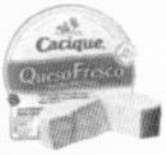

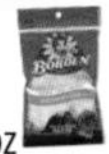

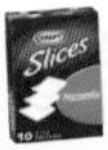

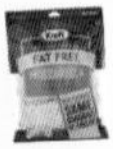

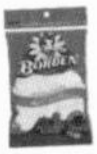

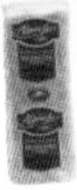

Per 1 oz Unless Indicated	C	F	Cb
Laughing Cow, Wedges:			
Creamy Asiago (1)	30	1.5	1
Creamy: Original (1)	50	4	1
Light (1)	30	1.5	1
Lifetime, Cholesterol Reducing,			
Fat Free, all varieties, 1 Slice, 1 oz	40	0	1
Limburger, 1 oz	95	8	0
Mascarpone, av., 1 oz	125	13	0.5
Mexican:			
Cacique: Asadero, sliced	70	4.5	1
Cotija	90	7	0
Enchilado; Manchego	90	7	0
Panela	80	8	0
Queso Blanco Fresco	80	6	0
Queso Quesadilla	90	7	0
Ranchero	80	6	0
Chi-Chi's, Salsa Con Quéso, Mild	45	3	4
El Mexicano: Cotija, 1 oz	90	6	0
Oaxaca, 1 oz	90	7	1
Kraft, Mexican Four Cheese; Taco,			
Shredded,	100	8	1
Sargento, 4 Cheese Mexican	110	9	2
Supremo, Quéso Chihuahua, 1 oz	100	8	0
Verole, Quéso Oaxaca, 1 oz	80	6	1
Monterey Jack:			
Regular, shredded, 1 oz	100	8	1
Land O Lakes, Co-Jack, 0.7 oz	80	7	0
Kraft, 1" cube, 1 oz	100	8	0
Mozzarella:			
Whole Milk: Average 1 oz	85	6.5	0.5
Land O'Lakes, String, 1 oz	80	6	2
Polly-O, Slice, average, 1 oz	80	6	1
Fat-Free,			
Kraft, Shredded, 1 oz	45	0	2
Reduced Fat,			
Kraft, 2% Milk Fat, Shredded, 1 oz	80	4	2
Part Skim:			
Borden, Shredded, 1 oz	90	6	2
Kraft, Shredded, 1 oz	80	5	2
Kraft, String, 1 oz	80	5	1
Polly-O, Shredded, 1 oz	80	5	0
Muenster:			
Alpine Lace, 1 oz slice	100	9	0
Wisconsin, 1 oz slice	100	8	0

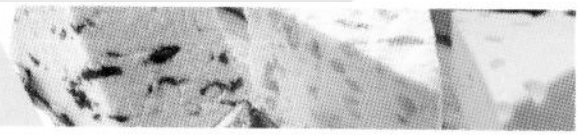

Cheese & Cheese Products (Cont)

Per 1 oz Unless Indicated	C	F	Cb
Parmesan:			
Fresh/Block, Dry, 1 oz 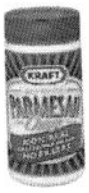	110	7.5	1
Grated (Packaged): 2 tsp	20	1.5	0
½ cup, 1.8 oz	215	14	2
Kraft: Shaker Bottle, 1 oz	110	8	1
Reduced-Fat Topping, 1 Tbsp	20	1	2
Philadelphia:			
Cream Cheese Brick:			
Original: 1 oz 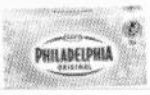	100	10	0.5
8 oz package	800	80	4
⅓ Less Fat, 1 oz	70	6	0.5
Flavored Spread:			
Chive & Onion, 1 oz	80	7	2
Cracked Pepper & Olive Oil, 1.1 oz	70	6	2
Smoked Salmon, 1.1 oz	70	5	2
Strawberry, 1.1 oz	80	6	5
⅓ Less Fat: Plain, 2 T., 1 oz	70	5	3
Neufchatel, 2 T., 1 oz 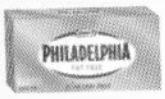	70	6	1
Fat-Free, Plain, 1 oz	30	0	3
Cheesecake Filling, 3 oz	240	17	18
Milk/White Chocolate:			
2 Tbsp, 1.27 oz 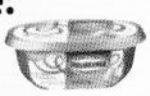	110	6	13
Dark Chocolate, 2 T., 1.23 oz	100	5	11
Whipped:			
Plain, 0.77 oz 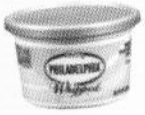	50	4	2
Mixed Berry, 0.77 oz	50	3	5
Port de Salut, 1 oz	100	8	0
Port Wine *(Kaukauna/WisPride):*			
10 oz Ball, 1 oz	100	7	5
10 oz Log, 2 Tbsp, 1 oz 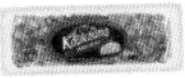	100	7	5
11.3 oz Tub, 0.85 oz	80	6	3
Provolone: Regular, 1 oz	100	7.5	0.5
Alpine Lace, Reduced-Fat, 1 oz	80	6	1
Sargento, 1 slice, 0.67 oz	70	5	0
Pub *(President)*, average all varieties	75	7	1
Quark: 40% fat 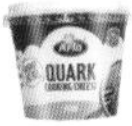	45	3	1
20% fat	30	1.5	1
Skim/Non-Fat	20	0	1.5
Rice Cheese Chunks *(Lisanatti),*			
average, 1 oz	60	3	2

Cheese & Cheese Products (Cont)

Per 1 oz Unless Indicated	C	F	Cb
Ricotta Cheese:			
Whole Milk: 1 oz 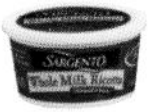	50	3.5	1
½ cup, 4.5 oz	215	16	4
Part Skim: 1 oz 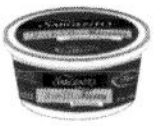	40	2	1.5
½ cup, 4.5 oz	170	10	6
Light/Low-Fat: 1 oz	25	1	1.5
½ cup, 4.5 oz 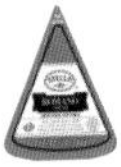	125	5	6
Fat-Free, ½ cup, 4.5 oz	100	0	10
Baked Ricotta, 2 oz	130	9	3
Romano: Block/Loaf	110	8	1
Grated: 1 oz 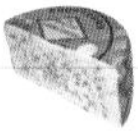	120	9	1
1 Tbsp, 0.2 oz	20	1.5	0
Roquefort, 1 oz	105	9	0.5
Sheep's Milk, (Manchego),			
Trader Joes/Wegman's, 1 oz	120	10	0
Soy Cheese:			
Trader Joe's, Mozzarella Style, 1 oz	70	4	3
Soya Kaas: Cheddar, 1 oz	50	2	8
Monterey Jack, 1 oz 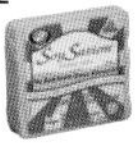	60	4	0
Soy Sation, Cheddar,			
1 slice, 0.67 oz	50	4	2
Smoked Cheddar, average, 1 oz	110	10	0
Stilton, average, 1 oz 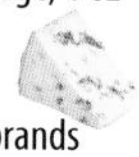	110	10	0
String:			
Regular, average all brands	80	6	0.5
Kraft: Twists/Strings,			
Mozzarella & Cheddar (1), 0.75 oz	60	4	0
Frigo, 1 oz 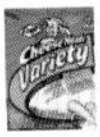	80	6	1
Light/Lite:			
Polly-O, String,			
2% Red-Fat, 1 oz 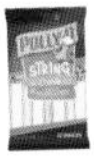	70	4.5	0
Sargento: 1 piece, 1 oz	80	6	1
Light, , 0.75 oz	50	2.5	1
Swiss: Regular, 1 oz	110	8	1.5
Alpine Lace, Reduced-Fat, 1 oz	90	6	1
Kraft, Slim Cut 2% Milk, 3 slices, 1.2 oz	110	7	0
Tilsit, 1 oz	100	7.5	0.5
Tofutti, Better Than Cream Cheese,			
all flavors, 2 Tbsp	60	5	2
Tybo, 1 oz	100	7	0.5
Velveeta *(Kraft)*: *Per Slice*			
Original, 0.74 oz	40	2	3
3 Cheese Blend, 0.74 oz	40	2	3
Jalapeno, 0.74 oz	40	2	3
Queso Blanco, Mild, 0.74	40	2	3

Dips/Spreads

Per 2 Tbsp, 1 oz, Unless Indicated

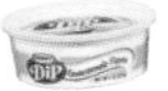
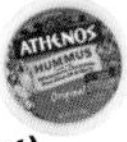
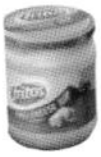
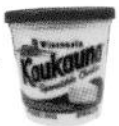
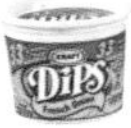
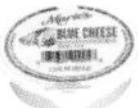
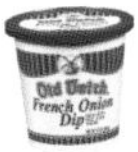

	C	F	Cb
Average All Brands			
Avocado/Guacamole	45	4	2
Baba Ghanoush (Eggplant/Sesame)	70	6	2
Cheese Fondue, ½ cup, 4 oz	260	15	4
French Onion Dip	60	4.5	3
Hummus: 2 Tbsp	50	1	5
½ cup, 4.5 oz	220	4.5	23
Tzatziki (Cucumber/Yogurt)	30	2.5	2
Clearman's, Original Spread	150	16	0
De La Casa, 5 Layer Party Dip	45	2.5	4
Fritos: *Per 2 Tbsp*			
Dips: Bean; Hot Bean w/ Jalapeno	35	1	5
Jalapeno Cheddar Cheese	40	2.5	3
Mild Cheddar	40	3	3
Great Value *(Walmart)*:			
Cheddar Jalapeno	60	4.5	4
Original Cheddar Cheese Dip	80	7	5
Melt & Dip, Easy Melt Cheese, 1 oz	80	6	3
Guiltless Gourmet,			
Black Bean/Spicy Black Bean Dip	40	0	7
Heluva Good Cheese,			
Jalapeno Cheddar; White Chedd. Bacon	60	4.5	3
Kaukauna *(Wisconsin)*:			
Spreadable Cheddar,			
Sharp/Smokey Cheddar	80	6	3
Kemps: *Per 2 Tbsp*			
Dips: French Onion; Ranch Style	60	5	2
Top The Tater,			
Taco Fiesta; Veggie Ranch, av.	60	5	3
Kroger, Dips, all varieties	60	5	2
Kraft: *Per 2 Tbsp*			
Dips: Average all varieties	60	5	3
Cheez Whiz: Orig., 1.2 oz	80	5	6
Salsa Con Queso ~ See Velveeeta			
Spreads: Light Cheez Whip, 1 Tbsp	30	1.5	2
Pimento, 1.1 oz	80	6	3
Old English Sharp; Roka Blue, av	90	7	0.5
Marie's: *Per 1.5 oz Cup,*			
Dips: Blue Cheese	250	27	1
Creamy Ranch	270	29	1
Marzetti:			
Dips: Chocolate Fruit, 2 oz Tub	180	2	36
Classic Caramel, 1.25 oz	140	4.5	24
Veggie: Dill; Ranch, 1.1 oz	80	7	2
French Onion; Spinach, 1.1 oz	80	7	3
Southwest Ranch, 1 oz	110	10	2
Old Dutch:			
Dips: French Onion, 1 oz	50	3	5
Mild Cheddar, 1 oz	40	3	2
Nacho Cheese, 1 oz	35	2.5	2

Dips/Spreads (Cont)

Per 2 Tbsp, 1 oz, Unless Indicated

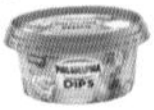
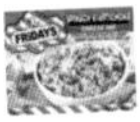
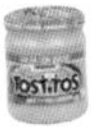
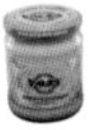

	C	F	Cb
On The Border,			
Dip, Salsa Con Queso, 2 Tbsp	45	3	4
Philadelphia: *Per 2 Tbsp, 1 oz*			
Dips:			
Buffalo Style with Celery	50	4	1
Caramelised Onion & Herb	60	5	2
Jalapeno & Cheddar,	70	6	2
Spinach & Artichoke	70	5	3
Spreads: Chive & Onion,	80	7	2
Honey Butter Cream Cheese	70	5	4
Whipped Mixed Berry, 0.78 oz	50	3	5
Price's: *Per 2 Tbsp*			
Dips: Fiesta; Green Chili, 1 oz	60	6	2
French Onion; Ranch Style, av., 1 oz	60	5.5	2
Spreads: French Onion, 1 oz	60	6	2
Pimiento Cheese , 1.1 oz	90	7	4
Stop & Shop: *Per 2 Tbsp*			
Dips: Veggie	100	10	3
Sour Cream French Onion	60	4.5	2
TGI Fridays,			
Spinach & Artichoke Cheese Dip, 1 oz	30	2	2
Toby's: Blue Cheesse Dip, 2 Tbsp	140	15	1
Honey Mustard, 2 Tbsp	120	10	5
Tostitos: *Per 2 Tbsp*			
Dips: Avocado Salsa, 1 oz	45	4	1
Salsa con Queso, 1.16 oz	40	2.5	5
Southwest Cheese & Corn, 1.3 oz	50	2.5	5
Wise: *Per 2 Tbsp*			
Dips: French Onion, 1.16 oz	60	5	3
Salsa con Queso, 1.2 oz	45	3	3

New Diet Aid
- The Refrigerator Air Bag!

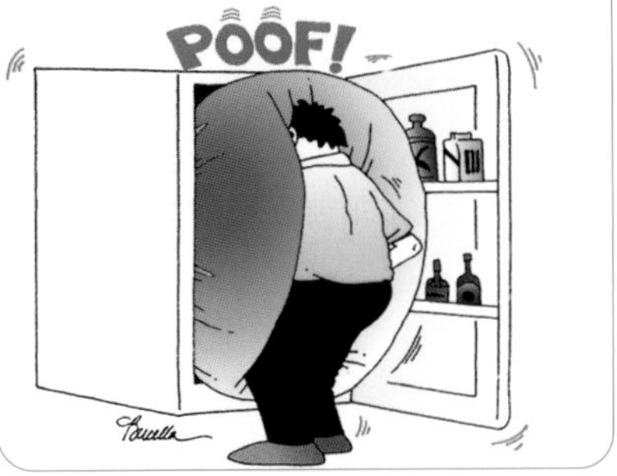

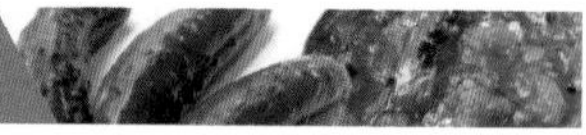

Condiments, Sauces

Average of Brands & Homemade	C	F	Cb
Apple Sauce:			
Sweetened, ¼ cup, 2.5 oz	55	0	13
Unsweetened, ¼ cup, 2 oz	25	0	7
Barbecue Sauce:			
Regular, av. all flavors, 2 Tbsp, 1 oz	40	0	10
Bull's Eye, Original, 1 oz	60	0	14
Bearnaise Sauce, ¼ cup, 2.5 oz	190	19	5
Buffalo Wing Sce: Hon. Mustard, 1 T.	40	3	3
Average other varieties, 1 Tbsp	25	2	2
Cheese, h/made, 1/4 cup, 2.5 oz	150	10	12
Chef-Mate, Hot Dog, ¼ cup	70	2.5	9
Chili Sauce *(Heinz)*, 1 Tbsp	20	0	5
Cocktail Sauce: ¼ cup	110	0	15
Walden Farms, Fat-Free, 1 Tbsp	0	0	0
Cranberry Sauce, av. all varieties: 2 T.	45	0	11
¼ cup, 2.5 oz	110	0	27
Demi Glaze Gold, 2 tsp	30	0.5	3
Honey Mustard *(French's)*, 2 Tbsp	60	0.5	12
Horseradish: 1 tsp	2	0	0
Kraft, 1 tsp	15	1.5	1
Ketchup: Regular, 1 Tbsp	15	0	4
Heinz: Reduced Sugar, 1 Tbsp	5	0	1
Simply Heinz, 1 Tbsp	15	0	4
Mole:			
Dona Maria, av. all varieties., 2 T.	150	10	10
Rogelio Bueno, 2 Tbsp, 1 oz	160	11	12
Mushroom Sce, ½ cup, 2 oz	50	2	5
Mustard, average, 1 tsp	5	0	0.5
Pesto Sauce, ¼ cup, 2 oz	270	28	2
Pizza Sauce, ¼ cup, 2 oz	30	0	6
Seafood Cocktail Sce, ¼ cup	60	0	15
Soy Sauce: Average all, 1 Tbsp	10	0	1
Kikkoman, Lite Soy, 1 Tbsp	10	0	1
Spaghetti Sce, ½ cup, 4.5 oz	135	6	19
Steak Sauce:			
Kraft, A1, 1 Tbsp, 0.5 oz	15	0	3
Lea & Perrins, 1 Tbsp, 0.5 oz	20	0	5
Strawb. Puree Sauce, Unsweet., 2 T.	10	0	2
Sweet & Sour Sauce:			
Contadina, 1.2 oz	40	1	8
Kraft, 1 Tbsp	60	0	13
Tabasco Sauce, 1 tsp	2	0	0
Taco Sauce, average all, 2 Tbsp, 1 oz	10	0	1
Tartar Sauce: *(Heinz)*, 2 Tbsp, 1 oz	120	11	4
Hellmann's, Regular, 2 Tbsp, 1 oz	80	7	4
McCormick, Fat-Free, 2 Tbsp, 1 oz	30	0	7
Teriyaki Sauce *(Kikkoman)*, 1 T., 0.5 oz	15	0	2
Vinegar, White or Wine, 2 T.	4	0	1
White Sauce, ½ cup, 5 oz	130	7	10
Worcestershire Sauce, 1 tsp	5	0	1

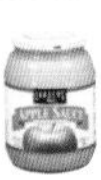
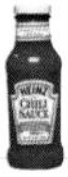
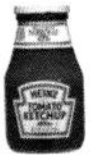
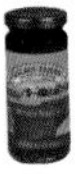
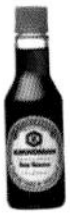
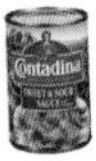
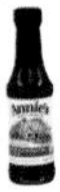

Pickles & Relish

Average All Brands	C	F	Cb
Bread & Butter Pickles, 4 sl.,1 oz	25	0	6
Chutney, 2 Tbsp, 1.25 oz	50	0.5	11
Dill Pickles:			
Slices, 4 slices, 1 oz	4	0	1
1 large, (3¾"x 1¼" diam.), 2.25 oz	12	0	3
Extra large (4"x 1¾" diam.), 5 oz	30	0	6
Halves: Small, 1 oz	3	0	0.5
Large, 2.5 oz	8	0	2
Gherkins, sweet, 1 medium, 1 oz	30	0	7
Green Chiles, chopped, 2 Tbsp	5	0	1
Horseradish, 1 Tbsp	10	0	2
Jalapenos, pickled (2), 2 oz	10	0.5	2
Jalapeno Relish, 1 Tbsp, 0.5 oz	5	0	1
Mustard, av. all brands, 1 tsp	5	0	0.5
Peppers, Hot/Mild (1), 1.5 oz	20	0	4
Pickled: Beets, ½ cup, 4 oz	75	0	19
Cocktail Onion, 1 onion	2	0	0
Red Cabbage, ½ cup, 3 oz	65	0	15
Pickles: Sweet, 2 Tbsp, 1 oz	35	0	8
Large (3" x ¾ diam.),1.25 oz	40	0	10
Pickle in a Pouch, 1 large	12	0	3
Relishes:			
Cranberry-Orange, 1 Tbsp	30	0	7
Hot Dog *(Heinz)*, 1 T., 0.5 oz	17	0	3
S'wich Spread, 1 tsp	20	1	5
Sweet Pickle, 1 Tbsp, 0.5 oz	20	0	5
Sweet Cauliflower, 1 oz	35	0	8
Sugar Free Relish, 1 tsp	5	0	1
Sweet Gherkins (2), 1 oz	5	0	1
Sauerkraut,			
Drained, 1 cup, 5 oz	25	0	6

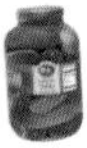
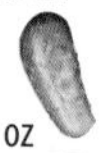
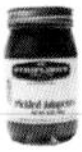
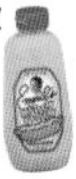
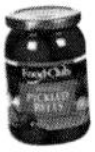
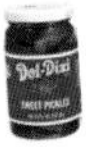
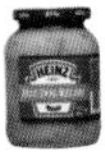
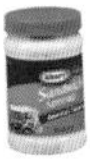
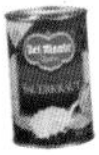
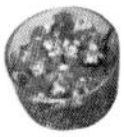

Salsa

Average all Types:	C	F	Cb
Regular, w/out oil, 2 T., 1 oz	15	0	3.5
Made with oil, 2 Tbsp, 1 oz	40	3	8
La Victoria, 2 Tbsp, 1 oz	10	0	2
Old El Paso, 1 Tbsp, 1 oz	10	0	3
TGI Friday's, 1.2 oz	15	0	4

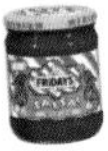
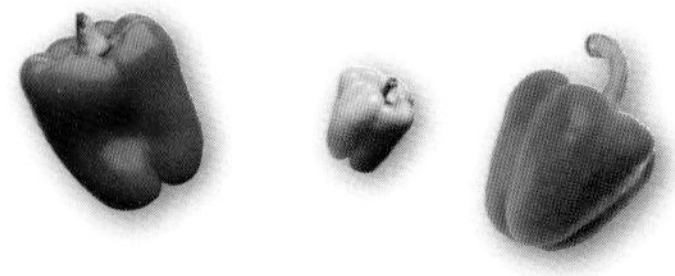

Quick Guide

Cookies:

Average All Brands: Per Cookie

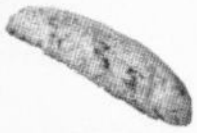
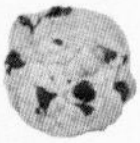
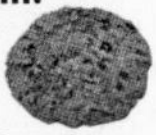
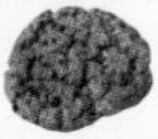
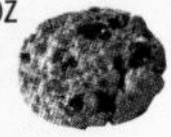

	C	F	Cb
Biscotti: Small, 0.5 oz	70	3	10
Regular, 1 oz	140	6.5	18
Chocolate Chip:			
Small/Thin, 0.5 oz	70	3.5	9
Regular, 1 oz	140	7	18
Large (*Mrs Fields*), 3 oz	350	17	45
Extra Large, 4 oz	555	28	73
Oatmeal/Oatmeal Raisin:			
Small/Thin, 0.5 oz	65	2.5	10
Regular, 1 oz	130	5	20
Large (*Mrs Fields*), 2.5 oz	330	14	44
Extra Large, 4 oz	510	20	78
Peanut Butter:			
Small/Thin, 0.5 oz	70	3.5	9
Regular, 1 oz	135	7	17
Large (*Mrs Fields*), 2.5 oz	330	17	41
Extra Large, 4 oz	540	27	67
Low-Fat Cookies:			
Choc Chip (Low-Fat), (1), 0.5 oz	65	2	10
Oatmeal Raisin (Fat-Free), (1), 1 oz	95	0.5	22
Peanut Butter (Low-Fat), (1), 1 oz	105	5	15

Quick Guide

Crackers

Average All Brands: Per Cracker Unless Indicated

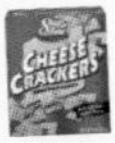

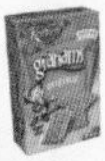
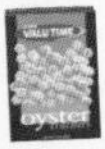

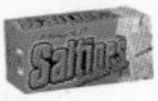

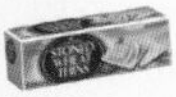

	C	F	Cb
Cheese Crackers:			
Plain: 1" square	5	0	0.5
Bag, single serving, 1 oz	140	7	16
Cheese/P'nut Butter filled	30	1.5	4
Crispbread, Rye	35	0	8
Grahams, 2½" square	30	0.5	5
Melba Toast, Plain, 1 piece	20	0	4
Matzo, Plain, 1 oz	110	0.5	23
Oyster/Soup, ½ cup	95	2	17
Rice: 1 crackers	70	1.5	11
Oriental Style, 1 oz	130	3.5	23
Saltines, 5 crackers	65	2	11
Snack-type, 1 round cracker	15	1	2
Soda Crackers (*Saltine*), 2	25	1	4.5
Water Cracker (*Carr's*), Original	15	0.5	2.5
Wheat:			
Wheat Thins	10	0.5	1.5
Cheese/Peanut Butter filled	35	2	4

Updated Nutrition Data ~ www.CalorieKing.com
Persons with Diabetes ~ See Disclaimer (Page 22)

Cookies & Crackers ~ Brands

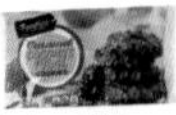
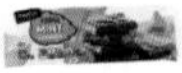
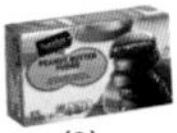
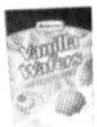
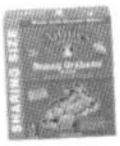
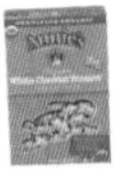
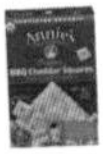
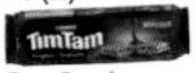

Per Cookie/Cracker, Unless indicated	C	F	Cb
Albertsons:			
Fresh Baked: PB Jumbo Cookie (1)	340	18	39
Rainbow Chip Jumbo Cookie (1)	320	14	46
Signature Select:			
Fudge:			
Caramel Coconut Stripes (2)	130	6	18
Graham (3), 1 oz	140	6	19
Mint (2)	180	9	25
Marshmallow (2)	150	5	25
Peanut Butter (2)	140	8	15
Stripes (3)	170	8	25
Swiss Milk Chocolate, (2)	130	6	17
Treasure Chips Chewy Cookie, (2)	140	6	20
Tuxedos, Double Flled Choc. (2)	140	6	21
Wafers: Chocolate Creme (3)	180	10	20
Strawberry Creme (3)	180	6	20
Vanilla (10)	140	5	22
Vanilla Creme (3)	180	10	20
Annie's (Organic):			
Bites, Choc. Chip Cookie (6)	150	8	19
Bunny Grahams:			
All Varieties, 1 oz	130	4.5	22
Gluten Free: Cocoa & Vanilla, 1 oz	120	4.5	23
SnickerDoodle, 1 oz	140	5	22
Sandwich Cookies, all varieties, (3)	160	7	24
Cheddar Bunnies Crackers:			
Regular (51), 1 oz	140	6	19
Super Cheesy (48), 1 oz	150	8	18
White Cheddar (48), 1 oz	150	7	17
Whole Wheat (51), 1 oz	140	5	20
Gluten Free, Bunny Tails (30), 1 oz	160	9	17
Squares: BBQ Cheddar (26), 1 oz	150	8	18
White Cheddar (26), 1 oz	150	7	18
Saltine Classics, (14), 1 oz	140	5	20
Arnott's:			
Tim Tams: Original; Chewy C'rml (2)	190	9	26
Classic Dark; Dark Mint (2)	190	10	25
Austin (Kellogg's):			
Sandwich Crackers: *Per Package*			
Cheese: with Cheddar Cheese	190	9	24
with Peanut Butter	190	9	24
Peanut Buter on Toasty Crackers	190	9	24

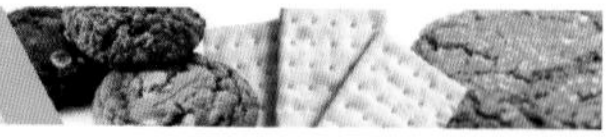

Cookies & Crackers ~ Brands (Cont)

Per Cookie/Cracker, Unless Indicated	C	F	Cb
BelVita *(Nabisco):*			
Breakfast Biscuits:			
Crunchy, 1 pack (4 biscuits), average	230	8	35
Soft Baked, 1 biscuit, average	200	8	32
Bites, (46), av., 1.8 oz	230	8	37

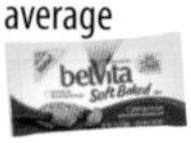

Blue Diamond:			
Nut Thins:			
Almond; Hint of Sea Salt (19), 1 oz	130	2	24
Average other varieties (19), 1 oz	130	3	24
Carr's:			
Crackers: Rosemary (4)	80	3.5	10
Toasted Sesame (4)	60	1.5	10
All other Varieties (4)	50	1	10

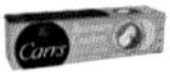

Cheez-It ~ *See Sunshine, Page 87*

Chips Ahoy! ~ *See Nabisco, Page 85*

Dr. Kracker:			
Crispbread: Klassic 3 Seed (2)	110	5	14
Multi Grain (2)	100	3.5	16
Pumpkin Seed Cheddar (2)	100	4.5	12
Flats: Robustica (4)	110	3.5	19
Roasted Red Pepper & Asiago (4)	100	3	18
Rosemary Parmesan (4)	110	4	17
Seed Power Snack Crackers, (8)	110	4	17
Seeds & Seasalt, (12)	120	4.5	19
Snackers, Pumpkin Seed Cheddar (8)	110	5	15

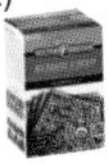

Ener-G Foods: (Gluten Free):			
Cinnamon Crackers, (7)	110	4.5	19
Flax Crackers, (9)	90	4.5	11

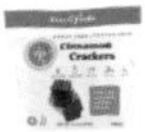

Erin Baker's:			
Original Breakfast: *Per 3 oz*			
Banana Walnut	310	8	55
Double Choc.; Oatmeal Raisin	300	7	57
Peanut Butter	320	11	51
Minis: Per 1 oz Cookie			
Caramel Apple, 1 oz	100	1.5	19
Double Chocolate, 1 oz	100	2.5	18
Grain free, Salted Choc. Cashew (2), 1 oz	130	9	14

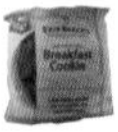

Famous Amos:			
Bite Size: Chocolate Chip (4)	150	7	0
Chocolate Chip & Pecans (4)	150	8	19
Double Chocolate Chip (3)	145	7	18

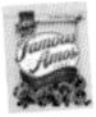

fifty50:			
Chocolate Chip, (4)	170	9	22
Hearty Oatmeal, (4)	160	7	24

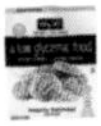

Fig Newtons ~ *See Nabisco, Page 85*

Per Cookie/Cracker, Unless Indicated	C	F	Cb
Gamesa:			
Arcoiris Marshmallow, 2 oz pkg, 6 cookies	220	5	38
Barras de Coco, 1 cookie	120	3	22
Chokis, Chocolate Chip, 1.4 oz pkg	190	8	27
Emperador: Chocolate, (1), 1.15 oz	160	6	23
Lime Flavor (3), 1.1 oz	140	5	23
Florentinas, (8), 1 oz	120	2	23
Giro, 3 cookies, 1 oz	140	6	20
Mamut, 1 cookie, 1 oz	130	5	21
Maravillas, (6), 1 oz	120	3.5	21
Marias, 8 cookies, 1 oz	120	2	23
Ricanelas, (2)	140	4.5	24
Sugar Wafers, (3), average, 1.2 oz	180	9	25

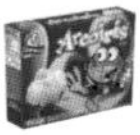

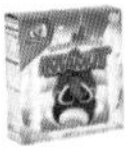

Girl Scouts Cookies:			
Caramel DeLites/Samoas, (2), av.	145	7	18
Girl Scout S'Mores, (2)	150	7	21
Peanut Butter S'wich, (3)	170	7	21
Shortbread, (4)	120	4.5	19
Thanks-A-Lo, (2)	140	6	22
Thin Mints, (4)	160	7	22
Trefoils, (5)	160	7	21

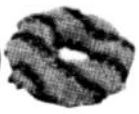

Goldfish Crackers ~ *See Pepperidge Farm, Page 86*

Goya:			
Lady Fingers , (4),1 oz	130	1	25
Marias, (5), 1 oz	130	3	23
Chocolate (5), 1 oz	130	3.5	23
Strawberry Wafers, (5), 1.15 oz	170	8	22

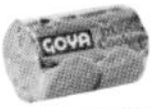

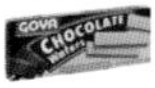

Grandma's *(Fritolay): Per Cookie*			
Chocolate Brownie	190	8	27
Chocolate Chip	200	10	25
Minis, 1 pkg	210	8	31
Oatmeal Raisin	180	7	26
Peanut Butter	190	10	22
Sandwich Cremes:			
Peanut Butter (4)	170	8	22
Vanilla (4)	170	7	23

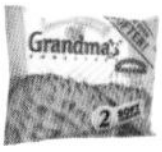

Great American Cookies: *Per Cookie*			
Chewy Choc. Supreme	200	9	29
Chewy Pecan Supreme	230	12	31
Double Fudge with Reese's	230	11	33
Original with Reese's or M&M's	240	12	31
Peanut Butter with M&M's	250	14	29
White Chunk Macadamia	250	14	30

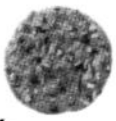

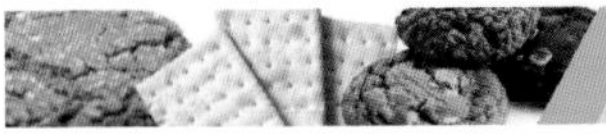

Cookies & Crackers ~ Brands (Cont)

Per Cookie/Cracker, Unless Indicated

	C	F	Cb
Great American Cookies (Cont): *Per Cookie*			
Double Doozies:			
Original, 5.3 oz	**690**	34	94
M&M Big Bite, 2.5 oz	**340**	17	46
Cookie Cakes:			
16", 3.5 oz	**460**	22	67
16" M&M, 4 oz	**500**	24	73
Heart Shaped, 3.5 oz	**440**	21	64
Great Value *(Walmart):*			
Caramel Coconut & Fudge, (2)	**130**	6	18
Chocolate Chip Chippers, Mini:			
Original, 1 Pack, 1 oz	**130**	6	18
Orange, 1 pack, 1 oz	**140**	7	21
Fudge: Grahams, (1)	**110**	5	16
Covered Peanut Butter Filled (2)	**160**	9	17
Striped Shortbread (3)	**170**	7	25
Iced Apple Oatmeal, Minis, 1 pack	**140**	6	21
Pecan Shortbread, (2)	**160**	9	19
Sandwich: Chocolate Cremes (3)	**160**	7	24
Vanilla (3)	**170**	7	26
Twist & Shout, Dble Choc Filled (2)	**140**	7	20
Snickerdoodle, (1)	**110**	5	15
Strawberry Filled Wafers, (4)	**160**	8	22
White Melting Wafers, (9)	**80**	4.5	10
Crackers:			
Buttery Smooth, (4), 0.5 oz	**70**	3	9
Cheddar Cheese, (28), 1 oz	**150**	8	18
Keebler:			
Animals, Frosted (8)	**160**	8	22
Chips Deluxe: Original (2)	**160**	8	19
With Peanut Butter (2)	**170**	9	20
Chocolate Lovers (2)	**170**	9	20
Chunk (2)	**170**	9	21
Coconut (2)	**160**	9	19
Deluxe Triple Choc (2)	**150**	8	20
Simply Made (2)	**140**	7	17
Soft Batch (2)	**150**	7	21
Soft 'n Chewy (2)	**150**	6	21
Rainbow, Choc. Chip wih M&M's (2)	**160**	8	21

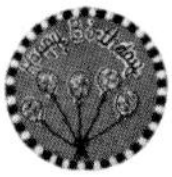

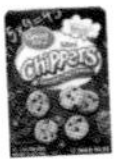

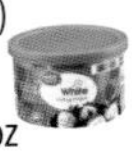

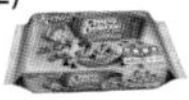

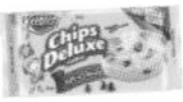

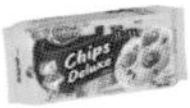

Per Cookie/Cracker, Unless Indicated

	C	F	Cb
Keebler (Cont):			
Danish Wedding, (5)	**160**	8	22
E.L. Fudge: Original (2)	**170**	7	25
Chocolate (2)	**170**	7	26
Double Stuffed (2)	**180**	9	24
Vanilla (2)	**180**	7	26
Fudge:			
Caramel Nut Dreams, (2)	**190**	11	20
Coconut Dreams Fudge Covered (2)	**170**	9	20
Deluxe Grahams (2)	**140**	7	18
El Fudge: Original Elfwich (2)	**170**	7	25
Double Stuffed (2)	**180**	9	24
Fudge Sticks:			
Original (3)	**150**	8	20
Fudge Stripes: Original (2)	**140**	7	19
Birthday (2)	**140**	6	19
Coconut Dreams (2)	**140**	8	17
Dark Chocolate (2)	**130**	6	20
Whoopsy!: (2)	**170**	8	23
Cookies & Cream (2)	**170**	8	23
Mint (2)	**170**	9	23
Grasshopper (4)	**150**	7	20
Peanut Butter Dreams (2)	**170**	11	16
Gripz, Chips Deluxe, 0.9 oz pouch	**120**	5	18
Oatmeal, Country Style (2)	**130**	6	19
Pitter Patter, P'nt Butter Creme (2)	**140**	6	19
Sandies Shortbread Cookies:			
Cashew (2)	**170**	9	19
Classic (2)	**160**	9	19
Pecan(2)	**170**	10	19
Simply Made Cookies:			
Butter (2)	**140**	7	18
Chocolate Chip (2)	**140**	7	17
Chocolate S'wich (2)	**140**	6	20
PB Chocolate Chip (2)	**140**	8	15
Vienna Fingers,			
Creme Filled (2)	**150**	6	22
Wafers, Vanilla Filled (4)	**150**	7	22

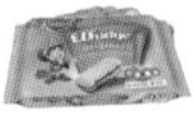

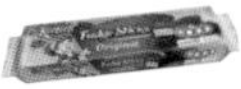

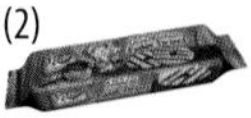

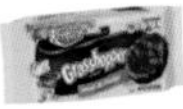

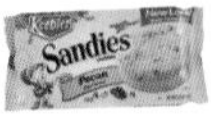

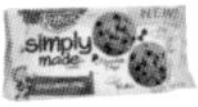

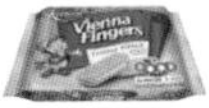

continued next page...

Updated Nutrition Data ~ www.CalorieKing.com
Persons with Diabetes ~ See Disclaimer (Page 22)

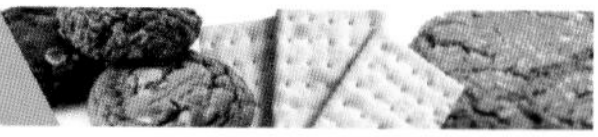

Cookies & Crackers ~ Brands (Cont)

Per Cookie/Cracker, Unless Indicated	C	F	Cb
Keebler (Cont):			
Crackers:			
Town House: Original (5)	80	5	9
Dippers, Original, (3)	70	3.5	8
Flatbread Crisps, all flavors (8)	70	2	11
Flip Side: Original (5)	70	3.5	10
Thins: Sea Salt (6)	70	3.5	10
Focaccia:			
Rosemary & Olive Oil (3)	70	3.5	9
Tuscan Cheese (3)	80	4	9
Pita:			
Mediterranean Herb (6)	70	2.5	12
Parmesan Cheese (6)	70	2.5	11
Kroger:			
Chip Mates: Original Choc. Chip (3)	130	6	17
Chewy Chocolate Chip (2)	150	7	20
Chunky Chocolate Chip (2)	140	7	18
Peanut Butter Chocolate Chunk (2)	130	7	15
White Chip Chocolate Chunk (2)	140	7	18
Sandwich Cookies:			
Kaleido: Original Chocolate (3)	160	6	25
Coconut Lime (3)	150	7	22
Salted Caramel (3)	140	6	21
Maple Creme, (2)	140	5	22
Olde Southern Pecan Shortbread, (2)	150	9	16
Vanilla Wafers, (8)	130	4	23
Crackers:			
Grahams, Orig.; Honey, (4)	130	3	24
Saltines, Original (5), 0.5oz	60	1.5	10
Lance: *Per Pack of 6 Cookies/Crackers*			
Nekot Cookies:			
Choc-O-Lunch/Van-O-Lunch, av.	220	8	34
Lemon Creme; Peanut Butter, av.	240	10	34
Crackers:			
Captain's Wafers:			
Cream Cheese & Chives	200	10	23
Grilled Cheese	190	9	25
PB & Honey	200	9	23
Cracker Sandwiches:			
Malt, with Peanut Butter Filling	180	8	20
Nip Chee, Cheddar Cheese	200	9	24
Toastchee, Peanut Butter	220	11	25
Toasty, Peanut Butter	190	9	21
Wholegrain: Cheddar Cheese	200	10	26
Peanut Butter	210	9	25

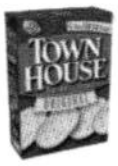

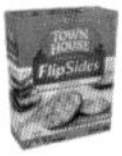

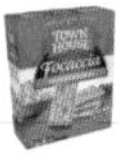

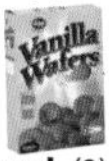

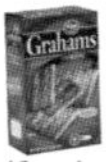

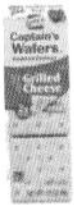

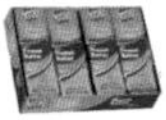

Little Debbie:	C	F	Cb
Choc. Chip Cream Pie, (1), 3 oz	380	16	58
Fudge Rounds, (1)	150	6	23
Marshmallow Pies, (1)	190	6	31
Nutty Buddy, (1)	120	7	12
Oatmeal Creme Pie, (1)	170	7	26
Big Size (1), 2.65 oz	330	12	52
Peanut Butter Cream Pies, (1)	170	7	25
Big Size (1), 3.1 oz	410	19	54
Star Crunch, (1)	150	6	22
Lu:			
Petit Ecolier: Dark Chocolate, (2)	130	7	15
Petit Ecolier, Milk Chocolate (2)	130	6	17
Pim's, Orange(2), 0.9 oz	100	3	17
Manischewitz:			
Crackers:			
Tam Tams: Original (10)	110	4	16
Everything; Garlic (10)	140	5	19
Mary's Gone Crackers:			
Chocolate Chip Cookies, (2)	130	6	19
Crackers:			
All Flavors, (13)	140	5	21
Super Seed:			
Rosemary; Lemon Dill (12)	140	6	17
Other Varieties (12)	150	7	16
Miss Meringue:			
Meringue Classiques:			
Cappuccino (4), 1 oz	110	0	26
Mint Choc. Chip (4), 1 oz	120	1.5	25
Triple Chocolate (4), 1 oz	120	1.5	25
Vanilla Rainbow/Van. (4), 1 oz	110	0	27
Meringue Minis, Low Fat:			
Mini: Chocolate Chip (12), 1 oz	130	1.5	27
Mint Chocolate Chip (12), 1 oz	120	1.5	26
Meringue Minis, Fat Free:			
Peppermint Crush (9), 1 oz	110	0	25
Rainbw Vanilla; Vanilla (13), 1 oz	110	0	27
Meringue Petites: Cafe au Lait (7)	100	0	25
Toasted Coconut (6)	120	2.5	23
Mother's:			
Circus Animal, (4), 1 oz	150	8	20
Chocolate Chips, (4), 1 oz	150	7	20
Coconut Cocadas, (4), 1 oz	140	7	17
Double Fudge, (1), 0.7 oz	100	4.5	14
English Tea, (2)	190	8	28
Oatmeal/Iced Oatmeal, (4), 1.2 oz	150	6	23
Peanut Butter Gauchos, (2), 1 oz	150	6	20
Taffy Dulce de Leche, (1), 0.7 oz	100	4.5	15

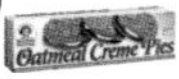

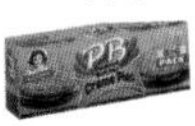

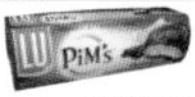

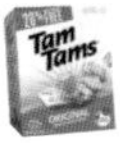

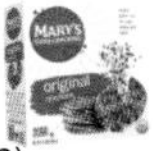

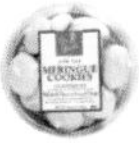

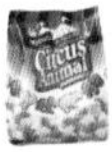

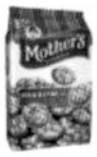

Mrs Fields Cookies ~ *See Page 219*

Cookies & Crackers ~ Brands (Cont)

Per Cookie/Cracker, Unless Indicated	C	F	Cb
Nabisco Cookies:			
Chips Ahoy!, Chocolate Chip:			
Original: 3 cookies, 1.2 oz	**160**	8	22
Single Serve, 2 oz	**280**	14	38
Reduced Fat (3), 1.2 oz 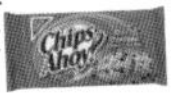	**150**	6	24
Mini Choc. Chips:			
Big Bag (5), 1oz	**150**	7	19
Chewy (4), 1.15 oz 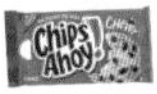	**140**	5	22
Go Pak (14), 1 oz	**150**	7	20
Snak Sak, Lunch Box (5), 1.1 oz	**160**	7	21
Chewy: Regular (2), 1.1 oz	**140**	6	21
Brownie Filled (1), 0.65 oz	**80**	3.5	12
Chunky: Choc. Chunk (2), 1.2 oz	**160**	8	20
Choco Chunky; White Fudge Choc. (1)	**80**	4	11
Hot Cocoa (2), 1.1 oz 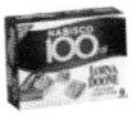	**150**	7	22
Oreo Creme, (2), 1.1 oz	**150**	7	21
Peanut Butter, (1), 0.7 oz	**90**	4	13
Lorna Doone: 100 Calorie Pack,			
Shortbread Cookie Crisps (6), 0.7 oz	**100**	3	16
Shorbreads: 1 oz pack	**140**	7	20
1.5 oz pack 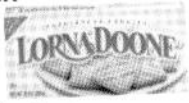	**210**	10	29
Mallomars (1), 1 oz	**120**	5	18
Newtons: 100% Whole Grain:			
Blueberry (2), 1 oz 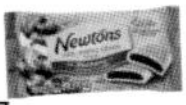	**110**	1.5	22
Fig (2), 1 oz	**110**	0	22
Strawberry (2), 1 oz	**100**	2	21
Original Fig: 1 cookie, 1 oz	**100**	2	21
Fat-Free, 1 cookie, 1 oz	**100**	0	24
Nilla Wafers: 8 Wafers, 1 oz 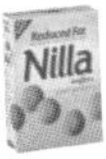	**140**	6	21
Reduced-Fat (8), 1 oz	**120**	1.5	24
Vanilla, 1 oz pkg	**120**	3	22
Nutter Butter:			
16 oz package, 2 cookies, 1 oz	**140**	6	19
4.8 oz package, 2 cookies, 0.8 oz	**120**	5	16
Bites, 1 package, 10 cookies, 1 oz	**150**	6	21
Snak Sak Lunch Box, 10 cookies	**150**	6	21
Wafer, 5 patties, 1.2 oz 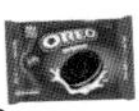	**160**	9	19
Oreo Chocolate:			
Regular; King Size (3), 1.2 oz	**160**	7	25
Mini, 1 oz pack	**130**	5	20
Snak Sak Mini Lunchbox (9), 1 oz	**140**	6	21
Apple Pie; Chocolate Mint (2), 1 oz	**140**	7	21
Blueberry Pie; Choco Chip (2), 1 oz	**140**	7	21
Coconut (4), 1 oz	**140**	6	21
Cookie Creme Filled S'wich, 3 oz pack	**360**	16	52
Double Stuff (2), 1 oz 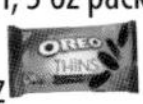	**140**	7	21
Thins, Choc. Creme (4), 1 oz	**140**	6	21
White Fudge Choc. Covered (1), 0.7 oz	**100**	5	13

Per Cookie/Cracker, Unless Indicated	C	F	Cb
Nabisco (Cont):			
Oreo Golden: Original (1) 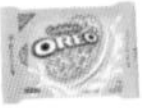	**55**	2.5	8
(3), 1.2 oz	**170**	7	25
Reduced Fat (3), 1.2 oz 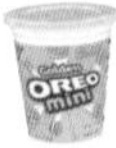	**150**	5	27
Mini (9), 1 oz Pack	**140**	6	21
15 oz Pack	**200**	8	30
Double Stuf (2), 1 oz 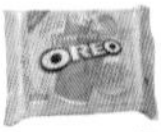	**150**	7	21
Fruity Crisps (2), 1 oz	**140**	7	21
Limeade (2), 1 oz	**140**	7	20
Lemon (2), 1 oz 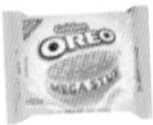	**150**	7	21
Mega Stuff (2), 1.3 oz	**180**	9	25
Thins, all flavors (4), 1 oz	**150**	6	21
Teddy Grahams: Cinnamon, 0.74 oz pkt	**90**	3	16
Single Serve, Honey (24), 1 oz	**120**	4	21
Nabisco Crackers:			
Barnum's Animals: 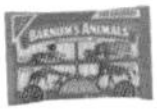			
1 oz Pack	**130**	4	21
Snack Saks (17), 1.2 oz Pack	**140**	4	24
Zoo Animals, 2 oz Pack 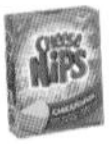	**250**	7	43
Cheese Nips:			
Cheddar: 29 pieces, 1 oz	**150**	6	19
Mini, Despicable Me, 1 oz Pack	**130**	4	19
Honey Maid: Chocolate 1 oz Pack	**140**	4.5	18
Grahams (8) average all varieties,	**130**	3	24
Bites, Snickerdoodle (24), 1 oz	**140**	4	18
Premium:			
Original: 5 crackers, 0.5 oz	**70**	1.5	12
Minis (17), 0.5 oz 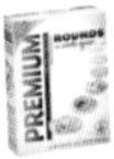	**70**	2	11
Unsalted Tops(5), 0.5 oz	**70**	1.5	13
Rounds: Original (6), 0.5 oz	**60**	1.5	12
Wholegrain (6), 0.5 oz	**60**	1.5	11
Soup & Oyster (22), 0.5 oz	**60**	1.5	11
Triscuit: Original (6), 1 oz 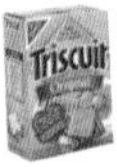	**120**	3.5	20
Av. other flav. (6), 1 oz	**120**	4	20
Reduced Fat (6), 1 oz	**110**	2.5	21
Brown Rice & Wheat (6),			
average all varieties 	**130**	3	22
Thin Crisps, Original (7)	**130**	4.5	21
Wheat Thins:			
Original (16); Big (11), 1.1 oz	**140**	5	22
Reduced Fat (16), 1 oz	**120**	3.5	22
Averae other flavors (14), 1.1 oz	**140**	5	21
Multigrain: Original (14), 1.1 oz	**130**	4	22
Toasted (13), 1 oz	**130**	5	19

Updated Nutrition Data ~ www.CalorieKing.com
Persons with Diabetes ~ See Disclaimer (Page 22)

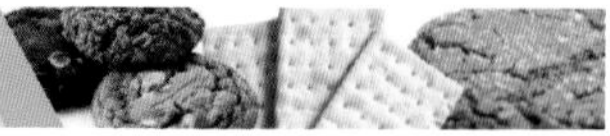

Per Cookie/Cracker, Unless Indicated

Nana's: *Per Cookie*	C	F	Cb
Choc. Chip Walnut; Dble Choc, av.	360	13	58
Oatmeal Raisin	360	12	58
Peanut Butter	360	18	46
Gluten Free: Chocolate	340	14	50
Ginger	340	10	62
Bags:			
Cacao Nib (2)	130	7	17
Coconut; Snickerdoodle (2)	130	6	19
Lemon (2)	120	5	19
Cookie Bars, average	150	6	23

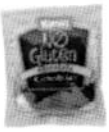

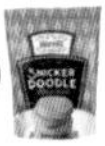

Newman's Own Organics:	C	F	Cb
Alphabet, all flavors (10)	110	3	20
Chocolate Chip: Original (5)	150	7	20
Double Choc Chip (5)	150	7	19
Oatmeal Chocolate Chip (2)	140	6	22
Orange Chocolate Chip (2)	150	7	20
Fig Newman's:			
Fat-Free (2)	90	0	21
Low Fat & Wheat/Dairy-Free (2)	100	1.5	20
Strawberry (2)	110	1.5	21
Wheat Free Non Dairy (2)	110	1	21
Newman-O's: Orig.; Hint O Mint (2)	130	5	19
Chocolate	120	5	18
Peanut Butter (2)	120	5	17
Wheat Free Non Dairy (2)	130	5	19

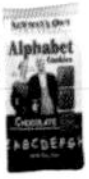

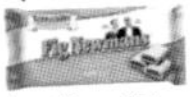

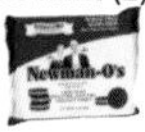

Nonni's:	C	F	Cb
Biscotti:			
Original, 1 piece, 0.8 oz	90	3	14
Av. other varieties, 1 piece, 0.8 oz	110	4	17
Cookie Bites, all flavors (5), average	150	10	17
THINaddictives: Cranb. Alm., 1 oz	130	4.5	20
Lemon Blueberry Almond, 1 oz	130	2.5	22
Pistachio Almond, 1 oz	140	6	18

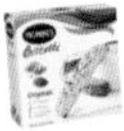

O Organics *(Signature Select)*	C	F	Cb
Animal Cookies, Chocolate (5)	120	4.5	20
Coconut Bites (1)	100	6	11
Koala Bites, 1 piece, 0.9 oz	130	7	16
Mini Chocolate Chip, 1oz Bag	140	7	19
Crackers:			
Mini Peanut Butter S'wich (12)	140	7	17
Rosemary Flatbread Crackers, with Sea Salt (3)	120	2	23
Water Crackers (8)	60	1.5	10

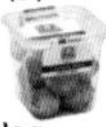

Oreo Cookies ~ *See Nabisco, Page 85*

Payaso:	C	F	Cb
Animalitos (19)	120	1.5	23
Esponjitas (4)	95	2	18
Marias (8)	120	2.5	22
Orejitas Finas (4)	100	5	13

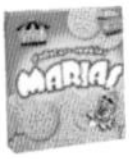

Per Cookie/Cracker, Unless Indicated

Pepperidge Farm:	C	F	Cb
Chunk: *Per Cookie*			
Chesapeake, Dark Chocolate Pecan	140	8	16
Lexington, Milk Chocolate, Toffee Almond	130	7	16
Monauk, Milk Chocolate	140	6	22
Nantucket, Dark Chocolate	130	7	17
Sausalito, Milk Choc. Macadamia	130	7	17
Tahoe, White Chocolate Macadamia	130	7	17
Disctinctive:			
Brussels; Geneva, av. (3)	150	8	20
Chessmen, Butter (3)	120	5	18
Gingerman (4)	130	3.5	22
Milano:			
Caramel Macchiato (2)	130	7	16
Dark Chocolate (2)	180	9	22
Double Milk Chocolate (2)	130	7	17
Irish Cream; Mint; Tstd M'shmallow (2)	130	7	16
Orange; Raspberry (2)	130	7	15
Salted Caramel (2)	120	6	15
Crackers:			
Cracker Trio (3)	60	2	9
Golden Butter (4)	70	2.5	11
Harvest Wheat (3)	80	3.5	11
Goldfish Crackers (Baked):			
Cheddar; Colors (55), 1 oz	140	5	20
1.5 oz Pack	200	7	28
Flavor Blasted, Sour Cream & Onion (57)	140	5	19
Parmesan (60)	140	5	20
Pizza (55)	140	5	20
Pretzel (43)	130	2.5	24
Veggie, Sweet Carrot (56), 1 oz	140	5	21
Whole Whole Grains, Cheddar (55)	140	5	19

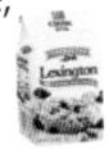

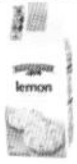

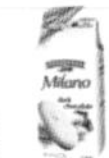

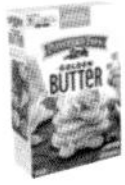

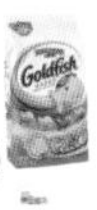

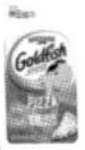

Ritz:	C	F	Cb
Originals: Orig.;Bacon (5)	80	4.5	10
Roasted Vegetable (5)	80	3.5	10
Whole Wheat (5)	70	2.5	10
Bits: Cheese (13)	160	9	19
Peanut Butter (12)	150	8	18
Crisp & Thins, all varieties (21)	130	4.5	21
Toasted Chips: Original (13)	130	4	20
Cheddar; Sour Crm & Onion (12)	130	6	19
Multigrain (13)	130	5	19
Vegetable (13)	120	4.5	20

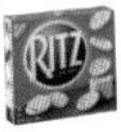

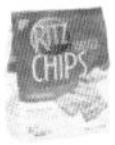

Sedano's:	C	F	Cb
Cinnamon (5)	160	6	24
Maria (5)	120	3	22

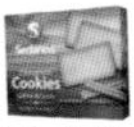

Shar Gluten Free ~ *See CalorieKing.com*

Cookies & Crackers ~ Brands (Cont)

Per Cookie/Cracker, Unless Indicated	C	F	Cb
Snackwell's Cookies:			
Choc. Creme S/wich, 1 pack (4)	210	6	38
Devil's Food Cake, 2 cookies, 32g	120	3	24
Vanilla Creme S/wich, 2 cookies, 24g	100	3	19
Special K:			
Cracker Chips, Sea Salt, 1 cup, 2 oz	190	1	46
Popcorn Chips, White Cheddar (25)	120	3	22
Stella D'Oro:			
Almond Delight (1)	140	7	18
Almond Toast (2)	110	1	24
Breakfast Treats (1), av. all varieties	90	2.5	15
Lady Stella Assorted (3)	120	4	19
Margherite: Chocolate (2)	130	6	19
Vanilla (2)	120	4	20
Original (1)	90	2	15
Swiss Fudge (3)	180	9	23
Trinkets (4)	150	7	19
Crackers:			
Breadsticks: Original (1)	40	1	7
Sesame (1)	50	2	6
Streit's:			
Flavored Wafers:			
Chocolate (3)	160	9	19
Vanilla (3)	170	11	18
Sunshine:			
Cheez-It Crackers:			
Original (27)	150	8	17
Reduced Fat (27)	140	6	19
Duos: C'rml Popcorn & Cheddar, 1 oz	130	6	18
Average other flavors (25), 1 oz	150	7	18
Extra BIG (14)	150	8	17
Four Cheese; White Cheddar (20)	150	7	18
Whole Grain (12)	150	8	17
Grooves: Orig. Cheddar (9)	140	6	19
Zesty Cheddar Ranch (9)	140	6	19
Snack Mix, Classic, ½ cup, 1 oz	130	4.5	20
Trader Joe's:			
100 Calorie Packs, av.	100	2.5	18
Almond Windmill (2)	140	6	18
Charmingly Chewy Choc Chip (2)	130	5	20
Cherry Granola (2)	110	4	18
Chocolate Chip: Small (4)	140	7	18
Large, singles, 1.7 oz	280	14	35
Deep Dish: 1/10 cookie, 1.6 oz	200	9	28
¼ Cookie, 4 oz	500	23	70
Vegan (1)	130	6	18
Caramel Cashew (3)	140	7	16
Crispy Crunchy Choc. Chip (12)	150	9	19
Crispy Oatmeal Choc. Chip (12)	150	7	19
Dark Choc Chunks w/ Almonds (3)	140	7	17
Dunkers: Chocolate Chip (2)	160	7	21
Choc. Coated Choc. Chip (2)	190	9	25

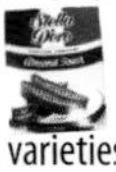
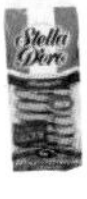
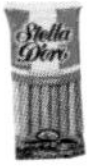
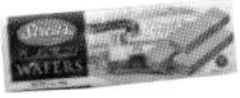
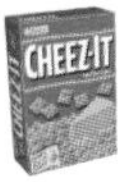
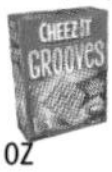
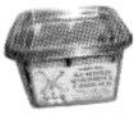
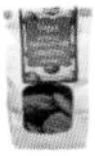

Per Cookie/Cracker, Unless Indicated	C	F	Cb
Trader Joe's (Cont):			
Ginger Snaps, Gluten Free (5)	140	6	21
Highbrow Chocolate (2)	140	7	17
Joe Joe's S'wich Cremes,			
Chocolate/ Vanilla (2)	130	6	19
Macarons A La Parisienne (2)	90	3	10
Meringues, Vanilla (4)	110	0	27
Oatmeal Raisin, 1.8 oz	270	12	35
Pecan Southern Style (4)	150	9	15
Thins: Meyer Lemon (9)	130	4.5	22
Toasted Coconut (8)	130	4.5	22
Triple Choc Chunk, 1 oz	140	7	20
Ultimate Vanilla Wafers (5)	120	6	15
Way More Chocolate Chip (3)	160	11	14
Crackers:			
Multigrain (14)	150	6	22
Savory Thin Edaname (38)	120	2	21
Water (4)	60	1	12
Triscuits ~ *See Page 85*			
Voortman: *Per Cookie Unless Indicated*			
Almond Crunch (2)	140	5	21
Chocolate Chip (1)	90	4	13
Coconut (1)	100	5	9
Fudge Striped Oatmeal (1)	110	6	14
Oatmeal Cranberry Flaxseed (1)	90	4	12
Wafers, average all flavors (3)	150	7	22
Sugar Free:			
Wafers (3), average all flavors	140	8	18
Note: Carbohydrate Figure Contains 7 g Sorbitol			
Whole Foods (365 Organic):			
Butter Shortbread (2)	150	8	17
Chocolate Chip: Bites, 1 oz pkg	150	8	19
Two Bite(3)	130	6	18
Double Chocolate Chip (2)	150	8	19
Oatmeal Raisin (2)	140	6	20

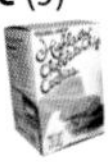
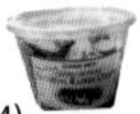
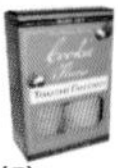
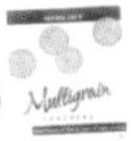
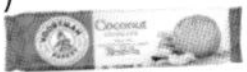
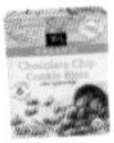

Cookie ~ Mixes

As Packaged	C	F	Cb
Betty Crocker: *Per 3 Tbsp (1 oz) Mix, Unless Indicated*			
Chocolate Chip	110	2.5	22
Double Chocolate Chunk	110	2.5	21
Snickerdoodle	110	1.5	24
Walnut Chocolate Chip	110	1.5	22
Limited Edition, Gingerbread	100	1.5	20
Snack Size, Sugar Cookie, 4 tbsp, 1 oz	120	2	23
Whole Foods (365 Organic): *Per 2 Tbsp Mix*			
Chocolate Chip, 2 tbsp	110	2.5	22
Gluten Free, ¼ cup, 0.74 oz	80	1.5	17

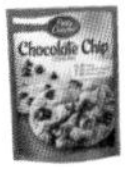

Thaw, Bake & Serve

Per Cookie/Cracker Unless Indicated

	C	F	Cb
Eat Pastry Vegan (Whole Food): *Per Cookie*			
Chocoholic Cookie Dough	50	2.5	8
Choc. Chip Cookie Dough	60	2.5	8
Gluten Free	60	2.5	8
Peanut Butter Choc. Chip	60	2.5	7
Pillsbury Cookies:			
Refrigerated Cookie Dough: *Per Cookie*			
Chocolate Chip Cookie, 1 oz	130	6	17
Peanut Butter, 1.1 oz	130	6	19
Sugar, 1 oz	120	5	18
Ready To Bake CookieDough: *Per 2 Cookies*			
Choc. Chunk & Chip Cookies, 1.34 oz	170	7	24
Chocolate Chip, 1.34 oz	170	7	24
Oreo Pieces, 1.34 oz	170	8	22
Rees'es PB, 1.34 oz	130	6	19
Shapes: Chick, 0.9 oz	110	4.5	16
Bunny; Hearts 0.9 oz	120	6	15
Sugar Cookies, 1.34 oz	160	7	23
Refrigerated Sweet Buns/Rolls ~ *See Page 67*			
Toll House (Nestle):			
Edible Batter, Fudge Brownie, 2 Tbsp	140	4.5	25
Edible Cookie Dough: Choc Chip, 2 T.	140	4.5	25
Funfetti, 2 Tbsp	140	4	25
PB Choc. Chip Monster, 2 Tbsp, 1.23 oz	140	5	21
Refrigerated Cookie Dough: *Per Cookie*			
Bars:			
P'B Chocolate Chip	80	4	11
Oatmeal Raisin	80	3	11
White Chip Macadamia	90	2	11
Chocolate Chip (1)	120	6	17
Chocolate Chip Lovers (1)	170	8	24
Peanut Butter (1)	130	7	15

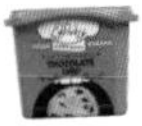
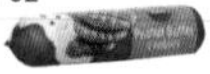
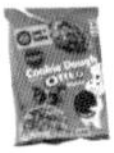
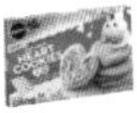
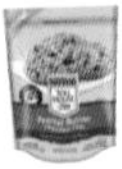
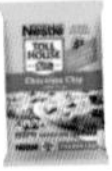

	C	F	Cb
Toll House (Nestle) Cont:			
Refrigerated Coookie Dough (Cont): *Per Cookie*			
Peanut Butter Chip, 1 oz	90	4.5	11
Pecan Turtle Delight (1)	180	10	21
Triple Chip, 1 oz	90	4.5	11

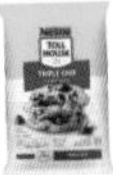

Crispbreads

Per Crispbread Unless Indicated

	C	F	Cb
Finn Crisp:			
Round: Multigrain	50	0	7.5
Original	40	0.5	8
Snacks, average all flavors, 1 oz	115	3.5	15
Thins, average all flavors	20	0.2	4
New York Flatbread Crisps,			
Everything, 3 pieces 1.1 oz	140	4	22
Ry-Krisp: Natural (2)	50	0	11
Seasoned (2)	50	0	11
Sesame (2)	50	0	9
Ryvita:			
Crispbreads: Original (4)	120	0	26
Sesame (4)	160	3	24
Thins: Caramelised Onion Flatbread (4)	120	2	21
Sweet Chilli Flatbreads (4)	110	1.5	21
WASA:			
Crispbread: Multigrain; Thin Rye (1)	35	0	8
Sourdough (1)	30	0	7
crisp'n light,			
7 Grains (3)	60	0	13
Thins: Rosemary & Sea Salt (2)	60	1.5	11
Sesame & Sea Salt (2)	60	2	10

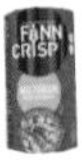
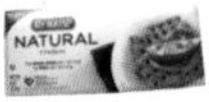

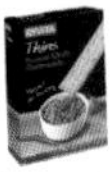
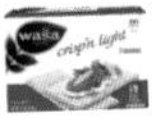
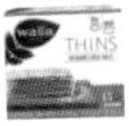

Matzos

	C	F	Cb
Manischewitz:			
Matzo: Original (1), 1 oz	110	0	24
Egg & Onion (1), 1 oz	80	0.5	17
Everything (1)	110	0.5	22
Thin Salted/Tea, average, 0.9 oz	95	0	20
Crackers:			
Tam Tams: Original (9), 1 oz	110	4	16
Unsalted (10)	120	4.5	17
Streit's:			
Matzos: Lightly Salted, (1)	110	0.5	23
Unsalted (1)	100	0	23
Moonstrips, Onion Poppy (1)	100	0.5	22

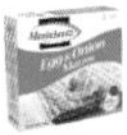
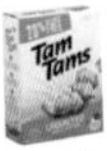

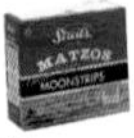

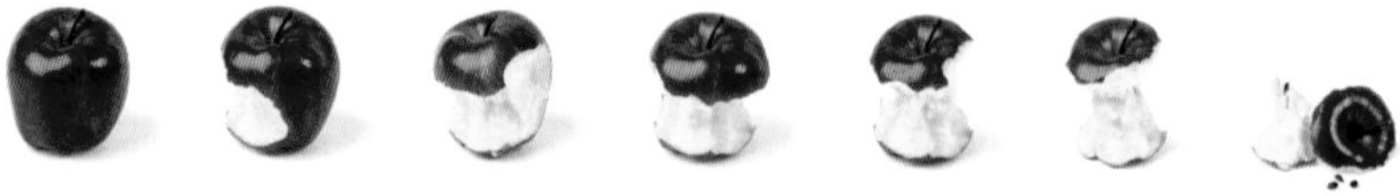

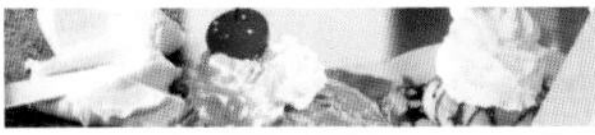

Quick Guide

	C	F	Cb
Cream			
Average All Brands			
Half & Half Cream:			
1 Tbsp, 0.5 oz	20	1.5	0.5
2 Tbsp, 1 oz	40	3	1
¼ cup, 2 oz	80	6	2
Light: Coffee/table (20% fat): 1 Tbsp	30	3	0.5
2 Tbsp, 1 oz	60	6	0.5
Sour Cream:			
Regular: 1 Tbsp, 0.5 oz	25	2.5	1
1 cup, 8 oz	445	45	7
Low-Fat/Light: 1 Tbsp, 0.5 oz	20	1.5	1
2 Tbsp, 1 oz	40	3	2
Fat-Free: Av., 2 Tbsp, 1 oz	20	0	3
Knudsen, 2 Tbsp, 1 oz	30	0	2
Kroger, 2 Tbsp, 1 oz	20	0	3
Sour Cream Substitute:			
Albertson's, 2 Tbsp, 1 oz	60	5	2
Tofutti, Sour Supreme, 2 Tbsp, 1 oz	85	5	9
Whipping Cream:			
Heavy, (37% fat):			
1 Tbsp fluid/2 Tbsp whipped	50	5.5	0.5
½ cup whipped	105	11	1
1 cup whipped	410	44	3.5
Light, (30% fat):			
1 Tbsp fluid/2 Tbsp whipped	45	4.5	0.5
½ cup fluid/1 cup whipped	350	37	3.5

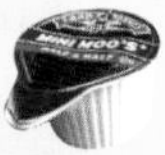
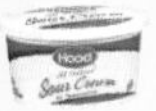
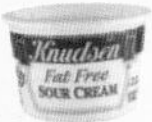
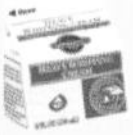

Coconut Cream/Milk

	C	F	Cb
Coconut Cream, (Canned):			
Plain/unsweetened: 2 Tbsp, 1 oz	75	6.5	3
½ cup, 4 oz	285	26	12
Sweetened:			
Coco Lopez: 1 oz	130	5	21
½ cup, 4 oz	520	20	84
Coconut Milk: (Canned):			
Thai Kitchen: Lite, ⅓ cup, 2 fl.oz	50	4.5	1
Premium/Organic, 2 fl.oz	115	10	4
Unsweetened, ⅓ cup	140	14	3
Coconut Water, (Center), 1 cup	45	0.5	9

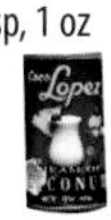
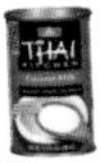

Whipped Toppings

	C	F	Cb
Average All Brands			
Cream (Pressurized): 2 Tbsp	20	1.5	1
¼ cup	40	3.5	2
Cream Topping, Lite, 2 Tbsp	20	1	3
Kraft: *Per 2 Tablespoons*			
Cool Whip: Original, 0.9 oz	25	1.5	3
Extra Creamy, 0.9 oz	25	2	2
Free, 2 Tbsp, 0.9 oz	15	0	3
Sugar Free, 0.9 oz	20	1	3

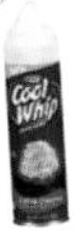
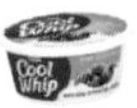

Whipped Toppings (Cont)

	C	F	Cb
Dream Whip Mix, ¹⁄₁₆ envolope,			
Reddi-wip:			
Original, 2 Tbsp, 0.18 oz	15	1	1
Extra Creamy, 2 Tbsp, 0.18 oz	15	1	1
Fat-Free, 2 Tbsp, 0.18 oz	5	0	1
Chocolate, 2 Tbsp, 0.18oz	15	1	1
Non Dairy: Almond, 0.18 oz	10	0.5	2
Coconut, 0.18 oz	10	0.5	2

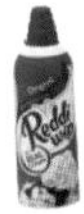

Creamers (Dairy)

	C	F	Cb
Natural Bliss: *Per Tbsp, 15 ml*			
Toasted Coconut	30	1	5
Other Flavors	35	1.5	5

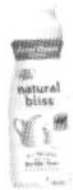

Creamers (Non-Dairy)

	C	F	Cb
Powder:			
Coffee-Mate/Cremora/N-Rich:			
Original: 1 tsp	10	0.5	1
Fat Free, 1 tsp	10	0	2
Flavors: All flavors, 0.10 oz	15	1	2
Sugar Free, all flavors, 0.07 oz	15	1	1
Liquid/Refrigerated:			
Per Tablespoon			
Baileys, Coffee Creamer,			
all flavors, 1 Tbsp, 15ml	35	1	6
Califia Farms, all flavors, 1 Tbsp	15	0	4
Coffee-Mate: *Per Tbsp, 15 ml Unless Indicated*			
Flavors: All flavors	35	1.5	5
Fat-Free, all flavors	25	0	5
Sugar free, all flavors	15	1	1
Shelf Stable, all flavors	35	1.5	5
Unflavored: Original	20	1	2
Fat-Free	10	0	1
Natural Bliss, all flavors	30	1	5
Hood, Country Creamer, 1 Tbsp	15	1	1
International Delight: *Per Tbsp*			
Regular, all flavors	35	1.5	5
Fat-Free, all flavors	30	0	7
Sugar-Free, all flavors	20	2	1
Singles, all flavors, 0.4 fl.oz	30	1	5
Kroger: *Per Tbsp*			
Coffee Creamers: Original	15	1	1
Hazelnut; White Choc Mocha	30	1	5
Fat-free, French Vanilla	25	0	5
Silk: Almond/Oat/ all flavors	25	1	4
Soy: Original	20	1.5	2
Vanilla	30	1.5	4

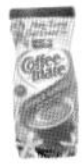
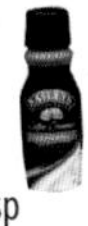
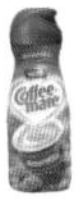
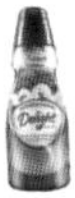
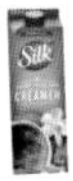

D Desserts ~ Puddings ♦ Gelatin

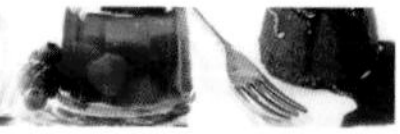

Ready-To-Serve

	C	F	Cb
Hunt's:			
Snack Pack Puddings:			
5.5 oz Container:			
Butterscotch	170	4	33
Chocolate	180	3.5	34
Vanilla	170	4.5	32
3.25 oz Container:			
Butterscotch	90	2.5	17
Choc.; M'maid Splashes; Unicorn Magic	100	2.5	19
Dragon Treasure	100	2	20
Tapioca	110	3	19
Vanilla	100	3	17
Sugar Free: Chocolate	70	3.5	14
Vanilla	60	3	11
Juicy Gels: All flav., 5.5 oz	160	0	39
All flavors, 3.25	90	0	21
Sugar Free, Cherry, 3.25 oz	5	0	1
Jell-O *(Kraft)*:			
Gelatin: Orig., av. all flav., 3.4 oz	70	0	17
Sugar Free, 3.2 oz	10	0	0
Puddings: *4 Packs*			
Choc. Vanilla Swirls, 3.5 oz	110	1.5	24
Strawberry Cheesecake, 3.5 oz	130	2	26
Sugar Free Puddings: *4 Packs*			
Chocolate Vanilla Swirls, 3.6 oz	60	1.5	10
Creme Brule Rice Pudding, 3.6 oz	70	2	12
Temptations: Lem. Meringue Pie, 3.4 oz	80	1.5	17
Strawberry Cheesecake, 3.5 oz	130	2.5	25
Kozy Shack:			
Flan, Creme Caramel, 1 cup, 4 oz	150	3	27
Original Puddings: *Per ½ Cup Unless Indicated*			
Chocolate, 4.6 oz	140	2.5	27
Cinn. Raisin Rice, 4.6 oz	140	2.5	26
French Vanilla Rice, 4.6 oz	140	2.5	24
Original Rice, 4.6 oz	130	2.5	24
Tapioca, 4.6 oz	130	2	25
Simply Well Puddings, average all flavors, 4 oz cup	90	1.5	14
Kroger:			
4 Pack Pudding Snacks: *Per 3.25 oz Cup*			
Butterscotch	90	2.5	17
Chocolate	100	2.5	19
Swiss Miss:			
Puddings: *Per 4 oz Cup*			
Butterscotch	130	3.5	22
Chocolate Vanilla Swirl	150	3.5	26
Creamy Milk Choc.	150	3.5	27
Tapioca; Vanilla	140	3.5	24
Triple Chocolate	160	4	27

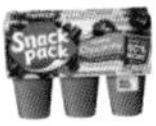
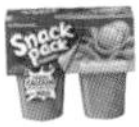
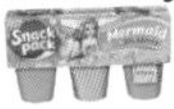
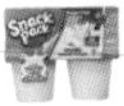
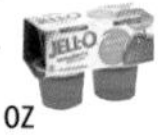
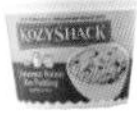
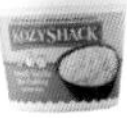
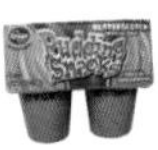
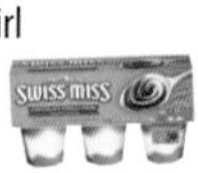

Homemade Puddings

	C	F	Cb
Apple Tapioca, ½ cup	150	0	32
Bread Pudding, ½ cup	250	8	40
Blancmange, ½ cup	140	5	19
Chocolate, ½ cup	190	6	30
Crème Brulée, ½ cup	400	35	16
Plum Pudding, 2 oz	170	3	32
Rice, with Raisins, ½ cup	200	4	38
Sponge Pudding, 3.5 oz	340	16	45
Tapioca Cream, ½ cup	110	4	15
Trifle, ½ cup	180	7	26

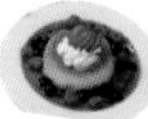
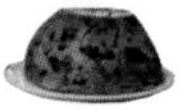
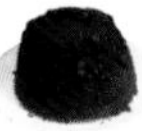

Custards

	C	F	Cb
Custard Mix *(Jello/Royal Flan)*, average:			
Dry, ¼ of 2.9 oz package, 0.7 oz	80	0	19
Prepared: whole milk, ½ cup	155	4	25
2% milk, ½ cup	140	2.5	25
Non-Fat milk, ½ cup	125	0	25
Home Made Egg Custard:			
With Whole Milk, ½ cup	170	8	18
With 2% Milk, ½ cup	155	6.5	18

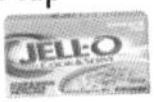

Gelatin • Parfait • Jell-O

	C	F	Cb
Jell-O:			
Gelatin Dessert Mix: *Dry Mix Only*			
All flavors, 0.8 oz	80	0	19
Sugar free, all flavors, 0.3 oz	10	0	0
Cook & Serve Pudding & Pie Filling: *Dry Mix Only*			
Banana Cream, 0.77 oz	80	0	20
Butterscotch, 0.85 oz	90	0	22
Chocolate Fudge, 1 oz	100	0	25
Coconut Cream, 0.77 oz	90	2.5	17
White Chocolate, 0.8 oz	100	0	23
Sugar free, Fat-Free:			
Chocolate var., 0.3 oz	30	0	8
Vanilla, 0.2 oz	20	0	5
Instant: Banana Cream, ½ pkt, 0.85 oz	90	0	22
Butterscotch, 0.88 oz	90	0	22
No Bake Dessert Mix: *Dry Mix Only*			
Cheesecake: Classic, 1.83 oz	210	5	42
Cherry, 2.2 oz	210	4	42
Home Style, 1.87 oz	220	4.5	43
Oreo, 2 oz	260	8	47
Ida Mae, Strawberry Parfait	90	2	18
Reser's, Parfaits, Rainb.;Rasp. 3.9 oz, av.	105	2	19

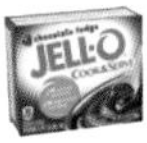
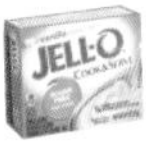

Meringues

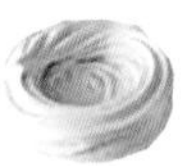

	C	F	Cb
Meringue Swirl, ½ oz	50	0	8
Meringue Shell, 1 oz	100	0	16

Chicken Eggs

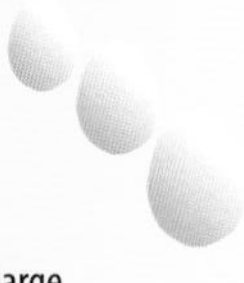

	C	F	Cb
Fresh Eggs:			
Raw:			
Small	55	4	0
Medium	65	4	0
Large	70	5	0
Extra Large	80	5.5	0
Jumbo	90	6	0
Egg Yolk, 1 extra large	55	4.5	0
Egg White, 1 extra large	17	0	0
Dried Egg Powder:			
Whole Egg: ¼ cup, 1 oz	170	12	0
1 Tbsp	30	2	0
Egg White, ¼ cup, 1 oz	105	0	0
Egg Yolk, ¼ cup, 1 oz	195	18	0

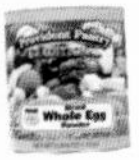

Egg Substitutes

¼ Cup (Equivalent to 1 Egg) ~ Zero Cholesterol

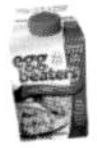

	C	F	Cb
All Whites *(Crystal Farms)*, 1.6 oz	25	0	0
Better 'n Eggs *(Crystal Farms):*			
Regular, 3 Tbsp	25	0	0
Egg Beaters *(ConAgra):*			
100% Egg White 3 Tbsp	25	0	0
Original, 3 Tbsp, 1.6 oz	25	0	0.5
Single Serve, 4 oz cup	50	0	1
Southwestern Style, 3 Tbsp, 1.6 oz	20	0	0.5
Egg Replacer *(Ener-g)*, 1.5 tsp	15	0	4
Naturegg *(Burnbrae Farms)*,			
Simply Egg White, ¼ cup, 2 oz	30	0	0
O-Organics *(Albertson's)*, Egg Whites	25	0	0
Vegan Egg Substitute:			
Aquafaba, ¼ cup, 2 oz	10	0	2

Liquid from cooked/canned beans or chickpeas. Replaces eggs and egg whites in recipes.

Extra Info: www.aquafaba.com

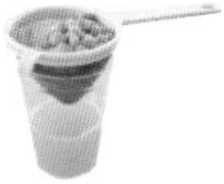

Other Eggs

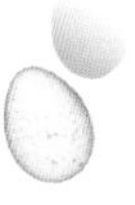

	C	F	Cb
Duck, 1 large, 2.5 oz	130	9.5	0
Goose, 1 large, 5 oz	280	19	0
Quail, 3 eggs, 1 oz	42	3	0
Turkey, 1 large, 3 oz	135	9.5	0
Turtle, 1 egg, 1.75 oz	75	5	0

Omega-3 Fat Enriched

	C	F	Cb
Egg•Land's Best, 1 large	60	4	0
Horizon Organic, 1 large	70	5	0

Note: Cholesterol content is the same as regular eggs.

Cooked Eggs

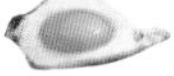

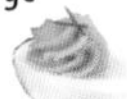

	C	F	Cb
Boiled Egg: *Same as Raw Egg*			
Hard-Cooked, Small, peeled	65	4	0
Fried Egg:			
With fat: 1 large egg	105	9	0.5
2 small eggs	175	13	1
No fat/nonstick pan, 1 large	75	5	0.5
Deviled Egg, 2 halves	145	13	0.5
Eggs Benedict, (2),			
on Toast or English Muffin	860	56	25
Eggs Florentine, (2),			
on Toast or English Muffin	890	59	25
Pickled Egg, 1 large	80	5.5	0
Poached Egg, 1 large	65	4	0
Quiche *(Homemade):*			
Egg & Bacon, 1 slice, 5.3 oz	580	43	27
Ham & Cheese, 1 slice, 5.3 oz	475	33	29
Scotch Egg, 1 egg	300	21	16
Scrambled Eggs:			
1 large egg:			
With 1 Tbsp milk + 1 tsp fat	120	9	1
With 1 Tbsp skim milk/no fat	85	5.5	1
2 large eggs:			
With 2 Tbsp milk + 2 tsp fat	260	20	2
With 2 Tbsp skim milk, w/o fat	180	11	2

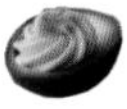

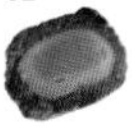

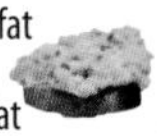

Omelets

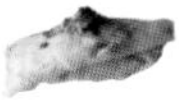

	C	F	Cb
1 Egg:			
Plain (with 1 tsp fat)	125	10	0.5
With: ½ oz cheese	175	15	0.5
½ oz cheese + ½ oz ham	200	16	0.5
2 Eggs:			
Plain (with 2 tsp fat)	250	20	1
With: 1 oz cheese	360	29	2
1 oz cheese +1 oz ham	410	32	2
3 Eggs:			
Plain (with 1 Tbsp fat)	360	29	1.5
With: 2 oz cheese	580	47	2.5
2 oz cheese+2 oz ham	680	53	2.5
Extras, Tomato/Onion/Veggies, 2 oz	20	0	4.5
Egg Substitute *(EggBeaters):*			
2 eggs (½ cup) + 1 tsp fat	100	4	2
3 eggs (¾ cup) + 2 tsp fat	160	8	3
Extras: 1 oz Cheese	110	9	1
1 oz Ham	50	3	1

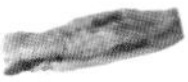

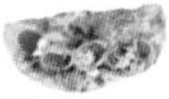

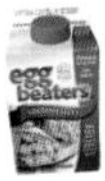

Egg Nog

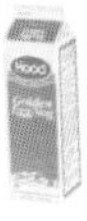

	C	F	Cb
Average all Brands,			
½ cup, 4 oz	170	8	18
Borden, Regular, 4 fl.oz	160	8	18
Hood, Golden, ½ cup, 4 fl.oz	180	9	22
Horizon, Low-Fat, 4 fl.oz	140	3	23

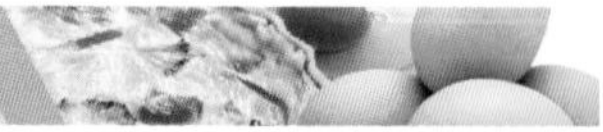

Breakfast Sides

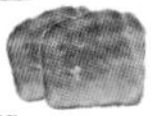
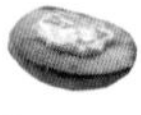
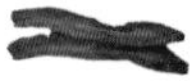
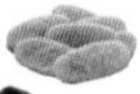
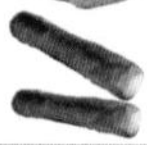

Breakfast Sides	C	F	Cb
Toast:			
Plain, 1 thick slice	85	1	13
With: 2 tsp butter/marg.	155	9	13
3 tsp/1 Tbsp fat	190	13	13
English Muffin:			
Plain, 2 oz	130	1	26
With 3 tsp fat	230	12	26
Bacon, 2 strips	70	5	0
Ham, lean, 2 oz	100	3	0
Hash Brown:			
½ cup, 3 oz	125	6.5	14
1 cup serving, 6 oz	250	13	28
Sausages, 2 oz link	180	16	1.5

Frozen Egg Breakfasts

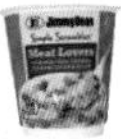
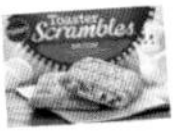
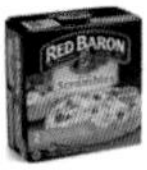

Frozen Egg Breakfasts	C	F	Cb
Jimmy Dean:			
Breakfast Sandwich: *Per Sandwich*			
Biscuit, Sausage, Egg & Cheese	410	28	27
Croissant, Sausage, Egg & Cheese	400	26	29
Muffin, Meat Lovers	480	32	30
Simple Scrambles:			
Bacon, 5.32 oz pkg	290	23	4
Meat Lovers, 5.32 oz pkg	290	22	2
MorningStar Farms,			
Breakfast Muffin Sandwich,			
Veggie Sausage, Egg & Cheese	200	8	20
Pillsbury: *Per Pastry*			
Toaster Scrambles:			
Bacon, 1.8 oz	180	10	19
Bacon & Sausage	180	10	19
Sausage	180	10	19
Red Baron:			
Biscuit Scrambles:			
Bacon (1), 5.85 oz	440	21	45
Sausage (1), 5.85 oz	410	19	46

Frozen Pancake/Waffles ~ *See Page 132*
Toaster Pastries ~ *See Page 64*

Frozen Egg Rolls

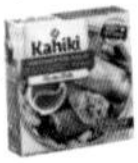
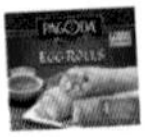

Frozen Egg Rolls	C	F	Cb
Kahiki: *Each*			
Chicken; Vegetable, av., 2.65 oz	150	3.5	24
Pork, 2.65 oz	150	4.5	23
Teriyaki Steak, 2.5 oz	170	6	23
Lotus Restaurant:			
Imperial, Chkn/Pork (1)	160	6.5	24
Vegetarian (1)	120	5	20
Pagoda Express: *Each*			
Chicken, 2.75 oz	160	4	24
Pork, 2.75 oz	180	8	20
Vegetable, 2.75 oz	130	4	21

Fast-Foods/Restaurants

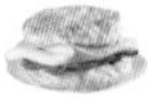
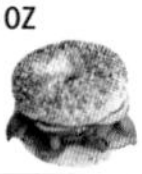
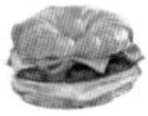

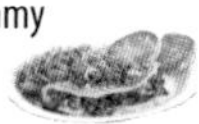
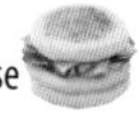
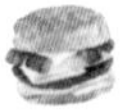
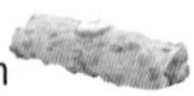
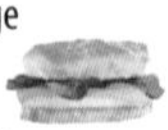

Fast-Foods/Restaurants	C	F	Cb
Arby's, Bacon, Egg & Cheese Croissant	440	27	29
Au Bon Pain, 2 Egg on Plain Bagel	390	11	51
Bob Evans:			
Omelets, Low Calorie: *Without Sides*			
Three Meat & Cheese	1210	94	21
Western	650	50	11
Bojangles: Cajum Filet Biscuit	570	27	57
Bacon, Egg & Cheese Biscuit	470	27	39
Bruegger's:			
Bagel: Egg & Cheese, 6.8 oz	450	14	62
Western, 9.2 oz	560	25	64
Burger King:			
Burrito, Breakfast	375	23	27
Croissan'wich:			
Bacon, Egg & Cheese	335	18	30
Dble Ssg., Egg & Cheese	710	52	31
Ham, Egg & Cheese	335	16	31
Carl's Jr:			
Biscuit, Beyond Sausage Egg & Cheese	660	42	46
Burrito: Bacon & Egg & Cheese	580	35	32
Big Country	660	40	55
Loaded Breakfast	760	48	46
Steak & Egg	600	33	37
Chick-fil-A, Chicken, Egg & Cheese, on Sunflower Multigrain Bagel	500	20	50
Del Taco, Bacon Breakfast Burrito	640	36	38
Denny's:			
Omelettes: MyHammy	600	42	4
Ultimate	710	60	5
Dunkin Donuts:			
Bagel, Bacon, Egg & Cheese	520	18	67
Croissant, Saus., Egg & Cheese	720	52	42
Eat 'N Park:			
Omelettes: Ham & Cheese	660	47	6
Meat Lovers	750	58	6
Hardee's:			
Biscuit: Loaded Omelet	630	41	46
Southwest Omelet	660	45	42
IHOP:			
Omelette: Country	880	69	14
Spinach & Mushroom	910	71	22
Jack in the Box:			
Burritos: Grand Sausage	1070	72	70
Meat Lovers	810	51	50
McDonald's:			
Biscuit, Bacon, Egg & Cheese, reg.	460	25	39
McMuffin, Egg	300	12	30
Whataburger, Breakfast Platter, with Bacon	615	39	36

Quick Guide

	C	F	Cb
Butter			
Average All Brands			
Regular: 1 tsp, 0.2 oz	35	4	0
1 Tbsp, 0.5 oz	100	11	0
2 Tbsp, 1 oz	205	23	0
1 Stick, ½ cup, 4 oz	810	92	0
1 Pound, 2 cups, 16 oz	3255	368	0
Light: Regular, 40% Fat			
1 tsp, 0.2 oz	30	3	0
1 Tbsp, 0.5 oz	70	7.5	0
2 Tbsp, 1 oz	140	15	0
Whipped Butter: Regular			
1 tsp, 0.1 oz	20	2.5	0
1 Tbsp, 0.3 oz	65	7.5	0
1 Stick, 2 .7 oz	545	62	0
Whipped Light Butter *(Land O Lakes):*			
1 tsp, 0.15 oz	15	1.5	0
1 Tbsp, 0.4 oz	45	5	0
2 Tbsp, 0.8 oz	90	10	0

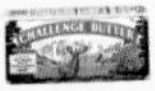
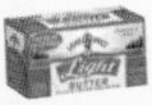
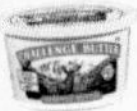
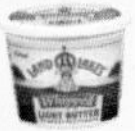

Unsalted ~ *Same as Salted*

Flavored Butter/Spreads

	C	F	Cb
Average All Brands			
Honey Butter, (60% Fat):			
1 Tbsp, 0.5 oz	90	8	4
Downey's, 2% Fat, 1 Tbsp, 0.5 oz	60	1	11
Garlic Butter, (80% Fat):			
1 Tbsp, 0.5 oz	100	11	0
Sweet Cream Butter:			
Land O Lakes: Reguar, 1 Tbsp	100	11	0
Honey Butter Spread, 1 Tbsp	70	6	4

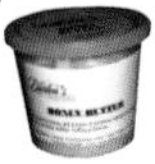
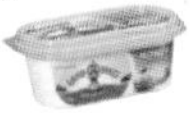

Butter & Butter Blends

	C	F	Cb
Per 1 Tablespoon			
Challenge: Stick, 0.5 oz	100	11	0
Tub, Whipped, 0.3 oz	70	7	0
Brummel & Brown,			
Spread Made with Yogurt, 0.5oz	45	5	0.5
Land O'Lakes:			
Sticks, Original, 0.5oz	100	11	0
Tubs, Butter With Olive Oil, 0.5 oz	90	10	0

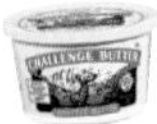
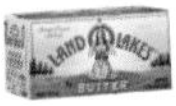

Ghee (Clarified Butter)

(Example ~ *Purity Farms*)
Note: Ghee is 100% fat compared to regular butter (80% fat + 20% water)

	C	F	Cb
1 tsp, 0.2 oz	45	5	0
1 Tbsp, 0.5 oz	120	14	0

Light & Reduced Fat Spreads

	C	F	Cb
Per Tablespoon			
bestlife, Buttery Spread, 0.5 oz	50	5	0
Benecol: Regular, 0.5 oz	70	8	0
Light, 0.5 oz	50	5	0
Blue Bonnet:			
Stick, Lactose Free, 0.5 oz	70	7	0
Tub, Orig. Soft Spread, 0.5 oz	50	6	0
Butter Buds:			
Butter Flavored: Mix, 1 tsp	5	0	2
Sprinkles, 1 tsp	10	0	2
Country Crock *(Shedd's)*: Stick, 0.5 oz	80	8	0
Tubs: Orig; Churn Spread, 0.5 oz	50	6	0
Light Spread, 0.5 oz	35	4	0
Plant Based,			
Almond/Avocado/Ol. Oil, 0.5 oz	100	11	0
Earth Balance, Original, 1 Tbsp	100	11	0
Fleischmann's,			
Olive Oil Spread, 0.4 oz	60	6	0.5
I Can't Believe It's Not Butter!:			
Tubs: Original Spread, 0.5 oz	60	6	0
Light, 0.5 oz	40	4	0
Olive Oil Spread, 1 Tbsp	60	6	0
Molly McButter, 1 tsp	5	0	1
Parkay:			
Spread: Original, 0.4 oz	60	6	0
Light, 0.5 oz	50	6	0
Stick, Original, 0.5 oz	70	8	0.5
Promise: Activ, Spread, 0.5 oz	45	5	0
Light Spread, 0.5 oz	45	5	0
Smart Balance:			
Tubs, Buttery Spread: Original, 0.5 oz	80	9	0
EVOO, 0.4 oz	60	7	0
Light EVOO, 0.4 oz	50	5	0
Light, with Flaxseed Oil, 0.5 oz	50	5	0
Omega 3, Light, 0.5 oz	50	5	0

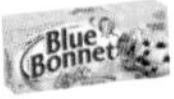

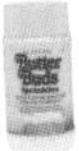
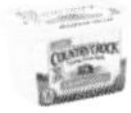
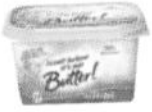
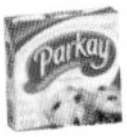

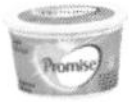
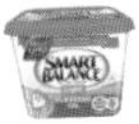

Animal Fats/Lards

	C	F	Cb
Average All Types			
Beef Tallow/Drippings, Lard (Pork), Chicken, Duck, Goose, Turkey:			
1 Tbsp, 0.5 oz	**115**	13	0
2¼ Tbsp, 1 oz	**255**	28	0
1 cup, 7.3 oz	**1850**	205	0
½ pound, 8 oz	**2040**	227	0

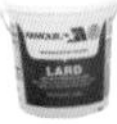

Ghee/Butter/ Oil ~ *See Page 93*

Vegetable Shortening

	C	F	Cb
Average All Types			
1 Tbsp, 0.5 oz	**115**	13	0
2¼ Tbsp, 1 oz	**250**	28	0
1 cup, 7.3 oz	**1810**	205	0

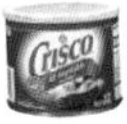

Vegetable Oils

Includes almond, avocado, canola, corn, coconut, flaxseed, grapeseed, linseed, mustard, olive, palm, peanut, rice bran, safflower, sesame, sunflower, soybean, wheat germ. Note: Oil is 100% fat.

	C	F	Cb
1 tsp, 0.2 oz	**45**	5	0
1 Tbsp, 0.5 oz	**120**	14	0
2 Tbsp, 1 oz	**240**	28	0
1 cup, 7.3 oz	**1930**	205	0

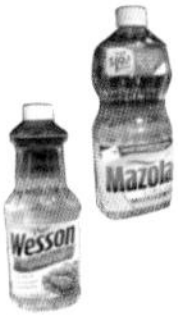

Fish Oils

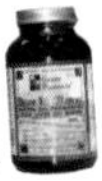

	C	F	Cb
Average All Types (Includes Cod Liver, Herring, Salmon, Sardines): 1 Tbsp, 0.5 oz	**125**	14	0

Cooking Sprays/Squeezes

Cooking Sprays: (PAM, Mazola, I Can't Believe It's Not Butter, Weight Watchers, Wesson):

	C	F	Cb
Pam: ¼ second spray	**2**	0	0
1-3 second spray	**6**	1	0
I Can't Believe It's Not Butter, Original Spray	**0**	0	0
Parkay, Buttery Spray	**0**	0	0

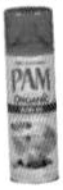

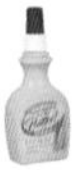

Olestra (Olean)

	C	F	Cb
Olestra *(Olean)*	**0**	0	0

Note: Olean is Proctor & Gamble's brand name for Olestra – a no-calorie cooking oil that gives snacks (like potato chips, tortilla chips and crackers) taste and texture without adding fat or calories.

Examples:

- *Frito-Lay,* Light Products (*Lays, Ruffles, Tostitos, Doritos)*
- *Pringles,* Fat-Free Potato Crisps

Quick Guide

Mayonnaise:	C	F	Cb
Regular: *Per 1 Tbsp, 0.5 oz Unless Indicated*			
Average All Brands	**90**	10	0
Best Foods; Hellman's; Kraft:			
Original/Real	**90**	10	0
½ cup, 4 oz	**720**	80	0
Hain, Safflower Mayonnaise	**100**	11	0
Spectrum, Canola Mayo	**100**	11	0
Light/Reduced Fat: *Per 1 Tbsp, 0.5 oz*			
Best Foods/Hellman's	**35**	3.5	1
Kraft, Light/Olive Oil	**35**	3	1
Smart Balance, Omega	**50**	5	0
Spectrum, Light Canola Mayo, Eggless	**35**	3.5	0.5
Fat Free:			
Kraft: Original, 1 Tbsp	**10**	0	2
½ cup, 4 oz	**80**	0	16
Sugar Free:			
Dukes Mayo, 1 Tbsp	**100**	12	0
Mayonnaise Style Dressing:			
Per 1 Tbsp, 0.5 oz			
Best Foods, Sandwich Spread	**60**	5	2
Kraft:			
Miracle Whip Dressing:			
Original	**50**	5	2
Light	**20**	1.5	2
Fat Free	**15**	0	3
Mayo:			
Homestyle Rich & Creamy; Real	**90**	10	0
Light	**35**	3	2
Horseradish	**50**	1	2
Nasoya, Egg & Dairy Free:			
Nayonaise: Regular/Whipped	**40**	3.5	1
Light	**20**	1.5	1
Sir Kensington's, Egg/Dairy Free			
Fabanaise (Vegan Mayo)	**90**	10	0

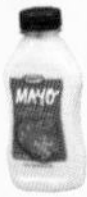

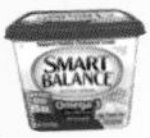

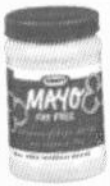

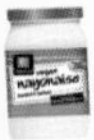

Quick Guide

Fresh Fish

Low Oil: *Less than 2.5% fat)*

White/Lightly-colored flesh. Examples:
Cod, Flounder, Haddock, Halibut, Mahi Mahi, Perch, Pike, Pollock, Snapper, Sole, Whiting.

	C	F	Cb
Raw, without bones, 4 oz	100	1	0
Steamed, broiled, baked, 4 oz	140	1.5	0
Fried: Lightly floured, 4 oz	210	8	3.5
Breaded, 4 oz	260	12	8
In Batter, 4 oz	320	16	27

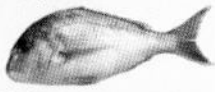

Medium Oil: *2.5-5% fat*

Lightly-colored flesh. Examples:
Bluefin Tuna, Catfish, Kingfish, Orange Roughy, Salmon (Pink), Swordfish, Rainbow Trout, Yellowtail.

	C	F	Cb
Raw, without bones, 4 oz	145	7	0
Baked/Broiled, 4 oz	195	8	0
Fried, 4 oz	230	11	8

High Oil: *Over 5% fat*

Darker-colored flesh. Examples:
Albacore Tuna, Mackerel,
Salmon (Atlantic/Chinook/Sockeye), Sardines, Trout.

	C	F	Cb
Raw, without bones, 4 oz	220	14	0
Baked/Broiled, 4 oz	275	17	0
Fried, 4 oz	340	23	12

Cooking Yields (Fin Fish):

4 oz Raw wt. = 3.5 oz Cooked weight
4 oz Cooked wt. = 5 oz Raw weight

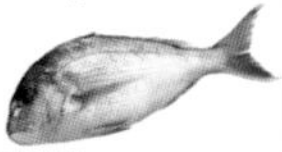

Calorie & Fat Variations:

The amount of fat/oil in fish varies with the species, season and locality. Within the same fish, fat/oil content is generally higher towards the head.

Fish & Shellfish

Edible Weights: (no bones/shell)

	C	F	Cb
Abalone: Raw, 3 oz	90	0.5	5
Fried, 3 oz	160	6	10
Ahi Tuna, grilled, 6 oz fillet (w/o fat)	235	2	0
Anchovy: Paste, 1 Tbsp, 0.5 oz	45	3	0
Canned in oil, drained, (5), 0.7 oz	40	2	0
Barracuda (Pacific), raw, 4 oz	130	3	0
Basa/Swai, raw, 4 oz fillet	70	2	0
Bass:			
Sea: Raw, 4.6 oz fillet	125	2.5	0
Baked, 3 oz	105	2	0
Striped: Raw, 1 fillet, 5.5 oz	150	3.5	0
Baked, 3 oz	105	3	0
Freshwater: Raw, 3 oz	95	3	0
Baked, 3 oz	125	4	0

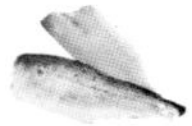

Fish & Shellfish (Cont)

Edible Weights: (no bones/shell)

	C	F	Cb
Calamari/Squid:			
Raw, 4 oz	100	1.5	3.5
Baked, 1 cup	190	6.5	5.5
Fried, 3 oz	150	6	7
Catfish:			
Farmed: Raw, 1 fillet 5.6 oz	190	9.5	0
Baked, 1 fillet 5 oz	205	10	0
Wild: Raw, 1 fillet, 5.6 oz	150	4.5	0
Baked, 1 fillet, 5 oz	150	4	0
Breaded, fried, 1 fillet, 3 oz	200	12	7
Caviar, black/red, 1 Tbsp, 16g	40	3	0.5
Clams: Raw (4 large/9 small), 3 oz	70	1	3
Breaded, fried (20 small), 6.6 oz	380	21	20
Canned, drained, ½ cup, 2.8 oz	115	1	0
Steamed (10 small), 3.3 oz	140	2	5
Cod:			
Atlantic: Raw, 4 oz	95	1	0
Baked, 3 oz	90	1	0
Canned, solids & liquid	90	0.5	0
Pacific: Raw, 4 oz	80	0.5	0
Baked, 3 oz	70	0.5	0
Crab:			
Alaska King,			
1 leg, cooked, 4.7 oz	130	2	0
Blue: Raw, 1 crab, 6 oz	150	1	0
Steamed, 3 oz	70	0.5	0
Canned, drained, 6.5 oz can	105	0.5	0
Dungeness: Raw, 1 crab, 5.8 oz	140	1.5	0
Steamed, 4.45 oz	140	1.5	0
Crab Cakes *(Capt. D's)*, (1), 2.8 oz	250	16	16
Crayfish:			
Farmed: Raw, 3 oz	60	1	0
Steamed, 3 oz	75	1	0
Wild: Raw 3 oz	65	1	0
Steamed, 3 oz	70	1	0
Cuttlefish, raw, 3 oz	70	1	1
Dolphinfish ~ *See Mahi-Mahi*			
Eel: Raw, 3 oz	155	10	0
Baked, 3 oz	200	13	0
Fish & Chips *(Red Lobster)*, battered, without condiments	700	33	61
Fish Sandwich *(Burger King)*, without Tartar Sauce	340	9	49
Fish Oil, 1 Tbsp, 0.5 oz	125	14	0
Flounder/Sole:			
Raw, 4 oz	80	2	0
Baked, 3 oz	75	2	0

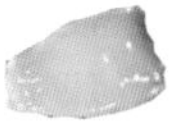
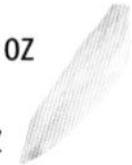
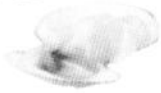
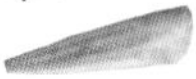
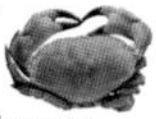
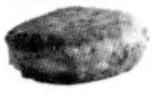
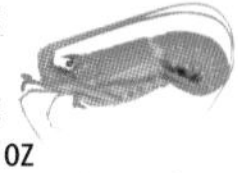
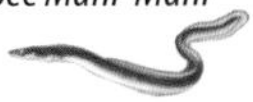
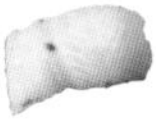

Frozen Fish ~ *See Pages 114-122*

Fish & Shellfish (Cont)

Edible Weights: Without Bones or Shell

Food	C	F	Cb
Haddock: Raw, 4 oz	**85**	0.5	0
Baked, 3 oz	**75**	0.5	0
Smoked, 3 oz	**100**	1	0
Halibut:			
Atlantic: Raw, 4 oz	**105**	1.5	0
Baked, ½ fillet, 5.6 oz	**175**	2.5	0
Herring:			
Atlantic, raw, 4 oz	**180**	10	0
Canned: Plain, drained, 3 oz	**130**	8	0
In Tomato Sauce, 3.5 oz	**140**	8	2
Pickled, 2 pieces, 1 oz	**75**	5	3
Smoked, kippered, 4 oz	**245**	14	0
Jellyfish: Raw, 4 oz	**30**	0	0
Dried, Salted, 1 cup, 2 oz	**20**	1	0
Ling, raw, 4 oz	**100**	0.5	0
Lobster, Northern:			
1.5 lb Whole Lobster, edible portion:			
Raw, 6.3 oz	**140**	1.5	0
Boiled, 5 oz	**140**	1	0
Lobster Salads, average, ½ cup	**220**	13	5
Lobster Newberg, average, ¾ cup	**360**	20	9
Lobster Thermidor, av., 1 serving	**370**	22	15
Lobster Tail (Rock),			
Red Lobster, grilled/roasted	**230**	6	2
Lox, Regular/Nova, 2 oz	**65**	2.5	0
Mackerel, Atlantic: Raw, 4 oz	**230**	16	0
Baked, 3 oz fillet	**225**	15	0
Pacific/Jack: Raw, 4 oz	**180**	9	0
Baked, 3 oz	**170**	9	0
Spanish: Raw, 4 oz	**160**	7	0
Baked, 3 oz	**135**	5.5	0
Mahi-Mahi/Dolphinfish:			
Raw, 4 oz	**95**	1	0
Baked, 4 oz	**125**	1	0
Monkfish: Raw, 4 oz	**85**	1.5	0
Baked, 3 oz	**80**	2	0
Mullet, Striped: Raw, 4 oz	**135**	4.5	0
Baked, 3 oz	**130**	4	0
Mussels:			
Raw: 4 oz (edible wt)	**100**	2.5	4
1 cup, 5.3 oz (edible weight)	**130**	3.5	5
Cooked, moist heat, 3 oz	**150**	4	6
Ocean Perch:			
Atlantic: Raw, 4 oz	**90**	2	0
Baked, 3 oz	**80**	1.5	0
Octopus:			
Common: Raw, 4 oz	**95**	1	3
Boiled, 3 oz	**140**	2	4
Orange Roughy:			
Raw, 4 oz	**85**	1	0
Baked, 3 oz	**90**	1	0

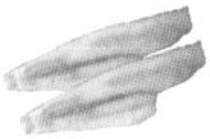
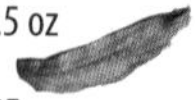
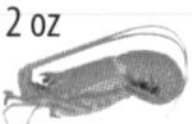
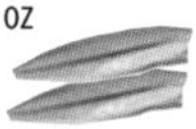
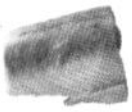
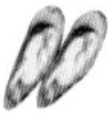
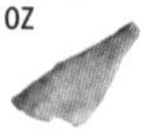
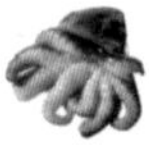
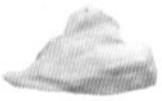

Fish & Shellfish (Cont)

Edible Weights: Without Bones or Shell

Food	C	F	Cb
Oysters, Common, Raw, 3 oz	**70**	2	4
Eastern:			
Farmed: Raw, 6 medium, 3 oz	**50**	1.5	5
Cooked, dry heat, 6 med., 2 oz	**45**	1.5	5
Wild: Raw, 6 medium, 3 oz	**45**	1.5	3
Cooked, dry heat, 6 med., 2 oz	**45**	1.5	3
Breaded & Fried, 6 med., 3 oz	**175**	11	10
Pacific: Raw, 1 medium, 1.8 oz	**40**	1	3
Steamed, 1 medium, 0.8 oz	**40**	1	3
Perch ~ *See Ocean Perch*			
Pike: Northern: Raw, 4 oz	**100**	1	0
Baked, 3 oz	**95**	1	0
Walleye: Raw, 4 oz	**105**	1.5	0
Baked, 3 oz	**100**	1.5	0
Pollock, Atlantic: Raw, 4 oz	**105**	1	0
Baked, 3 oz	**100**	1	0
Pompano, Florida, raw, 4 oz	**185**	11	0
Red Snapper ~ *See Snapper*			
Roe, raw, 2 Tbsp, 1 oz	**40**	2	0.5
Sablefish: Raw, 4 oz	**220**	17	0
Smoked, 3 oz	**220**	17	0
Salmon:			
Atlantic, Farmed: Raw, 4 oz	**235**	15	0
Baked, 3 oz	**175**	10	0
Steaks: Raw, 7 oz	**410**	27	0
Baked, 6 oz	**365**	22	0
Atlantic, Wild: Raw, 4 oz	**160**	7	0
Baked, 3 oz	**155**	7	0
Steaks: Raw, 7 oz	**280**	13	0
Baked, 6 oz	**310**	14	0
Chinook: Raw, 4 oz	**205**	12	0
Baked, 3 oz	**195**	11	0
Smoked, 3 oz	**100**	3.5	0
King: Raw, 3.5 oz	**185**	12	0
Kippered, 3.5 oz piece	**265**	16	0
Smoked & canned, 3.5 oz	**150**	6	0
Coho:			
Farmed: Raw, 4 oz	**180**	8.5	0
Baked, 3 oz	**150**	7	0
Wild: Raw, 4 oz	**165**	6.5	0
Steamed, 3 oz	**155**	6.5	0
Pink/Chum: Raw, 4 oz	**145**	5	0
Baked, 3.5 oz	**155**	5.5	0
Canned: Drained solids, 11 oz	**435**	16	0
Without skin & bones, 8.5 oz	**330**	10	0
Sockeye: Raw, 4 oz	**160**	6.5	0
Baked, 3 oz	**145**	5.5	0
Canned, Drained solids, 3 oz	**140**	6.5	0
Smoked, 3.5 oz	**205**	7.5	0
Salmon Cake (1), 3 oz	**240**	15	6

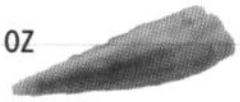
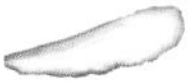

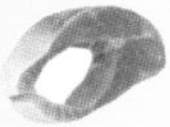
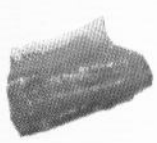
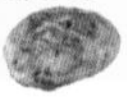

Fish & Shellfish (Cont)

	C	F	Cb
Sardines: *Canned, Average all Brands*			
Drained of Oil:			
¼ cup drained, 2.2 *oz*	130	9	0
3.75 oz can, drained, 3.3 oz	190	11	0
1 large/2 medium, ³⁄₅", 0.8 oz	50	3	0
in Tomato Sauce, 3.8 oz	150	8	3
Sashimi ~ *See Japanese Foods, Page 171*			
Scallops: Raw, 6 lge/15 small, 3 oz	65	0.5	3
Breaded, Fried (6), 5 oz 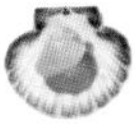	385	20	39
Steamed, 3 oz	95	0.5	0
Sea Bass ~ *See Bass*			
Seafood Salad, Deli Style,			
½ cup, 3.5 oz 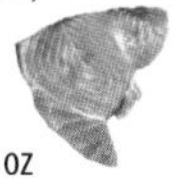	250	21	11
Shark: Raw, 4 oz	145	5	0
Baked, 4 oz	185	7	0
Batter-dipped, fried, 4 oz	260	16	7
Shrimp:			
Raw: Small/Medium (4), 0.8 oz	15	0	0
Large (4), 1 oz 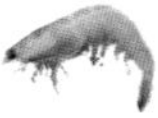	20	0	0
Breaded & Fried, 4.8 oz	395	24	27
Steamed, in shell, 3 oz	100	1.5	0
Canned, 1 can, 4.5 oz	130	2	0
Snapper: Raw, 4 oz 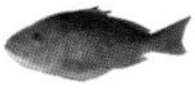	115	1.5	0
Baked: 3 oz	110	1.5	0
6 oz fillet	220	3	0
Sole: Raw, 4 oz 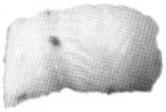	80	2	0
Baked, 3 oz	75	2	0
Squid ~ *see Calamari*			
Surimi, (Imitation Crab), 4 oz	110	0.5	17
Swai/Basa, raw, 4 oz 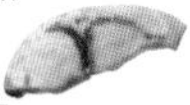	70	2	0
Swordfish: Raw, 4 oz	165	7.5	0
Medium Steak, 6 oz	250	11	0
Baked: Small Steak, 4 oz	205	7	0
Medium Steak, 6 oz	290	13	0
Tilapia: Raw, 4 oz 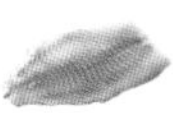	110	2	0
Baked: 3 oz	110	2.5	0
Trout, Rainbow:			
Farmed: Raw, 4 oz 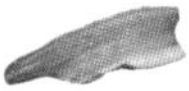	160	7	0
Baked, 3 oz	145	6.5	0
Wild: Raw, 4 oz	135	4	0
Baked, 3 oz	130	5	0
Tuna: 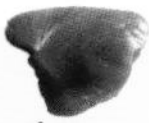			
Raw: Bluefin, 4 oz	165	5.5	0
Skipjack, Yellowfin, av., 4 oz	120	1	0
Baked: Bluefin, 3 oz	155	5.5	0
Skipjack, Yellowfin, av., 3 oz	110	1	0
Canned: *in Water, drained*			
Chunk Light: 2 oz	50	1	0
3 oz can 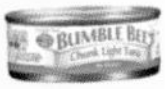	75	1.5	1
5 oz can	125	2.5	1.5

	C	F	Cb
Tuna (Cont): *in Water, drained (Cont)*			
Solid White: 2 oz	60	0.5	0
5 oz can 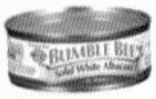	150	1.5	0
7 oz can	210	2	0
in Oil, drained:			
Chunk Light: 2 oz can	80	4	0
5 oz can 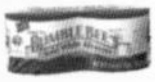	200	10	0
Solid White: 2 oz can	90	4	0
6 oz can	270	12	0
Whitefish: Raw, 4 oz 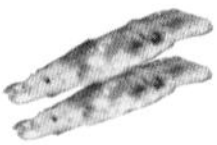	150	6.5	0
Baked, 3 oz	145	6.5	1
Smoked, 3 oz	90	1	0
Whiting: Raw, 4 oz	100	1.5	0
Baked, 3 oz	100	1.5	0
Yellowtail: Raw, 4 oz 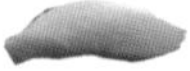	165	6	0
Grilled, 3 oz	160	6	0

Other Canned/Packaged Fish

	C	F	Cb
Bumble Bee: *Skinless, Boneless*			
Mackerel, in oil, drained, 1.9 oz	160	15	0
Pink/Red Salmon, av., 3 oz 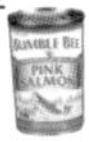	115	4.5	0.5
Sardines, in oil, drained, 2.6 oz	160	12	0
Tuna: *Drained*			
Chunk, Light, in water, 3 oz	60	0.5	0.5
Prime Fillets: Solid White, 4 oz	140	1.5	0
with Chipotle & Olive Oil, 2 oz	140	9	1
Pouch, in water, 5 oz	190	6	0
Solid White, in oil, drained, 4 oz	160	5	0
Snack Kits, per 2.5 oz Pouches:			
Cracked Pepper 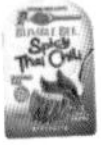	60	0.5	0.5
Jalapeno Seasoned	70	0	2
Spicy Thai Chili	90	1	8
Sun-Dried Tomato & Basil	60	0	2
Chicken of the Sea: *Drained*			
Pink Salmon: Skinless/boneless: 3 oz	80	2	0
Traditional, 14.75 oz can, 2.1 oz serve	90	5	0
Sardines, in oil, smoked, 3.75 oz can	150	10	0
Tuna: Chunk In Water, 5 oz can, 2 oz sv.	50	1	0
Solid in Water, 5 oz can, 2 oz serving	60	1	0
Starkist:			
Lunch To Go Kit, Tuna Salad, 4.1 oz	260	9	25
Pouch: *Per 2.6 oz Pouch*			
Albacore White Tuna in water	80	1.5	0
Pink Salmon in Water 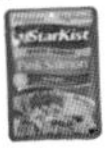	70	1	1
Ready To Eat Kit:			
Ranch Tuna Salad, 3.28 oz	130	3.5	13
Sweet & Spicy Tuna Salad, 2.75 oz	70	0.5	7
Salmon Creations: 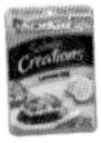			
Lemom Dill, 2.6 oz	70	1	0.5
Mango Chipotle, 2.6 oz	90	1	5
Tuna Creations: 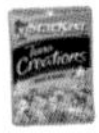			
Bold Thai Chili Style, 2.6 oz	90	1	7
Herb & Garlic, 2.6 oz	110	4	2

F Flours & Grains

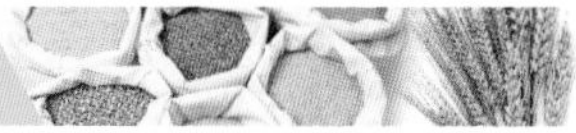

Flours & Grains

Food	C	F	Cb
Amaranth Flour *(Bob's Red Mill)*, ½ cup, 2.2 oz	220	4	40
Arrowroot Flour, ½ cup, 2.3 oz	230	0	56
Barley: Grain, regular, ½ cup, 2.6 oz	255	1	55
Pearled, raw, 3.5 oz	350	1	78
Buckwheat: Grain, ½ cup, 3 oz	290	3	61
Flour, whole-groat, ½ cup, 2 oz	200	2	42
Groats: Roasted, dry, ½ cup, 3 oz	285	2	62
Roasted, cooked, 3.5 oz	80	0.5	17
Bulgur: Dry, ½ cup, 2.5 oz	240	1	53
Cooked, ½ cup, 3.2 oz	75	0.5	17
Carob Flour, ½ cup, 1.8 oz	115	0.5	46
Coconut Flour, 2 Tbsp, 0.6 oz	60	3.5	10
Corn Kernels, cooked, av., ½ cup	80	0.5	18
Corn Bran, ½ cup, 1.3 oz	85	0.5	33
Corn Flour/Masa, ½ cup, 2 oz	215	2.5	43
Corn Grits:			
Dry, ½ cup, 2.8oz	290	1	62
Cooked, ½ cup, 4.3 oz	70	0.5	15
Corn Germ, toasted, ½ cup, 4 oz	100	1.5	22
Cornmeal, average all varieties:			
3 Tbsp, 1 oz	105	0.5	22
½ cup, 2.5 oz	255	1	54
Mixes, same as above	230	1	48
Cornstarch: 1 Tbsp, 0.3 oz	30	0	8
½ cup, 2.3oz	245	0	58
Couscous: Dry, 1 oz	110	0	22
Cooked, 1 cup, 5.5 oz	175	0.5	37
Farina: Dry, ½ cup, 3 oz	325	0.5	69
Cooked, ½ cup, 4 oz	55	0	12
Flaxseed: Whole, 1 T., 0.3 oz	45	3.5	2
Ground, 2 Tbsp, 0.3 oz	60	4.5	4
Garbanzo, (Chick Pea), ½ cup, 1.6 oz	180	3	27
Gluten Free Flour, 3 Tbsp	100	0	24
Hemp Flour, Wholemeal, ½ cup, 3.5 oz	300	10	5
Matzo Meal, ½ cup, 2.2 oz	230	0.5	48
Millet: Raw, ½ cup, 3.5 oz	380	4	73
Cooked, ½ cup, 3 oz	105	1	21
Oat Bran: Raw, ⅓ cup, 1 oz	75	2	21
Cooked, ½ cup, 3.8 oz	45	1	13
Oats, Rolled/Oatmeal:			
Dry/Groats, ½ cup, 1.5 oz	160	3	28
Cooked, ½ cup, 4.2 oz	75	1	13
Polenta ~ *See Cornmeal*			
Potato Flour, ½ cup, 2.8 oz	285	0.5	66
Psyllium Husks, 1 Tbsp, 0.2 oz	10	0	4
Quinoa: Dry, ½ cup, 3 oz	320	5	59
Cooked, ½ cup, 3.8 oz	130	2	24
Rice Bran, ½ cup, 2 oz	180	12	28
Rice Flour, ½ cup, 2.8 oz	290	1	63

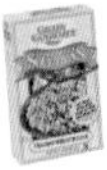
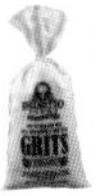
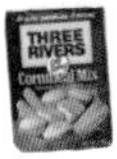
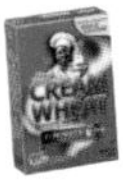
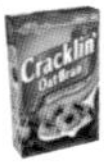
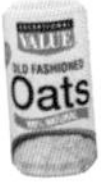
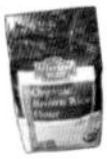

Flours & Grains (Cont)

Food	C	F	Cb
Rice Polish, ½ cup, 3.5 oz	360	0.5	80
Rye Flour:			
Dark, ½ cup, 2.3 oz	210	2	44
Light, ½ cup, 1.8 oz	190	1	41
Medium, ½ cup, 1.8 oz	180	1	40
Rye Grain: ½ cup, 3 oz	280	2	59
Flakes, ¼ cup, 1 oz	100	0.5	21
Semolina Flour, ½ cup, 3 oz	300	1	61
Sorghum, ½ cup, 3.4 oz	325	3	72
Soy Flour:			
Defatted, 1 cup, 3.5 oz	330	1	38
Low-Fat, 1 cup, 3 oz	325	6	33
Full-Fat, 1 cup, 3 oz	365	17	29
Soy Meal, defatted, 1 cup, 4.3 oz	415	3	49
Spelt Flour, ½ cup, 2 oz	190	1	41
Tapioca Pearl:			
Dry, ½ cup, 2.7 oz	270	0	67
3 Tbsp, 1 oz	100	0	25
Teff Seed Flour, 2 oz	215	2	42
Tortilla Flour Mix, ½ cup, 2 oz	220	6	37
Triticale:			
½ cup, 3.4 oz	325	2	70
Flour, wholegrain, ½ cup, 2.3 oz	220	1	48
Wheat Bran, unprocessed, ½ cup, 1 oz	65	1	19
Wheat Flakes, ½ cup, 1.5 oz	160	1	35
Wheat Germ:			
Raw, ¼ cup, 1 oz	105	3	15
Toasted, ¼ cup, 1 oz	110	3	14
Wheat Flour:			
White, All Purpose/Self-Rising:			
1 level Tbsp, 0.3 oz	30	0	6
½ cup, 2.2 oz	230	0.5	48
1 cup, 4.4 oz	455	1.5	95
Whole Wheat, 1 cup, 4.2 oz	405	2	87

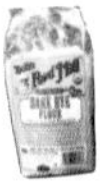
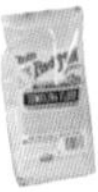
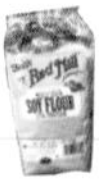
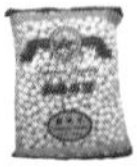
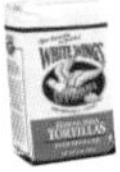
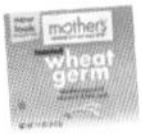
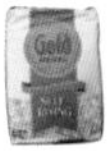

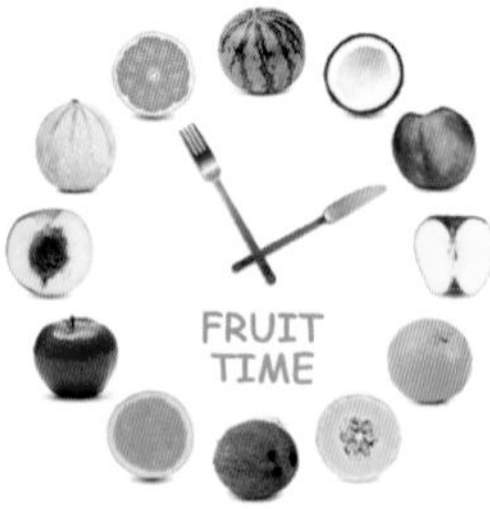

Fruit ~ Fresh

Weights As Purchased

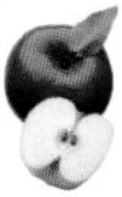
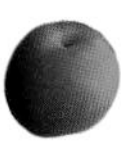
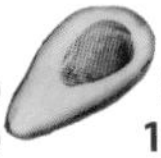
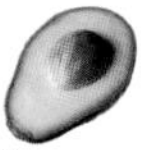

Food	C	F	Cb
Apples, all varieties, average:			
Whole, with skin:			
1 small, 4 oz	55	0	14
1 medium, 5.5 oz	75	0	19
1 large, 8 oz	110	0	28
1 extra large, 11 oz	145	0	36
Flesh only, no skin or core: 1 oz	15	0	3.5
Slices, 1 cup, 4 oz	55	0	14
Candy/Caramel Apple, 1 med., 6.5 oz	245	4	54
Chiquita, Apple Bites, 14 slices, 5 oz	80	0	20
Apricots: 1 small, 1.5oz	20	0	4
1 medium, 2 oz	25	0	6
1 large, 3 oz	40	0	10
1 extra large, 4 oz	50	0	12
Asian Pear, (Nashi Fruit), 1 med., 7 oz	85	0	21
Avocado:			
Fuerte (Florida) variety:			
¼ medium, 2.7 oz pulp	90	7.5	6
½ medium, 5.4 oz pulp	180	15	12
Mashed, 2 Tbsp, 1 oz	35	3	2
Hass variety (Californian/Mexican):			
Cubes, ½ cup, 2.5 oz	120	11	6
Mashed: 2 Tbsp, 1 oz	50	4	2
¼ cup, 2 oz	95	8	5
Pulp: ¼ medium, 1.5 oz	70	6.5	3
½ medium, 3 oz	140	13	7
1 medium (8.5 oz whole), 6 oz	280	26	14
Salad slices (3), 1 oz	50	4	2

Note: The fat of avocados is heart-healthy. Avocados are very low in carbs ~ most is fiber. This benefits blood sugar and cholesterol levels. Use in place of butter and other high-fat spreads.

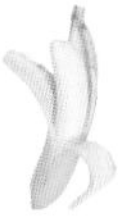
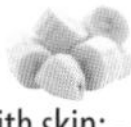
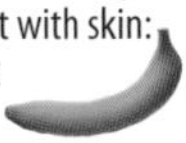
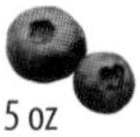

Food	C	F	Cb
Banana:			
Weight with skin:			
1 baby, 3 oz	50	0	12
1 small (5″), 4 oz	65	0	16
1 medium (7″), 5 oz	80	0	20
1 large (8″), 8 oz	120	0	30
1 extra large (9″), 9 oz	135	0	34
Flesh only, weight without skin:			
Mashed, ½ cup, 4 oz	100	0	25
Slices, ½ cup, 2.5 oz	65	0	16
Green Bananas, weight with skin:			
1 medium (7″), 5 oz	75	0	18
1 large (8″), 7 oz	110	0	27
Blackberries, 1 cup, 5 oz	60	0.5	14
Blueberries: ¼ cup, 1 oz	15	0	4
1 cup or ½ pint container, 5 oz	80	0	20
1 pint container, 10 oz	160	0	40

Weights As Purchased

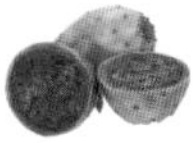
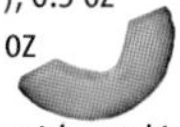

Food	C	F	Cb
Boysenberries, 1 cup, 4.5 oz	60	4.5	14
Breadfruit, ½ cup, 4 oz	115	0	30
Cactus Fruit:			
1 small, 2 oz	15	0	4
1 medium, 5 oz	40	0	9
1 large, 7 oz	55	0	13
Pulp, no skin, 1 cup, 5.3 oz	60	0	14
Cantaloupe: Flesh, without skin, 1 oz	10	0	2
Pieces/Balls, 1 cup, 5.5 oz	55	0	13
Slices, ½ circle, without rind:			
1 thin (buffet), ⅛″), 0.5 oz	5	0	1
1 medium (¼″), 1 oz	10	0	2
1 thick (½″), 2 oz	20	0	5
Wedges, length cut, without skin:			
1 thin, 1/16 medium, 2 oz	20	0	5
1 thick, ⅛ medium, 4 oz	40	0	9
Whole, weight with seeds and skin:			
½ small, 20 oz	195	1	46
½ medium, 28 oz	270	1.5	65
½ large, 2.5 lb	370	2	90
Cape Gooseberries, 1 cup, 5 oz	70	1	15
Cherimoya: Pulp, ½ cup, 3 oz	60	0	14
1 Fruit (11 oz), 8 oz edible	170	1	40

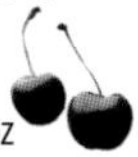
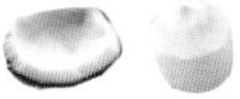
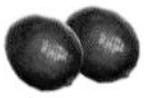
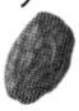
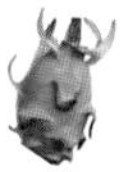

Food	C	F	Cb
Cherries, (Red/White), sweet, raw:			
6 medium or 4 large, 2 oz	30	0	7
1 cup, 4.5 oz	75	0	18
½ lb quantity	130	0	32
Sour, red, raw, 1 cup, 4 oz	50	0	12
Clementine, 1 medium, 2.6 oz	35	0	9
Coconut, raw:			
Young, sweet,			
Pieces: 1 piece (2″ x 2″), 1.5 oz	35	2	4
½ cup, 3.5 oz	80	5	9
Mature, hard, 1 piece (2″x 2″), 1.5 oz	160	15	6
Crabapples, slices, ½ cup, 2 oz	40	0	11
Cranberries,			
fresh, ¼ cup, 1 oz	25	0	6.5
Custard Apple ~ *See Cherimoya*			
Dates: Medium (1), 0.3 oz	20	0	5
Large Medjool (1), 0.5 oz	40	0	10
Extra Large Medjool (1), 0.9 oz	65	0	16
Chopped, ½ cup, 3 oz	240	0	58
Dragon Fruit, (Pitahaya):			
1 medium, 4″ long, 12 oz	60	0	12
1 large, 5″long, 16 oz	80	0	18
Durian, pulp, 4 oz	165	6	31
Elderberries, ½ cup, 2.5 oz	55	0.5	13

F Fruit ~ Fresh

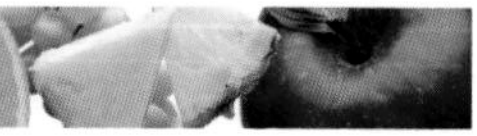

Weights As Purchased	C	F	Cb
Feijoa, (Pineapple Guava), 1 medium, 2 oz	30	0.5	5.5
Figs, green/black:			
1 medium, 2 oz	40	0	10
1 large, 3 oz	60	0	15
Gooseberries, raw, 1 cup, 5 oz	65	1	15
Grapefruit, all varieties, average:			
½ fruit, 10 oz (6 oz flesh)	55	0	13
1 cup sections w/ juice, 8 oz	75	0	18
Grapes: Average, 1 cup, 5.5 oz	105	0	28
1 small bunch, 4 oz	80	0	20
1 medium bunch, 7 oz	140	0	36
1 large bunch, 16 oz	315	0	82
Granadilla, pulp, 1/2 cup, 4 oz	110	0	27
Guanabana, pulp, 1/2 cup, 4 oz	75	0	19
Guava, 1 medium, 4 oz	80	1	16
Honeydew:			
1 slice, ¾" thick, 3 oz	30	0	7
1 wedge (⅛ of 7" diameter), 12 oz (with rind)	80	0	20
Cubes/Balls, 1 cup, 6 oz	60	0	14
½ small (4½ lb whole)	180	0.5	42
½ medium (6 lb whole)	230	1	56
Honey Murcots, 1 only, 5 oz	45	0	11
Jaboticaba, 1 cup, 5.5 oz	55	0	14
Jackfruit, flesh, ⅛, 4 oz	105	0	27
Kiwano, ½ medium, 5 oz	35	0	8
Kiwifruit:			
1 Medium, 2.7 oz	45	0	11
1 Large, 3.2 oz	55	0	13
Langsat, Duku, 1 medium, 2 oz	25	0	5
Lemons: 1 medium, 5oz	20	0	4
1 wedge, 1 oz	5	0	1
Limes, 1 medium, 2.4 oz	20	0	7
Loganberries, frozen, ½ cup, 2.5 oz	40	0	9
Longans, 5 fruit, 0.5oz	10	0	2.5
Loquats, 4 fruit, 2.3 oz	30	0	8
Lychees, 4 fruit, 2.3 oz	30	0	7
Mamey Apple, cubes, 1 cup, 6 oz	85	1	20
Mandarin Orange:			
1 small, 3 oz	35	0	9
1 medium, 4 oz	45	0	11
1 large, 6 oz	50	0	13
Mango:			
Slices, ½ cup, 3 oz	55	0	14
1 small mango, 7 oz	90	0.5	24
1 medium: 10 oz	130	0.5	34
Side cheek, 4 oz	60	0	14
1 large, 17 oz	220	1	58
1 extra large, 24 oz	310	1.5	82
Marionberries, 1 cup, 5 oz	75	1	15

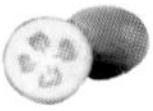
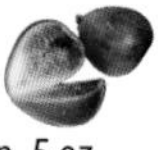
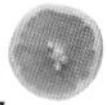
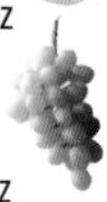
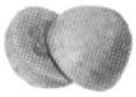
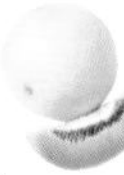

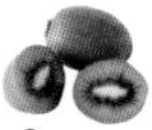
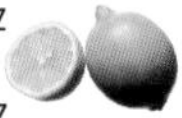
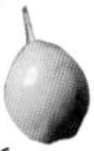
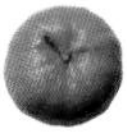
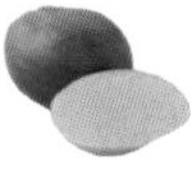
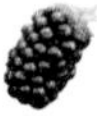

Weights As Purchased	C	F	Cb
Melons, all varieties, average, cubes/balls, 1 cup, 6 oz	60	0	14
Mulberries, 20 fruit, 1 oz	15	0	3
Nashi Fruit/Asian Pear, 1 med. 7 oz	85	0	21
Nectarines: 1 medium, 5oz	60	0	14
1 large, 7 oz	80	0	18
Oheloberries, ½ cup, 2.5 oz	20	0	5
Olives, Pickled: Green, 10 lge, 1.5 oz	60	6.5	1.5
Ripe, Greek Style, 10 medium, 1 oz	70	6	4
Ripe (Black) Californian:			
1 small/medium	5	0	0.2
1 large/extra large	6	0.5	0.5
1 jumbo	7	0.5	0.5
1 colossal	11	1	0.5
Oranges, all varieties, average, weights with skin:			
1 small, (2.5" diam.), 5 oz	45	0	11
1 medium (3") 7 oz	75	0	18
1 large, (3.5") 10 oz	105	0	25
1 extra large, (4"), 14 oz	130	0	30
Flesh/Pulp only, 1 cup, 6 oz	85	0	21
Peel, 1 Tbsp	0	0	0
California Navel (3"), 7 oz	70	0	17
California Valencia, 1 medium (2¾" diam.) 6 oz	60	0	14
Florida Orange, 1 med., 7 oz	70	0	17
Sunkist Navel, large, 14 oz	130	0	30
Papaya:			
1" pieces, 1 cup, 5 oz	60	0	15
1 medium, 16 oz	120	0	30
Green (unripe), ½ cup, 3.5 oz	20	0	5
Passionfruit:			
1 small, 1.5 oz	15	0	3
1 large, 2.7 oz	30	0	6
Pulp, ½ cup, 4 oz	110	0	27
Peaches: 1 baby/donut, 3 oz	30	0	7
1 small, 5 oz	50	0	12
1 medium, 6 oz	60	0	14
1 large, 7 oz	70	0	16
1 extra large, 9 oz	90	0	21
Pears, all varieties, average:			
1 mini, 2.5 oz	35	0	8
1 small, 5 oz	75	0	18
1 medium, 7 oz	100	0	25
1 large, 9 oz	130	0	33
1 extra large, 12 oz	170	0	42
Pepino, ½ medium, 4 oz	20	0	4
Persimmons: Native, 1 oz	35	0	9
Japanese (2½"d. x 2½"h), 7 oz	120	0	30
Maui, seedless, 1 medium, 5 oz	100	0	25

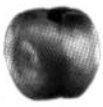

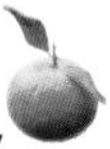
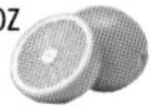
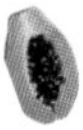
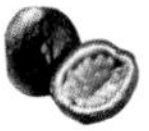
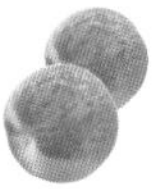
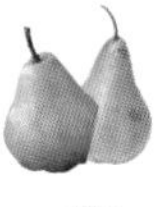
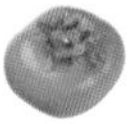

Weights As Purchased	C	F	Cb
Pineapple, average all varieties:			
Weights without skin:			
1 thin slice (½"), 2 oz 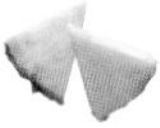	30	0	7
1 thick slice (¾"), 3 oz	40	0	10
1 cup, chunks, 6 oz	80	0	20
Whole fruit, wt with skin: 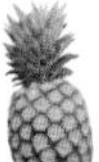			
Baby/Mini, 16 oz	150	0	39
Medium size, 3 lbs	450	1	118
Canned ~ *See Page 102*			
Pitanga, (Surinam-Cherry) (5), 1.2 oz	10	0	2
Plaintain:			
Fresh/Raw, weight with skin:			
1 medium, 10 oz 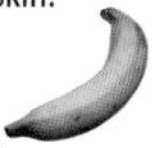	220	0	55
Slices, 1 cup, 5 oz	180	0	44
Cooked:			
Mashed, ½ cup, 3.5 oz	115	0	30
Slices, 1 cup, 5.5 oz	180	0	47
Fried in oil: 10 slices (¼"), 2 oz	160	6	26
1 cup, 4.2 oz	360	14	58
Plums, all varieties, average:			
1 mini/Damson, (1" diam), 0.5 oz	10	0	1.5
1 small (2"), 2.3oz	30	0	7
1 medium (2½"), 3.5 oz 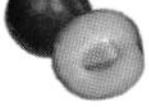	45	0	10
1 large (3"), 5 oz	60	0	14
Plumcot, 1 medium, 6 oz	75	0	18
Pomegranate:			
1 small (3"), 5.5 oz 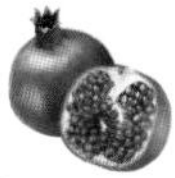	70	1	15
1 medium (3½"), 10 oz	125	2	27
1 large (4"), 16 oz	230	3	50
Seeds/Arils, ¼ cup, 2 oz	40	1	10
Pomelo, flesh, ½ cup, 3.5 oz	35	0	9
Prickly Pear ~ *See Cactus Fruit*			
Quince, 1 medium, 3.5 oz	55	0	14
Rambutan/Rambotang, 			
Red/Yellow, 1 medium, 2 oz	15	0	4
Raspberries: ½ cup, 2 oz	30	0	7
10 raspberries, 0.8 oz	10	0	2
1 cup, 4.3 oz 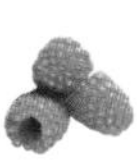	65	1	15
1 pint, 11 oz	160	2	37
Sapodilla: 1 medium, 6 oz	140	2	34
Pulp, 1 cup, 8.5 oz	200	2.5	45
Sapote:			
Black: 1 medium, 4.5 oz 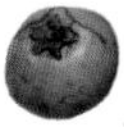	60	0	14
Pulp only, ½ cup, 4 oz	100	1	22
Mamey, piece, 1 cup, 6 oz	220	1	50
Satsuma Tangerine, 1 medium, 3 oz	45	0	11
Soursop, pulp, 1 cup, 8 oz	150	0.5	38
Starfruit, (Carambola):			
1 medium, (3½" long), 3 oz 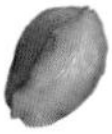	30	0	6
1 large (4½"), 4.5 oz	40	0	8
Strawberries: 1 cup, 5.5 oz	50	0.5	12
6 medium/3 large, 2 oz 	20	0	4
1 pint container, heaping, 16 oz	130	1	32
Chocolate dipped, 1 large	45	2.5	6

Weights As Purchased	C	F	Cb
Sugar-Apple (Sweetsop), 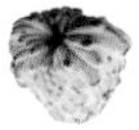			
pulp, ½ cup, 4 oz	120	0	28
Sugar Cane:			
Unpeeled, 1 baton (7" long), 4 oz	30	0	7
Peeled, 1 small stick (3"), 2 oz	35	0	8
Tamarillo, 1 medium, 3 oz 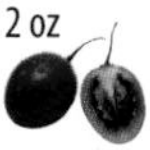	20	0	3
Tamarind: 1 fruit (3"x1")	5	0	1.5
Pulp, ½ cup, 2 oz 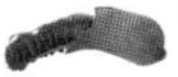	140	0.5	37
Tangelo: 1 small, 4 oz	55	0	13
1 medium, 5 oz 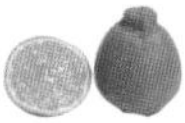	70	0	17
1 large, 7 oz	95	0	23
Tangerine, 1 med., (2½" diam.), 4 oz	50	0	13
Tangor, 1 medium, 4 oz	35	0	7
Tomatillos: 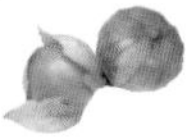			
3 medium, 3.5 oz	35	0.5	6
1lb (16 oz) quantity	160	2	27
Tomatoes:			
1 small (2¼" diameter), 3 oz 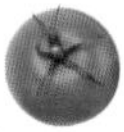	15	0	3
1 medium (2¾"), 5 oz	25	0	5
Sliced: 2 thin slices, 1 oz	5	0	1
2 thick (⅜"), 2 oz 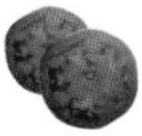	10	0	2
Wedge, ¼, 1.3 oz	6	0	1
1 large (3½"), 8 oz	40	0.5	9
1 extra large (4"), 12 oz	60	0.5	14
Cherry: 4 medium, 2 oz	10	0	2
1 cup, 5 oz 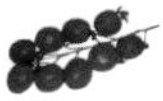	25	0	6
Grape, 5 medium, 2 oz	10	0	2
Yellow Tear Drop, 3 medium, 1 oz	5	0	2
Canned Tomatoes/Products ~ *See Page 144*			
Tree Tomato/Tamarillo, 3 oz	20	0	5
Ugli Fruit, Tangelo type, 5 oz 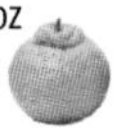	40	0	8
Watermelon:			
Flesh only, weights without skin:			
1 thin slice (½"), ¼ circle, 3 oz	25	0	6
1 thick slice (1"): ¼ circle, 6 oz	50	0	12
½ circle, 12 oz 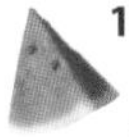	100	1	24
Buffet Slice, small, thin, 1 oz	8	0	2
Cubes or Balls, 1 cup, 5.5 oz	45	0	11
Round Seedless Melon, weight with skin:			
Medium size, 13 lb, (8" diam.):			
whole melon, 13 lb	1160	5	280
wedge, ⅛ whole, 26 oz	145	1	35
Mini size, 6 lb, (6.5" diam.): 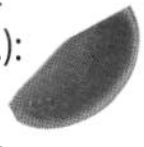			
whole melon, 6 lb	480	2.5	110
wedge, ⅛ whole, 12 oz	60	0	14

Dried Fruit

	C	F	Cb
Apples, 5 rings, 1 oz	**80**	0	19
Apricots, 8 halves, 1 oz	**65**	0	16
Banana Chips, ⅓ cup, 1 oz	**180**	9	16
Banana Flakes, 4 Tbsp, 1 oz	**80**	0	20
Cranberries *(Craisins):*			
Original, ¼ cup	**130**	0	33
Reduced Sugar, ¼ cup	**100**	0	31
Chocolate Covered, ¼ cup, 2 oz	**180**	8	28
Dates ~ *See Dates in Fresh Fruit*			
Figs, 3 medium figs, 1 oz	**90**	0	23
Goji Berries, 3 Tbsp, 1 oz	**100**	0	21
Mango Slices, 5 pieces, 1.4 oz	**25**	0	6
Papaya Spears, 2 pieces, 1.4 oz	**120**	0	30
Peaches, 2 halves, 1 oz	**60**	0	15
Pears, 3 halves, 2 oz	**140**	0.5	34
Plums *(Sunsweet)*, (5), 1.4 oz	**100**	0	24
Prunes/Dried Plums:			
with pits, 3 medium, 1 oz	**70**	0	17
without pits, 4 medium, 1 oz	**70**	0	17
Cooked: with sugar, ½ cup, 5 oz	**155**	0	38
without sugar, ½ cup, 4.5 oz	**135**	0	33
Raisins: 2 Tbsp, 1 oz pack	**85**	0	22
½ cup, (unpacked), 2.5 oz	**215**	0	56
White Mulberries, 1 oz	**90**	0.5	22

Candied/Glazed Fruit

	C	F	Cb
Apricot, 1 medium, 1 oz	**70**	0	17
Cherry, Maraschino (1)	**8**	0	2
Citron/Fruit Peel, 1 oz	**85**	0	20
Ginger, 1 oz	**90**	0	21
Pineapple, 1 slice, 1.3 oz	**120**	0	29
Tamarind, dried, sweetened, 1 oz	**70**	0	17

Fruit Leather Rolls

	C	F	Cb
Betty Crocker: Fruit By The Foot, 1 roll, 0.8 oz	**80**	0	17
Fruit Gushers, 1 oz	**90**	1	20
Fruit Roll-Ups, 1 roll	**50**	1	12
Stretch Island, Leathers, 1 pouch, 0.5 oz	**45**	0	12

Canned/Bottled Fruit

Solids & Liquids:
Per ½ Cup, 4½ oz Unless indicated

	C	F	Cb
Apricots/Peaches/Pears:			
in juice, light	**60**	0	15
in heavy syrup	**105**	0	28
in water/diet	**35**	0	8
Black/Blueberries:			
in heavy syrup	**120**	0	30
in light syrup	**110**	0	26

Canned/Bottled Fruit (Cont)

	C	F	Cb
Cherries, pitted:			
in heavy syrup	**105**	0	27
in light syrup	**85**	0	22
in water	**55**	0	15
Maraschino, 1 oz	**50**	0	12
Fruit Cocktail/Salad:			
in heavy syrup	**95**	0	25
in juice, light	**60**	0	16
in water/diet	**35**	0	10
Gooseberries, light syrup	**90**	0	24
Grapefruit, in light syrup	**75**	0	20
Lychees, ½ cup, 4.5 oz	**105**	0	26
Mixed Fruit: in fruit juices/light syrup	**70**	0	18
in heavy syrup	**90**	0	24
in water/diet	**40**	0	10
Pineapple: in heavy syrup, 4.3	**110**	0	26
in own juice, 4 oz	**60**	0	15
Prunes: with syrup, 3 oz	**90**	0	23
Stewed in water, ½ cup	**135**	0	35

Fruit Snack Cups

	C	F	Cb
Deli/Take-Out: Small, 6 oz	**70**	0	16
Large, 12 oz	**140**	0	32
Yogurt and Fruit Cup, 15 oz	**380**	4.5	75
Del Monte:			
Bubble Fruit, all flavors, 4 oz cup,	**60**	0	14
Fruit & Oats, average, 7 oz	**185**	2.5	36
Fruit Refreshers, average, 7 oz cup	**95**	0	23
Fruit Snack Cups: Average, 4 oz	**70**	0	17
No Sugar Added, average, 4 oz	**50**	0	14
Parfaits: Pineapple Coconut	**180**	7	31
Average other varieties, 6.25 oz	**200**	8	31
Dole:			
Fruit Bowls In 100% Juice:			
Diced Pears, 4 oz cup	**90**	0	22
Mixed Fruit, 4 oz cup	**70**	0	15
Fridge Packs In Juice: *Per 4.3 oz Container*			
Peach Slices	**80**	0	21
Pineapple Chunks	**70**	0	16
Other Fruits	**90**	0	21

Apple & Fruit Sauces

	C	F	Cb
Apple Sauce:			
Regular/sweetened, 2 Tbsp, 1 oz	**20**	0	6
Cranberry, Jellied, ¼ cup	**110**	0	25
Fruit Sauces & Purees:			
All fruit types, average: 2 Tbsp, 1 oz	**25**	0	6
½ cup, 4 oz	**100**	0	24
Mott's:			
Apple Sauce: Original, 4 oz	**60**	0	14
Unsweetened Mango Pineapple, 3.9 oz	**50**	0	13
Ocean Spray, Jellied Cranb. Sce, 2.5 oz	**110**	0	28

Quick Guide

Ice Cream

Average all Flavors:

Regular (10% fat):

Examples: Dreyer's Grand, Hood, Friendly's

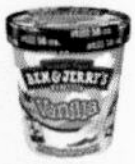

	C	F	Cb
½ cup, 4 fl.oz	**140**	7	16
1 cup, 8 fl.oz	**280**	14	32
1 pint, 16 fl.oz	**560**	28	64

Rich/Premium (16-17% fat):

Examples: Baskin Robbins, Ben & Jerry's, Haagen-Dazs

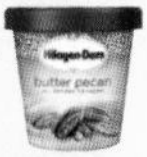

	C	F	Cb
½ cup, 4 fl.oz	**250**	16	24
1 cup, 8 fl.oz	**500**	32	48
1 pint, 16 fl.oz	**1000**	64	96

Reduced-Fat/Light (5% fat):

Examples: Breyers ½ The Fat, Friendly's Light, Hood Light

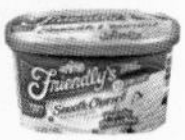

	C	F	Cb
½ cup, 4 fl.oz	**140**	5	21
1 cup, 8 fl.oz	**280**	10	42
1 pint, 16 fl.oz	**560**	20	84

Fat-Free:

Example: Breyers

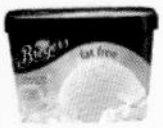

	C	F	Cb
½ cup, 4 fl.oz	**90**	0	21
1 cup, 8 fl.oz	**180**	0	42
1 pint, 16 fl.oz	**360**	0	84

Scoop Shops:

Average all Brands

Add extra for cone (see next column)

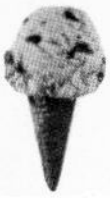

	C	F	Cb
Kids, 3 fl.oz	**125**	8	12
Regular, 6 fl.oz	**250**	16	24
Large, 9 fl.oz	**375**	24	36

Soft Serve:

Average all Brands

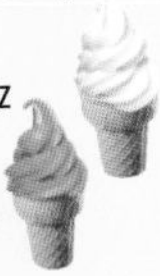

	C	F	Cb
Regular: ½ cup, 4 fl.oz	**255**	15	25
1 cup, 8 fl.oz	**510**	30	50
Light: ½ cup, 4 fl.oz	**145**	3	25
1 cup, 8 fl.oz	**290**	6	50

Quick Guide

Frozen Yogurt

Average all Brands

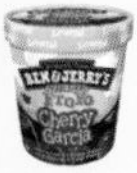

	C	F	Cb
Hard: Low-Fat, ½ cup	**110**	3	19
Non-Fat, ½ cup	**110**	0	24
Soft: Low-Fat, ½ cup	**120**	4	17
Non-Fat, ½ cup	**100**	0	30

Brands ~ *See Ice Cream & Novelties Section*

Quick Guide

Gelato/Ices/Frozen Custard

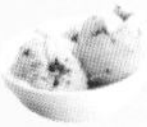

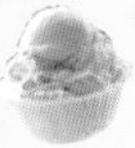

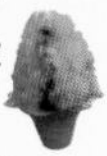

	C	F	Cb
Gelato: *Per ½ Cup*			
Milk base: Vanilla	**160**	6	25
Chocolate Hazelnut	**230**	15	21
Water base, ½ cup	**100**	0	26
Frozen Custard, Choc./Vanilla, av:			
½ cup	**210**	11	23
Single Scoop, 5 oz wt	**300**	15	38
Double Scoop, 10 oz wt	**600**	30	76
Ice (Milk base): *Average all flavors*			
Hard (4% fat), ½ cup	**100**	3	15
Soft Serve (3% fat), ½ cup	**110**	2	19
Shaved Ice, average, 12 fl.oz	**160**	0	40
Sherbet, average, ½ cup	**110**	1.5	22
Sorbet, Fruit, fat free, ½ cup	**70**	0	19
Fruit Ice Pops	**80**	0	20

Sundaes

Baskin Robbins:

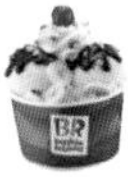

	C	F	Cb
Classic: Banana Royale	**690**	28	103
Choc. Chip Cookie Dough	**1130**	48	164
Made with Snickers	**1110**	43	165

Toppings ~ *See Page 195*

McDonald's:

Sundaes:

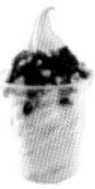

	C	F	Cb
Hot Caramel	**340**	8	60
Hot Fudge	**330**	10	52

Ice Cream Cones & Cups

Average all Brands

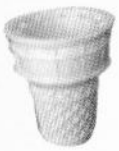

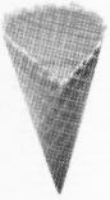

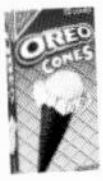

	C	F	Cb
Wafer Cone/Cup, average	**20**	0	4
Sugar Cone, average	**50**	0	14
Waffle Cone:			
Small	**50**	1	10
Large	**90**	0.5	19
Brands:			
Comet, Sugar Cone	**50**	0	11
Keebler, Sugar Cone	**50**	0	10
Oreo, Chocolate Cone	**50**	1	10

I Ice Cream & Frozen Yogurt

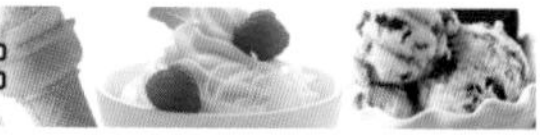

Ice Cream ~ Brands

Baskin-Robbins ~ *See Fast-Foods Section*

Ben & Jerry's:

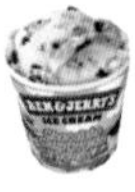
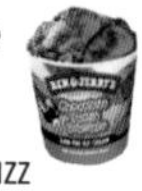
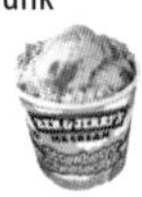

	C	F	Cb
Scoop Shop Ice Cream: *Hand Scooped, 3 oz Serving*			
Americone Dream	240	13	26
Boots on the Moooo'n	250	16	25
Butter Pecan	250	19	17
Cannoli	230	14	24
Chip Happens	240	14	24
Choc. Chip Cookie Dough	230	13	26
Chocolate Fudge Brownie	220	11	26
Chunky Monkey	240	15	24
Coconut Seven Layer Bar	250	16	24
Coffee, Coffee, BuzzBuzzBuzz	220	13	23
Mint Chocolate Chunk	220	14	22
Netflix & Chilll'd	250	15	25
New York Super Fudge Chunk	260	17	24
Salted Caramel Blondie	220	11	26
Strawberry Cheesecake	200	12	22
Sweet Cream & Cookies	210	12	23
Triple Caramel Chunk	220	12	26
Ice Cream, 1 Pint Tubs: *Per ⅔ Cup*			
Berry Sweet Mascarpone	350	22	32
Cannoli	360	21	38
Cherry Garcia	340	20	36
Chip Happens	390	24	40
Chocolate Therapy	330	18	38
Everything But The	420	26	40
Gimme S'more!	410	24	45
Netflix & Chilll'd	390	24	38
Peanut Butter Half Baked	370	20	43
Salted Caramel Almond	380	23	38
Strawberry Cheesecake	340	20	37
Triple Caramel Chunk	370	20	42
Vanilla Caramel Fudge	390	21	44
Core: Born Choclatta! Cookie	380	24	36
Peanut Butter Fudge	420	26	40
Salted Caramel	360	19	41
Light Ice Cream, 1 Pint Tubs: *Per ⅔ Cup*			
Chocolate Mint	190	6	30
Chocolate Cookie EnlightenMint	190	6	30
Mocha Fudge Brownie	200	4.5	36
P.B. Marshmallow Swirl	230	7	34
Non Dairy: *Per ⅔ Cup*			
Coffee Caramel Fudge	340	17	44
Creme Brulee Cookie	310	14	46
Choc. Salted 'n Swirled	320	15	44
Mint Chocolate Cookie	300	14	40
PB & Cookies	380	22	41
Fro Yo Frozen Yogurt: *Per ⅔ Cup*			
Cherry Garcia	230	4	44
Half Baked	230	3.5	45

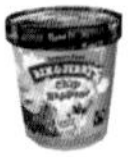
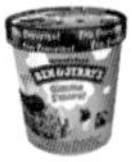
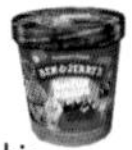
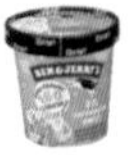
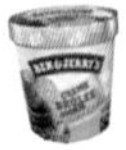

Blue Bunny:

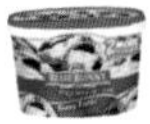
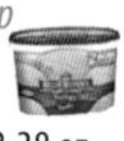
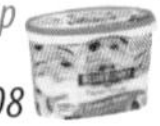

	C	F	Cb
Premium Ice Cream, 1 Pint Cont: *Per ⅔ Cup*			
Banana Split, 3.5 oz	220	9	30
Bunny Tracks, 3.35 oz	260	14	29
Chocolate, 3.1 oz	180	8	23
Cookies 'n Cream, 3.1 oz	200	10	26
Peanut Butter Party, 3.6 oz	280	16	29
Sweet Freedom: *Per ⅔ Cup*			
Bunny Tracks, 3.35 oz	180	9	30
Butter Pecan, 3.38 oz	140	6	25
Double Strawberry Swirl, 3.38 oz	120	3	26

Note: Carbohydrate figures include 5-10 g sugar alcohols

	C	F	Cb
Frozen Yogurt: *Per ⅔ Cup*			
Vanilla Bean, 3.17 oz	140	3	25

Bars/Pops ~ *See Page 108*

Breyers:

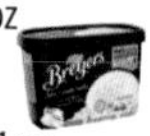
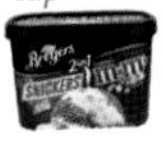

	C	F	Cb
Classics: *Per ⅔ Cup*			
Chocolate Chip/Mint, av., 3.1 oz	200	11	24
Other Choc. varieties, av., 3.1 oz	175	9	21
Natural Strawberry, 3.2 oz	150	7	20
Vanilla:			
Extra Creamy, 2.85 oz	140	4.5	24
Other Varieties, av., 3.1 oz	175	9	20
Carb Smart: Chocolate; Vanilla, 2.75 oz	110	6	17
Peanut Butter, 2.85 oz	150	9	17

Note: Carbohydrate figures include 7-8g sugar alcohol and 4g fiber

	C	F	Cb
Cookies & Candy: *Per ⅔ Cup*			
Oreo, 2.9 oz	170	6	27
Reeses, 3.1 oz	200	8	30
Snickers, 3.3 oz	210	8	32
2 in 1, Snickers & M&M's, 3.2 oz	200	7	30
Delights: *Per ⅔ Cup*			
Cookies & Cream, 3.3 oz	110	3	24
Creamy Chocolate, 3.2 oz	90	2.5	22

Note: Carbohydrate figures include 6g sugar alcohol

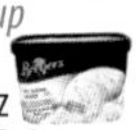

	C	F	Cb
No Sugar Added: *Per ⅔ Cup*			
Butter Pecan, 2.7 oz	130	7	17
Salted Cararmel Swirl, 2.7 oz	120	5	21
Vanilla Choc. Strawberry, 2.6 oz	110	4	17

Note: Carbohydrate figures include 8-12g sugar alcohol and 0-2g fiber

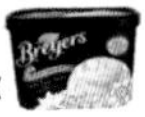

	C	F	Cb
Non Dairy: *Per ⅔ cup*			
Oreo Cookies & Crm, 2.9 oz	190	9	26
Van. P'nut Butter, 2.96 oz	190	11	21
Gelato: *Per ⅔ Cup*			
Raspberry Cheesecake, 3.7 oz	200	6	34
Vanilla Caramel, 3.7 oz	220	8	34

Bruster's: *Per Small Dish*

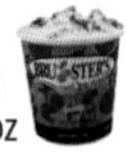

	C	F	Cb
Ice Cream: Banana, 4.93 oz	280	14	36
Butterscotch Ripple, 4.93 oz	310	15	40
Chocolate Mudslide, 4.93 oz	340	14	49
Non Dairy:			
Graham Central Station, 4.93 oz	260	5	52
Mint Chocolate Chip, 4.93 oz	230	7	40
Vanilla, 4.93 oz	160	2	36

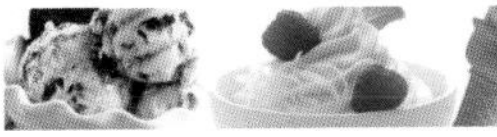

Ice Cream ~ Brands (Cont)

Carvel Ice Cream ~ *See Fast-Foods Section*
Coldstone Creamery ~ *See Fast-Foods Section*
Dairy Queen/Brazier ~ *See Fast-Foods Section*

Dannon: *Per ⅔ Cup, 3.88 oz*

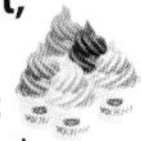

	C	F	Cb
Premium Frozen Yogurt,			
Average all flavors	155	4	25
Low Fat Frozen Yogurt:			
Chocolate Caramel Turtle	160	2	33
Cake Batter; Dulce De Leche	140	2	28
Fancy French Vanilla	130	0.5	27
Fudge Brownie Batter	150	0.5	33
No Sugar Added Nonfat Frozen Yogurt:			
Cheesecake	110	0	24
Praline	110	0	25
Raspberry	110	0	23
Strawberry Banana	110	0	24
Note: Carbohydrate figure includes 5-6g sugar alcohol			
Dairy Free Sorbet: Choc Fudge 2.9 oz	140	1	34
Average other flavors, 2.9 oz	110	0	20
Gelato, average all flavors, 3.88 oz	185	7	26

Dippin' Dots: *Per ⅔ Cup*

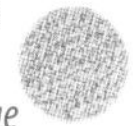

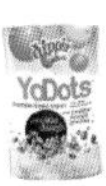

	C	F	Cb
Original Dots:			
Banana Split, 3.88 oz	180	9	22
Chocolate, 3.88 oz	190	9	25
Choc. Chip Cookie Dough, 3.5 oz	230	10	31
Cookies 'n Cream, 3.25 oz	210	10	26
Cotton Candy, 3.25 oz	170	9	20
YoDots: *Per 2.53 oz Package*			
Cookies 'n Cream	110	2	20
Cookie Dough	110	2	22
Cotton Candy	80	1	20

Dreyer's/Edy's:

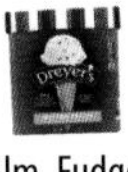

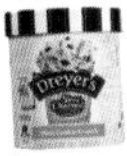

	C	F	Cb
Classic Ice Cream: *Per ⅔ Cup, 3 oz*			
Butter Pecan	200	11	20
Chocolate; Coffee, av.	175	9	21
Choc. Peanut Butter Cup	240	14	23
Mint Choc. Chip; Mocha Alm. Fudge	205	11	23
Rocky Road	210	11	24
Slow Churned Light Classics: *Per ⅔ Cup*			
Butter Pecan, 2.85 oz	170	7	22
Caramel Delight, 2.9 oz	160	4.5	26
Chocolate; Coffee, 2.8 oz	140	4.5	20
Double Fudge Brownie, 2.8 oz	160	4	26
Mint Cookie Crunch, 2.8 oz	150	3.5	26

Dreyers/Eddys (Cont):

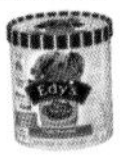

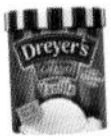

	C	F	Cb
Slow Churned No Sugar Added: *Per ⅔ Cup*			
Butter Pecan, 2.9 oz	150	6	21
Triple Chocolate, 2.9 oz	150	5	23
Vanilla Bean	130	4	19
Slow Churned Triple Filled: *Per ⅔ Cup*			
Choc. Fudge Cores, 3 oz	170	4	29
Crmy Chocolatey Cores, 3.1 oz	140	3	26
Rich Caramel Cores, 3.25 oz	200	6	33
Salted Caramel Cores, 3 oz	150	3.5	27

Gelati-da:

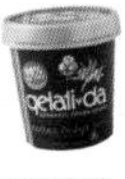

	C	F	Cb
Gelato: *Per ½ Cup, 4 oz*			
Amaretto Chocolate	150	4.5	23
Choc Mint Milano	120	2.5	22
Coffee Fudge Latte	130	2	22
Limoncello; Vanilla Marsala, average	120	2.5	21
Red Raspberry	130	1.5	25

Great Value *(Walmart): Per ⅔ Cup*

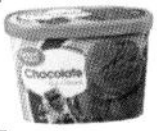

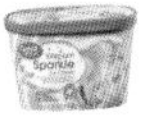

	C	F	Cb
Ice Cream: Butter Pecan, 3.5 oz	240	15	23
Cherry Chocolate, 5.4 fl.oz	190	10	22
Chocolate, 3.14 oz	180	8	23
Circus Cookie, 3.14 oz	200	11	24
Cookies & Cream, 3.14 oz	210	10	27
Mint Choc. Chip	140	8	17
Unicorn Sparkle, 3.2 oz	190	8	25
Vanilla Bean, 3.14 oz	170	9	21
Sherbet, av. all flav., ½ cup	110	0	26

Haagen-Dazs:: *Per ⅔ Cup*

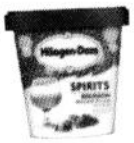

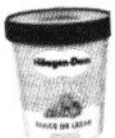

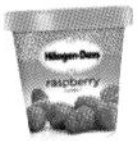

	C	F	Cb
Ice Cream, 14 fl.oz Tubs:			
Bourbon Praline Pecan	380	21	42
Caramel Cone	400	25	38
Cherry Vanilla	290	18	29
Chocolate Peanut Butter	450	29	36
Coffee Chip	340	22	30
White Chocolate Raspberry Truffle	360	20	41
Crispy Trio Layers:			
Coconut Caramel Chocolate	370	24	34
Belgian Choc. Van. & Blackberry	360	24	30
Decadent:			
Banana Peanut Butter Chip	440	30	33
Honey Salted Caramel Almond	350	22	33
Heaven: Choc Caramel Sea Salt	230	8	30
Cold Brew Espresso Chip	220	9	27
Non Dairy:			
Coconut Caramel	240	11	34
Raspberry Sorbet	170	0	42

Bars ~*See Page 109*

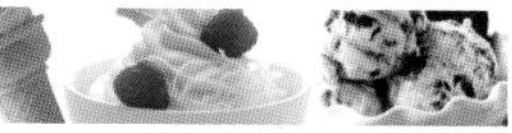

Ice Cream ~ Brands (Cont)

	C	F	Cb
Hood:			
Classic: *Per ⅔ Cup*			
Chocolate	**190**	9	25
Classic Trio	**180**	9	23
Coffee Cookies 'N Crm	**200**	10	26
Cookie Dough	**210**	10	28
Creamy Coffee	**180**	10	22
Fudge Twister	**190**	8	27
Golden Vanilla; Patchwork, av.	**190**	10	22
Maple Walnut Flavored	**200**	11	22
Churned, Light: *Per ⅔ Cup*			
Chocolate Chip	**170**	6	26
Coffee	**140**	4	24
Under The Stars	**210**	10	25
Vanilla	**140**	4	24
Frozen Fat-Free Yogurt: *Per ⅔ Cup*			
Chocolate; Strawberry, av.	**125**	0	26
Mocha Fudge	**130**	0	29
Salted Caramel Espresso	**150**	1.5	29
New England Creamery ~ *www.CalorieKing.com*			
Lucerne *(Vons): Per ⅔ Cup*			
Frozen Dairy Dessert: Chocolate	**130**	4	22
Cookies & Cream	**160**	5	26
Neapolitan	**130**	4	22
Orange Vanilla Swirl	**150**	3	30
Vanilla	**130**	3.5	21
Oberweis:			
Super Premium Ice Cream: *Per ⅔ Cup*			
Black Cherry, 3.8 oz	**280**	17	28
Chocolate Chip, 3.8 oz	**340**	22	33
Cookies & Cream, 3.8 oz	**300**	19	28
Cookie Dough P'nut Butter, 3.9 oz	**320**	19	35
Espresso Caramel Chip, 3.9 oz	**310**	18	36
Vanilla, 3.77 oz	**280**	19	24
Oikos ~ *see Dannon*			
Pinkberry:			
Frozen Yogurt: *Without Toppings*			
Original: Mini, 3.2 oz wt	**90**	0	19
Small, 4.9 oz wt	**150**	0	31
Medium, 8 oz wt	**240**	0	50
Large, 13 oz wt	**390**	1	81
Chocolate Hazelnut, 8 oz	**360**	9	59
Cookies & Cream, 8 oz	**320**	4.5	59
Passionfruit, 8 oz	**240**	0	50
Peanut Butter, 8 oz	**390**	16	49
Vanilla Latte, 8 oz	**240**	0	47
Red Mango (Stores):			
Frozen Yogurt: *1 Cup, 8 oz, Without Toppings*			
Original	**200**	0	46
Banana	**220**	0	50
Blueberry	**220**	0	48
Caribbean Coconut; Vanilla Bean	**260**	0	58
Dark Chocolate	**260**	1	60
Mango	**260**	0	58
Milk Chocolate; Raspberry, average	**260**	0	61
Peanut Butter	**300**	10	44
Pomegranate	**240**	0	54
Pomegranate Dark Chocolate	**240**	0	54
Fro-Yo Mashups: *Per ½ Cup, 4 oz*			
Brownie Brittle; Cookie Butter, av.	**140**	3	25
Cake Batter; Coffee	**120**	1	25
NY Cheesecake; Pistachio Mustachio	**130**	1.5	26
Vanilla Latte	**120**	1	25
White Chocolate	**140**	1	29
Bars ~ *See Page 110*			
So Delicious: *Per ⅔ Cup*			
Frozen Dessert:			
Cashew Milk:			
Bananas Foster, 4 oz	**240**	13	29
Chocolate Cookies & Cream, 4 oz	**250**	13	25
Creamy Chocolate, 3.88 oz	**220**	13	25
Dark Chocolate Truffle, 4.1 oz	**250**	15	30
Salted Caramel Cluster, 4 oz	**250**	13	32
Snickerdoodle, 4 oz	**240**	11	34
Very Vanilla, 3.67 oz	**240**	11	34
Coconut Milk: Chocolate, 3.8 oz	**200**	11	25
Choc. P'Nut Butter Swirl, 4.1 oz	**300**	20	29
Mocha Almond Fudge, 3.8 oz	**250**	15	28
No Sugar Added:			
Mint Chip, 3.84 oz	**160**	11	25
Vanilla Bean, 4 oz	**130**	9	24
Note: Carbohydrate Figure Includes 4-5g Sugar Alcohol			
Mousse: Mint Chip, 2.2 oz	**110**	4.5	22
Peanut Butter Swirl, 2.2 oz	**110**	5	20
Salted Caramel Swirl, 2.2 oz	**110**	4	23
Oatmilk: C'rmel Apple Crumble, 4.16 oz	**230**	10	36
P'nut Butter & Rasp., 4 oz	**250**	14	30
Soy Milk,			
Creamy Vanilla, 3.66 oz	**160**	4	31

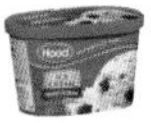
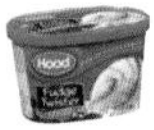
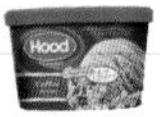
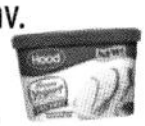
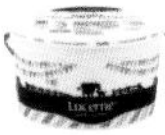
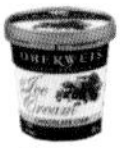
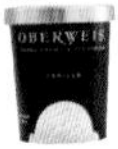
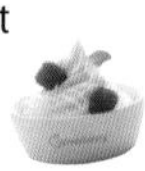

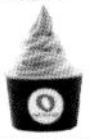

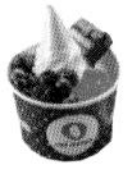
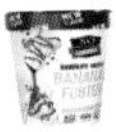
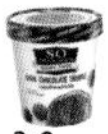
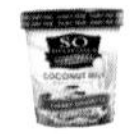
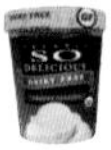

Ice Cream ~ Brands (Cont)

Stonyfield Organic:

Organic Frozen Yogurt: *Per ⅔ Cup*

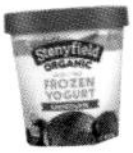

	C	F	Cb
Chocolate	170	4.5	28
Creme Caramel	210	5	35
Vanilla	170	4	27
Vanilla Fudge Swirl	190	3.5	33

Stop & Shop *(Ahold):*

Churn Style Ice Cream: *Per ⅔ Cup*

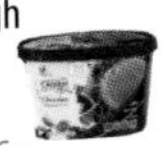

	C	F	Cb
Chocolate	135	4	23
Choc. Chip Cookie Dough	160	5	25
Cookies & Cream	160	5	27
Moose Tracks	200	8	28

Real Ice Cream: *Per ⅔ Cup*

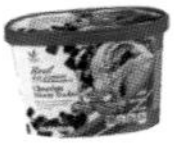

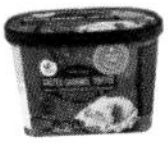

	C	F	Cb
Black Raspberry	180	10	22
Cafe Au Lait	130	6	16
Cherry Vanilla	140	7	18
Chocolate	200	11	23
Chocolate Moose Tracks	260	15	29
Cookies & Cream	200	10	26
Espresso Chip	210	11	26
Neapolitan	190	10	24
Salted Caramel Toffee	220	11	29

Tasti D-Lite:

Soft Serve: *Per 3 oz Wt*

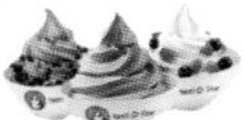

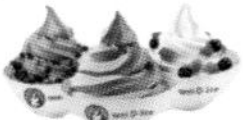

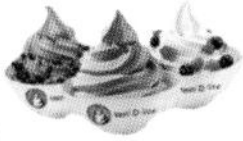

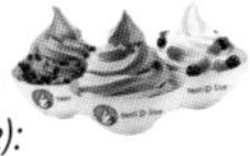

	C	F	Cb
Vanilla: Banana	70	1.5	14
Birthday Cake	80	1.5	14
Black Cherry	90	1.5	16
Brownie Batter	90	2	16
Butter Pecan	80	1.5	16
Cappuccino	80	1.5	15
Chocolate Mousse	80	1.5	16
Cinnamon Crunch	140	3	26
Creme Brulee; New York Chsecake	90	1.5	17
Mango	80	1.5	16
Mud Pie	100	2	19
Nutella Fusion	110	4	17
Oreo Mint	130	3	22
Peanut Butter	100	4	15

Tofutti *(Milk Free):*

Premium Pints: *Per ⅔ Cup*

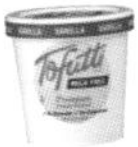

	C	F	Cb
Better Pecan	320	20	36
Chocolate	280	18	27
Vanilla	280	18	28
Vanilla Almond Bark	320	20	32
Van. Fudge; Wild Berry Supreme, av.	260	12	34

TCBY ~ *See Page 250*

Turkey Hill:

All Natural: *Per ⅔ Cup, 3.3 oz Unless Indicated*

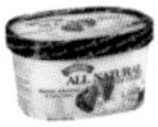

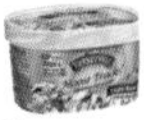

	C	F	Cb
Belgian Style Choc.	220	11	27
Butter Almond & Choc.	230	13	23
Raspberry Chocolate Chip	210	11	24
Salted Caramel	210	10	27
Vanilla Peanut Butter	250	16	21
Red. Fat, Moose Tracks, 2.9 oz	190	8	26
No Sugar Added,			
Vanilla Bean, 3.2 oz	100	0	26

Premium Ice Cream: *Per ⅔ Cup, 3 oz*

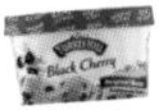

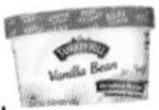

	C	F	Cb
Black Raspberry	170	8	23
Choco Mint Chip	200	11	23
Chocolate Peanut Butter Cup	230	13	24
Cookies 'n Cream; Tin Roof Sundae	200	10	25
Raspberry Cream Swirl	170	6	28
Vanilla Bean	170	9	21
Vanilla Chocolate Crunch	210	12	25
Stuff'd, average all flavors, ⅔ cup	195	8	29

Frozen Dairy Desserts: *Per ⅔ Cup, 3.2 oz*

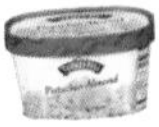

	C	F	Cb
Butter Pecan	170	6	24
Pistachio Almond	160	5	25
Rocky Road	180	4.5	32
Sherbet, Fruit Rainbow, 4 oz	160	1.5	36

Wawa:

Premium Ice Cream: *Per ½ Cup*

	C	F	Cb
Butter Pecan; Mint Choc. Chip, av.	180	10	20
Chocolate; Vanilla Bean, average	160	8	20
Cookies & Cream	180	9	21
Strawberry Shortcake	160	7	22

Wegmans: *Per ⅔ Cup Unless Indicated*

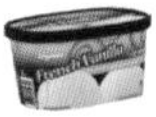

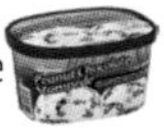

	C	F	Cb
Ice Cream: Choc. Peanut Butter Swirl	200	12	20
Coconut Almond Fudge	250	14	29
French Vanilla	200	9	26
Mint Chip	200	10	26
Neapolitan	180	9	23
Peanut Choc. Stampede	260	15	29
Vanilla & Chocolate	180	9	22
White Chocolate Raspberry	220	11	30

Light: *Per ⅔ Cup*

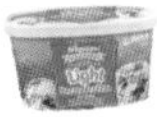

	C	F	Cb
Mint Chip	170	4	29
Pecan Praline	170	3.5	32

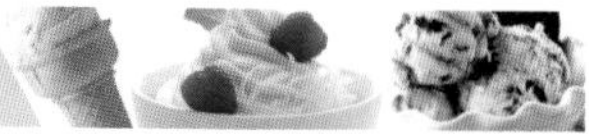

Ice Cream Bars & Pops ~ Brands

Per Bar/Serving Unless indicated	C	F	Cb
Ben & Jerry's:			
Pint Slices:			
Amer. Dream; Choc Chip Cookie Dough	280	18	30
Cherry Garcia	250	15	27
Choc Fudge Brownie	250	16	26
The Tonight Dough	290	18	31
Vanilla P'nut Butter Cup	300	22	24
Big Bear ~ *See Klondike*			
Blue Bunny:			
Big Alaska Bar	250	15	27
Sandwich Bars:			
Big: Bopper	400	16	61
Double Strawberry	230	6	42
Mississippi Mud	260	7	47
Single Bars: Chocolate Eclair	210	10	29
Cookies 'n Cream	250	12	32
Fudge Bar	40	0	9
Heath Bar	270	18	26
Nutt'n Better Bar	270	18	24
Strawberry Shortcake	200	10	26
Turtle Bar	360	23	33
Snacks, CMint Choc. Chip	150	5	24
Cones, 6 Pack:			
Caramel Lovers	310	16	38
Chocolate Lovers	270	12	36
Cookies 'n Cream	270	13	37
Big Dipper: Chocolate Lovers	260	12	36
Cookies 'n Cream	260	12	35
Breyers:			
Carb Smart, 6 Pack:			
Almond Bar, 2 oz	150	12	11
Caramel Swirl, 2 oz	60	2.5	11
Fudge Bar, 1.7 oz	60	3	10
Vanilla Ice Cream Bar, 2 oz	140	11	11

Note: Carbohydrate figure includes 4-5g sugar alcohol

	C	F	Cb
Butterfinger Bar ~ *See Nestle Page 110*			
Diana's Bananas:			
Banana Babies:			
Milk/Dark Chocolate (1)	130	6	18
Milk Choc. & Peanuts (1)	215	13	21
Banana Bites, (4), 1.5 oz	100	6	13

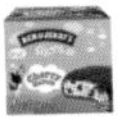
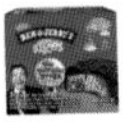
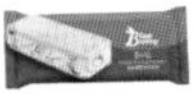
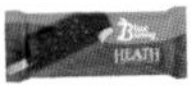
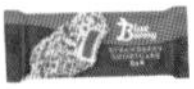
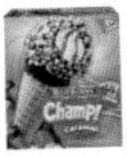

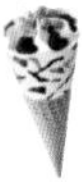
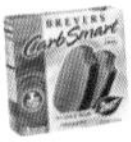
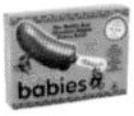

Per Bar/Serving Unless indicated	C	F	Cb
Dove:			
Single Bars: *Per 2.6 oz Bar*			
Milk Chocolate, Vanilla	250	16	24
Dark Chocolate, Choc.	250	16	26
Miniatures, Variety Pack, w/ Milk/Dark Choc., 1 piece	60	4	6
Sorbet Bars: Dark Chocolate Raspb.	150	8	19
Milk Chocolate Strawberry	150	7	20
Drumstick *(Nestlé):*			
Classic Sundae Cones: Banana	290	15	34
Banana with Fudge	300	15	38
Dulce de Leche	290	13	41
Strawberry with Fudge	300	15	38
Vanilla; Vanilla Fudge, average	300	5	37
Vanilla Caramel	310	15	39
Dipped: Choc. Cookie	280	13	38
Vanilla Caramel	290	14	32
Super Nugget: Strawberry	300	16	35
Vanilla	310	17	35
Vanilla Fudge	320	17	39
King Size: Triple Chocolate	340	14	50
Vanilla with Choc. Swirls	350	14	52
Lil' Drums: Choc. w/ Choc. Swirls	110	5	16
Vanilla with Choc. Swirls	120	5	17
Simply Dipped: Mint	260	12	37
Vanilla	270	12	38
Edy's ~ *See Dreyer's*			
Eskimo Pie ~ *See Nestle*			
Fudge Bar ~ *See Nestle*			
Fat Boy:			
Cones: Chocolate Fudge Brownie	300	15	40
Sundae Best	310	17	34
Other Flavors	310	15	40
Freeze Pops, Orange Cream	110	3	21
Sandwiches: Chocolate, 3 oz	210	8	32
Cookies 'n Cream, 3 oz	220	9	34
Mint Chocolate Chip, 3 oz	230	10	33
Premium Vanilla	210	8	32
S'mores, 3 oz	230	9	35
Strawberry, 3 oz	180	7	29
Sundae On A Stick: Caramel Pretzel	230	9	35
Cherry Cordial	230	16	20
Toffee Crunch	290	21	25
Vanilla Nut	270	18	25
Fudgsicle *(Breyers):*			
Fudge Bar: Original	80	3	14
Low Fat	60	1.5	11
No Sugar Added	80	2	18

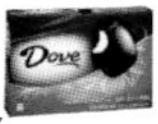

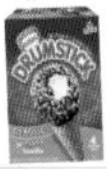
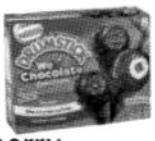
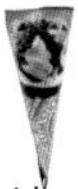
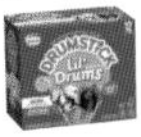
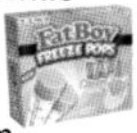
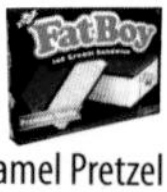
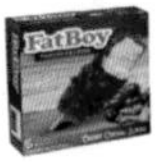

Ice Cream Bars/Pops ~ Brands (Cont)

Per Bar/Serving

Good Humor:	C	F	Cb
Cones:			
Single: Giant King Cone, Choc. & Vanilla, 5 oz	390	22	44
King Cone, Vanilla, 2.7 oz	230	14	25
4-Packs: Oreo Cone, 2.65 oz	200	9	29
King Cones, Vanilla, 3 oz	240	12	31
Dessert Bars, Singles:			
Original Vanilla, 2.8 oz	240	15	23
Birthday Cake, 2.6 oz	200	10	25
Chocolate Eclair, 2 oz	150	7	21
Creamsicle, 2.5 oz	100	2	20
Oreo, 1.8 oz	150	8	19
Reese's, 1.8 oz	180	11	20
Toasted Almond, 2 oz	160	9	18
Sandwiches:			
Single: Giant Neapolitan;Van., 3.6 oz	220	5	39
Choc. Chip Cookie, 2.7 oz	250	10	40
Stickless: *4 or 6-Pack*			
Reese's PB Dessert Cup, 2.43 oz	260	17	25

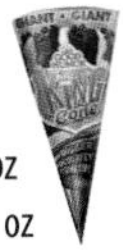
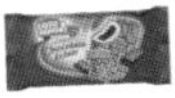
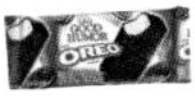

Haagen-Dazs:	C	F	Cb
Dark Chocolate Bar, Chocolate	280	20	22
Milk Chocolate Bars:			
Coffee & Almond Crunch	290	21	22
Vanilla & Almonds	290	21	21
Vanilla	270	19	22
Snack Size:			
Coffee & Almond Crunch	190	14	15
Vanilla & Almonds	195	15	13
Gelato, Vanilla Caramel Pizzelle	290	19	25
Healthy Choice: Fudge Bar	80	0.5	15
Smoothie Bars: Mango Peach	70	0.5	14
Raspberry	80	0.5	15
Strawberry	70	0.5	13
Hershey's:			
Bars, Gluten Free: Banjo	170	11	17
Fudjo	120	0	24
Orange Blossom	80	2.5	13
Cones: Incredible	290	14	38
Moose Tracks	480	28	52
P-Nutty	260	15	30
Low fat, Cookies & Cream; Crazy, av.	120	1.5	25

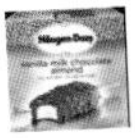
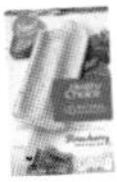
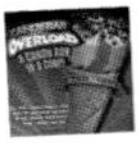

Per Bar/Serving

Hershey's (Cont):	C	F	Cb
Ice Pops, all flavors	35	0	10
Sandwiches:			
Vanilla Ice Cream, 4 oz	210	9	30
Giant:			
Andes Creme de Menthe, 6 oz	350	16	48
Neapolitan, 6 oz	280	12	40
Vanilla, 6 oz	300	12	43
Signature Bars: Chocolate Eclair	220	10	30
Salty Caramel Brownie	240	12	30
Strawb. Shortcake	240	11	32
Hood:			
Bars: Ice Cream Bar	130	7	14
Red Sox Sports Bar	250	16	26
Hoodsie:			
Cups, Chocolate; Vanilla, 3 oz	100	5	12
Sundae Cups, 3 oz	120	5	19
Sandwich: Av., 2.2 oz	175	6	29
Mini's, 1.2 oz	90	3.5	14

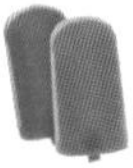
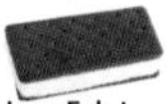
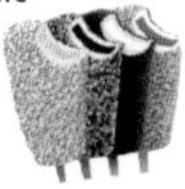
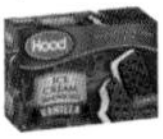

Klondike:	C	F	Cb
Bars:			
Single, Orig. Vanilla, 5.5 oz	300	17	34
4-Pack:			
Mint Choc. Chip, 2.8 oz	230	14	26
6 Pack: Cookies & Cream, 2.15 oz	200	10	24
Double Chocolate, 3 oz	240	14	27
Oreo, Cookies & Cream, 2.57 oz	250	15	27
Reeses, PB Cup , 2.75 oz	250	15	28
8-Count Snack Size: Orig., 1.4 oz	120	7	13
English Toffee, 2.6 oz	230	14	24
Choco Taco, Original, 4 oz	250	12	34
Kandy, Caramel & Peanuts, 2.7 oz	250	14	28
Sandwiches:			
Single: Mrs Fields, 3.9 oz	340	12	55
Oreo, 4.5 oz	220	7	37
4-Pack: Mrs Fields, 2.3 oz	210	8	34
Oreo, 2.4 oz	210	7	35
6-Pack, Vanilla, 2.7 oz	180	5	31

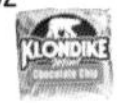
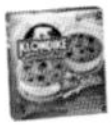
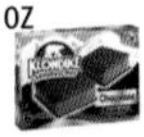

Kroger: *Per Bar*	C	F	Cb
Arctic Blasters:			
Fudge Bar	100	1	21
Ice Cream Bar	150	11	13
Orange Cream	100	2.5	18
Strawberry Shortcake	140	8	16
Toffee Bar	160	11	14
Mighty Pops, Grape Cherry, Orange (3)	140	0	33
Luigi's: *Per 6 fl.oz cup*			
Real Italian Ice: Blue Rasp. Lemon	130	0	27
Cherry; Lemon; Strawb.	100	0	26
Cherry & Lemon Swirl	120	0	30

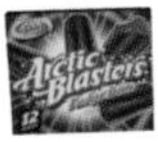

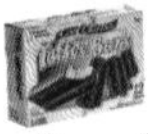
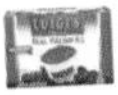

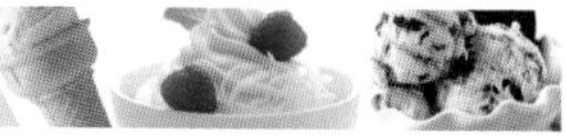

Ice Cream Bars/Pops ~ Brands (Cont)

Per Bar/Serving	C	F	Cb
M&M's:			
Cone, Single, 2.6 oz	250	12	32
Sandwiches: Choc. Ice Cream, 2.9 oz	240	10	36
Vanilla Ice Cream, 2.9 oz	240	10	37
Magnum:			
Singles: Almond 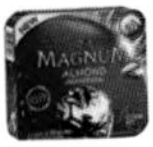	270	18	25
Dark Chocolate	240	16	23
Double Caramel	270	17	29
White	240	15	24
Double: Cookies & Cream	280	17	30
Raspberry 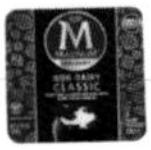	260	16	28
Minis, Almond	170	11	15
Non Dairy: Classic	230	14	26
Almond	250	16	25
Minute Maid, Juice Bars, 2.25 fl.oz	40	0	10
Nestlé:			
Bars: Butterfinger 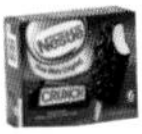	290	17	30
Cookies N' Cream	180	11	19
Crunch	150	9	15
Crushed It: Cookies N' Cream	170	9	21
Vanilla Fudge	180	9	22
Eskimp Pie 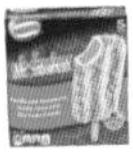	150	5	15
Fudge Bar	110	2	20
Strawberry Shortcake	140	6	20
Dibs, Crunch, 3.3 oz container	320	21	31
Drumsticks ~ See Page 108			
Push-Up Pops, all flavors	70	1	16
Sandwiches, Vanilla 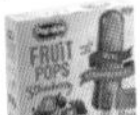	160	3	30
Popsicle:			
Fruit Pops: Strawberry	150	0	34
Average Other Fruit Flavors	165	0	40
Fruit Stacker, Banana, Orange, Strawb.	160	0	38
Fudgsicle, Low Fat	60	1.5	11
Scribblers, 2 Pops	60	0	14
Reeses Dessert Bar~*See Good Humor*			
Skinny Cow: *Per Item*			
Bars: Fudge; Chocolate Truffle, av.	120	3	19
Vanilla Almond Crunch 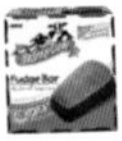	190	11	19
Cones, all flavors	170	5	28
Minis, Salted C'rmel Pretzel	90	6	9
Sandwiches, all flavors	160	3.5	29
Snickers:			
Bars: Milk/Dark Choc. 1.7 oz 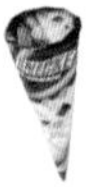	180	11	18
2.8 oz bar	250	15	25
Cone, 2.7 oz	250	13	31
Snow Cone *(Wonder)*, av. all, 7 fl.oz	60	0	15

Per Bar/Serving	C	F	Cb
So Delicious *(Turtle Mountain):*			
Almond Based:			
Bars, Mocha Alm. Fudge 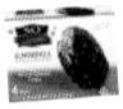	180	13	16
Sandwich, Vanilla, 1.3 oz	100	4	14
Cashewmilk:			
Dipped Bars: Dble Choc Delight, 2 oz	170	13	16
Salted Caramel Bar, 2 oz	180	13	17
Coconut Milk:			
Dipped Bar: Coconut Alm., 1.85 oz	190	14	15
Vanilla Bean, 1.8 oz	170	12	14
Fudge Bar, 2 oz 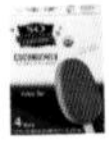	100	6	13
Sandwiches:			
Coconut, 1.3 oz	100	4	14
Vanilla Bean, 1.3 oz	100	4	14
Tampico, Freezer Pops, all var., 1.4 oz	30	0	7
Tofutti: *Per Item*			
Bars: Chocolate Fudge, 1.4 oz	30	0	6
Hooray Hooray, 1.4 oz 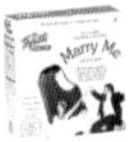	120	8	8
Marry Me, 1.4 oz	170	8	22
Totally Fudge Pops	95	1.5	19
Note: Carb figures include 0-7g sugar alcohols			
Cone, Yours Truly Sundae 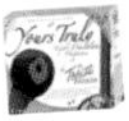	170	8	22
Cuties, average all flavors	130	6	18
Toll House *(Nestle):*			
Sandwiches:			
Chocolate Choc. Chip Cookie, 4 oz	380	16	54
Vanilla Choc. Chip Cookie, 2.1 oz	210	8	32
Mini, Vanilla 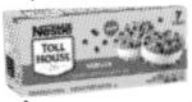	105	4	16
Turkey Hill:			
Sandwiches: Double Decker	200	8	31
Vanilla Bean 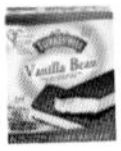	190	7	30
Reduced Fat	170	3	33
Sundae Cone, Van. Fudge	360	22	35
Twix:			
Cookies & Cream, 2.4 oz	250	14	29
Vanilla Ice Cream Bar: 3 fl.oz	250	14	28
1.6 fl.oz Bar 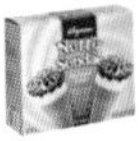	160	9	18
Wegmans:			
Bars: Organic Fudge	190	12	16
Chocolate Sundae Crunch	180	10	22
Strawberry Sundae Crunch	180	9	22
Sandwiches: Vanilla, 3.5 fl.oz	160	5	27
Light Vanilla, 3.5 fl.oz	160	3	29
Weight Watchers: *Per Item*			
Bars: Dark Choc. Raspberry 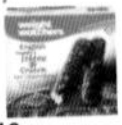	70	2	11
English Toffee	80	3.5	11
Giant Bar, Chocolate Fudge	90	1	21
Snack Bars: Cookies & Cream	90	3	15
Divine Triple Chocolate	90	3	14
Salted Caramel	90	2.5	14

Canned & Packaged Meals ~ Brands

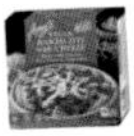
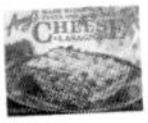

Amy's:	C	F	Cb
Frozen:			
Bowls: *Per Package*			
Asian Dumplings, 8.5 oz	370	13	47
Baked Ziti, 9.5 oz	380	13	54
Brocc. & Cheeze Bake, 9.5 oz	450	22	55
General TSO's, 8 oz	270	11	36
Meatless Pepperoni Mac & Cheese, 9 oz	490	21	52
Pesto Tortellini, 9.5 oz	530	22	63
Vegan Tortilla Casserole, with Cheese, 9.4 oz	360	15	48
Entrees: Cheese Enchilada, 9 oz	490	29	36
Cheese Lasagna, 10.3 oz	410	17	42
Greek Red Rice & Veggies, 8.65 oz	500	29	50
Macaroni & Cheese, 9 oz	450	18	55
Mex. Veggies & Black Beans, 8.5 oz	270	10	36
Sweet & Sour Asian Noodle, Light, 8 oz	260	4	47
Vegan Tortilla Casserole w/ Chse, 9.4 oz	380	15	49
Vegetable Pakoras, 9.5 oz	340	16	40
Pot Pie, Vegetable, 7.5 oz	470	27	46
Snacks: Chse & Bean Nachos, 5-6 pcs	230	9	28
Pizza: Cheese, 6 pieces	220	9	25
Meatless Pepperoni Pizza, 6 pcs	220	10	22
Veggie Burger Patties,	130	4	18
Wraps:			
Indian Samosa, 5 oz	270	12	32
Teriyaki, gluten free, 5.5 oz	250	6	38

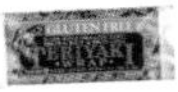
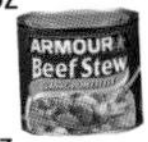

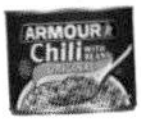

Armour-Star:	C	F	Cb
Beef Stew, 9 oz	230	12	21
Chili: Orig., with Beans, 7 oz	350	14	33
No Beans, 8.5 oz	320	17	20
Corned Beef, 2 oz	120	7	1
Corned Beef Hash, 7 oz	420	26	22
Potted Meat, Chicken/Pork, 2.1 oz	170	16	0

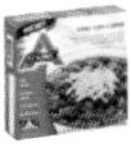
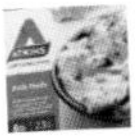

Atkins: *Per 9 oz Tray/Bowl*	C	F	Cb
Frozen:			
Beef Merlot; Chsy Chkn Risotto, av.	305	20	9
Chicken & Broccoli Alfredo	290	18	10
Chili Con Carne	340	23	11
Crustless Chkn Pot Pie	300	19	9
Meatloaf, with Portobello Mshrm Gravy	330	21	12
Mongolian-Style Beef	270	18	10
Pork Verde	300	20	10
Shrimp Scampi	290	19	19

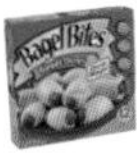

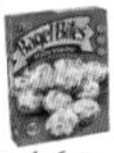

Bagel Bites: *Per 4 Pieces*	C	F	Cb
Frozen:			
Bagel Dogs	200	10	19
Pizza Snacks:			
Cheese & Pepperoni	210	6	33
Cheese, Sausage & Pepperoni	210	6	32
Cheesy Garlic Bread	220	8	27
Extreme Beef Nacho, Mini	190	5	27
Three Cheese	200	5	32

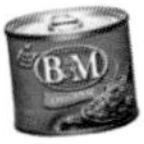

B&M:	C	F	Cb
Baked Beans: *Per ½ cup, 4.6 oz*			
Original; Maple Flavor, av.	160	1	32
Bacon & Onion; Boston's Best, av.	185	1	36
Country Style	170	1	35
Homestyle	190	1.5	39
Vegetarian	160	0.5	32
Brown Bread, Orig., 1 slice (½"), 2 oz	130	0.5	28

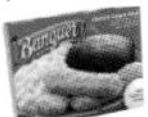

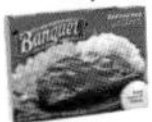

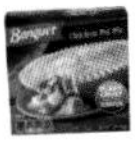

Banquet:	C	F	Cb
Homestyle Bakes: *1 Cup, Prepared*			
Creamy Cheesy Chicken Alfredo	330	15	37
Creamy Chicken & Biscuits	420	18	53
Frozen:			
Backyard BBQ & Mshd Potato, 8 oz	290	11	35
Chicken: Fingers w/ Mac & Chse, 6.5 oz	310	12	33
Fettuccine Chicken Alfredo, 9 oz	220	6	31
Chicken Fried Chicken, 10.1oz	330	14	40
Parmesan, 8.5 oz	320	11	41
Strip Meal, 10 oz	340	17	32
Homestyle Patty, 10 oz	340	17	32
Lasagna with Meat Sauce, 7.5 oz	250	9	31
Mac & Cheese, 8 oz	240	9	32
Pepper Steak, 10 oz	320	13	39
Rigatoni & Italian Sausage, with Meatballs, 8 oz	300	12	35
Salisbury Steak w/ Mshd Pot., 9.5 oz	350	14	44
Spaghetti & Meatballs, 10 oz	320	14	34
Swedish Meaballs, 10.45 oz	370	17	39
Turkey, 10 oz	280	11	29
Family: Gravy & Meat Loaf, 4 oz	120	6	9
Salisbury Steak & Gravy, 4.5 oz	170	12	8
Zesty Marinara Sauce & M'balls, 5 oz	170	10	11
Pot Pie: Beef	380	23	36
Chicken	350	19	33
Chicken & Broccoli	330	18	31
Salisbury Steak Deep Dish, 7 oz	400	23	40
Turkey	320	18	31

Barilla:	C	F	Cb
Entrees: *Per Container* 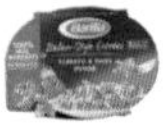			
Chicken Alfredo, 8.5 oz	310	18	22
Marinara/Tom. & Basil Penne, av., 9 oz	305	4	62
Meat Sauce Gemelli, 9 oz	320	3.5	63
Betty Crocker:			
Chicken Helper: *Per ½ Cup As Packaged*			
Chicken Fettuccine Alfredo, 1.26 oz	140	1.5	28
Chicken Fried Rice, 1.2 oz	110	0	24
Hamburger Helper: *As Packaged*			
Bacon Chsebgr; Beef Pasta, av., 1 oz	95	0.5	21
Cheesy Enchilada, 1.4 oz	145	2	29
Del. Beef Strog.; Four Chse Lasag 1. oz	100	1	21
Philly Cheesesteak, 1.26 oz 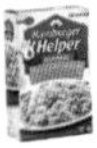	130	2	25
Potato Stroganoff, 0.9 oz	90	0	21
Potatoes: *As Packaged*			
Casserole: Cheddar & Bacon, 1 oz	100	0	22
Julienne, 0.9 oz 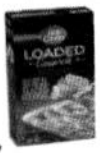	80	0	20
Other flavors, 0.9 oz	90	0	21
Mashed Potatoes, all, 0.8 oz	90	2	16
Tuna Helper: *As Packaged*			
Cheesy Pasta; Creamy Pasta, 1.1 oz	110	1	21
Creamy Broccoli; Fett. Alfredo, 1.3 oz	130	1	26
Birds Eye:			
Frozen:			
Chef's Favorites, Asian Medley, 3 oz	60	2	9
Power Blends: *Per Bag*			
Chickpea & Spinach, 10 oz	320	7	51
Quinoa & Spinach, 10 oz 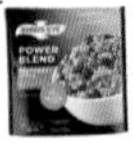	310	5	57
Southwest Style, 12.7 oz	470	5	85
Steamfresh Sides: *Per Bag*			
Garlic Butter Rotini & Vegetables	290	3.5	53
Pasta & Broccoli w/ Cheese Sauce	210	3.5	35
Voila!: Alfredo Chicken, 7.5 oz	240	9	25
Cheesy Chicken Riced Cauli, 8.6 oz	240	13	16
Cheesy Ranch Chicken, 6.7 oz	220	4.5	31
Chicken Stir Fry, 8.5 oz	230	3	36
Garlic Chicken, 6.2 oz 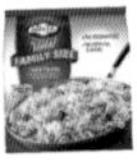	220	7	28
Garlic Shrimp, 6.7 oz	230	7	31
Selects: Beef Lo Mein, 8 oz	270	5	42
Shrimp Scampi, 9 oz	210	4	34

Boca:	C	F	Cb
Bowls, average all flavors, 9 oz bowl	290	9	42
Burger Patties: *Per 2.5 oz Patty*			
Original: All American 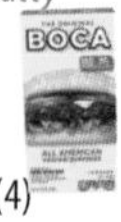	110	4.5	7
Original Chik'n	130	4	13
Original Vegan Veggie	70	1	6
Chik'n Nuggets, all flavors (4)	160	5	16
Crumbles, 2 oz	60	0	5
Falafel Bites, average all flavors (4)	150	5.5	23
Boston Market:			
Frozen Dinners: *Per Pkg* 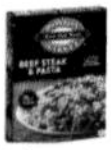			
Beef Steak & Pasta	380	9	49
Carver's Cut:			
Herb Seasoned Grilled Chicken	350	13	22
Roadhouse Beef Meatloaf	520	27	44
Chicken Parmesan 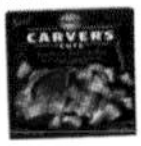	480	14	66
Country Fried Beef Steak	490	27	43
Meatloaf	430	23	37
Salisbury Steak	530	32	40
Swedish M'balls, 13 oz 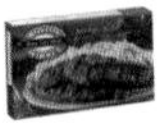	520	22	53
Pot Pie, Chicken	470	34	35
Buitoni:			
Refrigerated:			
Ravioli, Four Cheese, 3.3 oz 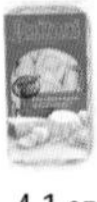	180	9	39
Tortellini: Herb Chkn, 3.9 oz	320	8	51
Mixed Cheese, 3.7 oz	300	8	47
Tortelloni, Sweet Italian Ssg., 4.1 oz	320	8	52
Other Pasta Dishes ~ *See Page 133*			
Bush's Best: *Per ½ cup, 4.6 oz*			
Baked Beans: Orig,; Vegetarian, av.	135	0.5	29
Country Style 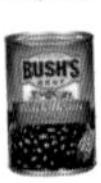	170	1	33
Maple & Cured Bacon	150	1.5	27
Black Beans	120	0.5	23
Dark Red Kidney Beans	130	0	24
Garbanzo Beans (Chick Peas)	130	2	21
Pinto Beans	100	0	18
Bush's Best (Cont): *Per ½ Cup, 4.6 oz*			
Grillin' Beans,			
Bourbon & Br. Sugar; Smokehouse	170	0.5	35
Refried Beans, Traditional, 4.4 oz	140	3	21
Campbell's: 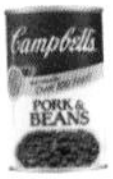			
Pork & Beans, 11 oz can,			
½ cup, 4.6 oz serving	130	0.5	27
Spaghetti O's: *Per 1 Cup* 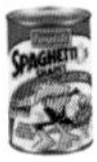			
Original, 8.9 oz	170	1	33
With Meatballs, 8.9 oz	230	7	31
With Franks, 8.9 oz	220	7	29

Chef Boyardee:	C	F	Cb
Canned: *Per Cup*			
Beefaroni, 8.8 oz	250	9	32
Ravioli: *Per 1 Cup*			
Beef, Tom. & Meat Sauce, 8.7 oz	220	7	33
Cheese, in Tomato Sauce, 9 oz	210	2	40
Ital. Sausage, overstuffed, 9.2 oz	240	6	38
Spaghetti: with Meatballs, 9 oz	260	11	31
Mini Rings & Meatballs, 8.6 oz	250	11	29
Microwaveable: *Per 7.5 oz Bowl*			
Beefaroni; Lasagna, average	215	8	28
Ravioli: Beef In Tom. & Meat Sce	200	7	28
Cheese in Tomato & Meat Sauce	190	5	28
Mini Micro Beef	160	4	25
Boxed Pizza Maker Kits: *Single Kits*			
Pepperoni, ⅛ package, 4 oz	280	7	43
Traditional, ⅛ package, 4 oz	250	3.5	45
Pizza Sauce, w/ Cheese, ¼ c., 2 oz	35	1.5	4
Dennison's Chili: *Per 15 oz Can*			
Chili Con Carne:			
Original: with Beans	340	14	34
without Beans	260	14	17
Chunky, with Beans	330	13	33
Hot, with Beans	340	14	34
Turkey with Beans	220	3.5	32
Vegetarian, 99% fat free	280	1.5	52
Devour ~ *See Heinz Page 114*			
Dinty Moore *(Hormel):*			
Big Bowl (Microwave): *Approx. ½ of 15 oz Bowl*			
Beef Stew, 8.3 oz	200	10	17
Chicken & Dumplings, 8.5 oz	220	7	29
Can, Chicken & Dunplings, 8.5 oz	200	7	24
Microwave:			
Cup, Scalloped Pot, with Ham, 7.5 oz	260	16	20
Tray, Beef Stew, XL, 12.5 oz	330	17	29
Dr. McDougall's:			
Asian Noodles, Pad Thai, 2 oz	200	1.5	43
Lentil Quinoa Salad, 2 oz	220	3.5	40
Sesame Chkn Rice Noodle, 1.3 oz	130	1	26
Eden Foods (Organic):			
Black Beans & Quinoa Chili, 8.8 oz	190	2	35
Brown Rice & Pinto Beans, 4.6 oz	120	1	24
Curried Rice & Green Lentils, 4.6 oz	130	1	21
Kidney Beans & Kamut Chili, 8.8 oz	220	1.5	41
Mexican Rice & Black Beans, 4.6 oz	110	1	22

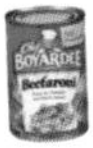
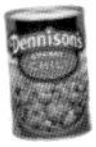
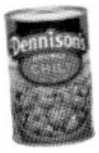
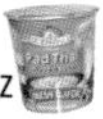

Farmhouse: *Per 1 Cup Prepared*	C	F	Cb
Pasta: Fettuccine Alfredo	460	22	51
White Cheddar	380	14	51
Rice: Long Gr., & Wild Herbs & Butter	250	7	43
Mexican	230	5	42
Roasted Chicken Flavor	230	5	44
French's:			
French Crispy Fried Onions:			
Original; White Cheddar:2 Tbsp	40	3.5	3
¼ cup, 0.5 oz	80	7	6
1 cup, 2 oz	320	28	24
GardenBurger:			
Veggie Burger: *Per 2.5 oz Burger*			
Original	110	3.5	17
Black Bean Chipotle	90	3	16
Portabella	90	2	16
Garden Lites: *Per Package*			
Bakes: Broccoli Cheddar Bake	190	6	25
Butternut Squash Souffle	180	1	38
Roasted Vegetable Bake	150	3	24
Spinach	140	3	22
Zucchini	150	2.5	25
Cakes: Mac & Cheese (1)	80	3	9
Veggie Bacon Mac & Cheese (1)	90	3	10
Frittata: Mushroom & 3 Cheese, 2 oz	80	4	6
Spinach Egg White, 2 oz	70	4	5
Veggie, Bacon & Potato, 2 oz	80	4.5	6
Gorton's:			
Frozen:			
Delicious Classics:			
Clams, Crunchy Breaded, 15 pieces	210	10	22
Flounder, Crispy Batt. Fillets (2)	250	13	25
Pollock: Beer Battered Fillets (2)	230	12	23
Crispy Battered Fillets (2)	230	11	23
Crunchy Breaded Fish Sticks (4)	230	10	26
Potato Crunch Fillets (2)	230	11	24
Popcorn Shrimp, 3.5 oz	370	15	23
Everyday Gourmet:			
New England Cod: Baked (1)	250	13	16
Fish Sticks, Crunchy Panko (4)	270	13	26
Simply Bake:			
Roasted Garlic Butter Salmon (1)	140	2.5	8
Shrimp Scampi (9)	180	7	5
Tilapia, with Seasoning (1)	130	3	6

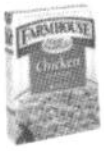
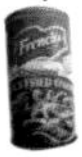
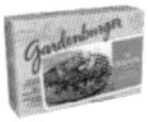
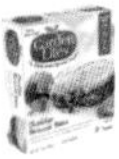
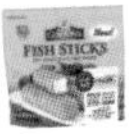
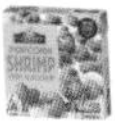

continued nex page...

Gorton's (Cont):	C	F	Cb
Frozen:			
Smart Solutions: *Per Fillet*			
Haddock, Signature Grilled (1)	**70**	1	0
Pollock: Cajun Style (1)	**90**	2.5	1
Italian Herb Grilled (1)	**80**	2	2
Lemon Butter Grilled (1)	**70**	0.5	0
Tilapia: Roasted Garlic & Butter (1)	**100**	3	1
Signature Grilled (1)	**100**	4	1
Great Value *(Walmart)*:			
Frozen:			
Breakfast Bowls: Meat Lovers, 7 oz	**430**	30	14
Sausage & Gravy, 7 oz	**340**	25	14
Meals: Beef Shepherd's Pie, 6.4 oz	**190**	10	15
Beef Stroganoff with Noodles, 10 oz	**380**	18	37
Butter Chicken, 10 oz	**260**	11	24
Cheese Ravioli Pasta, 8 pieces	**250**	4	43
Lasagna with Meat Sauce, 7.5oz	**250**	9	30
Rstd Orange Chkn & Veggie, 10 oz	**180**	4.5	18
Spinach Pesto Chkn & Veggie, 10 oz	**240**	10	21
Steam Meal, Lem. Herb Chicken, 12 oz	**360**	6	51
Healthy Choice:			
Frozen:			
Cafe Steamers:			
Beef Teriyaki, 9.5 oz	**280**	5	42
Chicken & Noodles, 10 oz	**260**	7	31
Crustless Chicken Pot Pie, 9.6 oz	**300**	6	40
General Tso's Spicy Chicken, 10.3 oz	**290**	3.5	47
Grilled Chkn Pesto with Veg., 9.6 oz	**290**	7	36
Sweet & Sour Chicken, 10 oz	**390**	8	65
Gluten Free: Beef Merlot, 9.5 oz	**180**	4	20
Cajun Style Chkn & Shrimp, 9.6 oz	**220**	2.5	35
Vegetarian, Portab. Spin. Parmesan	**230**	5	38
Classics: Chicken Parmigiana, 11.6 oz	**320**	9	44
Lemon Pepper Fish, 10.7 oz	**280**	3.5	48
Power Bowls: *Per Bowl*			
Adobo Chicken	**330**	8	38
Chicken Feta & Farro	**310**	9	34
Cuban Inspired Pork	**340**	8	46
Italian Chicken Sausage & Peppers	**290**	9	36
Vegetatian/Vegan:			
Cauliflower Curry, 10 oz	**290**	3.5	50
Falafel & Tahini, 9.6 oz	**360**	13	49
Simply Steamers: *Per Package*			
Beef & Broccoli, 10 oz	**280**	7	32
Beef Chimichurri, 9 oz	**220**	6	24
Chicken & Vegetable Stir Fry, 9.2 oz	**190**	4	15
Gr. Chicken & Broc. Alfredo, 9.15 oz	**190**	5	8
Meatball Marinara, 10 oz	**280**	6	36

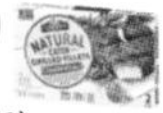
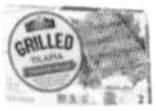

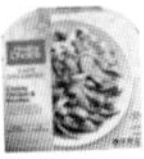
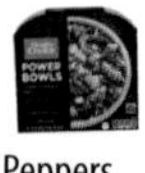
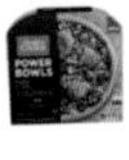

Heinz:	C	F	Cb
Beans, Baked in Tom. Sauce, 4.6 oz	**100**	0	18
Frozen:			
Devour Meals: *Per Package*			
Bacon Topped Meatloaf w/ Ketchup	**510**	29	38
Buffalo Chicken Mac & Cheese	**620**	31	56
Cajun Syle Alfredo w/ Ssg & Chkn	**410**	19	34
Loaded Potato w/ Beef & Bacon	**330**	14	31
Pesto Ravioli w/Spicy Italian Ssg	**670**	37	55
Pulled Chicken Burrito Bowl	**450**	15	47
White Chedd. Mac & Cheese w/ Bacon	**710**	41	54
Bowls: Creamy Alfredo Mac & Chse	**350**	12	50
Hot & Melty Nacho Mac & Cheese	**400**	13	60
Sharp Chedd. Mac & Chse w/ Bacon	**350**	10	49
Sandwiches: Buffalo Chkn Gr. Cheese	**520**	19	60
Philly Cheesesteak Grilled Cheese	**480**	17	62
Turkey & Bacon w/ Ranch Gr. Cheese	**550**	23	59
Hormel:			
Chili with Beans: *Per 8.7 oz Cup*			
Regular; Hot; Chunky, av.	**265**	9	32
Turkey, 98% Fat-Free	**220**	3	29
Vegetarian, 99% Fat Free	**200**	1.5	35
Chili No Beans: *Per 8.3 oz Cup*			
Regular	**260**	14	19
Hot; Chunky, average	**255**	13	19
Turkey, 98% Fat-Free	**190**	3	16
Compleats, Comfort Classics: *Per 7.5 oz Pkg*			
Beefy Mac	**230**	4	37
Chicken & Noodles,	**180**	6	20
Dumplings & Chicken	**190**	3.5	32
Noodles & Beef	**170**	2	28
Spaghetti & Meat Sauce	**220**	6	31
Compleats, Homesyle: *Per Package*			
Beef Pot Roast	**200**	6	20
Chicken Alfredo	**350**	18	30
Chkn Brst, Gravy & Mashed Potatoes	**220**	4	28
Meatloaf, Gravy & Mashed Potates	**300**	14	28
Salisbury Steak	**300**	16	27
Swedish Meatballs	**280**	13	26
Refrigerated Entrees: *Per Package*			
H'style Meat Loaf & Tom. Sce, 5 oz	**220**	9	14
Sliced Rstd Turkey Brst & Gravy, 5 oz	**110**	2.5	3
Slow Simm. Beef Tips w/ Gravy, 4.3 oz	**170**	10	3
Side Dishes: Bacon Mac & Chse, 8.2 oz	**340**	11	45
Chipotle Chedd. Mac & Chse, 8.2 oz	**340**	14	41
Tamales: Beef in Chile Sauce, 7.5 oz	**190**	9	22
Beef, Hot & Spicy in Chile Sce, 7.5 oz	**180**	8	22

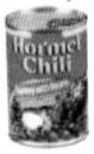

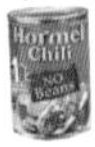

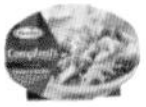
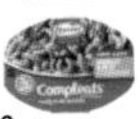
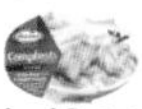
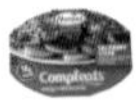

Hot Pockets:

Item	C	F	Cb
Sandwiches: *Per Sandwich*			
Big & Bold: Cheesy Sriracha Steak	440	18	56
Chicken Bacon Ranch	460	17	59
Crispy Buttery Crust:			
BBQ Recipe Beef	300	11	42
Cheddar Cheeseburger	290	10	41
Chicken Broccoli & Cheddar	270	9	37
Ham & Cheddar	270	9	39
Crispy Crust:			
Five Cheese Pizza	310	14	35
Pepperoni Pizza	330	17	34
Croissant Crust:			
Chicken Broccoli & Cheddar	300	13	36
Hickory Ham & Cheddar	300	13	36
Philly Steak & Cheese	310	14	37
Breakfast:			
Bacon, Egg & Chse	310	14	35
Sausage, Egg & Cheese	290	14	33
Flaky Crust, Chicken Pot Pie	230	8	31
High Protein:			
Crispy Butter Crust:			
Chicken Bacon Cheddar Melt	280	10	33
Steak & Cheddar	310	13	33
Garlic Buttery Crust,			
Four Meat & Four Cheese Pizza	310	14	32
Stuffed Pretzels: Cheesy Jalapeno	130	3.5	19
Chorizo Queso Fundido	140	4.5	19

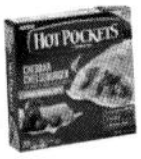

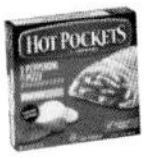

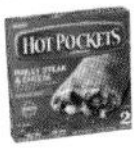

Hungry Jack:

Item	C	F	Cb
Casserole Potatoes: *Prepared*			
Au Gratin	140	4.5	24
Cheddar & Bacon	140	4.5	24
Cheesy Scalloped	140	4.5	24
Hashbrowns: *Prepared*			
Original, ⅓ cup	100	4.5	14
Black Pepper & Onions, ¼ cup	80	3	13
Cheesy, ½ cup	140	7	17
Mashed Potatoes,			
Dry Mix, ⅓ cup, prepared	170	7	24

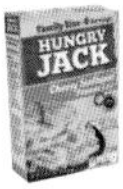

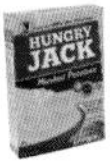

Hungry Man: *Per Package*

Item	C	F	Cb
Bowls: Double Chicken Bacon Ranch	570	29	30
Double Meat Angus Meatloaf	580	35	37
Dinners: Backyard BBQ	690	24	91
Country Fried Chicken	530	27	54
Roasted Carved White Meat Turkey	410	11	61
Salisbury Steak	580	32	51

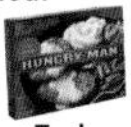

Hungry-Man (Cont):

Item	C	F	Cb
Selects: *Per Package*			
Classic Fried Chicken	970	59	59
Golden Battered Chicken w/ Fries	690	32	73
Mexican Style Fiesta Enchiladas	640	19	103

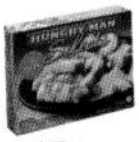

José Olé:

Item	C	F	Cb
Breakfast Burritos: *Per 4 oz Burrito*			
Egg, Cheese & Bacon	260	10	30
Egg, Sausage & Cheese	240	10	28
Burritos: *Per Burrito*			
Beef & Cheese	350	15	41
Beef & Jalapeno	320	12	40
Chicken Monterey	270	7	39
Chimichangas: *Per Chimichanga*			
Beef & Cheese	390	20	40
Chicken & Cheese	330	13	42
Chipotle Chicken	330	13	42
Loaded Beef Nacho	420	25	36
Queso Chicken Nacho	330	16	33
Minis & Bites:			
Beef & Cheese (5)	230	11	24
Queso Chicken Nacho (5)	220	10	24
Taquitos: Beef, Corn tortillas (3)	230	12	26
Beef & Cheese, Flour Tortillas, (2)	250	13	25
Chicken, Corn Tortillas, (3)	220	9	26
Chicken & Cheese, Flour Tortillas, (3)	220	10	25

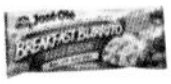

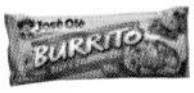

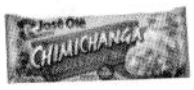

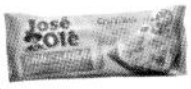
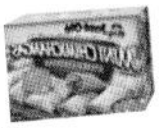

Kashi:

Item	C	F	Cb
Bowls: *Per Package*			
Black Bean Mango	310	8	55
Chimichurri Quinoa	240	7	41
Creamy Cashew Noodle	360	14	46
Mayan Harvest Bake	330	8	56
Sweet Potato Quinoa	270	6	48

Kid Cuisine: *Per Meal*

Item	C	F	Cb
All Star Chicken Breast Nuggets	420	16	54
Bikini Bottom Chkn Brst Nuggets	440	19	55
Bug Safari Chkn Breast Nuggets	430	13	62
Carnival Mini Corn Dogs	490	15	75
Friends Forever Mac & Cheese	380	11	54
Popstar Popcorn Chicken	470	18	65

Updated Nutrition Data ~ www.CalorieKing.com
Persons with Diabetes ~ See Disclaimer (Page 22)

Kraft:	C	F	Cb
Macaroni & Cheese:			
Original (7.25 oz Box),			
2.5 oz (makes 1 cup) 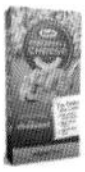	250	3	47
Whole Grain (6oz Box),			
2.5 oz (makes 1 cup)	260	3	51
Deluxe:			
Orig./4 Cheese/Broccoli/Bacon, average:			
¼ box, 3.5 oz (makes 1 cup)	315	10	42
White Cheddar, Galic & Herbs,			
¼ box, 3.5 oz (makes 1 cup	270	8	38
Microwave Cups: Star Wars, 1.8 oz	210	4	37
Average all flavors, 2 oz	220	4	41
Big Cups: Original, 4.1 oz	430	7	79
Triple Cheese 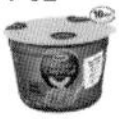	440	7	79
Velveeta: *Per Container*			
Cheesy Bowls: Bacon Mac & Chse	330	13	39
Chicken Alfredo 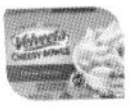	300	9	35
Lasagna with Meat	340	15	35
Ultimate Cheeseburger Mac	360	15	38
Shells & Cheese Cups:			
Original, 5 oz 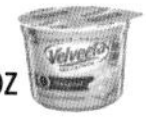	480	16	65
2% Milk Cheese, 2.2 oz	180	3	31
Queso Blanco, 2.4 oz	210	7	30
Kroger:			
Frozen: 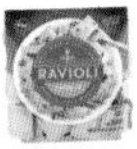			
Cheese Ravioli, 5.1 oz	280	6	43
Chicken Fried Rice, 1 cup, 4.23 oz	220	5	32
Flame Broiled Meatballs:			
Homestyle, 3 oz	200	13	7
Italian Style: Beef & Pork, 3 oz	230	17	5
Italian Style, 3 oz	190	13	7
Meat Lasagna, Party Size, 1 cup	280	10	34
Sweet & Spicy BBQ Pulled Pork, 1 cup	320	12	32
Microwaveable: *Per Container*			
Beef Stew	160	8	15
Cheeseburger with Bacon	430	21	39
Chicken & Dumplings 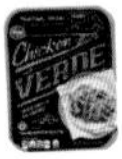	170	5	22
Refrigerated:			
Beef Barbacoa, 5 oz	200	10	2
Chicken Verde, w/ Cilantro Lime Rice	560	3.5	97
Creamy Mac & Cheese, 8.8 oz	400	17	45
Pork Burnt Ends in BBQ Sauce, 5 oz	190	3.5	21

Lean Cuisine:	C	F	Cb
Bowls: *Per Bowl* 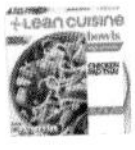			
Balsamic Glazed Chicken	370	9	46
Chicken Pad Thai	390	5	65
Chicken Teriyaki 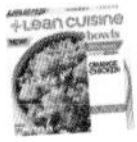	310	5	45
Orange Chicken	370	9	55
Four Cheese Tortelloni w/ Pesto Sce	330	9	44
Korean Style Rice & Vegetables	370	7	64
Mango chicken with Coconut Rice	360	6	55
Panko Chicken Romano 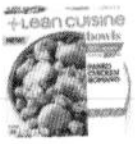	400	8	59
Peanut Chicken Stir Fry	400	10	56
Roasted Turkey & Vegetables	300	8	38
Savory Sesame Chicken & Veggies	370	9	54
Sesame Stir-Fry with Chicken	350	7	46
Shrimp Alfredo	320	9	41
Spice Market Chicken & Cauliflower	220	4	26
Spicy Baja-Style Chicken 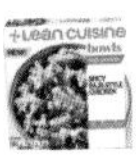	320	4	47
Sticky Ginger Chicken	320	5	51
Sweet & Sour Chicken	400	8	66
Unwrapped Chicken Burrito	340	7	44
Favorites: *Per Package*			
Alfredo Pasta with Chkn & Brocc.	280	5	39
Asian-Style Pot Stickers 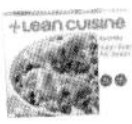	270	4	51
Cheese Ravioli	250	6	39
Classic: Five Cheese Lasagna	330	7	49
Macaroni & Beef	260	5	39
Fettuccini Alfredo 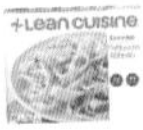	290	5	49
Five Cheese Rigatoni	360	10	54
Four Cheese Cannelloni	240	8	32
French Bread Pepperoni Pizza	300	7	44
Glazed Turkey Tenderloins 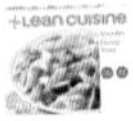	300	6	47
Penne Rosa	280	7	43
Santa Fe-Style Rice & Beans	300	4	54
Spaghetti w/ Meatballs 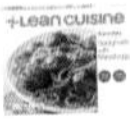	290	5	45
Spicy Penne Arrabbiata	250	6	39
Swedish Meatballs	300	6	44

Lean Cuisine (Cont):	C	F	Cb
Features: *Per Package*			
Butternut Squash Ravioli	290	6	49
Cheese & Fire Roasted Chile Tamale	330	9	55
Chicken, Spinach & Mushroom Panini	320	8	41
Chicken Tikka Masala	300	4	48
Garlic Chkn Spring Rolls	180	8	21
Maple Bourbon Chicken	350	9	50
Meatloaf with Mshd Potatoes	240	7	25
Mushroom Mezzaluna Ravioli	270	8	40
Philly-Style Steak & Cheese Panini	330	9	42
Ricotta Cheese & Spinach Ravioli	250	6	40
Spinach, Artichoke & Chkn Panini	340	10	44
Tortilla Crusted Fish	310	8	45

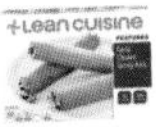
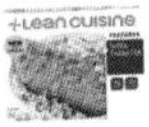

Pizzas ~ *See Page 137*

Extra Product Listings ~ *www.CalorieKing.com*

Lean Pockets:	C	F	Cb
Sandwiches: *Per Single Pocket*			
Garlic & Herb Seasoned Crust:			
Caprese; Chicken Parmesan	250	5	41
M'balls & Mozzarella	280	9	41
Pepperponi Pizza	280	8	42
Pretzel Bread:			
BBQ Recipe White Meat Chicken	240	3.5	42
Chicken Japalpeno & Cheese	250	7	35
Roasted Turkey, Bacon & Cheese	270	9	35
Uncured Ham & White Cheddar	270	7	39
Seasoned Crust:			
Philly Steak & Cheese	260	7	41

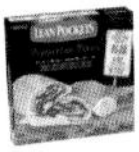
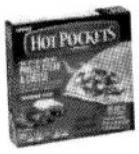

Lightlife (Meatless):	C	F	Cb
Frozen:			
Burger Patty, 4 oz	250	16	8
Gimme Lean Sausage, 2.3 oz	60	0.5	7
Smart Bacon, 1 oz	60	3	2
Smart Deli, Turkey, 4 sl.	100	3.5	5
Smart Ground, Zesty Italian, 2 oz	80	1.5	5
Smart Menu, Meatballs (3)	100	1	10
Smart Tenders, 3 oz	90	1	9
Tempeh: Original, 3 oz	160	4.5	12
Smoky Strips, 4 slices	140	5	10

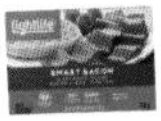
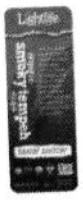

Updated Nutrition Data ~ www.CalorieKing.com
Persons with Diabetes ~ See Disclaimer (Page 22)

Lunchables: *Per Package*	C	F	Cb
Without Drink:			
Bologna, Am. Chse & Choc Chip Cookie	320	17	32
Ham & Cheddar with Crackers	260	13	22
Nachos, Cheese Dip & Salsa	370	20	42
Pepperoni Pizza	420	19	49
Turkey & Cheddar with Crackers	260	13	22
Lunchmakers *(Armour)*: *Per Package*			
Bologna Cracker Crunchers	240	14	21
Chkn Cracker Crunchers	200	9	21
Nachos	210	10	28
Pepperoni Flav. Sausage Pizza	220	10	25
Turkey Cracker Crunchers	210	10	22

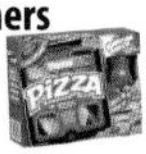

Marie Callender's:	C	F	Cb
Frozen:			
Beef: *Per Container*			
Beef Pot Roast	200	4.5	26
Meat Loaf & Gravy	380	13	45
Salisbury Steak	400	17	40
Spaghetti w/ Meat Sce	350	7	54
Slow Roasted Beef	260	9	32
Bowls: *Per Bowl*			
Creamy Vermont Mac & Cheese	570	22	71
Red Chili Grilled Chicken Burrito	360	10	44
Spicy Buffalo Style Chkn Mac & Chse	540	25	53
Sweet & Savory Sesame Chicken	470	14	68
Chicken/Turkey: *Per Container*			
Cheesy Chicken & Rice	430	14	54
Grilled Chkn Alfredo Bake	420	16	42
Honey Roasted Turkey Breast	260	6	31
Sweet & Sour Chicken	550	15	88
Pasta: *Per Container*			
Fettuccini Alfredo & Garlic Bread	610	31	59
Fettuccini, Chicken & Broccoli	440	20	38
Grilled Chicken Alfredo Bake	460	19	45
Pot Pies: *Per 1 Cup, 7 oz*			
Beef	400	21	40
Brocc. & Cheddar Potato	680	40	69
Cheesy Chicken & Bacon	510	32	41
Chicken Corn Chowder	460	28	38
Chili with Beans	420	23	43
Creamy:			
Mushroom Chicken	430	25	39
Parmesan Chicken	430	26	36
Turkey	480	28	46

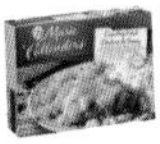
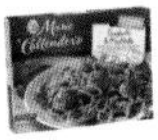
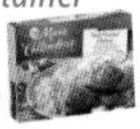
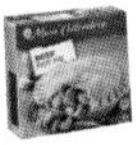
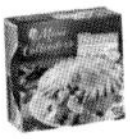
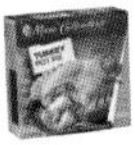

Maruchan:	C	F	Cb
Bowls, all var., 3.3 oz	380	16	50
Ramen Noodle Soup,			
average all, 3 oz pkg	380	15	52
Instant Lunch,			
average, 1 container	290	11	39
Yakisoba: *Per 4 oz Pkg*			
Chicken/Teriyaki Beef Flavor, av.	500	19	69
Cheddar Cheese Flavor	540	24	68

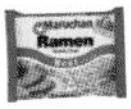
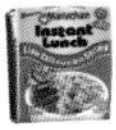

Michael Angelo's:	C	F	Cb
Frozen:			
Calzones: Meatball (1)	300	10	39
Primo Supreme (1)	330	12	40
Gourmet Bowls: Chicken Cavatappi	290	7	37
Gnocchi Alfredo with Bacon	260	10	40
Meat Lasagna Bolognese w/ Ssg.	340	14	34
Organic: Chicken Parmigiana, 10 oz	310	6	47
Eggplant Parmigiana, 10 oz	240	12	22
Lasagna with Meat Sauce, 10 oz	370	16	37
Signature: Baked Ziti w/ M'balls, 11 oz	480	20	51
Chicken Parmesan, 10 oz	400	15	44
Manicoti w/ Sauce, 11 oz	440	19	41
Shrimp Scampi, 10 oz	580	28	61
Vegetable Lasagna, 11 oz	350	13	40

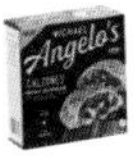
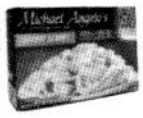

Minute Rice:	C	F	Cb
Ready To Serve: *Per 4.4 oz Container, Prepared*			
Brown/Chicken Rice	220	3	43
Fried/Yellow Rice Mix, average	220	2.5	45
Quinoa, Red & White	160	2	34

Morningstar Farms (Meatless):	C	F	Cb
Burgers: Grillers Original (1)	130	5	8
Mediterranean Chickpea (1)	120	4.5	13
Spicy Black Bean (1)	170	5	26
Chik'n:			
Nuggets: Regular (4)	200	9	20
BBQ (4)	200	8	23
Patties, Buffalo (1)	160	6	19
Veggitizers:			
Mini Corn Dogs, 4 pieces	170	4.5	27
Popcorn Chik'n, 12 pieces	200	8	23
Wings: Buffalo (5)	200	8	21
Parmesan Garlic (5)	190	8	19

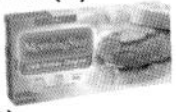
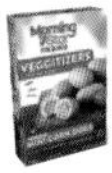

Nissin:	C	F	Cb
Chow Mein: *Per 4 oz Package*			
Chicken	490	22	65
Pad Thai; Shrimp Flavor, average	555	29	64
Teriyaki Beef Flavor	510	24	63
Cup Noodles:			
All flavors, 1 cup	290	11	41

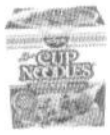

Nissin (Cont):	C	F	Cb
Cup Noodle Stir Fry,			
average all flavors	370	13	55
Top Ramen: *Per Package With Soy Sauce*			
Beef; Chicken, average	390	14	57
Shrimp	450	22	54

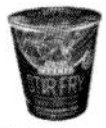
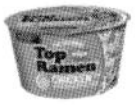

Old El Paso:	C	F	Cb
Dinner Kits: *Per 2 Tortillas, Sauce & Seasoning Only*			
Caribbean Inspired Jerk; Fajita, av	185	5	32
Fiesta Taco	160	6	18
Korean Inspired BBQ	210	6	34
Rice & Beans:			
Cheesy Mex. Rice, 2.6 oz	270	0.5	59
Spanish Rice, 2.6 oz	260	0.5	58
Traditional Refried Beans, 4.23 oz	110	2.5	14

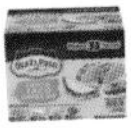

Ortega: *Per ½ cup, 4.6 oz*	C	F	Cb
Black Beans	110	0	20
w. Diced Jalapeños	130	2	23
Refried Beans:			
Traditional	130	2.5	21
w. Diced Green Chiles	140	2.5	22
Fat Free Refried Beans	120	0	21
Vegetarian Refried Beans	120	0	21
Meal Kits: *Per Serving*			
Bakeable Tortilla Bowl	120	2	22
Fiesta Flats Taco	160	6	22
Hard & Soft Grande Taco	230	3.5	41
Soft Taco	230	3.5	42
Taco Dinner	140	6	21
Taco Pizza	200	4.5	35

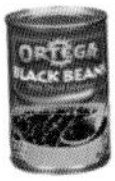
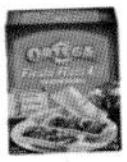
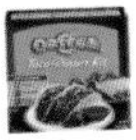

Pasta Roni: *Per Cup, Prepared*	C	F	Cb
Angel Hair with Herbs	310	12	42
Butter & Herb Italiano; Chkn Flav., av.	300	12	40
Chicken & Broccoli	360	15	47
Fettuccine Alfredo	440	24	48
White Cheddar & Broccoli	310	13	39

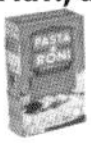

P.F. Chang's: *Per ½ Package, 11 oz*	C	F	Cb
Frozen:			
Entrees: Beef with Broccoli, 9.47 oz	270	10	25
General Chang's Chicken, 10.8 oz	370	11	50
Kung Pao Chicken, 10.6 oz	210	8	17
Mongolian Style Beef, 8.57 oz	230	5	31
Sesame Chicken, 10.2 oz	230	10	17
Sweet & Sour Chicken, 9.2 oz	280	6	44
Ramen: Chicken Tonkotsu, 6.17 oz	230	10	20
Veggie Shoyu, 6.63 oz	160	2	28
Sides, Chang's Signature Rice, 8 oz	290	2	61

Prego:	C	F	Cb
Ready Meals: *Per Pouch*			
Creamy Three Cheese Alfedo Rotini	370	19	37
Creamy Tomato Penne	400	15	57
Marinara & Italian Sausage Rotini	350	9	55
Roasted Tomato & Vegetables Penne	300	4	55

Rice-A-Roni:	C	F	Cb
Classic Favorites: *Per Cup, Prepared*			
Beef	**310**	9	51
Chicken & Broccoli	**230**	4	41
Chicken & Garlic	**250**	8	41
Mexican Style	**250**	8	41
Rice Pilaf	**310**	8	52
Single Serve Cups:			
Cheddar Broccoli	**230**	4.5	41
Chicken Flavor	**190**	1	41
Creamy Four Cheese	**240**	6	43

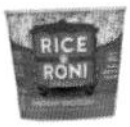

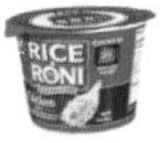

Rosarita:	C	F	Cb
Black Beans, 4.5 oz	**110**	0.5	19
Pinto Beans, 4.5 oz	**120**	0	22
Refried Beans:			
Traditional, 4.5 oz	**120**	2.5	18
No Fat, 4.5 oz	**100**	0	18
Restaurant Style, 4.4 oz	**90**	2.5	13
Vegetarian, 4.5 oz	**120**	2	19

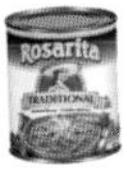

Safeway Select *(Albertsons)*:	C	F	Cb
Frozen:			
Signature Select: *Per Container*			
Beef & Broccoli Power Bowl	**330**	7	46
Cheesy Scramble	**180**	6	20
Chicken Teriyaki	**250**	3.5	42
Chicken with Basil Cream Sauce	**310**	8	35
Chicken with Peanut Sauce	**260**	6	31
Roasted Turkey	**270**	8	34
Sweet & Sour Chicken	**270**	4.5	42

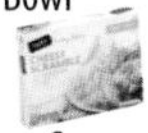
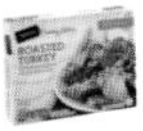

S & W: *Per ½ Cup, 4.6 oz*	C	F	Cb
Chili, average	**125**	1	22
Classic, average	**110**	0	21
Flavored Savory Sides:			
Indian Style Savory Sides	**150**	3.5	24
Jalapeno Black Beans	**130**	1.5	22
New Orleans Style Savory	**160**	4	23
Southwest Style	**110**	0	22
Tuscan Style Savory	**130**	2	21

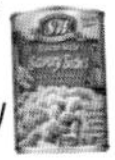

Seapak ~ *See www.calorieking.com*

Simply Asia: *Per Container*	C	F	Cb
Noodles & Broth:			
Japanese: Ramen Noodles	**200**	1	42
Ramen Soy Chicken Broth	**40**	1	2
Udon Noodles	**190**	0.5	41
Noodle Bowls: Roasted Peanut	**460**	12	75
Sesame Teriyaki	**420**	3.5	87
Soy Ginger	**440**	6	86

Smart Ones *(Weight Watchers)*:	C	F	Cb
Frozen:			
Indulgence, Cavatapppi Bolognese	**280**	6	41
Smartmade: *Per Package*			
Black Beans & Cheese over Cilantro Rice	**320**	6	49
Chicken Fried Cauliflower Rice Bowl	**150**	2.5	16
Chicken with Spinach Fettuccine	**230**	6	20
Grilled Sesame Beef & Broccoli	**220**	5	31
Lemon Garlic Chicken Fettuccini	**200**	4	23
Mexican Style Chicken Bowl	**260**	5	33
Mexican Style Pulled Pork Bowl	**320**	9	33
Roasted Turkey & Veggies	**240**	2.5	37
Rosemary Grilled Beef & Veggies	**270**	8	30
White Wine Chicken & Couscous	**190**	2.5	23
Smart Ones: *Per Package*			
Angel Hair Marinara	**200**	2.5	37
Chicken Enchiladas Suiza	**290**	6	46
Chicken Fettuccine	**300**	4.5	44
Chicken Parmesan	**280**	6	35
Creamy Basil Chicken with Broccili	**170**	3.5	15
Creamy Rigatoni w/ Broccoli & Chkn	**260**	4	40
Crustless Chicken Pot Pie	**190**	3.5	20
Fettuccine Alfredo	**250**	4	42
General Tso's Chicken	**320**	7	48
Homestyle Beef Pot Roast	**180**	3.5	18
Macaroni & Cheese	**260**	2	50
Meatloaf	**220**	8	19
Meat Sauce Lasagna	**330**	12	41
Pasta with Swedish Meatballs	**290**	5	41
Ravioli Florentine	**210**	3.5	37
Santa Fe Rice & Beans	**260**	6	39
Sesame Noodles with Vegetables	**270**	3	51
Slow Roasted Turkey Breast	**170**	3.5	16
Spaghetti with Meat Sauce	**280**	5	45
Three Cheese Ziti Marinara	**300**	8	43
With Meatballs	**340**	13	39
Traditional Lasagna w/ Meat Sauce	**330**	12	41

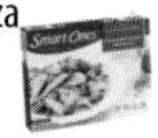
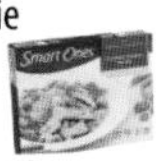
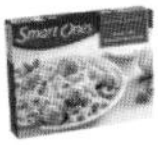
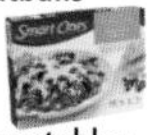
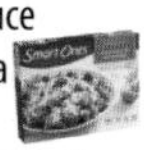

Stagg:	C	F	Cb
Chili with Beans, 15 oz Can: *Per Cup*			
Classic, 8.7 oz	**290**	13	26
Dynamite Hot, 8.7 oz	**340**	16	33
Laredo, 8.7 oz	**300**	17	23
Silverado Beef, 8.7 oz	**250**	9	25
Turkey Ranchero	**260**	6	32
Vegetarian Garden 4-Bean Chili	**200**	2	37

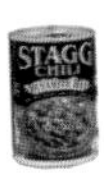

Stouffer's:

Frozen:

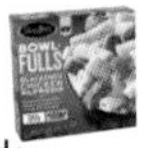

Bowl-FULLS: *For One*	C	F	Cb
Blackened Chicken Alfredo	**580**	25	59
Cheesy Chicken Parmesan	**520**	16	67
Chicken Bacon Ranch Pasta	**610**	26	58
Chicken Mac & Cheese Broccoli	**590**	24	63
Classic Pub Meatballs & Potatoes	**470**	20	42
Fried Chicken & Mashed Potatoes	**470**	19	51
Philly Cheese Steak Mac & Cheese	**550**	25	54
Slow Roasted Steak & Potatoes	**370**	15	36
Southwest Style Mac & Cheese	**520**	25	47
Spicy Italian Sausage Pasta	**660**	35	63

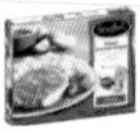

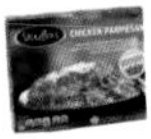

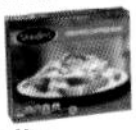

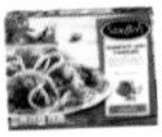

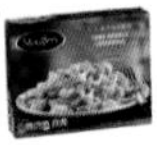

Classics: *For One*	C	F	Cb
Baked Chicken	**240**	8	17
Baked Macaroni & Cheese	**500**	23	52
Cajun Style Chicken	**290**	2	45
Cheddar Potato Bake	**270**	17	21
Chicken a la King	**360**	12	44
Chicken & Mushroom Marsala	**300**	7	40
Chicken Parmesan	**410**	14	47
Creamed Chipped Beef	**140**	7	11
Escalloped chicken & Noodles	**450**	22	43
Fettuccini Alfredo	**630**	35	63
Fish Fillet with Mac & Cheese	**400**	19	35
Five Cheese Lasagna	**370**	14	49
Four Cheese Mac with Bacon	**440**	19	47
Fried Chicken	**340**	16	28
Green Pepper Steak	**240**	4	32
Macaroni & Cheese	**340**	16	33
Meat Lovers Lasagna	**420**	19	41
Romano Crusted Chicken	**470**	19	51
Salisbury Steak	**340**	16	26
Spaghetti w/ Meatballs	**360**	12	45
Three Cheese Ravioli	**360**	11	43
Tuna Noodle Casserole	**450**	20	45
White Meat Chicken Pot Pie	**670**	38	64

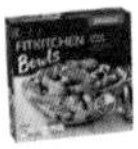

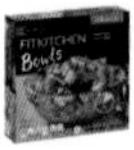

Fit Kitchen Protein Bowls: *Per Package*	C	F	Cb
Beef with Broccoli	**360**	9	50
Bourbon Steak	**290**	5	41
Broccoli with Beef	**360**	3	50
Oven Roasted Chicken	**250**	3	35
Steak Fajitas	**340**	8	44
Teriyaki Chicken	**390**	6	60

Swanson:

Frozen:

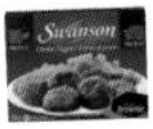

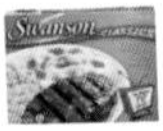

Dinners: *Per Package*	C	F	Cb
Chicken Nuggets	**590**	25	71
Chicken Parmigiana	**450**	23	45
Chicken Strips	**480**	19	61
Fried Chicken	**520**	26	54
Meatloaf	**450**	23	45
Rib Style Boneless Pork	**540**	23	71
Salisbury Steak	**450**	22	44
Turkey	**330**	9	45

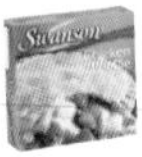

	C	F	Cb
Meat Pies: Beef	**430**	26	37
Chicken	**370**	20	37
Turkey	**400**	23	38

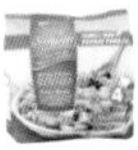

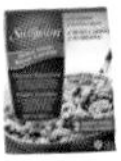

Skillets: *For Two*	C	F	Cb
Alfredo Chicken	**370**	12	42
Beef Lo Mein	**360**	6	55
Chicken Florentine	**310**	7	40
Chicken Parmesan	**430**	14	60
Creamy Cheddar Chicken	**360**	8	52
Garlic Chicken	**420**	15	51
Garlic Shrimp	**390**	14	49
Teriyaki Chicken	**290**	2.5	51

Tasty Bite:

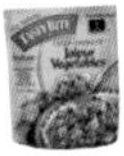

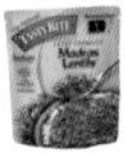

Mains: *Per ⅔ Cup*	C	F	Cb
Bombay Potatoes, 4.9 oz	**130**	5	18
Channa Masala	**160**	6	28
Coconut Vegetables	**130**	7	13
Jaipur Vegetables	**180**	12	12
Jodhpur Lentils	**120**	4	14
Kashmir Spinach	**120**	9	6
Madras Lentils	**140**	6	17
Mushroom Masala	**100**	4.5	13
Punjab Eggplant	**110**	5	12

TGI Friday's:

	C	F	Cb
Buffalo Style Chicken Wings, with Sauce, 4.5 oz	**240**	16	10
Cheddar & Bacon Potato Skins (1)	**190**	13	15
Cheeseburger Sliders w/ BBQ Sce	**250**	13	24
Honey BBQ Chicken Wings, 3 oz	**290**	15	24
Mozzarella Sticks, with Marinara Sauce (1)	**100**	5	12
Poppers, Crm Chse Stuffed Jalapeno (3) with Raspberry Habanero Dip	**250**	14	27

Thai Kitchen:	C	F	Cb
Curry & Noodle Kits (Gluten Free):			
Pad Thai	260	1	58
Thai Peanut	200	4	37
Noodle Carts (Gluten Free):			
Pad Thai, 9.77 oz	440	2.5	98
Thai Peanut, 9.77 oz	540	12	96

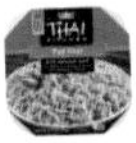

Trader Joe's:			
Baked Beans, Organic, av., ½ cup	140	0	29
Black Beans:			
Regular, ½ cup	110	0	19
Cuban Style, ½ cup	100	0.5	19
Black Bean & Jack Cheese Burrito	600	20	77
Chicken Chili with Beans, 1 cup	290	9	32
Potatoes: Garlic Mashed, ½ cup	150	7	19
Cheddar Cheese Au Gratin, ½ cup	140	5	21
Turkey Chili w/ Beans, 1 cup	240	4.5	30
Frozen:			
Black Beans & Chse Taquitos (2)	190	7	26
Butternut Squash Mac & Cheese, 8 oz	250	8	38
Chicken Quesadilla, (1), 6 oz	320	16	26
Fiery Chicken Curry, 9.5 oz	360	13	40
Mac & Cheese: Regular, 1 cup, 7 oz	360	15	42
Reduced Guilt, 7 oz	270	6	40
Pies: Chicken Pot Pie, ½ pie, 8 oz	360	22	28
Shepherd's Pie, 1 cup, 8 oz	170	3	22
Plant Based Protein Patties:			
Burger Patties (1), 4 oz	290	20	11
Turkeyless Patties (1), 4 oz	240	14	7
Spaghetti & Beef Meatballs, 1 cup, 9 oz	380	13	48
Spicy Beef & Broccoli, 1¾ cups	430	13	64
Trad. Carnitas, Mexican Style, 3 oz	200	14	1
Veggie & Sobda Noodle Stir Fry, 1 cup, 3 oz	80	1.5	14

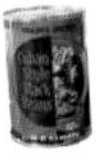

Tyson:			
Any'tizers Snacks:			
24 oz Bags Boneless Chicken Bites:			
Buffalo Style, 3 oz	180	9	12
Honey BBQ, 3 oz	210	9	20
Homestyle Chicken Fries, 3.2 oz	260	16	16
Popcorn Chicken, 3 oz	170	7	14
Wings, Tequila Lime flavored, 3 oz	170	11	3

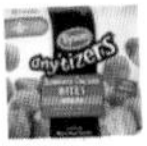

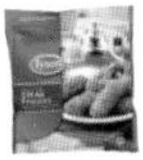

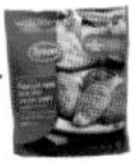

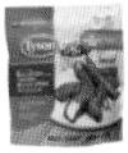

Tyson (Cont):	C	F	Cb
Frozen:			
Beef:			
Country Fried Steak (1)	300	21	15
Steak Fingers, 2.5 oz	250	18	14
Breaded Chicken: *Per 3 oz Unless Indicated*			
Crispy Chicken Strips	210	10	17
Fun Nuggets 2.7 oz	180	11	10
Honey Batt. Breast Tender	210	13	13
Nuggets, 3.2 oz	270	17	15
Parm. Herb Encrusted Crispy Strips	210	10	13
Southern Breast Tenderloins, 3 oz	180	9	12
Spicy Breast Patties, 2.7 oz	200	13	10
Grilled Chkn Breasts: Blackened, 3 oz	110	3	1
Breast Fillets, 3.5 oz	130	4.5	2
Fajita Strips, 3 oz	100	2	2
Oven Roasted, Diced, 3 oz	100	2.5	1
Sweet Teriyaki Chicken Fillets, 3 oz	140	6	4
Meal Kits: Chipotle Chicken, with Honey Lime Glaze, 4.5 oz	160	5	3
Instant Pot:			
Cajun Style Chicken & Rice, 7 oz	330	10	41
Teriyaki Chicken & Rice, 7.2 oz	410	8	63

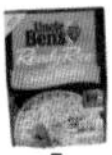

Uncle Ben's:			
Flavored Grains: *Dry Mix Only*			
Average all flavors, ¼ cup	155	1	31
Long Grain Varieties, ¼ cup	200	0.5	42
Flavor Infusions, dry mix, av., 1.7 oz	155	0.5	34
Ready Rice: *Per Pouch Unless Indicated*			
Butter & Garlic Flavored	370	6	73
Creamy Four Cheese Flavored Rice, with Vermicelli, 1 cup, 5.65 oz	220	5	40
Garden Vegetable Rice, 1 c., 5.1 oz	210	2.5	42
Jambalaya Rice, 1 cup, 5 oz	200	2	40
Risotto: Cheese	430	10	76
Mushroom	420	8	77
Roasted Chicken Flavored, 1 c., 5 oz	210	3	42
Spanish Style Rice, 1 cup, 5 oz	200	2.5	40

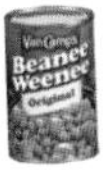

Van Camp's:			
Baked Beans: Orig., ½ cup, 4.8 oz	150	0.5	30
Bacon, ½ cup, 4.8 oz	160	1	30
Beanee Weenee: Original, 7.75 oz	260	8	33
Barbecue, 7.75oz	280	8	39
Smoked Hickory, 7.75 oz	320	8	48
Chili, with Beans, 9 oz	410	24	34
Pork & Beans, in Tom. Sce, 4.6 oz	120	1	23

Van De Kamp's:	C	F	Cb
Frozen:			
Fillets: Beer Battered, 3.8 oz	210	10	21
Cracked Black Pepper Salmon, 4.5 oz	230	8	20
Crispy, 3.8 oz	210	10	21
Crunchy, 3.8 oz	240	12	24
Fish Sticks:			
Crunchy, 3.6 oz	220	10	20
Nacho, 3 oz	200	10	18
Ranch (4), 3 oz	200	10	18
Whole Foods (365):			
Macaraoni & Cheese, 1 c. prepared	400	17	50
Plant-Based:			
Chicken-Style: Breaded Patties (1)	130	5	12
Meatballs (4), 2 oz	170	11	9
Nuggets (4)	140	6	13
Tradtnl Burgers, 1 Patty	80	3	7
Pasta Rings in Tom. Sauce, 7.5 oz	140	0	30
Worthington/Loma Linda *(Vegan):*			
Big Franks, 1 link, 1.8 oz	110	6	3
Burger, 1.94 oz	70	1.5	3
Chili, 1 cup, 8.10 oz	280	10	25
Choplets, 2 slices, 3.2 oz	90	1	4
Complete Meal Solution:			
Chipotle Bowl, 5 oz	130	0	23
Hearty Stew, 10 oz	270	2	47
Italian Bolognese, 5 oz	90	3	10
Medit. Tom. & Olive with Pasta, 5 oz	100	3	12
Pad Thai, 5 oz	130	4	18
Southwest Chunky Stew, 5 oz	125	2	19
Thai Red Curry, 5 oz	130	6	12
Thai Green Curry, 5 oz	155	5	23
Tikka Masala, 5 oz	125	3	19
Linketts (1), 1.3 oz	70	4	1
Nutolene, 2 slices, 3 oz	230	20	2
Redi-Burger, 3 oz slice	120	2.5	7
Saucettes (1), 1.34 oz	90	6	1
Sloppy Joe, ⅓ cup, 1.62 oz	40	0.5	6
Swiss Stake with Gravy, 3.25 oz	120	6	7
Tuno: In Spring Water, 2 oz	40	0	2
Lemon Pepper, 2 oz	55	1	5
3 oz pouch	80	2	7
Sesame Ginger, 3 oz pouch	87	1	13
Sriracha, 2 oz	70	3	6
Thai Sweet Chili, 3 oz pouch	90	0.5	13
Vege-Burger, ¼ cup, 1.9 oz	60	0.5	2
Veja-Links (1)	45	1.5	3

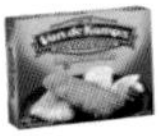
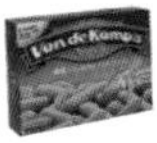
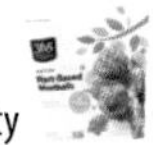
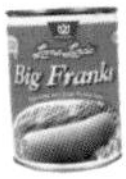

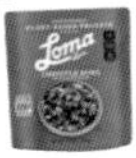
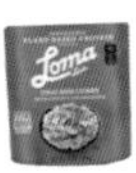
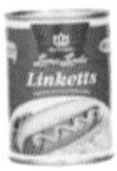

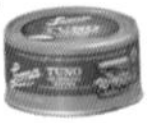
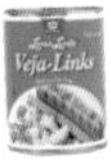

Yves Veggie Cuisine *(Meatless):*	C	F	Cb
Appetizers:			
Balls, Falafel (3)	150	7	17
Bites: Broccoli (4)	80	3	11
Kale & Quinoa (4)	90	2.5	13
Sweet Potato & Chickpea (4)	100	3	17
Burger Patties:			
Gluten Free Veggie (1)	110	6	5
Kale & Root Vegetables (1)	110	6	5
Deli Veggie Slices:			
Bologna (3)	60	1	2
Ham (5)	80	1	5
Pepperoni (10)	45	1	3
Salami (5)	80	1	5
Turkey (5)	80	1	4
Veggie Dogs:			
Good Dog, 1.35 oz	45	1	2
Regular (1)	50	0.5	2
Jumbo (1), 2.7 oz	110	2	4
Tofu (1)	50	1	2
Ground Rounds:			
Original Veggie, 1.9 oz	60	0.5	5
Garden Veggie Crumble, 1.95 oz	80	1.5	9
Other Vegan Plant Based Meals ~ *See Page 124*			
Zatarain's:			
Rice Mixes New Orleans Style: *Per Dry Mix Only*			
Creole Piiaf Mix, with Long Grain & Wild Rice, 2 oz	220	1	46
Jambalaya Mix, 1.74 oz	170	0.5	37
Red Beans & Rice, 2.5 oz	250	1	50
Red. Sodium: Dirty Rice, 1.74 oz	180	0.5	39
Red Beans & Rice, 2.5 oz	250	1	50
Frozen Entrees: *Per Single Serve*			
Blackened Chicken Alfredo, 10.5 oz	500	22	54
Blackened Chkn w/ Yellow Rice, 10.5 oz	540	17	77
Bourbon Chicken Pasta, 10.5 oz	460	18	52
Creamy Cajun Style Pasta, 10.5 oz	420	16	48
Dirty Rice with Beef & Pork, 10 oz	430	13	64
Jambalaya Flavored w/ Ssg, 12 oz	440	7	86
Red Beans & Rice with Sausage, 12 oz	480	14	78
Sausage & Chicken Gumbo with Rice, 12 oz	310	10	45
Shrimp Alfredo, 10.5 oz	490	17	62
Shrimp Scampi with Pasta, 10.5 oz	350	10	47

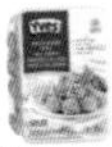
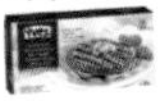
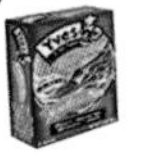
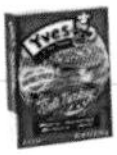
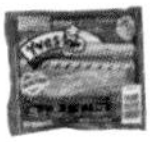
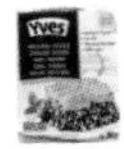

Note: Cooking reduces weight of meat by 20-45% due to water and fat losses. Average weight loss is 30%. Actual loss depends on cooking method and cooking time.

Examples:

4 oz raw weight = approx. 3 oz cooked weight

4 oz cooked weight = approx. 5½ oz raw weight

What 3 oz Cooked Meat Looks Like:

- Rectangular piece (4" x 2½" x ½" thick)
- Deck of cards (3½" x 2½" x ⅝" thick)

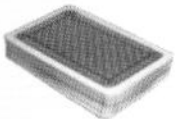

Quick Guide

Sirloin (Choice Grade):
External fat trimmed to ½"
Broiled, Edible Portion (no bone)

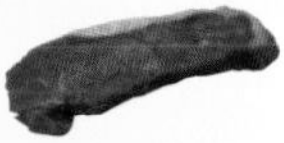

	C	F	Cb
Small/Regular Serving, 3 oz, cooked weight:			
(from 4-4½ oz raw)			
Lean + external fat (⅛"), 3 oz	**220**	13	0
Lean + marbling, 3 oz	**185**	9	0
Lean only, 3 oz	**160**	6	0
(No external fat or marbling)			
Medium Serving, 5 oz, cooked weight:			
(from approximately 7 oz raw)			
Lean + external fat (⅛"), 5 oz	**365**	22	0
Lean + marbling, 5 oz	**310**	15	0
Lean only, 5 oz	**265**	10	0
Large Serving, 8 oz, cooked weight:			
(from approximately11-12 oz raw)			
Lean + external fat (½"), 8 oz	**585**	36	0
Lean + marbling, 8 oz	**500**	24	0
Lean only, 8 oz	**425**	15	0
Extra Large Serving, 12 oz, cooked weight:			
(from approximately 16-17 oz raw)			
Lean + external fat (⅛"), 12 oz	**875**	54	0
Lean + marbling, 12 oz	**745**	36	0
Lean only, 12 oz	**640**	22	0
Pan Fried:			
Sirloin (Choice), medium serving,			
Lean + external fat (⅛"), 5 oz	**445**	30	0

Other Steaks

	C	F	Cb
Filet Mignon (Tenderloin):			
1 Medium steak, 6 oz raw weight:			
Broiled, with ¼" fat trim:			
Lean + fat (¼"), 4 oz	**360**	27	0
Lean only, 3.5 oz	**230**	12	0
New York/Club Steak:			
Top Loin/Short Loin:			
1 steak, regular (9.25 oz raw, ¼" fat):			
Broiled: Lean + fat (¼"), 6.3 oz	**580**	43	0
Lean + marbling, 5.5 oz	**400**	25	0
Lean only, 5.25 oz	**360**	20	0
Porterhouse Steak:			
1 Medium, 6 oz raw weight, w/out bone, broiled:			
Lean + fat (¼"), 4.3 oz	**410**	33	0
Lean only, 3.5 oz	**210**	11	0
1 Large ,12 oz raw weight, without bone, broiled:			
Lean + fat (¼") 8.5 oz cooked	**820**	66	0
Lean only, 7 oz cooked	**420**	22	0
T-Bone Steak: *Broiled or Grilled*			
Medium Size: *8 oz raw weight, without bone*			
Approximately 6 oz cooked:			
Lean + Fat (¼"), 5 oz	**400**	28	0
Lean only, 4 oz	**265**	12	0
Large Size: *12 oz raw weight*			
Approximately 9 oz cooked:			
Lean + fat (¼"), 7 oz, without bone	**560**	39	0
Lean only, 6 oz, without bone	**400**	18	0
Extra Large Size: *20 oz raw weight*			
Approximately 16 oz cooked:			
Lean + Fat (¼"), 12 oz, without bone	**960**	66	0
Lean Only, 10 oz, without bone	**660**	30	0

Also See Fast-Foods & Restaurants Section ~
Lone Star Steakhouse; Outback Steakhouse

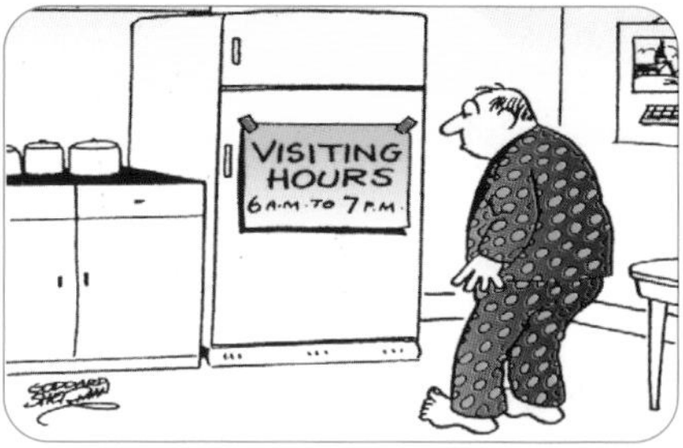

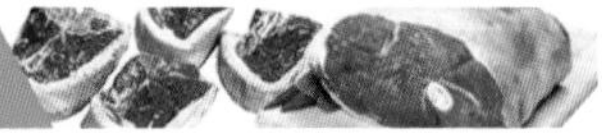

Beef – Individual Cuts

Average All Grades
Edible Weight, Without Bone

	C	F	Cb
Brisket, whole, braised:			
Lean + fat (¼" trim), 3 oz	330	27	0
Lean + marbling, 3 oz	250	17	0
Lean only, 3 oz	185	9	0
Chuck Blade, braised:			
Lean + fat (¼"), 3 oz	310	24	0
Lean + marbling, 3 oz	295	22	0
Lean only, 3 oz	245	13	0
Flank: Raw, 4 oz	175	8	0
Braised, 3 oz	225	14	0
Broiled, 3 oz	155	6	0
Round, bottom, braised:			
Lean + marbling, 3 oz	190	7.5	0
Lean only, 3 oz	185	6.5	0
Round, eye/tip, rstd:			
Lean + fat (¼"), 3 oz	205	11	0
Lean, w/ marbling, 3 oz	150	5	0
Round, top: *Per 3 oz, Cooked Weight*			
Braised, Lean + fat	210	10	0
Lean only	170	4	0
Broiled, Lean + fat	180	8	0
Lean only	160	5	0
Pan-fried, Lean + fat	235	13	0
Lean only	195	7	0

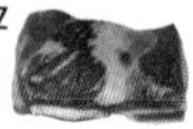
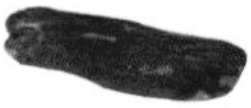
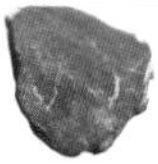
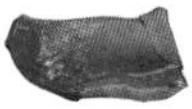

Beef Ribs

Back Ribs: *7" long, visible fat trimmed to ¼"*
10.3 oz raw w/ bone or 3.5 oz cooked, braised, w/o bone

	C	F	Cb
1 average rib	410	34	0
3 ribs	1230	102	0

Short Ribs: *2½" long, visible fat trimmed to ¼"*
6 oz raw with bone or 2.52 oz cooked, braised, w/o bone

	C	F	Cb
1 average rib	320	28	0
3 ribs	960	85	0

Ground Beef

	C	F	Cb
Ground Beef, Raw: *Per 4 oz*			
70% lean (30% fat)	380	34	0
75% lean (25% fat)	335	29	0
80% lean (20% fat)	290	23	0
85% lean (15% fat)	245	17	0
90% lean (10% fat)	200	12	0
95% lean (5% fat)	155	6	0
Baked/Broiled: Regular (70%), 3 oz	230	16	0
Lean (80%), 3 oz	215	14	0
Extra lean (90%), 3 oz	185	10	0
Pan-Broiled:			
Regular (70%), 3 oz	230	15	0
Lean (80%), 3 oz	210	14	0
Extra lean (90%), 3 oz	195	10	0
Ground Beef Patties: *Average, 23% Fat*			
Raw, 4 oz	330	25	0
Broiled, 3 oz (from 4 oz raw)	250	19	0

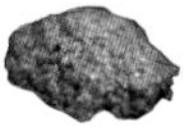
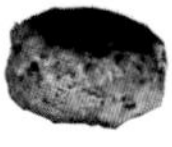

Quick Guide

Roast Beef

Round (Eye/Tip, average): *Average All Cuts*

	C	F	Cb
Small/Regular Serving: *3 oz*			
(2 thin slices/1 thick slice)			
Lean + fat (⅛" fat trim)	180	9	0
Lean only	145	4	0
Medium Serving: *5 oz*			
(3-4 thin slices)			
Lean + fat (⅛" fat trim)	300	15	0
Lean only	245	6.5	0
Large Serving, 8 oz: *3 thick slices*			
Lean + fat (⅛" fat trim)	480	24	0
Lean only	385	11	0
Beef Kebab: Cooked			
Beef & Veggies, 2 oz	160	10	4
If very lean meat	100	4	4

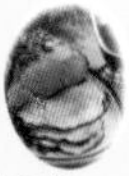
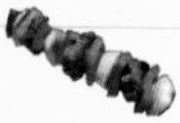

Meat Alternatives (Vegan)

	C	F	Cb
Beyond Meat:			
Beyond: Burger Patty, 4 oz	260	18	5
Cookout Classic, Burger Patties	290	22	4
Crumbles: Beefy, 1.94 oz	90	3	2
Fiesty Crumbles, 1.94 oz	90	2.5	2
Ground Beef, 4 oz	260	18	5
Sausage: Original Brat, 2.9 oz	190	12	5
Hot/Swseet Italian (1), cooked, 2.7 oz	190	12	5
Gardein:			
Beefless: Burger Patty, 3 oz	130	4.5	7
Sliders (1) with Bun, 2.5 oz	130	2.5	20
Tips, ¾ cup, 3.5 oz	170	7	8
Chick'n: BBQ Wings, w/o Sce, 2.5 oz	120	5	5
Crispy Patty (1), 3.1 oz	160	7	12
Mandarin Crispy, w/out Sce, 2.68 oz	150	7	6
Fishless: Golden Filet (2), 3.38 oz	180	10	14
Mini Crabless Cakes (3), 2.65 oz	130	6	11
Meatless Meatballs, (3), 3.17 oz	150	7	9
Porkless, Sweet & Sour Bites, 2.47 oz	120	3	9
Quorn:			
Meatless: Buffalo Dippes, 3.7 oz	230	10	21
Chipotle Cutlets (1), 3.5 oz	205	9	24
Fillets (1), 2.2 oz	70	1	7
Fishless Sticks, 3.5 oz	200	8	30
Pieces, 3.9 oz	120	3	11
Spicy Patties, 2.3 oz	130	5	14
Tofurky:			
Burger Patty, (1), 4 oz	250	16	7
Crumbles: Beef Style, 1.94 oz	100	5	4
Chorizo, 1.94 oz	130	9	5
Ham Style Roast, 3.2 oz	170	6	8
Roast w/ Wild Rice Stuffing, 5.2 oz	290	10	17

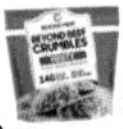

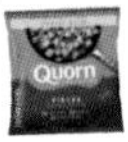

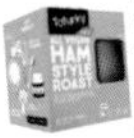

Yves Veggie Cuisine/Loma Linda ~ *See page 122*

Lamb

	C	F	Cb
Choice Grade:			
Leg (Whole), roasted:			
Lean + fat, 3 oz	220	14	0
Lean only, 3 oz	160	7	0
Leg (Sirloin Half), roasted:			
Lean + fat, 3 oz	250	18	0
Lean only, 3 oz	175	8	0
Leg (Shank Half), roasted:			
Lean + fat, 3 oz	190	11	0
Lean only, 3 oz	155	6	0
Loin Chop, broiled:			
1 chop (raw weight,4.25 oz):			
Lean + fat (2.25 oz edible)	180	12	0
Lean only (1.6 oz edible)	85	3.5	0
Rib Chop, broiled:			
1 chop (raw wt., 3.5 oz):			
Lean + fat (2.5 oz edible)	255	21	0
Lean only (1.75 oz edible)	105	6	0
Shoulder (Arm/Blade):			
Braised: Lean + fat, 3 oz	295	21	0
Lean only, 3 oz	240	12	0
Broiled: Lean + fat, 3 oz	240	17	0
Lean only, 3 oz	170	8	0
Roasted: Similar to Broiled			
Cubed Lamb (Leg/Shoulder):			
For stew or kebab:			
Braised, lean only, 3 oz	190	8	0
Broiled, lean only, 3 oz	160	6	0

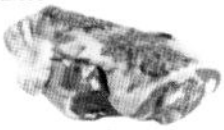
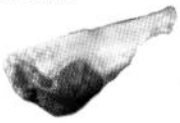
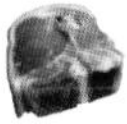
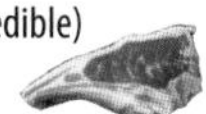
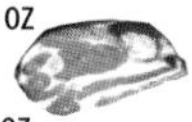
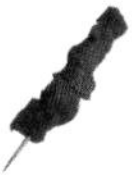

Veal

	C	F	Cb
Edible Weights:			
Leg (Top Round):			
Braised: Lean + fat, 3 oz	180	6	0
Lean only, 3 oz	175	5	0
Pan-fried, breaded:			
Lean + fat, 3 oz	195	8	9
Lean only, 3 oz	185	6	9
Pan-fried, not breaded:			
Lean + fat, 3 oz	180	7	0
Lean only, 3 oz	155	4	0
Roasted: Lean + fat, 3 oz	135	4	0
Lean only, 3 oz	130	3	0

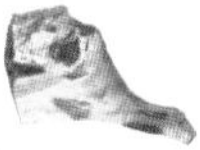
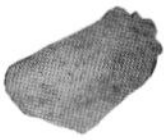
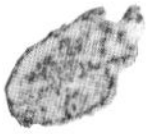
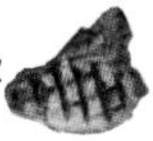

Veal (Cont)

	C	F	Cb
Loin Chop: *1 chop, 7 oz raw weight*			
Braised: Lean + fat, 3 oz	240	15	0
Lean only, 3 oz	190	8	0
Roasted: Lean + fat, 3 oz	185	11	0
Lean only, 3 oz	150	6	0
Rib, roasted: *Lean + fat, 3 oz*	195	12	0
Lean only, 3 oz	150	7	0
Shoulder, Arm/Blade, roasted:			
Lean + fat, 3 oz	155	7	0
Lean only, 3 oz	140	5	0
Sirloin, roasted:			
Lean + fat, 3 oz	170	9	0
Lean only, 3 oz	145	6	0
Cubed for Stew, braised:			
Leg/Shoulder, lean only, 3 oz	160	4	0
(1 lb raw yields approximately 9.25 oz cooked)			

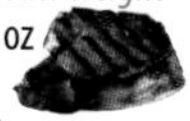
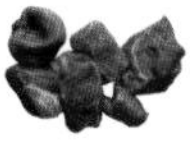

Pork

Fresh Pork: *Cooked Weight, without bone): 4 oz raw weight = approx. 3 oz cooked weight*

	C	F	Cb
BBQ, Pulled:			
2 oz	90	2.5	10
4 oz	180	5	20
8oz	360	10	40
Blade Steak, broiled:			
Lean + fat, 3 oz	220	15	0
Lean only, 3 oz	190	11	0
Country Style Ribs, broiled/roasted:			
Lean + fat, 3 oz	280	22	0
Lean only, 3 oz	210	13	0
Spareribs, braised: *Lean & fat, 6 oz*			
(from 1 lb raw weight)	675	52	0
Leg (Ham), whole, roasted:			
Lean + fat, 3 oz	230	15	0
Lean only, 3 oz	180	8	0
Loin Chops, broiled: *Average*			
(From 1 chop: 5 oz raw weight with bone or 4 oz raw weight, without bone)			
Lean + fat, 3 oz	200	11	0
Lean only, 3 oz	165	7	0
Loin Roast, roasted:			
Lean + fat, 3 oz	210	13	0
Lean only, 3 oz	180	8	0
Rib Chops, (Boneless), broiled:			
Lean + fat, 3 oz	220	14	0
Lean only, 3 oz	185	9	0
Rib Roast:			
Lean + fat, 3 oz	215	13	0
Lean only, 3 oz	180	9	0

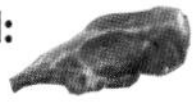
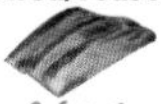
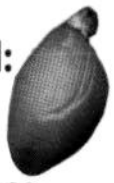
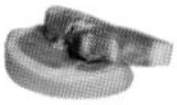
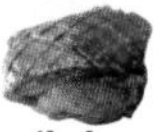
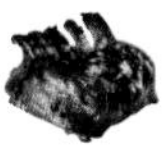

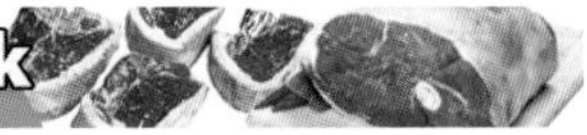

M Meat ~ Lamb ◆ Veal ◆ Pork

Pork (Cont)

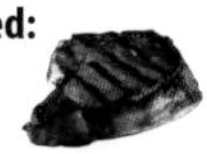
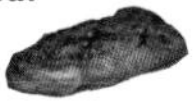
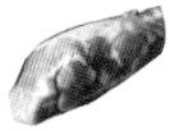
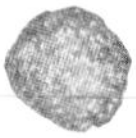

	C	F	Cb
Sirloin Chop, broiled:			
Lean + fat, 3 oz	**180**	8	0
Lean only, 3 oz	**165**	6	0
Sirloin Roast, roasted:			
Lean + fat, 3 oz	**175**	8	0
Lean only, 3 oz	**170**	7	0
Tenderloin (Boneless), roasted:			
Lean + fat, 3 oz	**125**	4	0
Lean only, 3 oz	**120**	3	0
Ground Pork:			
Raw, average, 1/4 lb, 4 oz	**300**	24	0
Broiled, 3 oz	**250**	18	0
Pan-fried, drained, 3 oz	**260**	19	0

Bacon

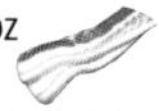
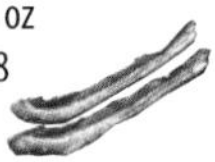
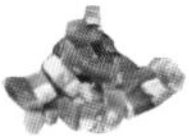

	C	F	Cb
Raw: 1 med. slice, 0.75 oz	**95**	9	0
1 thick slice, 1.3 oz	**175**	17	0
(1 lb raw yields approximately 5 oz cooked)			
Broiled/Pan-Fried:			
1 medium slice, 0.3 oz	**40**	3	0
3 medium slices, 0.8	**125**	10	0
2 thin slices, 0.5 oz	**75**	6	0
1 thick slice, 0.9 oz	**65**	5	0
Canadian Bacon:			
Cooked: 1 slice, 1 oz	**45**	2	0.5
2 slices, 2 oz	**90**	4	1
Bacon Bits, 1 Tbsp, 0.3 oz	**35**	2	0
Breakfast Strips, Broiled, 1 sl., 0.4 oz	**50**	4	0

Ham

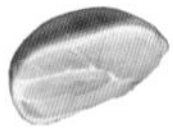
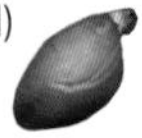

	C	F	Cb
Boneless Ham, cooked:			
Regular, (approximately 13% fat):			
Roasted, 3 oz	**150**	8	0
Extra Lean (5% fat),			
Roasted, 3 oz	**125**	5	0
Whole Ham, cooked:			
Lean + fat (as purchased)			
Roasted, 3 oz	**210**	15	0
Lean only, Roasted, 3 oz	**135**	5	0
Canned Ham: *Similar to boneless ham*			
Chopped, canned, 3 oz	**200**	16	0
Ham Patties, cooked, (1), 2.3 oz	**220**	20	1
Ham Steak, extra lean, 2 oz	**70**	2.5	0

Lunch Slices ~ *See Deli Meats, Page 128*

Game & Other Meats

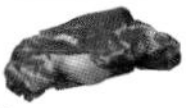
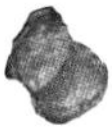
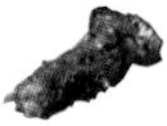
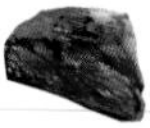
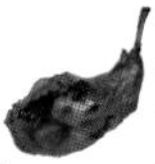

	C	F	Cb
Bison Steak,			
lean, 6 oz (raw)	**205**	4	0
Boar (wild), roasted, 3 oz	**140**	4	0
Buffalo Steak,			
New West Foods, 4 oz	**70**	3	0
Caribou, roasted, 3 oz	**140**	4	0
Deer/Venison, roasted 3 oz	**135**	3	0
Goat (Capretto):			
Raw, 3 oz	**95**	2	0
Roasted, 3 oz	**120**	2.5	0
Ostrich:			
Blackwing Ostrich Meats:			
Sausage Patties, 4 oz	**110**	1.5	0
Strip Filet, 6 oz	**160**	1.5	0
New West Foods:			
Ground Ostrich, 4 oz	**165**	7	0
Ostrich Steak, 4 oz steak	**130**	2.5	0
Rabbit: Roasted, 3 oz	**165**	7	0
Stewed, 1 cup, diced, 5 oz	**290**	12	0

Variety & Organ Meats

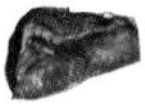
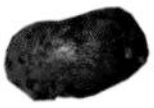
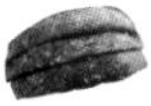
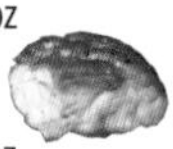
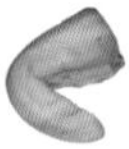

	C	F	Cb
Brain (Lamb): Braised, 3 oz	**125**	9	0
Pan-fried, 3 oz	**230**	19	0
Chitterlings, pork, simmered, 3 oz	**260**	25	0
Ears, pork, simmered, 1 ear, 4 oz	**185**	12	0
Feet, Pork: Simmered, 3 oz	**200**	14	0
Cured, pickled, 3 oz	**170**	14	0
Hormel, 2 oz	**80**	6	0
Head Cheese (Pork Snouts/Ears/Vinegar/Spices), 1 oz slice	**50**	4	0
Heart, Beef, braised, 3 oz	**140**	4	0
Jowl, pork, raw, 4 oz	**750**	80	0
Kidneys, braised, 3 oz	**140**	5	0
Liver (beef): Raw, 4 oz	**150**	4	4
Braised, 3 oz	**140**	4	3
Pan-fried, 3 oz	**185**	7	7
Pancreas, pork, braised, 3 oz	**185**	8	0
Pork Cracklins, 0.5 oz	**80**	6	0
Pork Hocks, 1 piece, 6 oz	**340**	23	0
Scrapple, pork, 2 oz	**120**	8	8
Spleen, pork, braised, 3 oz	**130**	3	0
Stomach, pork, raw, 4 oz	**185**	12	0
Sweetbreads:			
Beef,/Lamb, cooked, 3 oz	**125**	9	0
Tail, pork, simmered, 3 oz	**340**	31	0
Tongue: Raised Veal, 3 oz	**170**	9	0
Beef/Lamb/Pork, av., 3 oz	**235**	17	0
Tripe, beef, raw, 3 oz	**85**	3.5	0

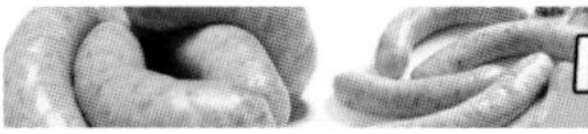

Quick Guide

	C	F	Cb
Franks & Weiners			
Average All Brands			
Regular (Pork Mix): *Per Frank*			
Regular, 1.5 oz	140	13	1
Bun Length/Jumbo, 2 oz	185	17	2
Extra Long, 2.75 oz	255	24	2
Small/Cocktail, each	30	3	0.5
Beef Franks: *Per Frank*			
Regular, 1.5 oz	140	13	2
Bun Length/Jumbo, 2 oz	175	17	2.5
1/4 lb Dog, 4 oz	375	33	5

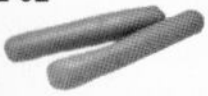

Franks & Weiners

	C	F	Cb
Ball Park: *Per 2 oz Frank Unless Indicated*			
Angus Beef:			
Orig.; Bun Size, 1.76 oz	160	15	2
Bun Size, 1.76 oz	70	5	2
Beef: Original; Bun Size, 1.8 oz	180	15	4
Deli Style, Regular, 1.76 oz	160	15	2
Grillmaster, Hearty, 2.9 oz	260	24	3
Lean, 1.76 oz	80	5	2
Classic: Cheese (1), 1.76 oz	120	10	2
Chicken & Pork(1); Bun Size, 1.9 oz	130	11	2
Turkey, (1), 1.76 oz	110	7	6
Foster Farms, Chicken; Turkey, 1.5 oz	110	9	1
Hebrew National: *Per Frank*			
Beef: Regular, 1.7 oz	150	13	2
All Natural, 1.7oz	140	12	2
Bun Length, 2 oz	170	15	2
Jumbo, 3 oz	260	23	3
97% Fat-Free, 1.6 oz	45	1	2
Reduced Fat, 1.6 oz	100	8	2
Jennie-O: *Per Frank*			
Turkey Franks:			
1.2 oz	70	6	1
Jumbo, 2 oz	120	9	2
Turkey Bratwurst, 3.85 oz	150	8	0
Uncured Breast Frank, 1.83 oz	90	6	0
Oscar Mayer: *Per Frank*			
Angus Beef:			
Bun Length; Jumbo, 1.76 oz	170	15	0
Beef, Classic, 1.48 oz	130	12	0
Cheese, 1.48 oz	120	10	0
Weiners, Classic, 1.48 oz	110	10	0
Shelton's: *Per Frank*			
Chicken, uncured, 1.2 oz	80	7	0
Turkey, 1.2 oz	60	4.5	1
Zacky Farms, Chkn; Turkey, av, 2 oz	115	10	4

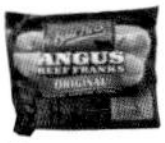

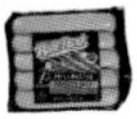

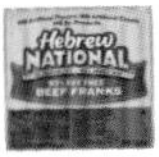

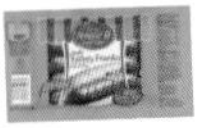

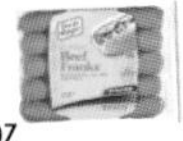

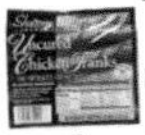

Quick Guide

	C	F	Cb
Fresh Sausages			
Pork/Beef: *Average All Types*			
Small: Raw, 4" link, 1 oz	85	7.5	0
Broiled/Pan-fried	80	7	0
Medium: Raw, 2 oz	170	15	0
Broiled/Pan-fried	165	14	0
Large: Raw, 3 oz	255	22	0
Broiled/Pan-fried	245	21	0
Italian: Raw, 3.2 oz	315	28	1
Cooked, 2.4 oz	230	18	3
Chorizo: Beef Chorizo, 2.5 oz piece	250	23	5
Pork Chorizo, 2 oz piece	250	23	5

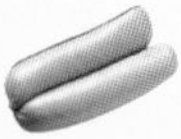

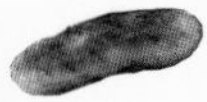

Note: Fat is lost in broiling/pan frying.
Cooked weight = approx. 60-70% raw weight

Smoked Sausages

	C	F	Cb
Per Link:			
Butterball, Turkey, 2 oz	100	5	5
Eckrich:			
Original, Natural Casing, (1)	180	15	4
Skinless Rope: Beef (1), 2 oz	180	15	5
Cheddar (1), 2 oz	180	16	3
Turkey (1), 2 oz	110	7	5
Hillshire Farm:			
Basil Pesto Chicken, 2 oz	110	7	3
Beef, 2 oz	170	14	3
Cheddarwurst, 2 oz	180	16	2
Chicken, Roasted Garlic, 2 oz	100	6	3
Hot Smoked, 2 oz	180	16	3

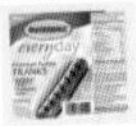

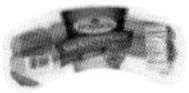

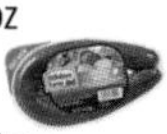

Johnsonville ~ *See CalorieKing.Com*

Breakfast Sausages/Patties

	C	F	Cb
Butterball: *Fully Cooked*			
Turkey: B'fast Sausage Links (3), 2 oz	90	5.5	0
Patties (2), 2 oz	90	5.5	0
Jimmy Dean: *Fully Cooked*			
Heat 'N Serve Sausage Links:			
Pork, Regular (3), 1.9 oz	210	19	2
Turkey (3), 2 oz	130	8	2
Heat 'N Serve Sausage Patties:			
Pork, Original (2), 1.8 oz	200	17	2
Turkey (2), 1.8 oz	120	8	1
Maple Pork Sausages,(3), 2.4 oz	280	26	4
Pork Patties, (2), 2.4 oz	280	27	1
Breakfast Sandwiches ~ *See Page 92*			
Jones Dairy Farm:			
Golden Brown Sausages: *Fully Cooked*			
Mild/Maple Pork (3), average, 2 oz	250	24	2

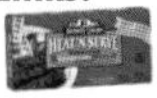

Vegetarian Patties:

Boca ~ *See Page 112*
GardenBurer ~ *See Page 113*

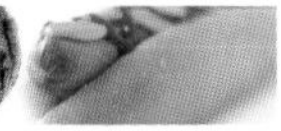

Bagel, Corn & Hot Dogs

	C	F	Cb
Hot Dogs, Ready-To-Go:			
Includes Ketchup/Relish			
Regular, 1.5 oz frank, 1.5 oz bun	260	15	22
Bun Length, 2 oz frank, 1.5 oz bun	290	18	21
Jumbo Dog, 2 oz frank, 2 oz bun	360	20	36
¼ lb Beef Dog, 2 oz bun	480	15	36
Mile Long Dog, 2.6 oz dog, 1.5 oz bun	360	24	23
Corn Dogs:			
Beef/Pork Frank, average, 2.6 oz	170	10	16
Foster Farms:			
Corn Dogs:			
Cheese & Jalapeno (1)	180	8	20
Honey Crunchy:			
Regular (1), 2.7 oz	180	9	18
Mini (4), 2.7 oz	220	13	19
Gluten Free, 2.7 oz	180	9	20
State Fair: *Per Dog*			
Beef Corn Dog, 2.7 oz	240	13	26
Classic Corn Dog: Regular (2), 4 oz	330	11	34
Mini (5), 3.3 oz	270	14	29
Bagel Dogs:			
Hebrew National:			
Beef Bagel Dogs, 4 pieces, 2.75 oz	240	13	22
Schwanns: Classic Corn Dog (1), 2.7 oz	230	11	25
Mini Corn Dogs (4), 2.7 oz	220	13	21
Vienna Beef,			
Mini Bagel Dogs,(5), 4.6 oz	310	18	31
Hot Dog Toppings/Extras:			
American Cheese, 1 slice, 1 oz	110	9	1
Chili Con Carne, ¼ cup	50	2	5.5
Ketchup, 1 Tbsp	15	0	4
Mustard, 1 Tbsp	20	0	1
Onions, chopped, 1 Tbsp	5	0	1
Pickle Relish, 1 Tbsp	20	0	5
Sauerkraut, ½ cup	20	0	5

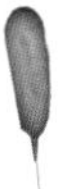
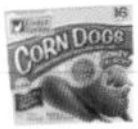
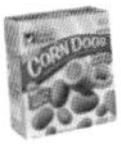
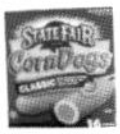
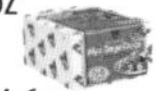
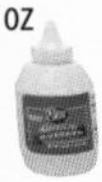
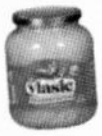

Deli/Lunch Meats & Sausage

	C	F	Cb
Beef Jerky/Meat Snacks,			
Berliner (pork/beef), 1 oz	65	5	1
Beerwurst (Beef):			
Small (2¾"diam), 1/16" slice	20	2	0
Large (4" diam), ⅛ " slice	75	7	0.5
Beerwurst (Pork):			
Small (2.75"diameter), 1/16" slice	15	1	0
Large (4"diameter), ⅛" Slice	55	4	0.5
Blood Sausage, 1 oz	100	9	0.5

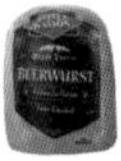
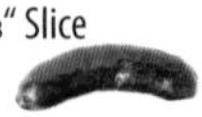

Deli/Lunch Meats & Sausages (Cont)

Bologna:	C	F	Cb
Beef Bologna: 1 slice, 1 oz	90	8	0
Light, 1 slice, 1 oz	60	4	2
Oscar Mayer: Regular, 1 oz	90	8	0
Light, 1 slice, 1 oz	60	4	1
Chicken & Pork Bologna,			
Oscar Mayer, with added Beef, 1 oz	80	7	0
Pork Bologna: 1 Slice, 1 oz	65	6	1
Fat-Free, 1 slice, 1 oz	20	0	2
Pork & Beef,			
Boar's Head, 2 oz	150	13	1
Turkey Bologna, av., 1 oz	60	5	0.5
Oscar Mayer, 1 oz	50	4	0
Bratwurst, average, 1 oz	80	7	1
Braunschweiger, (Pork/Liver/Sausage),			
Oscar Mayer, Liver, 2 oz	190	14	0
Chicken, average:			
1 thick or 2 thin slices, 1 oz	30	1	1
2 oz slice	60	2	2
Hillshire Farm,			
Rotisserie S'snd Chicken Breast, 2 oz	60	1	3
Corned Beef, average, full fat, 1 oz	60	5	0.5
Ham, Sliced: *Per 1 oz Slice*			
Baked/Broiled	35	1	1
Honey/Brown Sugar, average	35	1	1
Oscar Mayer, Honey Ham	60	1.5	1
Prosciutto, average	70	5	0
Ham & Cheese Loaf, average, 1 oz	70	5	1
Oscar Mayer, 1 oz	70	4.5	1
Italian Sausage, 2.6 oz	250	20	3
Kielbasa: Polish Sausage, 2 oz	65	5	1
Beef, 2 oz link	190	17	1
Knockwurst, av., 1 oz	90	8	0.5
Linguica *(Gaspar's),* 2 oz	130	9	1
Liverwurst, 1 oz	65	5	2
Liver Pate, fresh, average, 1 oz	90	8	1
Mortadella: 1 oz	105	9	0
Boar's Head, 6 slices	160	14	0
Olive Loaf: Average, 1 oz	70	5	3
Oscar Mayer, 1 oz	80	6	1
Pancetta, *Boars Head, 0. 5 oz slice*	50	4.5	0

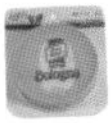
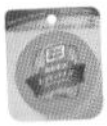
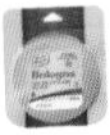
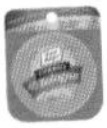
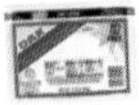
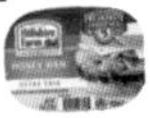

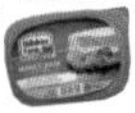
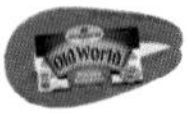
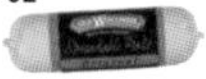
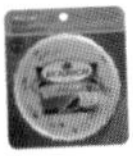

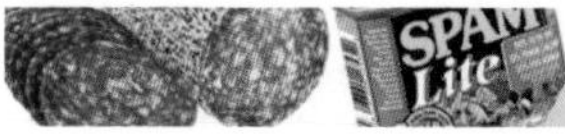

Deli/Lunch Meats & Sausages (Cont)

	C	F	Cb
Pastrami (Beef): 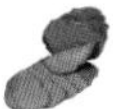			
Boar's Head:			
1st cut Pastrami Brisket, 2 oz	**90**	4	2
Top Round Pastrami, 2 oz	**80**	3	0.5
Hillshire, Deli Select, 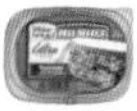			
Ultra Thin. 2 oz	**60**	1.5	0.5
Peppered Beef, 1 oz slice 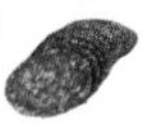	**40**	2	1
Pepperoni, 5 slices, 1 oz	**140**	13	0
Pickle Loaf, average, 1 oz	**70**	5	5
Pickle & Pepper Loaf, 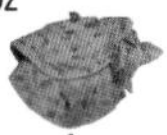			
Boars Head, 2 oz	**150**	13	2
Proscuitto/Proscuitti, av., 1 oz	**70**	5	1
Roast Beef, Lean, 1 oz	**40**	2	0
Salami:			
Beef, average, 1 oz 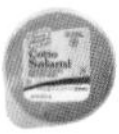	**80**	7	1
Beef Chicken Pork,			
Oscar Mayer: Cotto, 1 slice, 1 oz	**50**	4	0
Beer Salami, average, 1 oz	**50**	4	0.5
Pork: Genoa, sliced, average, 1 oz	**100**	8	1
Boarshead, 2 oz	**190**	15	1
Fortuna's Stick, 1 oz	**110**	8	1
Pork & Beef: 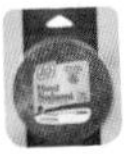			
Dry, Hard, av., 1 oz	**100**	8	1
Boar's Head, 5 slices	**110**	9	1
Oscar Mayer: Hard: 1 slice, 1.8 oz	**100**	8	0.5
Cracked Black Pepper, 1 oz	**110**	9	0
White Cheddar Cheese, 3.45 oz	**400**	27	7
SPAM (Hormel): *Per 2 oz*			
Classic: 2 oz serving 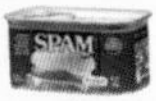	**180**	16	1
7 oz can	**630**	56	3.5
12 oz can	**1080**	96	6
Spam Lite: 2 oz 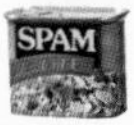	**110**	8	1
12 oz can	**660**	48	6
Other Spam Products: *Per 2 oz Unless Indicated*			
Hickory Smoke Flavor	**180**	16	1
Hot & Spicy 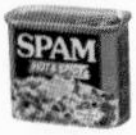	**160**	14	2
Oven Roasted Turkey	**80**	4.5	1
Spam Fries, 3 oz	**300**	23	14
Spam Spread	**160**	12	5
Spam with Bacon 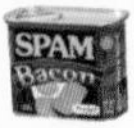	**180**	16	1
Spam with Cheese	**170**	15	1
25% Less Sodium	**180**	16	1
Spam Singles: *Per 3 oz* 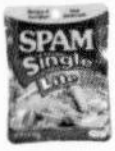			
Classic, 2.5 oz package	**210**	18	2
Lite, 2.5 oz package	**130**	9	2

Deli/Lunch Meats & Sausages (Cont)

	C	F	Cb
Summer Sausage:			
Armour, Beef, 2 oz 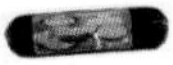	**190**	17	2
Hillshire Farm, 2 oz	**190**	16	1
Treet *(Armour),* Luncheon Loaf,			
Original, 2 oz 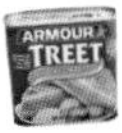	**140**	11	4
Turkey, average: 1 oz slice	**30**	1	0.5
0.8 oz slice	**22**	0.5	0.5
Turkey Breast: 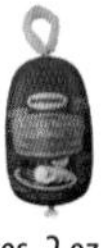			
Butterball, Oven Roasted:			
1 slice 1 oz	**30**	0.5	1
Deli Inspirations,			
Extra Thin Slices, 4 slices, 2 oz	**50**	1	3
Hillshire, Deli Select,			
Oven Roasted, 6 slices, 2 oz	**50**	0.5	2
Turkey Ham, 1 slice, 1 oz	**35**	1.5	0.5
Turkey Loaf, 1 oz 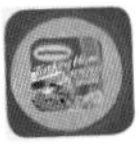	**30**	1	0.5
Turkey Pastrami, 1 oz	**35**	1.5	1
Turkey Roll, 1 oz	**40**	2	0.5

Vegetarian Deli ~ *See Page 118*

Meat Spread

	C	F	Cb
Average All Brands:			
Chicken, white meat, 2oz	**140**	11	2
Corned Beef, 2 oz 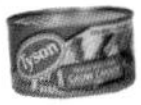	**140**	11	1
Ham, Deviled, 2 oz	**180**	15	1
Liverwurst, 2 oz	**160**	13	4
Roast Beef, 2 oz 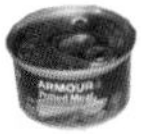	**130**	10	2
Turkey, 2 oz	**110**	7	2
Underwood: *Per 2 oz*			
Deviled Ham 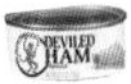	**180**	15	1
Liverwurst	**160**	13	4
Roast Beef	**140**	10	2
White Meat Chicken 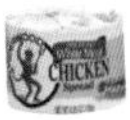	**130**	8	3

Paté

	C	F	Cb
Les Trois Petit Cochons: *Per 8 oz Package*			
Pate: au Poivre Noir, 2 oz 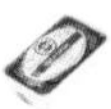	**210**	19	2
de Campagne 2 oz	**240**	22	2
de Canard a l'Orange, 2 oz	**210**	18	3
Paysan, 2 oz	**160**	13	2
Rustique, 2 oz 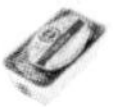	**240**	22	2
Wild Boar, 2 oz	**180**	15	4
Old Wisconsin Pate,			
Braunschweiger, 2 oz 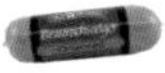	**210**	18	3

Nuts

Per 1 oz Unless Indicated

	C	F	Cb
Acorns, raw 1 oz	110	7	12
Almonds: Dried/Dry Roasted:			
Whole: 12 medium size, 0.5 oz	85	7.5	3
23-25 medium size, 1 oz	170	15	6
½ cup, 2.5 oz	420	37	13
Ground, 1 cup, 3.4 oz	545	47	20
Sliced, ½ cup, 1.6 oz	260	22	10
Slivered, ½ cup, 2 oz	310	27	12
Chocolate Coated (5-6), 1 oz	150	10	15
Honey Roasted, 1 oz	170	14	8
Oil Roasted (*Blue Diamond*), 1 oz	170	16	5
Brazil Nuts, 8 medium, 1 oz	185	19	3.5
Cashews, dry or oil roasted:			
14 large/18 med./26 small: 1 oz	165	14	9
½ cup, 2.4 oz	375	31	20
Honey Roasted, 1 oz	165	13	10
Chestnuts:			
Average, dried, 1 oz	105	1	22
Raw/Fresh, 5-6 nuts, 1 oz	60	0	13
Canned, water chestnuts, sliced/whole/drained, 1 oz	30	0	7
Coconut, Fresh:			
1 piece, 2"x2"x ½ ", 1 oz	185	18	7
Shredded, fresh, ½ cup, 1.4 oz	140	13	6
Dried (Desiccated):			
Sweetened: Shredded, 1 oz	145	10	14
Grated, ½ cup, 1.3 oz	185	13	18
Unsweetened, 1 oz	185	18	7
Cream (canned), ½ cup, 5.2 oz	285	26	12
Milk (canned), unsweetened, ¼ cup, 2 fl.oz	100	10	3
Water (center liquid), ½ cup, 4.3 oz	25	0	4.5
Filberts or Hazelnuts:			
Shelled, 18-20 nuts	180	17	4.5
Chopped, ¼ cup, 1 oz	180	18	5
Ground, ¼ cup, 0.6 oz	120	12	3
Ginkgo Nuts, canned, 14 med., 1 oz	32	0.5	6.5
Hickory, 30 small nuts, 1 oz	200	18	5
Macadamia Nuts, Shelled:			
Raw or Dry Roasted, avg:			
12 small or 8 med., 1 oz	200	21	4
6-7 large, 1 oz	200	21	4
½ cup, 2.3 oz	480	51	10
Mixed Nuts: Raw, 18-22 nuts, 1 oz	170	15	7
Oil Roasted, all types	170	16	6
Sweet Roasts, 26 pieces, 1 oz	160	12	10
Planters, Dry Roasted/Honey, 1 oz	150	11	11
Nut Toppings, chopped, 1 Tbsp, 0.3 oz	40	4	1.5

Per 1 oz Unless Indicated

	C	F	Cb
Peanuts:			
Dry or oil roasted, average:			
Small handful, 0.5 oz	85	7	3
⅕ cup, 1 oz	165	14	6
½ cup, 2.5 oz	415	35	15
3 oz bag	500	42	18
7 oz bag	1160	98	42
Raw: Shelled, 1 oz	160	14	4.5
In shell, 1 oz	115	110	3
Planters:			
Cocktail, all varieties	170	14	5
Honey Roasted	160	13	7
Spanish Redskins	170	15	4
Sweet N' Crunchy	140	8	15
Japanese Style Peanuts, Coated in Crunchy Shell	150	8	13
Pecans, roasted:			
10 halves, 0.5 oz	95	10	2
20 Halves, 1 oz	195	20	4
1 cup, halves, 3.5 oz	680	71	14
Pilinuts, dried, 1 oz	215	24	1
Pine Nuts, dried, 1 Tbsp, 0.3 oz	70	7	1.5
Pistachios, raw:			
Shelled, 45 nuts, 1 oz	160	13	8
Unshelled, 2 oz	165	14	7
Lance, Roasted, 1.5 oz	120	9	6
Sesame Nut Mix, 1 oz	160	13	9
Soy Nuts: Dry Roasted	130	6	9
½ cup, 3 oz	390	18	28
Revival, Chocolate Covered, 2 oz	200	12	20
Trail Mix *(Planters):*			
Dessert Mixes: Banana Sundae, 1 oz	150	10	13
Oatmeal Raisin Cookie, 1 oz	140	7	17
Turtle Sundae, 1 oz	160	11	13
Energy Mix, 1.4 oz	240	19	14
Peanut Butter Chocolate, 1.15 oz	180	12	13
Spicy Nuts & Cajun Sticks, 1 oz	150	11	11
Sweet & Salty, 1.1 oz	150	9	15
Tropical Fruit, 1.1 oz	150	9	15
Walnuts, average all types:			
7-10 halves, 0.5 oz	90	9	2
15-20 halves, 1 oz	175	17	3
Chopped, ½ cup, 2.2 oz	380	36	6
Ground, ¼ cup, 0.7 oz	130	13	3

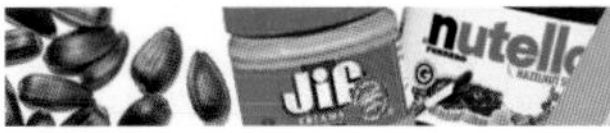

Quick Guide

	C	F	Cb
Peanut Butter: *Average All Brands*			
1 level tsp, 0.2 oz	35	3	1
1 level Tbsp, 0.6 oz	100	8.5	3.5
1 oz Quantity	165	14	6
1/2 cup, 5 oz	835	72	29

Peanut Butter ~ Brands

	C	F	Cb
Jif: Regular, all varieties, 2 Tbsp	190	16	8
Honey Varieties, 2 Tbsp	190	15	10
No Added Sugar, 2 Tbsp	200	17	7
Reduced Fat, all varieties, 2 Tbsp	190	12	15
Laura Scudder's:			
Natural: Smooth; Nutty, 2 Tbsp	190	16	7
Smooth, Unsalted, 2 Tbsp	190	16	7
Organic, Smooth; Nutty, 2 Tbsp	180	16	5
Peter Pan:			
Just Peanuts: Creamy/Crunchy, 2 T.	210	17	6
Honey Roast Creamy, 2 Tbsp	200	16	6
Natural, Creamy/Crunchy, 2 Tbsp	210	17	6
Planters, Creamy/Crunchy, 2 Tbsp	180	15	8
Smucker's, Goober,			
Grape/Srawberry, av., 3 Tbsp. 2 oz	220	11	30
Skippy: *Per 2 Tbsp*			
Blended with Plant Protein, all var.	210	16	6
Creamy; Super Chunky	190	16	6
Reduced Fat, Creamy/Crunchy	190	12	14
Roasted Honey Nut, Creamy	200	16	6

Peanut Butter & Jelly Sandwich

	C	F	Cb
1 sandwich: *With 2 oz Bread*			
Thin Spread, 1 Tbsp Peanut Butter + 1 Tbsp Jelly	310	10	48
Thick Spread, 2 Tbsp Peanut Butter + 2 Tbsp Jelly	480	19	67

Nut & Chocolate Spread

	C	F	Cb
Nutella:			
1 Tbsp, 0.7 oz	110	6	11
2 Tbsp, 1.3 oz	200	11	22

Note: Nutella contains approx. 50% sugar & 13% hazelnuts

Other Nut & Seed Butters

	C	F	Cb
Per 1 Tbsp, 0.5 oz			
Almond Butter	100	10	3.5
Cashew Butter	95	8	4.5
Hazelnut Butter; Pecan Butter	110	10	2
Pistachio Butter	90	6.5	4.5
Sesame Butter (Tahini)	90	8	3
Soy Nut Butter	75	5	4

Seeds

	C	F	Cb
Alfalfa Seeds, sprouted, ½ cup, 0.5 oz	5	0	1
Caraway/Fennel, 1 tsp	7	0.5	1
Chia Seeds: 1 Tbsp, 0.4 oz	45	3	4
3 Tbsp, 1 oz	140	8.5	12
Cottonseed Kernels, roasted, 1 Tbsp	50	3.5	2
Flaxseeds, 3 Tbsp, 1 oz	140	9	9
Hemp Seeds, 3 Tbsp, 1 oz	160	14	3
Lotus Seeds, dried, ½ cup, 0.5 oz	55	0.5	10
Poppy Seeds, 1 tsp	15	1	1
Pumpkin/Pepita Seeds, whole:			
Roasted/Tamari: 1 oz	150	12	4
½ cup, 4 oz	590	48	15
Dried (hulled), ¼ cup, 1 oz	155	13	5
Safflower Kernels, dried, 1 oz	150	11	10
Sesame Seeds:			
Dried, 1 Tbsp, 0.3 oz	50	4.5	2
Roasted/Toasted, 1 oz	160	14	7.5
Sunflower Kernels/Seeds:			
Dried, ¼ cup w/out hulls, 0.3 oz	200	18	7
Dry Roasted: 1 Tbsp, 0.3 oz	45	4	2
¼ cup, 1 oz	165	14	7
Oil Roasted, ⅕ cup, 1 oz	170	14	6.5
Watermelon Seeds, dried, ¼ cup, 1 oz	150	13	4

Nut eaters are healthier and live longer, say scientists.

Nuts are a nutritious source of protein, vitamins, minerals, fiber, healthy fats, and antioxidants.

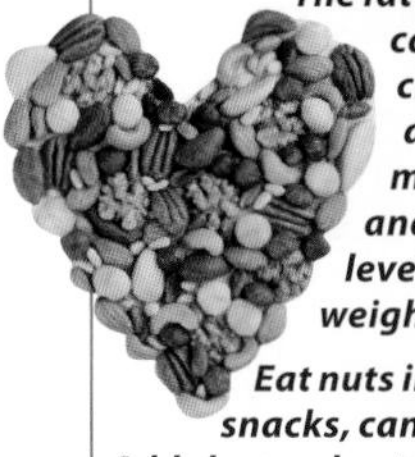

The fat and fiber of nuts can help reduce blood cholesterol. Their protein and fiber also promotes meal satiety (fullness) and reduces hunger levels – of benefit in weight control.

Eat nuts instead of high-sugar snacks, candy and soft drinks. Add chopped nuts to breakfast cereals.

P Pancakes & Waffles

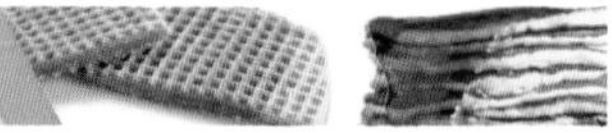

Quick Guide

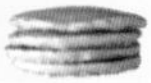
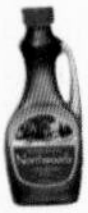
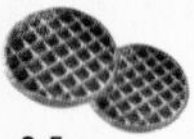

	C	F	Cb
Pancakes:			
Plain: *Average All Types*			
Small (3" diameter), 0.8 oz	50	2	6
Medium (4" diameter), 1.3 oz	85	3.5	11
Large (6" diameter), 2.5 oz	175	7.5	22
Add Extra for Syrups/Butter			
Pancake Syrup: Regular, 1 Tbsp	50	0	12
¼ cup, 4 Tbsp	185	0	49
Lite, 1 Tbsp	25	0	6.5
¼ cup, 4 Tbsp	100	0	27
Butter/Margarine:			
Regular, 1 Tbsp	100	11	0
Whipped, 1 Tbsp	65	7.5	0
Waffles:			
Homemade, 7" waffle, 2.5 oz	220	11	25
Frozen + Toasted, (4" diam.), 1 oz	105	3	16

Pancake Brands

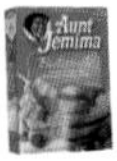
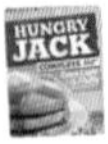
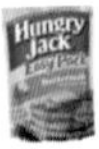
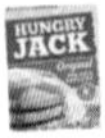

	C	F	Cb
Prepared as Directed			
Aunt Jemima: *Prepared*			
Mixes: *Makes 4" Pancakes*			
Original (2)	190	5	30
Buttermilk (2)	180	5	30
Whole Wheat Blend (3)	200	5	30
On The Go, average, 2 oz mix	225	4.5	42
Bisquick: *Prepared with Water*			
Pancake/Waffle Mix: *Makes 3 Pancakes*			
Complete Whole Grain, ½ cup, 2 oz	210	3	40
Hungry Jack: *Just Add Water*			
Pancake & Waffle Mixes: *Makes 3 4" Pancakes*			
Complete Mixes:			
Buttermilk, 1.9 oz	190	1	39
Chocolate Chip, 1.9 oz	190	2.5	39
Extra Light & Fluffy, 1.8 oz	180	1	38
Easy Packs:			
Buttermilk, 1.9 oz	190	1	39
Chocolate Chip, 1.9 oz	190	2.5	39
Traditional:			
Original, 1.7 oz	160	1	34
Buttermilk, 1.7 oz	160	1	34
Extra Light & Fluffy, 1.6 oz	150	1	32
Northern Pines, Just Add Water,			
Premium Mix (3), prepared	200	3.5	38

Frozen Breakfasts

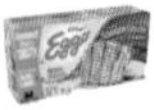
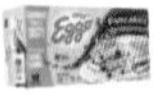
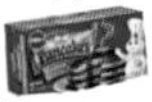

	C	F	Cb
Eggo *(Kellogg's):*			
Cinna-Toasts, Cinnamon Roll			
1 slice (set of 4), 1.4 oz	110	4	18
French Toast, Thick & Fluffy:			
Blueberry (1)	160	6	24
Classic (1)	120	2.5	21
French Toaster Sticks:			
Original (2)	210	6	35
Cinnamon (2)	220	6	38
Pancakes:			
Blueberry (3)	250	7	42
Chocolatey Chip (3)	260	8	42
Bites, Chocolatey Chip, 1.7 oz pouch	130	3.5	24
Minis, Buttermilk Pancakes, (11)	270	9	44
Pillsbury:			
Pancakes,			
Buttermilk; Homestlye, (3)	230	4	45

Frozen Waffles

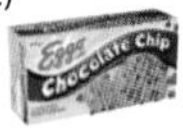
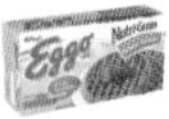
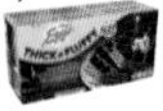
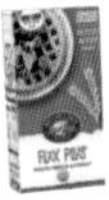
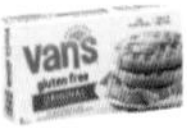
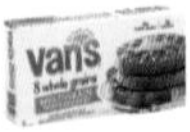

	C	F	Cb
Eggo *(Kellogg's):*			
Blueberry; Strawberry (2)	180	6	29
Buttermilk (2)	180	6	28
Chocolatey Chip (2)	200	7	32
Homestystyle (2)	180	5	30
Nutri-Grain:			
Blueberry (2)	180	6	30
Whole Wheat , low fat (2)	140	2.5	27
Thick & Fluffy:			
Original (1)	160	7	22
Cinnamon Brown Sugar (1)	170	7	25
Double Chocolately (1)	160	6	25
Nature's Path:			
Ancient Grains (2)	180	6	30
Buckwheat Wildberry (2)	190	7	33
Chia Plus; Homestyle (2)	210	7	34
Dark Chocolate Chip (2)	220	7	34
Flax Plus (2)	200	8	30
Maple Cinnamon (2)	180	6	28
Van's:			
Original, (2)	160	6	26
Blueberry, (2)	210	7	27
Gluten Free: Original (2)	210	7	34
Apple Cinnamon (2)	200	6	35
Blueberry (2)	210	7	34
Homestyle, (2)	190	8	29
Mini Chocolate Chip, (12)	210	6	35
Multigrain, (2)	160	5	29

Spaghetti/Pasta

- Pasta includes all shapes and sizes; (e.g. spaghetti, fettuccini, elbows, shells, twists, sheets, cannelloni, linguini, tubes, ziti).
- All regular pasta products have the same cals/fat/carbs on a weight basis.
- 1 oz Dry = approximately 2.5 -3 oz cooked.

Dry Spaghetti/Pasta

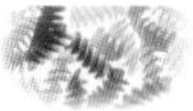
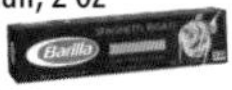
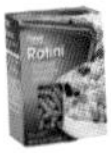

	C	F	Cb
1 oz quantity	105	0.5	21
1lb box/pkg, 16 oz	1685	7	339
Elbows, 1 cup, 4 oz	380	2	80
Shells, small, 1 cup, 3.3 oz	330	1.5	69
Spirals, 1 cup, 3 oz	305	1.5	64
Barilla:			
Blue Box: Angel Hair, 2 oz	200	1	42
Fettuccini, 2 oz	200	1	42
Other varieties, 2 oz	200	1	42
Great Value:			
Angel Hair, 2 oz	200	1	41
Penne Rigate, 2 oz	200	1	42
Rigatoni, 2 oz	200	1	41

Cooked Spaghetti/Pasta

	C	F	Cb
Plain, All Types (no added fat):			
Firm/Al Dente (8-10 minutes), 1 oz	42	0.5	8.5
Medium (11-13 minutes), 1 oz	37	0.5	7.5
Tender (14-20 minutes), 1 oz	32	0.5	7
Longer cooking increases water absorbed			
Spaghetti: ½ cup, 2.5 oz	90	0.5	18
Medium serving, 1 cup, 5 oz	225	1.5	44
Large serving, 2 cups, 10 oz	450	3	88
Extra large, 3 cups, 15 oz	675	5	132
Elbows/Spirals, 1 cup, 5 oz	220	1.5	43
Small Shells, 1 cup, 4 oz	180	1	36
Protein-fortified:			
Dry, 1 c., 3.4 oz	350	2	63
Cooked, 1 cup, 5 oz	230	0.5	45
Spinach/Vegetable:			
Dry, 1 cup, 3 oz	310	1	61
Cooked, 1 cup, 5 oz	180	0.5	38
Whole-wheat:			
Dry, 1 cup, 3.8 oz	365	1.5	79
Cooked, 1 cup, 5 oz	175	1	37

Fresh Pasta (Refrigerated)

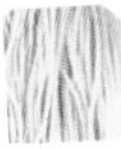
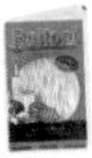
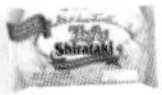
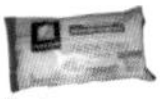

	C	F	Cb
Average All Brands:			
Plain/Spinach/Tomato:			
As purchased, 4.5 oz	370	3	70
Cooked, 1 cup, 5 oz	185	1.5	35
Home-made, w/o egg, cooked, 1 c. 5 oz	175	1	35
Buitoni:			
Cut Pasta:			
Angel Hair, 2.8 oz	220	1.5	45
Fettuccine/Linguine, av., 3 oz	235	1.5	46
House Foods:			
Tofu Shirataki Noodles:			
Angel Hair/Fettuccini, Macaroni/Spaghetti, 4 oz	20	1	6
Nasoya,			
Shirataki Spaghetti, Pasta Zero, ⅔ cup, 4 oz	15	0	4

Macaroni & Cheese

Packaged (Kraft) ~ *See Page 116*

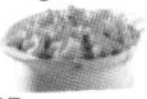

	C	F	Cb
Restaurant: *Average*			
Side Serve, 6 oz	265	13	26
Medium serve, 1 cup, 9 oz	350	17	34
Large serve, 2 cups, 18 oz	700	34	68

Noodles

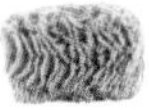
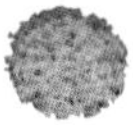
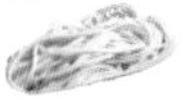
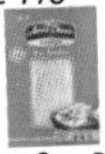

	C	F	Cb
Plain/Egg: Dry, 1 oz	110	1.5	20
1 cup, 1.4 oz	145	1.5	27
Cooked: ½ cup, 2.8 oz	110	1.5	20
1 cup, 5.5 oz	220	3.5	40
Stir-Fried: 1 cup, 5.5 oz	270	9	40
2 cup serving, 11 oz	540	18	80
Low Carb Noodles, Quest Pasta, 4 oz	10	0	3
Note: Carbs are from glucomannan fiber			
Yolk Free (Cooked):			
Manischewitz, Yolk Free, 2 oz	200	1	41
Chinese: Cellophane/Rice, dry, 1 oz	100	0	25
Chow Mein/hard, dry, 1 oz	150	9	16
Japanese: Soba: Dry, 1 oz	95	0.5	21
Cooked, 1 cup, 4 oz	115	0.5	24
Somen: Dry, 1 oz	100	0.5	21
Cooked, 1 cup, 6 oz	230	0.5	49
Japanese Style Pan Fried,			
Yaki-Soba (*Maruchan's*), av., 5.6 oz	260	3	50
Ramen Noodles ~ *See Page 118*			
Rice Noodles: Dry, 3.5 oz	365	0.5	83
Cooked, 1 cup, 6.2 oz	190	0.5	44
Annie Chun's, 2 oz	190	0	43

Simply Asia/Thai Kitchen ~ *See Pages 119 & 121*

Egg Roll/Won Ton Wrappers

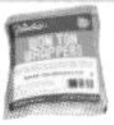

	C	F	Cb
Egg/Spring Roll (1), 0.8 oz	65	0	15
Won Ton Wrapper (1), 0.3 oz	20	0	4

Quick Guide

	C	F	Cb
Fruit Pies: *Average All Brands, 9″ Pie*			
Apple; Blueberry; Cherry:			
Small Serving,			
⅛ pie, 4.8 oz	350	16	49
Medium Serving,			
⅙ pie, 6.5 oz	465	22	65
Large Serving			
¼ pie, 9.5 oz	700	33	98
Whole Pie (9″), 38 oz	2800	131	392
Other Pies: *Per Serving, 1/6 of 9″ Pie*			
Chocolate Cream Pie	345	22	38
Custard: Egg Pie	220	12	22
Coconut Pie	330	18	35
Lemon Meringue Pie	305	10	53
Peach Pie	260	12	39
Pecan Pie	440	23	57
Pumpkin Pie	315	14	41
Shoo-Fly Pie	400	13	70

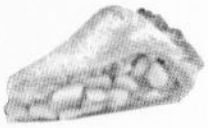
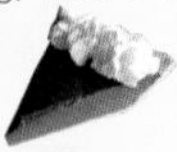
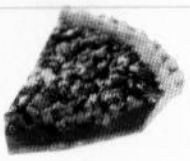

Dessert/Fruit Pies ~ Brands

	C	F	Cb
Hostess:			
Apple, 4.5 oz	450	19	65
Cherry Pie, 4.5 oz	480	20	69
Marie Callender's:			
Key Lime Pie, 4.5 oz	490	19	72
Lattice Cherry Pie, 4.5 oz	380	16	56
Peach Cobbler Pie, 4 oz	330	16	43
Peanut Butter Pie, 4.7 oz	620	46	43
Southern Pecan Pie, 4 oz	530	30	60
Turtle, 4.7 oz	560	36	55
Mrs Smith's:			
Cobblers: Blackberry, 4 oz	240	8	38
Peach, 4 oz	240	8	39
Flaky Crust: *Per 1/8 Pie*			
Apple, 4.6 oz	330	18	41
Cherry, 4.4 oz	340	17	43
Peach, 4.6 oz	330	18	41
Sara Lee: *Per Slice*			
Creme Pies:			
Chocolate, ⅕ pie, 3.9 oz	440	27	46
Coconut, ⅙ pie, 4.5 oz	370	20	44
Key Lime, ⅕ pie, 4.8 oz	410	17	59
Fruit Pies: Apple, 4.27 oz	320	13	44
Cherry, 4.27 oz	310	14	44
Peach, 4.27 oz	300	13	42
Raspberry, 4.27 oz	320	13	48
Seasonal Pies: Pumpkin, 4.27 oz	260	11	38
Sweet Potato, 4.27 oz	260	9	43
Tastykake: Baked Apple Pie (1)	300	12	45
Orange Kream-Cicle Pie (1)	320	15	42

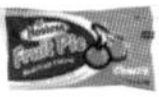
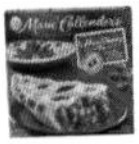
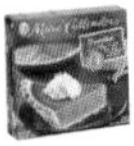
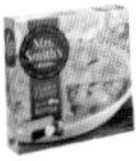
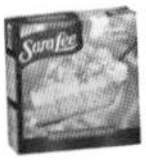
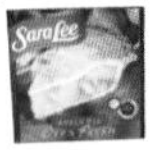

Croissants

	C	F	Cb
Average all Brands			
Plain/Butter/Cheese: Mini, 1 oz	115	6	13
Small, 1.5 oz	170	9	19
Medium, 2 oz	230	12	26
Large, 2.5 oz	290	15	32
Sweet Croissants:			
Almond Filled, 3 oz	330	18	39
Chocolate Filled, 3 oz	360	19	43
Dunkin' Donuts, Plain Croissant	340	19	37

Croissant Sandwiches ~ *See Page 165*

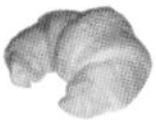
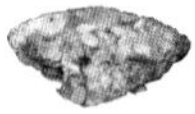

Pastry & Pie Crust

	C	F	Cb
Pie Crust, Baked, 9″ diameter shell:			
1 Pie Shell, 6.5 oz	970	64	87
2-crust Pie, 9″, 11.3 oz	1660	109	150
Filo Pastry: 4 sheets, 2.5 oz	210	2.5	40
Athens, Phyllo Dough, 5 sheets, 2 oz	180	1	36
Puff:			
Pepperidge Farms: Sheets, 1.5 oz	160	10	16
Bake & Fill Shells, 1.7 oz	180	11	18
Arrowhead Mills,			
Graham Cracker Pie Crust, ⅛ of 9″	110	4.5	15
Keebler:			
Ready Crust: *Per ⅛ of 9″ Crust*			
Chocolate	100	4.5	14
Graham	100	4.5	13
Low Fat	100	3.5	15
Shortbread Crust	100	5	14
Marie Callenders,			
Pastry Pie Shell, ⅛, 1 oz	130	8	13
Mrs Smith's,			
Deep Dish Pie Crust, ⅛ pie, 1 oz	130	8	14
Nabisco:			
Honey Maid,			
Graham Cracker Crust,⅛ pie, ¾ oz	110	5	14
Nilla, Pie Crust,			
⅛ of Pie, 0.75	100	3	16
Pillsbury, Pie Crusts,			
Refrigerated, ⅛ pie, 0.9 oz	100	6	12
Trader Joe's, Pie Crust, ⅛ pie, 1.37oz	190	13	17

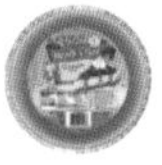
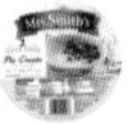
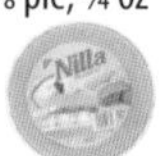

Pie Fillings ~ Canned

	C	F	Cb
Apple/Blueb./Cherry/Strawb., average:			
Sweetened: ⅓ cup, 3.2oz	90	0	22
1 cup, 9.5 oz	270	0	66
1 can, 21 oz	600	0	150
Light/Lite, ⅓ cup, 3.2 oz	60	0	15
Unsweetened, ⅓ cup, 3.2 oz	35	0	8
Lemon Crm/Creme, ⅓ cup, 3.2 oz	130	1.5	28

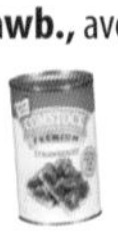

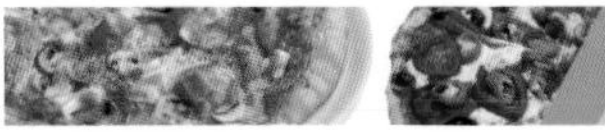

Pizzas ~ Ready to Eat

Figures Based On Pizza Hut

Cheese

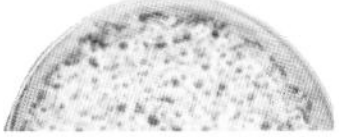

Medium Size (12"):	C	F	Cb
Hand Tossed Crust:			
⅛ Pizza (1 slice)	**210**	8	26
½ Pizza (4 slices)	**840**	32	104
Whole Pizza (8 slices)	**1680**	64	208
Original Pan: ⅛ Pizza (1 slice)	**240**	10	28
½ Pizza (4 slices)	**960**	40	112
Whole Pizza (8 slices)	**1920**	80	224
Thin 'N Crispy Crust:			
⅛ Pizza (1 slice)	**190**	7	22
½ Pizza (4 slices)	**760**	28	88
Whole Pizza (8 slices)	**1520**	56	176

Ham & Pineapple

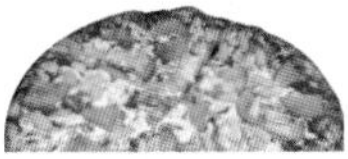

Figures Based On Domino's

Medium Size (12"):	C	F	Cb
Hand Tossed Crust:			
⅛ Pizza (1 slice)	**190**	7	23
½ Pizza (4 slices)	**760**	28	92
Whole Pizza (8 slices)	**1520**	56	184
Handmade Pan: ⅛ Pizza (1 slice)	**290**	14	29
½ Pizza (4 slices)	**1160**	56	116
Whole Pizza (8 slices)	**2320**	112	232
Thin Crust:			
⅛ Pizza (1 slice)	**140**	7	13
½ Pizza (4 slices)	**560**	28	52
Whole Pizza (8 slices)	**1120**	56	104

MeatZZA

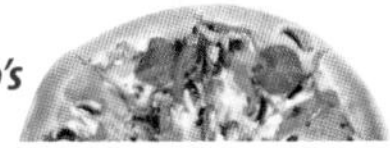

Figures Based On Domino's

Medium Size (12"):	C	F	Cb
Hand Tossed Crust:			
⅛ Pizza (1 slice)	**270**	13	24
½ Pizza (4 slices)	**1080**	52	96
Whole Pizza (8 slices)	**2160**	104	192
Handmade Pan: ⅛ Pizza (1 slice)	**360**	20	29
½ Pizza (4 slices)	**1440**	80	116
Whole Pizza (8 slices)	**2880**	160	232
Thin Crust: ⅛ Pizza (1 slice)	**220**	14	14
½ Pizza (4 slices)	**880**	56	56
Whole Pizza (8 slices)	**1760**	112	112

Pepperoni

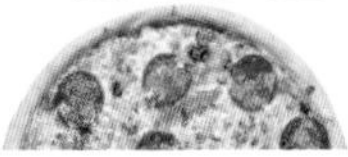

Figures Based On Pizza Hut

Medium Size (12"):	C	F	Cb
Hand Tossed Crust:			
⅛ Pizza (1 slice)	**220**	9	25
½ Pizza (4 slices)	**880**	36	100
Whole Pizza (8 slices)	**1760**	72	200
Original Pan: ⅛ Pizza (1 slice)	**250**	11	28
½ Pizza (4 slices)	**1000**	44	112
Whole Pizza (8 slices)	**2000**	88	224
Thin 'N Crispy: ⅛ Pizza (1 slice)	**210**	9	22
½ Pizza (4 slices)	**840**	36	88
Whole Pizza (8 slices)	**1680**	72	176

Large Pizzas

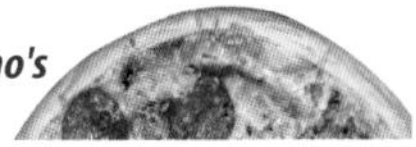

Figures Based On Domino's

Large (14")	C	F	Cb
Hand Tossed Crust:			
ExtravaganZZa: ⅛ Pizza (1 slice)	**390**	19	36
½ Pizza (4 slices)	**1560**	76	144
MeatZZA: ⅛ Pizza (1 slice)	**370**	18	34
½ Pizza (4 slices)	**1480**	72	136
Pepperoni: ⅛ Pizza (1 slice)	**280**	12	31
½ Pizza (4 slices)	**1120**	48	124

Extra Large NY, Single Slice

Figures Based On Sbarro	C	F	Cb
Cheese	**430**	15	51
Classic Hawaiian	**470**	15	57
Sausage	**520**	24	50
Spinach & Tomato	**370**	15	42

Individual Personal Pan Pizzas

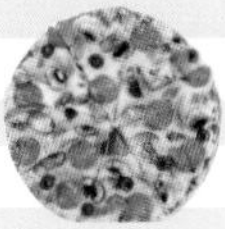

Pan (6"): Figures Based On Pizza Hut	C	F	Cb
Buffalo Chicken	**640**	20	88
Cheese	**600**	24	68
Pepperoni	**600**	28	68
Supreme	**680**	32	72
Veggie Lovers	**560**	20	72
Chicago-Style Deep Dish: *Per Individual, 6 slices*			
Figures Based On Uno Pizzeria			
Cheese & Tomato	**1680**	78	108
Chicago Classic	**2160**	156	114
Prima Pepperoni	**1680**	190	108

Frozen Pizzas

	C	F	Cb
Amy's: *Per ⅓ Pizza*			
Cheese	290	12	33
Margherita	270	12	31
Meatless Pepperoni	340	16	34
Mushroom & Olive	260	11	31
Pesto & Artichoke	300	16	34
Gluten-Free, Roasted Vegetable	320	11	51
Spinach	300	12	36
Vegan: Meatless Pepperoni, gluten free	320	15	40
Pesto & Rstd Artichoke, ½ pizza	370	20	45
Supreme, ⅓ pizza	290	12	37
California Pizza Kitchen: *Per ⅓ Pizza*			
Cauliflower: Artisanal Style Cheese	270	12	29
Pepperoni, Mushroom & Sausage	300	15	28
Crispy Thin Crust: BBQ Recipe Chkn	290	11	33
Four Cheese; Margherita, average	320	16	29
Sicilian Recipe	350	17	31
Signature Pepperoni	330	17	29
White Recipe	280	11	31
Gluten-Free:			
BBQ Recipe Chicken, **½** pizza	290	9	37
Margherita, ⅓ pizza	190	8	21
Single Serve: BBQ Recipe Chicken	300	11	31
Five Cheese & Tomato	280	12	29
Celeste: *Per Pizza*			
Pizza For One: Original 4 Cheese	380	16	48
Deluxe	360	15	47
Pepperoni	370	16	46
Sausage	370	16	47
Daiya *(Vegan)*:			
Cheese Lovers, ⅓ pizza, 5,22 oz	400	15	60
Meatless: Meat Lover's, ¼ pizza, 4.8 oz	340	14	48
Pepperoni, ⅓ pizza, 5.53 oz	410	17	61
M'shrm & Rstd Garlic, ¼ pizza, 4.27 oz	290	11	45
Supreme, gluten free, ¼ pizza	310	11	45
DiGiorno:			
Bacon & Cheese Stuffed Crust:			
Bacon Me Crazy, ¼ pizza	410	21	34
Better with Bacon ⅕ pizza	330	17	28
Cheese Stuffed Crust:			
Bacon Cheeseburger, ⅕ pizza	330	17	29
Buffalo Style Chkn, ¼ pizza	380	16	40
Five Cheese; Pepperoni, av., ⅕ pizza	315	15	29
Three Meat; Supreme, av., ⅕ pizza	355	18	31

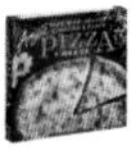
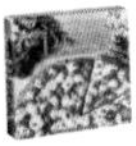
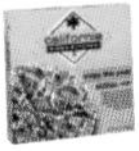
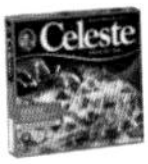

DiGiorno (Cont):	C	F	Cb
Crispy Pan: *Per ⅕ Pizza*			
Cheesy Garlic	410	20	40
Four Cheese	430	22	40
Pepperoni	430	22	39
Croissant Crust: *Per ⅕ Pizza*			
Four Cheese	370	18	36
Pepperoni	380	20	35
Three Meat	410	22	36
Rising Crust: *Per ⅙ Pizza*			
Four Cheese; Spicy Chkn Supreme, av	300	10	38
Hawaiian Style	280	8	39
Italian Sausage	340	13	48
Small Pizzas: *Per Pizza*			
Cheese Stuffed Crust:			
Four Cheese	650	29	67
Pepperoni; Supreme	660	31	66
Thin Crispy Crust:			
Pepperoni	580	25	68
Supreme	580	23	68
Traditional Crust:			
Four Cheese	690	29	83
Pepperoni	750	34	83
Freschetta:			
Brick Oven: *Per ⅕ Pizza Unless Indicated*			
5 Cheese, ¼ Pizza, 5.2 oz	370	17	39
Pepperoni, 4.55 oz	330	17	32
Spinach & Roasted M'shrms, 4.5 oz	270	10	34
Three Meat, 4.6 oz	340	18	32
Supreme, 4.6 oz	310	14	33
Naturally Rising:			
4 Cheese, 5 oz	370	14	48
Canada Style Bacon P'apple, 4.5 oz	290	9	41
Pepperoni, 4.55 oz	330	13	40
Supreme, 5.2 oz	350	15	41
Great Value *(Walmart)*:			
Deep Dish Minis: Cheese (1)	400	16	48
Supreme (1)	410	19	47
Three Meat (1)	400	17	47
Rising Crust:			
Cheese, 4.6 oz	300	10	41
Supreme, 5.11 oz	330	12	42
Three Meat, 4.6 oz	320	11	41
Thin Crust: Four Cheese, 5.15 oz	370	18	33
Pepperoni, 5.43 oz	410	22	34

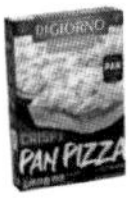

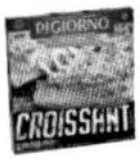

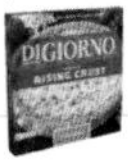

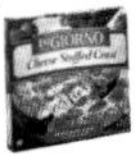
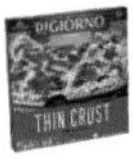

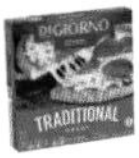

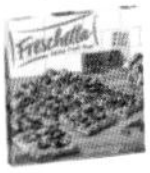

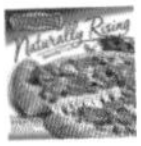

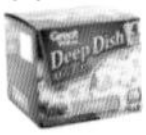

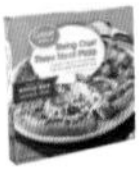

Frozen Pizzas (Cont)

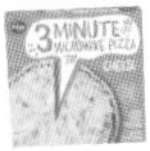

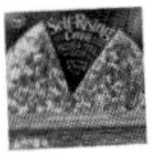
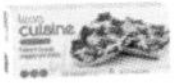
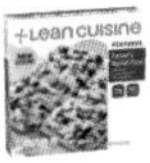
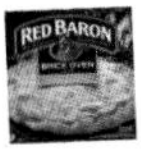

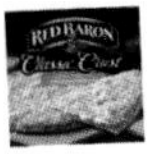
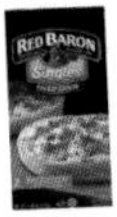
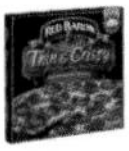

	C	F	Cb
Kroger:			
3 Minute Microwave: *Per 7.2 oz Pizza*			
Cheese	480	18	62
Pepperoni	540	25	63
Three Meat	510	21	64
Self Rising Crust: *Per ⅙ pizza*			
Double Bacon	300	9	43
Four Cheese	300	8	43
Supreme	330	12	42
Three Meat	340	13	44
White Chicken	310	11	41
Lean Cuisine:			
Favorites: *Per Package*			
French Bread Pepperoni	300	7	44
Features: *Per Package*			
Farmer's Market	340	9	50
Four Cheese	360	7	55
Margherita	330	8	51
Pepperoni; Supreme. av	395	8	60
Deep Dish: Spinach & Mushroom	360	8	54
Three Meat	390	9	56
Thick Crust, BBQ Recipe Chicken	340	5	54
Red Baron:			
Brick Oven: *Per ¼ Pizza*			
Cheese Trio, 4.4 oz	320	15	34
Meat-Trio, 4.6 oz	320	15	35
Pepperoni, 4.5 oz	330	17	33
Classic Crust: *Per ¼ Pizza*			
Four Cheese, 5.25 oz	380	17	40
Sausage & Pepp.,4.4 oz	320	16	32
Supreme, 4.7 oz	310	15	33
Deep Dish Minis:			
Cheese, 4 pieces, 5.4 oz	380	15	48
Pepperoni, 4 pieces, 5.6 oz	430	20	48
Deep Dish Singles: *Per Pizza*			
Hawaiian Style, 5.6 oz	370	14	48
Meat-Trio, 5.6 oz	400	18	47
Sausage, 5.8 oz	440	20	49
Scrambles: Bacon, 5.85 oz	440	21	45
Sausage, 5.85 oz	410	19	46
Thin & Crispy Crust: *Per ⅓ Pizza*			
Five Cheese, 5 oz	350	16	38
Pepperoni, 5.3 oz	390	20	38
Supreme, 4.4 oz	300	15	31

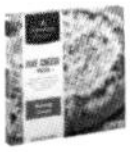
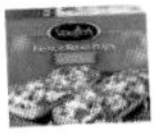
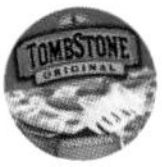

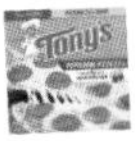

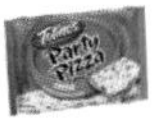

	C	F	Cb
Signature Select *(Albertsons):*			
Rising Crust: *Per ⅙ Pizza*			
Five Cheese	330	12	41
Pepperoni	380	17	41
Supreme	360	15	41
Ultra Thin Crust: *Per ⅓ Pizza*			
Italian Sausage; Sausage, average	345	19	27
Smart Ones *(Weight Watchers):*			
Thin Crust: Cheese	290	6	42
Pepperoni Pizza, 4.37 oz	310	10	39
Stouffer's:			
French Bread Pizzas:			
Two Per Box:			
Cheese (1)	360	15	43
Deluxe (1)	430	21	44
Three Meat (1)	470	25	43
Nine Per Box, Pepperoni (1)	430	21	44:
Tombstone:			
Original: *Per ¼ Pizza*			
Canadian Bacon, 4.9 oz	300	12	33
Deluxe; Supreme, av.	345	16	35
Five Chees; Hamburger	340	15	34
Pepperoni;Pepperoni & Sausage, av.	350	17	34
Pepperoni & Sausage	340	16	34
Sausage; Sausage & Mushroom	350	16	35
Veggie	300	12	35
Half & Half: *Per ¼ Pizza*			
Pepperoni & Sausage/Cheese	350	17	34
Garlic Bread Crust,			
Pepperoni; Supreme, av., ⅙ pizza	340	14	37
Tony's:			
Pizzeria Style Crust: *Per ¼ Pizza*			
Cheese, 4.7 oz	330	13	41
Meat Trio, 5 oz	360	16	41
Pepperoni, 4.7 oz	330	14	40
Sausage & Pepperoni, 4.83 oz	350	15	41
Supreme, 5.1 oz	350	15	41
Totino's:			
Crisp Crust Party Pizza: *Per ½ Pizza*			
Canadian Bacon	330	16	37
Cheese	320	16	37
Hamburger	360	19	38
Pepperoni & Bacon	340	17	37
Trader Joe's:			
Cauliflower Crust Cheese, ⅓ pizza	250	12	24
Org. Six Cheese & Tomato, ¼ pizza	340	16	35

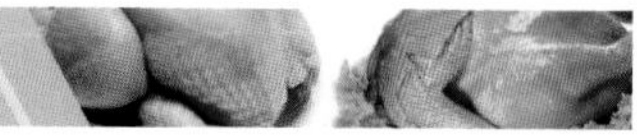

Quick Guide

	C	F	Cb
Chicken			
From 3lb ready-to-cook chicken			
Breast/Wing Quarter:			
Roasted: with skin	300	15	0
without skin	185	5	0
Fried, batter dipped	530	30	17
Leg Quarter:			
Thigh & Drumstick:			
Roasted: with skin	270	16	0
without skin	185	8	0
Fried, batter dipped	435	25	15
KFC ~ *See Fast-Foods Section*			

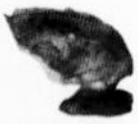
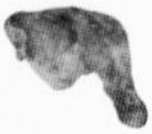

Per 4 oz Edible Portion

	C	F	Cb
Average of Light Meat: *Per 4 oz without Bone*			
Roasted: with skin	250	12	0
without skin	175	4.5	0
Stewed: with skin	230	12	0
without skin	180	4.5	0
Fried: Batter-dipped, with skin, 4 oz	315	17	11
Flour-coated, with skin, 4 oz	280	14	2
Average of Dark Meat: *Per 4 oz without Bone*			
Roasted: with skin	290	18	0
without skin	235	11	0
Stewed: with skin	265	17	0
without skin	220	10	0
Fried: Batter-dipped, with skin, 4 oz	340	21	11
Flour-coated, with skin, 4 oz	325	19	5

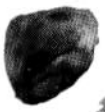
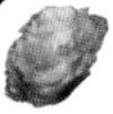
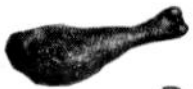
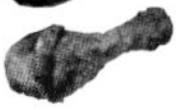

Chicken Parts

	C	F	Cb
Broilers or Fryers: *Edible Weights (no bone)*			
Breast: *Per 1/2 Breast*			
Raw: with skin, 5 oz	250	14	0
without skin, 4.25 oz	140	3	0
Roasted: with skin, 3.5 oz	195	8	0
without skin, 3 oz	140	3	0
Stewed: with skin, 4 oz	200	8	0
without skin, 3.3 oz	145	3	0
Fried: Batter-dipped, w/ skin, 5 oz	365	19	13
Flour-coated, with skin, 3.5 oz	220	9	2
Drumstick: *Per Drumstick*			
Roasted: with skin, 2 oz	115	6	0
without skin, 1.5 oz	75	2.5	0
Stewed: with skin, 2 oz	115	6	0
without skin, 1.5 oz	80	3	0
Fried: Batter-dipped, w/ skin, 2.5 oz	195	11	6
Flour-coated, with skin, 1.8 oz	120	7	1

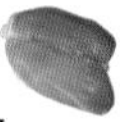
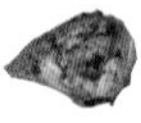
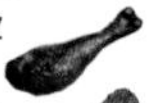
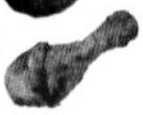

Chicken Parts (Cont)

	C	F	Cb
Broilers or Fryers (Cont): *Edible Weights (no bone)*			
Thigh Portion:			
Raw: with skin, 3.3 oz (4 1/4 oz with bone)	200	14	0
without skin, 2.4 oz	80	3	0
Roasted: with skin, 2.3 oz	155	10	0
without skin, 2 oz	110	6	0
Stewed: with skin, 2.5 oz	160	10	0
without skin, 2 oz	105	5	0
Fried: Batter-dipped, with skin 3 oz	240	14	8
Flour-coated, with skin, 2.3 oz	165	9	2
Wing: *Per Wing, Bone In*			
Raw Weight, 3.2 oz			
Raw: with skin	110	8	0
without skin	35	1	0
Roasted: with skin	100	7	0
without skin	45	2	0
Fried: Batter-dipped, with skin	160	11	5
Flour-coated, with skin	105	7	1
Stewed, with skin, 4 oz	100	7	0
Buffalo Wings ~ *See Fast-Foods Section*			
Neck: Simmered, with skin	95	7	0
without skin	30	2	0
Skin Only: *Skin from 1/2 Chicken*			
Raw skin, 3 oz	275	26	0
Roasted skin, 2 oz	255	23	0
Stewed skin, 2.5 oz	260	24	0
Fried, flour-coated, 2 oz	280	24	5
Fried, batter-dipped, 6.8 oz	750	55	44
Roasters: *Average of Light & Dark Meat*			
Roasted: with skin, 4 oz	250	15	0
without skin, 4 oz	190	8	0
Dark Meat, without skin	200	10	0
Light Meat, without skin	175	5	0
Stewing Chicken: *Per 4 oz, average of Light & Dark Meat*			
Stewed: with skin	325	22	0
without skin	270	14	0
Dark Meat, without skin	290	17	0
Light Meat, without skin	240	9	0
Capon Chicken:			
Roasted: with skin, 4 oz	260	13	0
1/2 Chicken, with skin, 22.5 oz	1460	74	0
Chicken Offal & Stuffing:			
Giblets: Simmered, 1 Cup	230	7	0.5
Fried, flour-coated, 1 Cup	400	20	6
Gizzard, simmered, 1 Cup	210	4	0
Heart, simmered, 1 Cup	270	12	0.2
Liver: Raw, 4 oz	130	5.5	0
Simmered, 1 Cup	215	8.5	1
Liver Pate, fresh, 1 Tbsp, 0.5 oz	30	2	1
Stuffing, average, 1/2 Cup	180	9	22

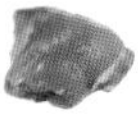
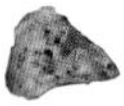
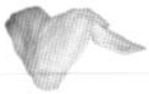
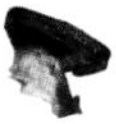
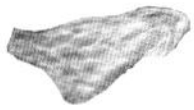
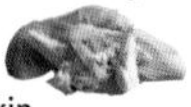
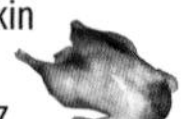
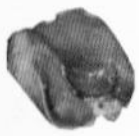

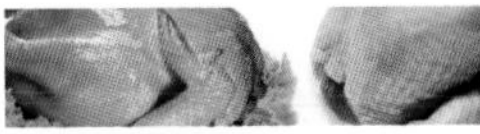

Poultry ~ Chicken ♦ Turkey (P)

Chicken Products

	C	F	Cb
Bumble Bee:			
Chicken In Water: *Per 2 oz Drained*			
Premium White	70	1.5	0
Premium Breast	70	1	1
Foster Farms:			
Chicken Breast Strips, grilled, 3 oz	100	2	1
Wings: Chipotle, 3 wings, 3 oz	190	13	4
Honey BBQ Glazed, 3 wings, 3 oz	190	11	7
Hot 'n' Spicy, 3 wings, 3 oz	190	14	1
Tyson:			
Anytizers, Frozen:			
Wings:			
Hot Wings, Buffalo Style (3)	190	13	1
Honey BBQ Seasoned (3)	190	12	8
Wyngz, Boneless:			
Buffalo Style, 3 pieces, 3 oz	150	7	8
Sweet Garlic Glazed, 3 pcs, 2.8 oz	130	5	10

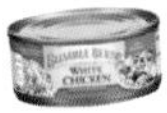
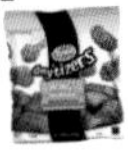

Duck, Goose, Quail

	C	F	Cb
Duck, Roasted:			
with skin, 3 oz	290	24	0
without skin, 3 oz	170	10	0
½ duck, with skin, 13.5 oz	1290	108	0
Goose: Roasted with skin, 3 oz	260	19	0
without skin, 3 oz	200	11	0
Pheasant, cooked, 3 oz	210	10	0
Quail, cooked, 1 whole, 6 oz	385	24	0

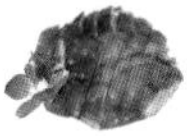
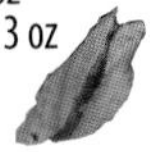

Turkey

	C	F	Cb
Fryer-Roasters: *Per 3 oz Serving*			
Roasted:			
Light Meat: with skin	140	4	0
without skin	120	1	0
Dark Meat: with skin	155	6	0
without skin	140	4	0
½ of Whole Turkey: (Approx. 3.3 lbs raw weight without neck and giblets; 1.8 lbs cooked weight)			
Roasted: with skin	1650	74	0
without skin	1125	31	0
Ground Turkey, raw: (4 oz raw wt. = 3 oz cooked wt.)			
85% lean, regular, 4 oz	170	10	0
93% lean: Average, 4 oz	160	8	0
Jennie-O, 4 oz	170	8	0
Trader Joe's, 4 oz	150	8	0
94% lean, *Foster Farms*, 4 oz	150	7	0
Breast, no skin, 4 oz	115	1	0
Patties: Small, 3 oz	130	7	0
Medium, 4 oz	170	10	0

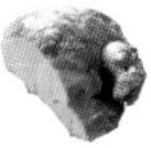
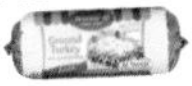
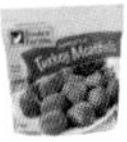

Turkey Parts

	C	F	Cb
Roasted, Edible Weights, without bone:			
Breast, (½), (from 17.3 oz raw weight with bone):			
with skin, 12 oz (no bone)	525	11	0
without skin, 10.8 oz	415	2	0
Back (½): with skin, 4.5 oz	265	13	0
without skin, 3.5 oz	165	6	0
Leg (Thigh & Drumstick): (from 1 lb raw weight with bone)			
with skin, 8.5 oz (without bone)	410	13	0
without skin, 7.8 oz (w/out bone)	355	8.5	0
Wing: (From 7.3 oz raw weight)			
with skin, 3 oz (without bone)	185	9	0
without skin, 2 oz (w/out bone)	100	2	0
Neck: Simmered, 1 neck, 9 oz (with bone)	275	11	0
Giblets, simmered, 1 Cup, 5 oz	240	7	3

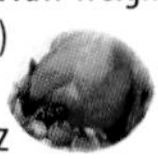
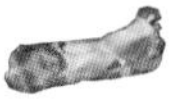

Young Hens (Roasted)

	C	F	Cb
Light Meat:			
with skin, 3 oz	175	8	0
without skin, 3 oz	135	3	0
Dark Meat: with skin, 3 oz	200	11	0
without skin, 3 oz	165	7	0
Young Toms ~ *Similar to Young Hens*			

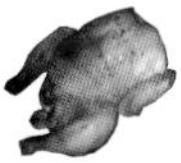

Turkey Products

	C	F	Cb
Foster Farms:			
Raw: Breast Cutlets, 4 oz	120	0.5	0
Ground Turkey, 85% lean, 4 oz	230	17	0
Tenderloins, Island Teriyaki, 4 oz	120	1	5
Hormel, Canned Turkey Breast, 97% Fat Free, in water, 2 oz	50	1	0
Jennie-O:			
Cooked: Meatballs, Italian, 3 oz	180	13	2
Home Style, 3 oz	180	13	3
Raw: Bacon, raw, 1 slice,	30	2.5	0
Bratwurst, lean, 1 link, 3.85 oz	150	8	0
Patties, 93% Lean All Natural, 4 oz	150	8	0
Spam, Oven Roasted Turkey, 2 oz	80	4.5	1
Valley Fresh, 100% Natural, Canned White Turkey Breast, in water, 2 oz	50	1	0

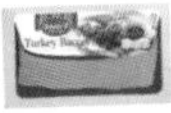
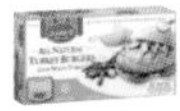

R Rice & Rice Dishes

White Rice

	C	F	Cb
Raw:			
Glutinous, 1 Cup, 6.5 oz	685	1	151
Long Grain, 1 Cup, 6.5 oz	675	1	148
Short Grain, 1 Cup, 7 oz	715	1	158
Wild Rice, 1 Cup, 5.5 oz	570	2	120
Cooked Rice: *Boiled/Steamed*			
Short/Medium Grain:			
½ Cup, 3.3 oz	140	0	30
1 Cup (½ Pint), 7.2 oz	265	0.5	59
2 Cups (1 Pint), 13 oz	480	1	106
Long Grain: ½ Cup, 2.8 oz	100	0	22
1 Cup, 5.5 oz	205	0.5	44
Glutinous/Sticky, 1 Cup, 6 oz	170	0.5	37
Parboiled, ½ Cup, 3 oz	105	0.5	22
Precooked/Instant:			
Dry, ½ Cup, 3.5 oz	380	1	82
Cooked, ½ Cup, 3 oz	95	0.5	21
Wild Rice,			
Cooked, 1 Cup, 5.8 oz	165	0.5	35

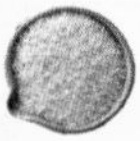
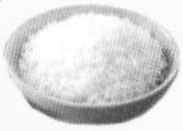
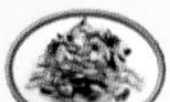

Brown Rice

	C	F	Cb
Average of Short or Long Grain			
Raw/Dry: ½ Cup, 3.3 oz	340	2.5	71
1 Cup, 6.5 oz	685	5.5	143
Cooked: ½ Cup, 3.5 oz	110	1	22
1 Cup, 7 oz	220	2	46

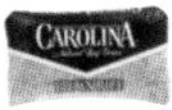

Rice Dishes

	C	F	Cb
Chinese Fried Rice:			
½ Cup, 2.5 oz	140	4.5	21
1 Cup, (½ Pint), 5 oz	280	9	42
2 Cups, (1 Pint), 10 oz	565	18	84
Mexican Style Rice:			
Taco Time, Seasoned, 4.6 oz	200	3	40
Rice-A-Roni ~ *See Page 119*			
Rice with Raisins/Pinenuts, 1 Cup	400	11	60
Rice Pilaf: Restaurant, 1 Cup	275	7.5	46
O'Charley's, side dish, 1 portion	160	4	27
Rice Pudding,			
Kozy Shack, Original, 1 pudding cup	130	2.5	24
Risotto, 1 Cup	420	12	70
Saffron Rice, 4 oz	175	7	25
Spanish Rice: 1 Cup, 5 oz	390	9	72
El Pollo Loco, Small, 4.5 oz	160	1.5	32
Sticky Rice, 1 Cup, 5 oz	155	0.5	34
Sushi Rice: 1 Tbsp	25	0	5
1 Cup, 5.2 oz	390	0	77
Other Packaged Rice Products:			
Uncle Ben's / Zatarain's ~ *See Page 121*			

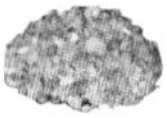
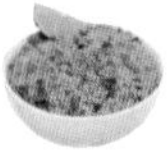

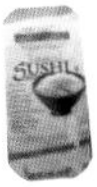

CalorieKing.com Recipes

See the CalorieKing website for a salubrious selection of healthy recipes – all analyzed for calories, fat, protein, carbohydrate, fiber and sodium.

Choose from:

- ***Starters/Appetizers***
- ***Salads***
- ***Entrees: Meat, Fish and Chicken***
- ***Vegetarian***
- ***Desserts***
- ***Cakes, Cookies***
- ***Drinks***

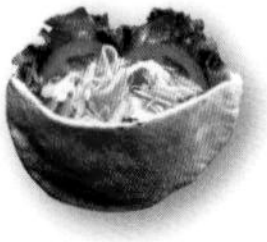

www.CalorieKing.com/recipes

HEALTHY RECIPE TIPS

- **Use non-fat milk** in place of whole or 2% milk
- **Use low-fat yogurt** in place of sour cream
- **Skim fat** from surface of soups and casseroles after cooling
- **Add extra vegetables** to soups and hot entreés
- **Cakes/cookies/muffins:** Replace most or all the fat/oil with applesauce and/or prune puree (Example, *Sunsweet Lighter Bake*)
- **Drinks:** Replace sugar with no-calorie sweeteners such as *Equal, Stevia, Splenda and Sweet 'N Low*

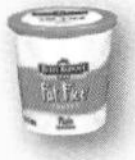
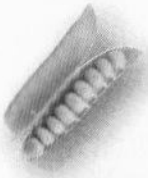
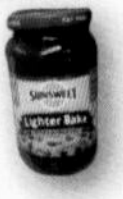
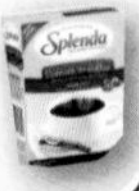

Deli Salads

	C	F	Cb
Average All Outlets			
Antipasto Salad, ½ Cup	135	8	13
3-Bean Salad, ½ Cup	90	4.5	12
Bulgur Salad, ½ Cup	70	2	12
Caesar Salad, Classic, 1 Cup	200	14	15
Side Salad, without Dressing	25	0	6
Carrot Raisin: with Dressing, ½ Cup	135	12	6
without Dressing, ½ Cup	20	0	5
Chef's Salad: Regular, w/o Dressing	620	37	8
with 2 oz Thousand Island Drssng	860	61	8
Chicken Salad, ½ Cup/scoop, 4 oz	280	21	2
Coleslaw: Traditional, ½ Cup	150	8	18
w/ Low Cal Dressing, ½ c.	50	2	8
Corn, Mexican, ½ Cup	240	12	33
Cucumber: Non-Oil Dressing, ½ Cup	60	0	14
with Oil Dressing, ½ Cup	140	12	8
Eggplant Salad, ½ Cup	75	5	7
Fettucini, with veges, ½ Cup	135	6	16
Garden Salad, without Dressing, 1 Cup	10	0	2
Greek Salad, 1 Cup	105	8	7
Greek Vegetables, 1 Cup	110	8	6
Lobster Salad, ½ Cup, 4 oz	250	21	11
Macaroni Salad, ½ Cup, 5 oz	360	26	26
Nicoise, 1 Cup	450	32	18
Pasta Salad, ½ Cup	200	11	19
Potato Salad: Dijon, 3 oz	120	7	13
with Mayonnaise, ½ Cup, 4 oz	215	15	17
Lowfat, ½ Cup	110	1.5	21
Rice Salad, ½ Cup	150	10	13
Saffron Rice, 4 oz	175	7	25
Spinach Salad, 1 Cup	180	13	13
Tabouli, ½ Cup	125	7	13
Three Bean Salad, ½ Cup	90	4.5	12
Tomato & Mozzarella, ½ Cup	180	14	10
Tortellini, with Basil Pesto, ½ Cup	150	9	15
Waldorf, with Mayo, ½ Cup	110	7	12
Signature Salads: *Per 6 oz Serving* (Supplied to Deli's and Institutions)			
Antipasto Salad	510	50	4
Artichoke Salad, marinated	400	41	8
California Medley	120	7	15
Cheese Agnolotti	250	8	23
Chicken Salad	420	33	11
Crabmeat Flavored	450	38	20
Egg Salad	300	23	14
Fresh Button Mushroom	190	16	6

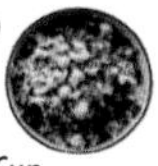
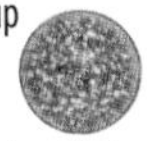
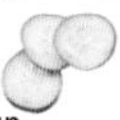
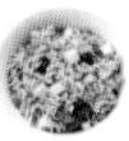
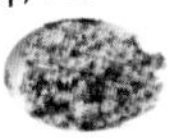
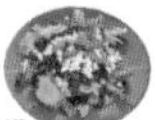
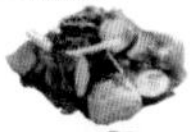
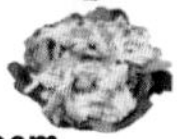

Updated Nutrition Data ~ www.CalorieKing.com
Persons with Diabetes ~ See Disclaimer (Page 22)

Signature Salads (Cont): *Per 6 oz*	C	F	Cb
Fresh Button Mushroom	190	16	6
Ham Salad	400	32	14
Prima Pasta Salad	360	30	18
Seafood Pasta Del Mar	170	10	21
Seafood, Crab & Shrimp	420	34	20
Shrimp Salad	360	32	8
Tuna Salad	450	36	14

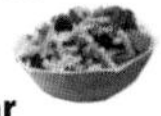
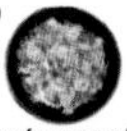

~ Also See Fast-Foods & Restaurants Section

Fresh Salad Packs

	C	F	Cb
Pre-Packaged (Supermarkets):			
Dole:			
Kits: *Per 3.5 oz, with Dressing*			
Blueberry Bliss	170	12	13
Caesar: Classic	150	13	8
Ultimate	170	13	10
Chopped Kits: Bacon & Bleu	150	13	6
BBQ Ranch	140	10	11
Sesame Asian	140	10	12
Salad Blends: *Per 3 oz, Without Dressing*			
American	15	0	3
Arugula; Baby Spinach	20	0	3
Field Greens; Very Veggie	20	0	4
Fresh Express:			
Chopped Salad Kits: *Per Serving*			
Twisted Asian Caesar, 3.84 oz	190	15	13
Twisted Greek Caesar, 3.72 oz	90	6	7
Gourmet Kits: *Per Container*			
Chef Salad	300	23	10
Grilled chicken Caesar	170	29	13
Saute Kits: *Per 3.9 oz Serving*			
Lemon Garlic Spinach	160	13	9
Tuscan Kale with Genovese Pesto	120	8	10
Ready Pac:			
Bistro Bowls: *Per Container*			
Apple Bleu Pecan, 4.5 oz	220	14	23
Caprese, 5 oz	210	17	12
Complete Chopped Salad Kits: *Per 3.5 oz*			
Asian,	100	6	11
Kale Cranberry Pecan	200	14	17
Mediterranean	130	10	11

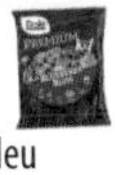
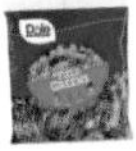
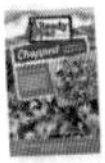

Salad Toppings

	C	F	Cb
Bac'n Pieces, *McCormick*, 1Tbsp, 0.3 oz	30	1	2
Bacon Bits *(Hormel)*, 1Tbsp	25	1.5	0
Bac-Os, Bits *(Betty Crocker)*, 1 Tbsp	30	1	2
Chow Mein Noodles, dry, ½ Cup	120	7	13
Croutons, 2 Tbsp, 0.3 oz	40	1	7
Salad Toppins, *McCormick*, 4 tsp	35	1.5	3
Sunflower Seeds, 1 Tbsp, 0.3 oz	45	4	1.5
Toasted Sliced Almonds, 2 T., 0.5 oz	85	7	3

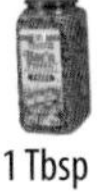
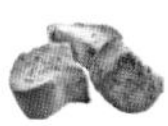

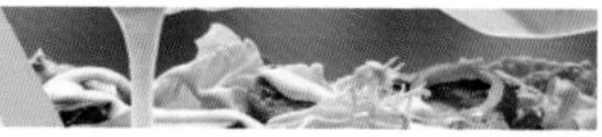

Quick Guide

Salad Dressings

Average All Brands: *Per 2 Tbsp, Approx 1 fl.oz*

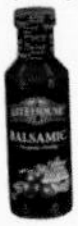
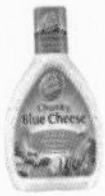
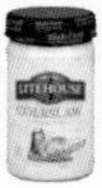
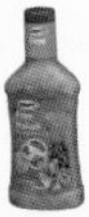
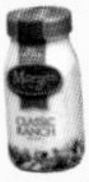
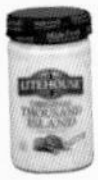

	C	F	Cb
Balsamic Vinaigrette:			
Regular	90	9	3
Light, 2 Tbsp	45	4	2
Fat Free, 2 Tbsp	25	0	6
Blue Cheese: Regular, 2 Tbsp	145	15	1.5
Regular, 1/4 cup, 2 oz	280	30	3
Light, 2 Tbsp	30	1	4
Caesar: Regular, 2 Tbsp	165	17	1
Regular, 1/4 cup, 2 oz	310	34	2
Light, 2 Tbsp	35	1.5	5.5
Coleslaw: Regular, 2 Tbsp	125	11	8
Regular, 1/4 cup, 2 oz	245	21	15
Light, 2 Tbsp	110	7	14
French: Regular	145	14	5
Regular, 1/4 cup, 2 oz	260	25	9
Light, 2 Tbsp	65	4	9
Fat/Oil-Free, 2 Tbsp	40	0	10
Italian: Regular, 2 Tbsp	85	8.5	3
Regular, 1/4 cup, 2 oz	165	16	6
Light, 2 Tbsp	55	5.5	2
Fat/Oil-Free, 2 Tbas	15	0	2.5
Ranch: Regular, 2 Tbsp	145	16	2
Regular, 1/4 cup, 2 oz	290	30	4
Light, 2 Tbsp	60	4	6.5
Fat-Free, 2 Tbsp	35	0.5	8
Thousand Island: Reg., 2 T.	115	11	4.5
Regular, 1/4 cup, 2 oz	210	20	9
Light, 2 Tbsp	60	3.5	7
Fat-Free, 2 Tbsp	40	0.5	10

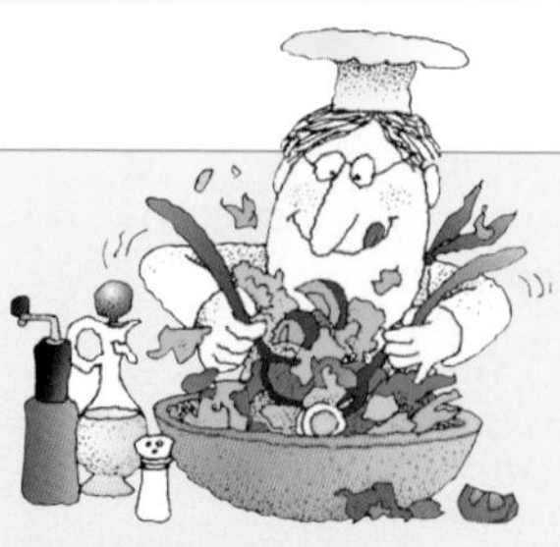

Enjoy a healthy salad but don't drown it in high-fat salad dressings.

Use 'light' dressings to halve the fat and calories.

Brands ~ Salad Dressings

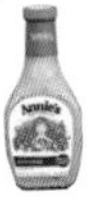
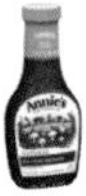
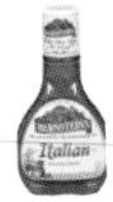
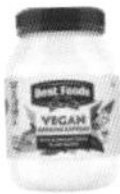
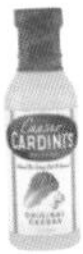
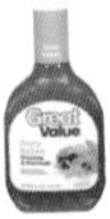
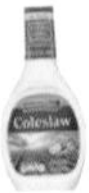

	C	F	Cb
Annie's Naturals: *Per 2 Tbsp*			
Organic: Goddess Dressing	120	12	2
French	110	10	3
Original Caesar	100	11	2
Papaya Poppy Seed	90	8	5
Vinaigrettes:			
Red Wine & Olive Oil	140	14	1
Sesame Ginger	90	8	4
Shiitake & Sesame	130	13	2
Bernstein's: *Per 2 Tbsp*			
Creamy Caesar	120	13	1
Herb Garden French	130	12	6
Italian	90	9	2
Restaurant Recipe Italian	120	12	1
Fat-Free, Cheese & Garlic Italian	10	0	2
Light Fantastic: Cheese Fantastico	30	1.5	3
Roasted Garlic Balsamic	45	3.5	3
Best Foods: *Per 1 Tbsp Unless Indicated*			
Mayonnaise: Real	100	11	0
Light	35	3.5	1
Organic	100	11	0
Olive Oil	60	6	1
Sunflower Oil	60	7	0.5
Vegan Dressing & Spread	70	8	0.5
Cardini's: *Per 2 Tbsp*			
Caesar: 80 Calorie	80	8	1
Original	140	15	0.5
Garlic Lemon	150	16	1
Red Jalapeno	140	15	0.5
Three Cheese; Vinaigrette	140	15	0.5
Vinaigrette, Balsamic:			
Regular	100	8	5
Lite Greek	50	4.5	2
Great Value (Walmart): *Per 2 Tbsp Unless Indicated*			
Creamy: Caesar	120	12	2
Thousand Island	120	12	4
Light Mayo, 1 Tbsp	35	3.5	1
Ranch: Buttermilk	110	11	2
Classic	130	14	1
Traditional Italian	80	7	5
Hidden Valley: *Per 2 Tbsp*			
Creamy: Coleslaw	150	15	4
Southwest Chipotle	100	10	2
Greek Yogurt: Cucumber Dill	60	5	3
Ranch	60	5	3
Spinach & Feta	60	5	3
Light, Butterilk Ranch; Ccumber, av.	65	5	3

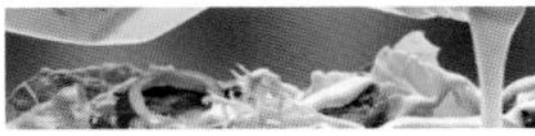

Brands ~ Salad Dressings (Cont)

Item	C	F	Cb
Hidden Valley (Cont): *Per 2 Tbsp*			
Ranch: Bacon; Cheddar & Bacon	100	11	2
Buffalo	110	11	2
Simply Ranch: Buttermilk	110	12	2
Chili Lime	120	12	2
Classic Ranch	110	12	2
Kraft: *Per 2 Tbsp*			
Balsamic Vinaigrette	70	5	5
Regular Dressings:			
Asian Toasted Sesame	80	6	7
Buttermilk Ranch	120	12	2
Catalina Classic	90	6	9
Classic Caesar	120	12	2
Chunky Blue Cheese	120	12	2
Creamy Italian	90	8	1
Creamy Italian	80	8	2
Cucumber Ranch	110	11	3
Honey Mustard	90	6	3
Roka Blue Cheese	80	7	2
Viva Italian	50	4.5	2
Zesty Catalina	80	6	5
Zesty Italian	60	4.5	3
Fat Free: Catalina	50	0	11
Thousand Island	60	0	12
Zesty Italian	15	0	3
Lite: Catalina	60	1	11
House Italian	35	1	5
Raspberry Vinaigrette	30	1	5
Zesty Italian	25	1	4
Seven Seas, Green Goddess	100	8	5
Marie's: *Per 2 Tbsp*			
Classics:			
Chunky Blue Cheese	160	17	1
Creamy: Caesar	120	13	1
Chipotle Ranch	170	19	1
Italian Garlic	180	19	1
Ranch	180	19	1
Original Coleslaw	140	13	7
Thousand Island	150	15	3
Vinaigrette: Blue Cheese	120	11	4
Garlic Parmesan	110	11	2
Mango Chardonnay	120	11	6
Raspberry	50	3	7
White Balsamic Shallot	120	11	4

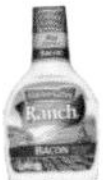
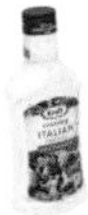
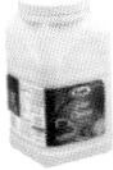
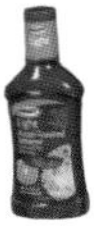
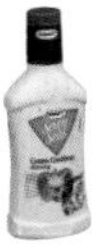
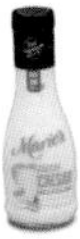
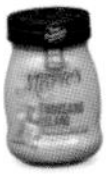
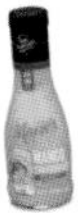

Item	C	F	Cb
Marzetti's: *Per 2 Tbsp*			
Classic Refrigerated:			
Asiago Peppercorn	150	16	2
Cilantro Avocado	110	12	1
Honey French	160	12	11
Supreme Caesar	140	15	0.5
Simpoly 60:			
Balsamic Vinaigrette	60	3.5	6
Dijon Honey Mustard Vinaigrette	60	4.5	4
Other Flavors	60	6	2
Simply Dressed: Blue Cheese	130	13	1
Caesar	120	12	1
Ranch: Regular	110	12	1
Cucumber	80	8	2
Vinaigrette: Lemon	90	9	2
Strawberry Poppyseed	120	10	6
Tastefully Dressed:			
Asiago Caesar & Black Garlic	140	15	1
Superfruit w/ Acai Bery & Pomegr.	110	11	5
Newman's Own: *Per 2 Tbsp*			
Oils: Caesar, Avoc. & Extra Virgin O. Oil	160	18	0
Greek, Avoc. & Extra Virgin O. Oil	150	16	1
Regular: Balsamic	110	11	2
Creamy Caesar	160	18	1
Family Recipe Italian	120	13	1
Honey Mustard	90	7	7
Poppy Seed	140	13	5
Light: Balsamic Vinaigrette	45	4	2
Caesar	70	6	2
Italian	60	6	0
Wish-Bone: *Per 2 Tbsp*			
Creamy: Buffalo Ranch	130	13	2
Caesar	190	20	1
Chunky Blue Cheese	130	14	1
French	120	11	5
Ranch	130	13	1
Russian	110	6	14
Thousand Island	120	11	5
Fat Free, Chunky Blue Cheese			
Light, ParmesanPeppercorn Ranch	60	5	2
Vinaigrettes:			
Balsamic	60	5	4
Jalapeno Lime	80	8	3
Lemon Herb	60	5	3
Red Wine	70	5	6
Strawberry Balsamic	50	4.5	3

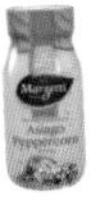
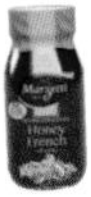
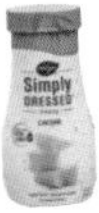
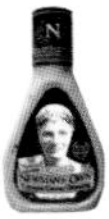
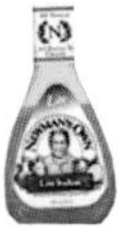
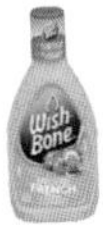
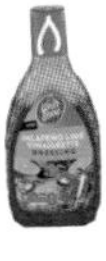

S Sauces & Gravy

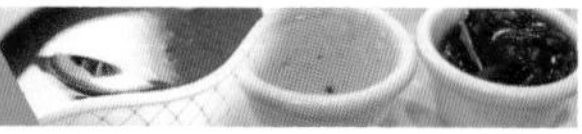

Gravy

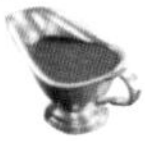

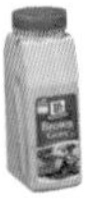

Gravy	C	F	Cb
Homemade Gravy, average:			
Thin, little fat,			
2 Tbsp, 1 oz	20	1	3
Thick: 2 Tbsp, 1.3 oz	50	2	9
1/4 cup, 2.5 oz	100	4	18
McCormick:			
Brown, 1 Tbsp	20	0.5	4
Turkey, 1 Tbsp	20	0.5	4

Gravy-In-Jars

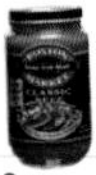

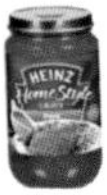

Gravy-In-Jars	C	F	Cb
Boston Market,			
Classic Beef, 1/4 cup, 2 oz	30	1	4
Campbell's,			
Beef/Chicken/Turkey, 1/4 cup, 2 oz	30	1	4
Heinz: *Per 1/4 Cup, 2 oz*			
Homestyle: Bistro Au Jus	15	0	2
Classic Chicken	30	2	3
Mushroom; Pork	20	0.5	3
Roasted Turkey	25	2	3
Savory Beef	25	1	3
Safeway, Chicken, 1/4 cup, 2 oz	40	2.5	3

Tomato Products

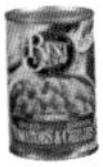

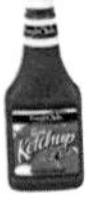

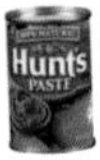

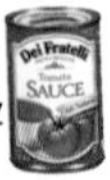

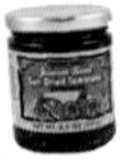

Tomato Products	C	F	Cb
Whole/Chopped/Crushed/Diced:			
Regular: 1 Cup, 8.5 oz	50	0	10
In Aspic, 1/2 Cup	50	0	12
with Green Chili, 1 c., 8.5 oz	60	0	16
Stewed, 1/2 Cup, 1.7 oz	40	1.5	7
Wedges in Tomato Juice, 1 Cup	70	0.5	18
Salsa, average, 2 Tbsp, 1 oz	25	0	6
Tomato Ketchup:			
Regular: 1 Tbsp, 0.5 oz	15	0	4
Single Serve, 1 packet	10	0	3
Heinz, Simply Heinz			
1 Tbsp, 0.5 oz	15	0	4
Tomato Paste:			
Regular: 2 Tbsp, 1 oz	25	0	6
3/4 cup, 6 oz	140	1	32
Tomato Puree, 1/2 Cup, 4.5 oz	50	0	10
Tomato Sauce:			
Regular, 1/2 Cup, 4.4 oz	50	0	11
Spanish Style, 1/2 Cup, 4.3 oz	40	0	9
with Mushr., 1/2 Cup, 4.3 oz	45	0	10
with Onions, 1/2 Cup, 4.3 oz	50	0	12
Tomato Seasoning, 3 tsp	20	0	4
Sundried Tomatoes:			
Natural, 5-6 pieces, 0.4 oz	20	0	5
In Oil, drained, 6 pieces, 0.5 oz	40	2.5	4

Sauces ~ Brands

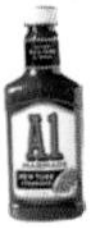

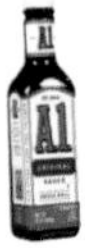

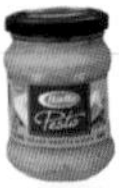

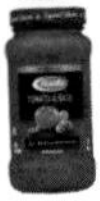

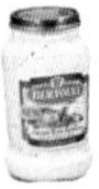

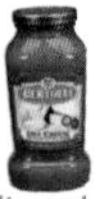

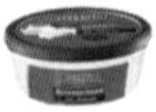

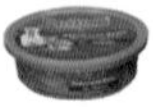

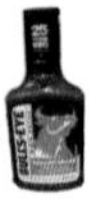

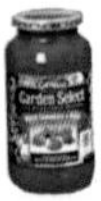

Sauces ~ Brands	C	F	Cb
A-1 *(Kraft):*			
Marinades: *Per Tbsp, ½ oz*			
Chicago Steakhouse	20	1	2
Classic	15	0	4
New Orleans Cajun	25	0	6
New York Steakhouse	20	0	5
Sauce: Original	15	0	3
Bold & Spicy	20	0	4
Smoky Black Pepper	30	0	6
Spicy Chipotle	30	0	7
Sweet Chili; Thick & Hearty	25	0	6
Sweet Hickory	25	0	5
Barilla:			
Pesto: *Per ¼ cup*			
Creamy: Genovese Pesto	310	29	8
Ricotta & Arugula	270	26	7
Rustic Basil	200	19	5
Sun-Dried Tomato	130	10	7
Regional: *Per ½ Cup*			
Fire Roasted Marinara	45	1	9
Marinara; Tomato Basil	50	1	11
Roasted Garlic; Savory Tomato, av.	60	1	11
Tomato Rosa	80	3	8
Bertolli:			
Alfredo Sauces: *Per ¼ Cup*			
Creamy Basil	100	10	2
Four Cheese Rosa	110	10	5
Garlic with Parmesan	100	10	2
Rustic Cut Marinara,			
with Traditonal Vegetables	100	6	10
Traditional: *Per ½ Cup*			
Five Cheese w/ Ricotta	90	3	12
Portobello Mushroom	70	2.5	9
Vodka	140	10	10
Buitoni: *Per ¼ Cup Unless Indicated*			
Pasta Sauces:			
Alfredo: Regular	140	13	3
Light	70	5	4
Marinara, 1/2 Cup	70	3	9
Pesto: With Basil	290	27	5
Reduced Fat	230	18	8
Bull's-Eye: Per 2 Tbsp			
BBQ Sauce: Original	50	0	4
Hickory Smoke	60	0	5
Regional, average all varieties	50	0	4
Catelli: *Per 1/2 Cup*			
Garden Select Pasta Sauce:			
Country Mushroom	45	1	9
Garlic & Onion	45	1	9
Meat Sauce	50	1.5	8
Pizza Sauce, all varieties	60	1.5	11

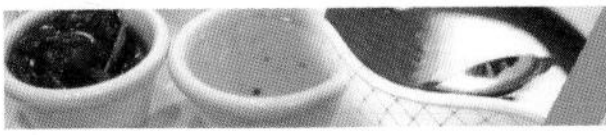

Sauces ~ Brands (Cont)

Item	C	F	Cb
Cento:			
Arrabbiata, ½ Cup	60	3.5	6
Italiano, ¼ cup	25	0	6
Marinara, ¼ cup	60	3.5	6
Porcini, ½ Cup	70	4	7
Puttanesca, ½ Cup	70	4.5	7
Vodka, ½ Cup	100	5	8
Classico:			
Alfredo: *Per ¼ Cup*			
Creamy, 2 oz	50	3.5	3
Roasted Garlic, 2 oz	45	3.5	3
Family Favorites: *Per ½ Cup*			
Meat, 4.4 oz	60	1	10
Parm. & Romano, 4.4 oz	70	2	10
Traditional, 4.4 oz	80	2.5	13
Contadina: *Per ¼ Cup*			
Pizza Sauce: Four Cheese, 2.2 oz	30	0	6
Tomato, 2.2 oz	30	0	6
Tomato Sauce, average	20	0.5	4
Crosse & Blackwell:			
Meat: Ham Glaze, 1 Tbsp	25	0	6
Mint Meat Sauce, 1 tsp	5	0	2
Mincemeat: *Per ¼ Cup*			
Regular	140	0	35
Rum & Brandy	140	0	36
Seafood: *Per ¼ Cup*			
Cocktail Sauce, 2.5 oz	90	0	21
Shrimp Sauce, 2.5 oz	90	0	21
Dave's Gourmet:			
Pasta Sauce: *Per ½ Cup*			
Butternut Squash	100	4	16
Creamy Parmesan Romano	120	8	9
Hearty Marinara	70	3.5	9
OrganicRed Heirloom	70	2.5	9
Rstd Garlic & Sweet Basil	70	4.5	8
Spicy Heirloom Marinara	45	1.5	7
Vegan Bolognese	80	4	8
Del Monte:			
Pasta Sauces: *Per ½ Cup*			
Four Cheese; Traditional, av.	60	1	12
Mushroom	60	1	11
Average other varieties	60	1	13
Sloppy Joe Sauce: *Per ¼ cup*			
Hickory	60	0	14
Original	60	0	13

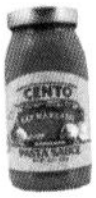

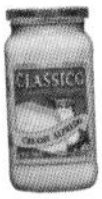

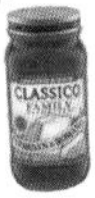

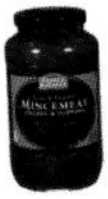

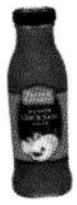

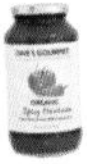

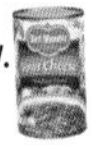

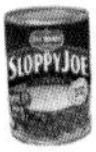

Item	C	F	Cb
Emeril's:			
Alfredo, Four Cheese Sauce, ¼ cup	60	5	4
Pasta Sauces: *Per ½ Cup*			
Homestyle Marinara	90	3	14
Kicked Up Tomato	80	3.5	11
Roasted Gaaahlic	80	3.5	12
Roasted Red Pepper	70	3.5	9
Vodka Sauce	110	7	12
Francesco Rinaldi:			
Alfredo, all flavors, ¼ cup	90	8	2
Cheese,			
Three Cheese, ½ Cup	70	1	15
Garden, all var., ½ Cup	60	1	12
Meat: Meat Flavored, ½ Cup	70	2.5	13
Sicilian Family, Sausage, ½ Cup	70	2.5	11
Pizza, ¼ cup	20	0	4
Tomato, Marinara, ½ Cup	60	1	12
French's,			
Worcestershire Sauce, 1 tsp	0	0	1
Heinz: *Per 1 Tbsp*			
57 Steak Sauce	20	0	4
Chili Sauce	20	0	5
Cocktail Sauce, Original, ¼ cup, 2.2 oz	70	0	18
Horseradish Sauce, tsp, 5 ml	25	2	1
Tartar Sauce, 2 tbsl	120	11	5
Tomato Ketchup: Regular	20	0	5
No Sugr Added	10	0	1
Worcestershire Sce, tsp	0	0	0
House of Tsang:			
Bangkok P'nut Sce, 1.16 oz	80	5	8
Classic Stir Fry Sauce, 0.6 oz	25	0.5	5
Ginger Sriracha Sce, 1.23 oz	15	0	4
General Tsao, 0.67 oz	45	0.5	10
Green Thai Curry Sauce, 1.1 oz	60	4	6
Korean BBQ Sauce, 0.67 oz	25	0	6
Oyster Flavored Sauce, 0.63 oz	30	0	7
Saigon Sizzle Sauce, 0.63 oz	40	1	7
Sweet & Sour Sauce, 0.63 oz	30	0	7
Hunt's:			
BBQ Sauces, average, 2 Tbsp	70	0	16
Pasta Sauce: *Per ½ Cup*			
Four Cheese	60	1	11
Garlic & Herb	40	0.5	8
Mushroom	60	0.5	11
Zesty & Spicy	60	1.5	11

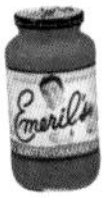

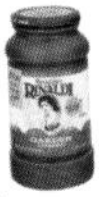

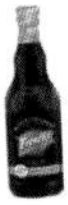

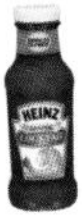

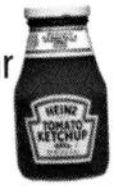

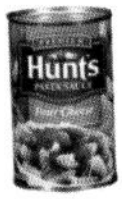

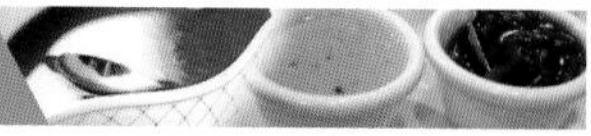

Brands (Cont)

	C	F	Cb
Kikkoman: *Per Tablespoon*			
Marinade: Gourmet Teriyaki	25	0	6
Roasted Garlic & Herbs	15	0	3
Toasted Sesame	40	0.5	7
Asian Authentics: *Per Tbsp, Unless Indicated*			
Katsu	20	0	5
Kotteri Mirin	50	0	12
Plum Sauce, 2 Tbsp	90	1	21
Sukiyaki	25	0	5
Tempura	5	0	1
Unagi Sushi	40	0	10
Wasabi, 1 tsp	10	1	0.5
Knorr: *Dry Mix Only*			
Classic Sauce Mix:			
Bernaise, teaspoon	10	0	2
Creamy Pesto, 1 Tbsp	25	0	5
Four Cheese, 1 Tbsp	30	1	4
Hollandaise, teaspoon	10	0	2
Pesto, 1 tbsp	20	0	3
Kraft:			
Horseradish, 2 Tbsp	100	9	4
Mesq. Smoke BBQ Sauce, 2 T.	60	0	15
Tartar, 1 Tbsp	70	6	4
Las Palmas: *Per ¼ Cup*			
Green Enchilada Sauce, all varieties, 2 oz	25	1.5	3
Red Chili Sauce	15	0.5	3
La Victoria,			
Red/Green Enchilada Sauce, av., 2 oz	25	1.5	3
Lawry's:			
30 Minute Marinade: *Per Tbsp*			
Baja Chipotle	10	0	2
Caribbean Jerk with Papaya	20	0	4
Chipotle Molasses	30	0	7
Herb & Garlic; Lemon Pepper	10	0	2
Honey Bourbon	20	0	5
Mesquite, w/ Lime Juice	10	0	2
Sesame & Ginger	20	0	5
Steakhouse	10	0	2
Teriyaki with Pineapple Juice	15	0	4
Sweet Asian	20	0	4
Lea & Perrins:			
Marinade, Chkn; Rstd Garlic, 1 T.	15	0	4
Tradit. Steak Sauce, 1 Tbsp	20	0	5
Worcestershire Sauce:			
Original, 1 tsp, 5 ml	5	0	1
Reduced Sodium, 1 tsp, 5 ml	5	0	1

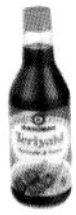

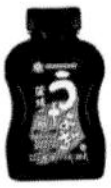

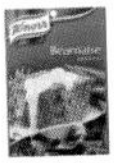

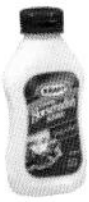

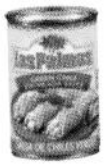

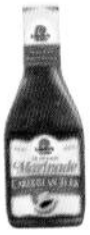

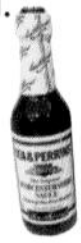

	C	F	Cb
McCormicks:			
Cooking, Tomato, Garlic & Wine, 1 T.	15	0	3
Seafood Sauces: *Per 2 Tbsp*			
Asian; Santa Fe Style, av.	50	2	7
Cajun Style	15	0	3
Lemon Butter Dill	100	9	4
Lemon Herb	80	8	0
Scampi	160	17	2
Mrs. Dash			
Marinades: *Per 1 Tbsp*			
Garlic Herb	15	0	3
Lime Garlic	15	0	3
Sweet Teriyaki	35	0	9
Newman's Own: *Per ½ Cup Inless Indicated*			
Pasta Sauce: Alfredo, 2.1 oz	50	4.5	3
Italian Sausage & Peppers	90	3.5	10
Marinara; Sockarooni	70	1	12
Roasted Garlic	60	1.5	11
Tomato & Basil Bombolina	70	2	11
Vodka	140	9	11
O Organics (Von's): *Per ½ Cup Unless Indicated*			
Enchilada, average, ¼ cup	20	0.5	4
Pasta: Arrabiata	60	1.5	10
Classic Alfredo	70	7	3
Marinara; Roasted Garlic, av.	60	1.5	11
Portobello Mushroom	45	1.5	7
Old El Paso: *Per ¼ Cup*			
Creamy: Queso, 1 Tbsp	20	1.5	2
Salsa Verde, 1 Tbsp	40	3.5	1
Enchilada Sauce:			
Green Chile, 2.15 oz	25	1.5	4
Red, all, 2.1 oz	20	0	4
Taco Sauce, all, 1 Tbsp	5	0	1
Pace: *Per 2 Tbsp*			
Picante Sauce, all varieties	10	0	2
Queso,			
Salsa: Regular, all varieties	10	0	3
Salsa con Queso	40	3	3
Prego: *Per ½ Cup, Unless Indicated*			
Alfredo, all varieties, ¼ cup	70	6	3
Basil Pesto Italian	200	19	4
Classic Italian: Chnky Tom. & Greens	70	1.5	11
Italian: Chunky Zucchini	60	1.5	10
Rstd Garlic Parm.; Three Chse, av.	70	1.5	13
Spicy Sausage Meat	110	4	15
Favorite:			
Italian: Flavored with Meat	90	3	13
Fresh Mushroom	70	1.5	12
Sausage & Garlic Meat	90	3	12
Premier Japan, Hoisin; Teriyaki, 1 T.	15	0	3

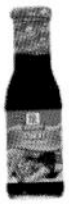

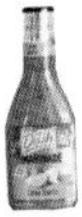

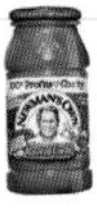

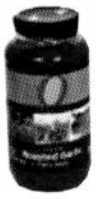

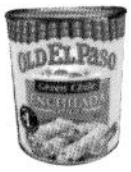

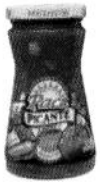

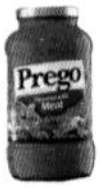

Brands (Cont)

Ragu:

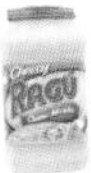

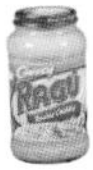

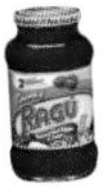

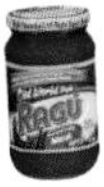

	C	F	Cb
Cheese Sauce: *Per ¼ Cup*			
Butter Parmesan	60	5	2
Classic/Creamy Alfredo, av.	90	9	2.5
Double Cheddar	100	9	3
Light Parmesan Alfredo	60	4	2
Roasted Garlic Parmesan	90	8	3
Chunky Sauce: *Per ½ Cup*			
Garden Combination	90	2.5	14
Mama's Special Garden	90	2.5	15
M'shrm & Green Peppers	80	2	13
Parmesan & Romano	80	2.5	13
Six Cheese	90	2.5	14
Super Chunky Mushroom	80	2	14
Old World Style: *Per ½ Cup*			
Flavored with Meat	90	4	12
Marinara; Mushroom, av.	75	2	11
Traditional	60	1	11
Pizza: Homemade Style, ¼ Cup	30	1	5
Margherita, ¼ Cup	25	0.5	3
Snack Sauce, Traditional, ¼ Cup	45	1.5	6
Simply Pasta Sauce: *Per ½ Cup*			
Chunky Marinaraa	70	1.5	11
M'shrm; Rstd Garlic; Traditional, av.	60	1.5	11
Safeway Select: *Per ½ Cup Unless Indicated*			
BBQ, Carolina Style Gold, 2 Tbsp	60	1	13
Pasta Sauce: Marinara; Rstd Garlic, av.	60	1.5	11
Portobello Âushroom	45	1.5	7
Vodka	150	10	10
Simmer Sauce: Butter Chicken	160	13	11
Lemon Butter	190	15	13
Thai Coconut Curry	140	9	10
Tikka Masala	90	6	7
White Wine & Mushroom	100	5	8
Taco Bell, Creamy Jalapeno Sauce, 1 Tablespoon, 0.5 oz	70	7	1
Tony Roma's:			
Original, 2 Tbsp	50	0	12
Carolina Honey BBQ Sce, 2 Tbsp	70	0	18
Trader Joe's, Kansas City Style BBQ Sauce, 2 Tbsp	45	0	11
Walnut Acres,			
Organic Pasta Sauces, average all var., ½ Cup, 4.5 oz	50	1	10

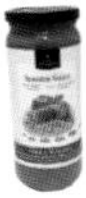

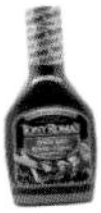

Seasonings & Flavorings

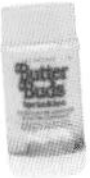

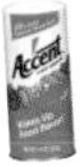

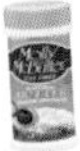

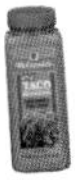

	C	F	Cb
Auromatic Bitters *(Angostua)*, 1 tsp	15	0	4
Bacon Bits, average, 1 Tbsp	35	2	2
Bacon Chips *(Durkee)*, 1 Tbsp	30	1	2
Bac-Os *(Betty Crocker)*, 1Tbsp	30	1.5	2
Blends *(Mrs Dash)*, 1 tsp	0	0	0
Butter Buds, 1 tsp	5	0	2
Flavor Enhancer *(Accent)*, 1 tsp	0	0	0
Flavor Sprinkles *(Molly McButter)*, Natural/Cheese, 1 tsp	5	0	1
Garlic Bread Sprinkle, 1 tsp	8	0.5	1
Garlic Salt, 1 tsp	2	0	0
Italian Seasoning, 1 tsp	4	0	1
Lemon Pepper Seasoning, 1 tsp	7	0	1
Meat Tenderizer, av., 1 tsp	7	0	1
Salad Crunchies *(McCormick)*, 1 tsp	10	0.5	2
Salt, Reg., Sea Salt, Lite Salt	0	0	0
Seasoning *(Old Bay)*, ¼ tsp	0	0	0
Seasoning Mix *(Vegit)*, ¼ tsp	0	0	0
Seasoning Mixes, av., ¼ pkg	70	1	9
Taco Seasoning, av., ¼ pkg	30	0.5	4
Bragg's, Liquid Aminos	0	0	0
Old El Paso: Chili Season. Mix, 1 Tbsp	8	0.5	1.5
Cheesy Taco Seasoning Mix, 1 Tbsp	10	0.5	2
Taco/Burrito Seasoning Mix, 2 tsp	15	0	4
Fajita Seasoning Mix, 1 tsp	5	0	1.5

Spices & Herbs

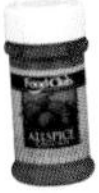

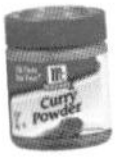

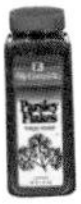

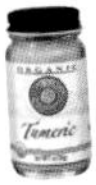

	C	F	Cb
Average all types, 1 tsp	5	0	1
All Purpose, 1 tsp	0	0	0
Allspice, ground	5	0	1
Chili Powder	8	0	1
Cinnamon, ground	6	0	2
Curry Powder	6	0	1
Garlic Powder	9	0	2
Nutmeg, ground	12	0	1
Onion Powder	7	0	2
Parsley, dried	4	0	1
Pepper, average	6	0	1
Saffron	2	0	0
Salt-Free Blends, 1 tsp	0	0	0
Tumeric, ground	8	0	1
Seeds: Fenugreek	12	1	2
Mustard, Poppyseed	15	1	1
Other varieties, average	7	0	1

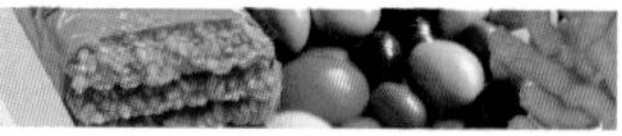

Home-Popped Popcorn

	C	F	Cb
Popping Corn Kernels, 2 Tbsp, 1 oz (makes approximately 5 Cups)	110	1	26
Air-popped, without oil: Plain, 1 oz	110	1	22
1 Cup, 0.2 oz	20	0	5
Oil-popped: Plain, 1 oz	145	8	16
1 Cup, 0.4 oz	55	3	6
Popcorn Oil, 1 Tbsp	120	14	0

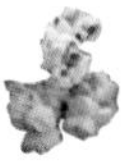

Microwave Popcorn

	C	F	Cb
Average all Brands: *Per 1 Cup Popped, Unless Indicated*			
Butter: Regular, 1 Cup	35	2	4
Light, 1 Cup	25	1	4
Act II Popcorn:			
Butter,			
Microwave, 2.75 oz bag	130	6	19
Butter Lovers: 1 Cup	30	1.5	4.5
4.5 Cups	140	7	20
Movie Theatre Butter/ Buttery Kettle Corn:			
1 Cup	35	2	4.5
4.5 Cups	150	8	19
Xreme Butter: 1 Cup	30	2	4
5 Cups	160	9	20
BodyKey *(Amway)*, Slim Popcorn, Sea Salt, 1 bag, 0.7 oz	110	7	10
Jolly Time:			
Blast O Butter, 1 Cup	45	3	4
Crispy 'n White Light, 1 Cup	25	1	4
Xtra Butter: 1 Cup	40	2.5	4
4 Cups	160	10	16
Newman's Own: *Per 3½ Cups*			
Microwave: Butter Flav.	150	8	16
Tender White	150	9	16
Sea Salt	150	9	16
Organic Butter	150	4.5	23
Orville Redenbacher's:			
Butter: 4½ Cups	170	12	17
Light, 6 Cups	160	6	27
Movie Theater Butter, 5 Cups	160	10	18
Ultimate Butter, 4½ Cups	160	9	19
Naturals, Simply Salted, 4½ Cups	170	11	18
Sweet & Savory:			
Cheddar Cheese, 4½ Cups	190	13	18
Melt On Caramel, 3 Cups	180	8	26
Pop Secret: *Per Cup*			
94% Fat-Free, Butter	20	0	3
Double Butter	40	2	3
Skinnygirl *(Orville Redenbacker's)*, **Butter/ Lime & Sea Salt,** 6 cups	160	6	28

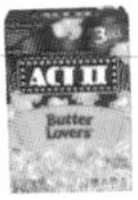
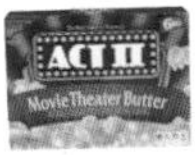
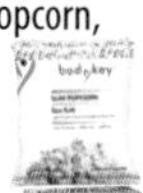
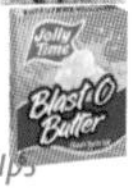
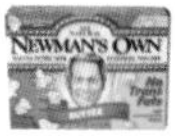
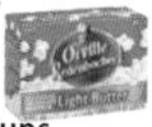
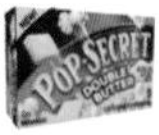

Bagged Popcorn

	C	F	Cb
Average All Brands (Ready-to-Eat)			
Regular/Plain: ½ oz package	80	5	8
1 oz package	160	10	16
4 oz package	640	40	64
2 oz Box (store/airport)	320	16	32
3 oz Bag (9" high x 5" wide)	480	24	48
Caramel Popcorn, with nuts, 1 Cup, 1.5 oz	230	12	39

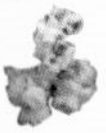

Bagged Popcorn ~ Brands

	C	F	Cb
Boston's, Lite, 3½ Cups, 1 oz	140	4.5	20
Cracker Jack: Original, 1 Cup, 2 oz	240	4	46
Chocolate & Caramel, 1 Cup, 2 oz	220	1	50
Crunch 'N Munch:			
Buttery Toffee: ⅔ cup, 1.1 oz	150	5	24
1 Cup, 1.65 oz	225	7.5	36
Caramel: ⅔ cup, 1.1 oz	160	7	22
1 Cup, 1.65 oz	240	10	33
fiddle faddle:			
Butter: ⅔ Cup	130	2	26
1 Cup	195	3	39
Caramel: ⅔ Cup	120	2	24
1 Cup, 2 oz	180	3	36
Popcorn Indiana:			
Kettlecorn: Maple, 1 oz	160	11	14
Sweet & Salty, 1 oz	130	7	16
Popcorn:			
Aged White Cheddar, 1 oz	130	10	12
Movie Theater, 1 oz	140	11	11
Sea Salt, 1 oz	150	9	15
Poppycock:			
Bags: Cashew Lovers, ½ Cup, 1 oz	150	6	20
Pecan Delight, ½ Cup, 1 oz	150	6	22
Cannisters, Orig./Pecan Delight, av:			
½ Cup, 1.1 oz	155	7	21
1 Cup, 2.2 oz	310	14	42
Skinny Pop:			
Original/Cheddar, avg., ¼ bag, 1 oz	150	10	15

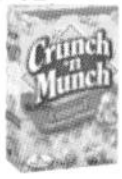
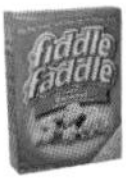
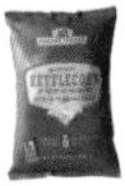
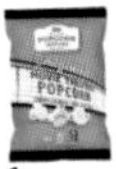

Movie Theater Popcorn

	C	F	Cb
Small, (7 Cups): Plain	385	21	44
with Butter (3 pumps, 0.8 oz)	570	42	44
Medium, (15 Cups): Plain	825	45	94
with Butter (4 pumps, 1 oz)	1075	73	94
Large, (20 Cups): Plain	1100	60	124
with Butter (6 pumps, 1.5 oz)	1485	102	124
Butter: 1 Pump, 0.3 oz	65	7	0
4 Pumps (2 Tbsp), 1 oz	250	28	0

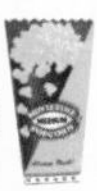

Corn & Tortilla Chips

	C	F	Cb
Average All Brands			
Corn Chips:			
Average all types: 1 oz	150	8	18
8 oz bag	1200	64	144
Fritos, Original, 32 chips, 1 oz	160	10	16
Tortilla Chips: Average, 1 oz	140	7	18
(1 oz = approx. 12 chips or 13 strips)			
Doritos: Original, 1 oz	140	7	18
Nacho Chse; Salsa Verde, av., 1 oz	145	8	18
Popchips: Barbecue, 1 oz	130	4.5	20
Buffalo Ranch, 1 oz	120	4	20
Snyder's:			
El Restaurante, all flavors, 1 oz	150	8	17
Yellow Corn/White, av., 1 oz	135	5	21
Tostitos:			
Average all flav., 1 oz	145	7	19
Baked! Scoops, 1 oz	120	3	22
Utz, Bar-B-Q Flavor Corn Chips	150	9	16

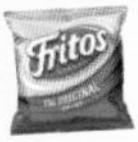

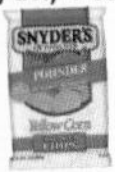

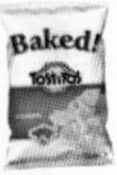

Potato Chips/Crisps

	C	F	Cb
Average All Brands			
Regular:			
Plain or flavored, (4 chips)	30	2	3
1 oz package (20 chips)	150	10	15
4 oz quantity	600	40	60
14 oz package	2100	140	210

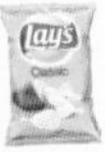

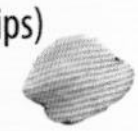

Chips/Crisps ~ Brands

	C	F	Cb
Hippeas, Chick Pea Puffs,			
average all flavors, 0.78 oz	90	4	11
Lay's *(Fritolay):*			
Classics; Wavy Originals, 1 oz	160	10	15
Kettle Cooked, Original, 1 oz	150	9	17
Pringles:			
All Flavors: 1 oz	150	9	16
Large can, 6 oz	900	54	96
Reduced Fat, Original, 1 oz	140	7	18
Ruffles: Regular, av. all flavors, 1 oz	150	9	15
Double Crunch, all flavors, 1 oz	150	8	17
Simply7, Hummus/Lentil Chips,			
average all flavors, 1 oz	135	5	19
Sun Chips: Original, 16 crisps, 1 oz	140	6	19
Whole Grain, Garden Salsa, 1 oz	140	6	19

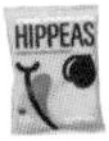

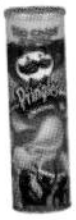

Pretzels

	C	F	Cb
Average All Brands			
Hard-Baked Pretzels: *Each*			
1 oz quantity	110	1	23
Sticks, thin, 2¼" (9/oz)	12	0	3
Twists, thin, ¼" thick, (5/oz)	25	0	5
Dutch (2¾"x 2⅝"), 0.5 oz	55	1	11
Snyders, Sourdough, 1 oz	110	0	23
Soft Pretzel Twists, average: *Each*			
Plain: Small, 2 oz	210	2	43
Medium, 4 oz	390	3.5	80
Large, 5 oz	485	4.5	100
Big Cheese, 1.8 oz	130	3	22
New York Street Vendors, 7 oz	660	6	135
Trader Joe's, Peanut Butter filled, 1 oz	140	8	14
Snyder's: Milk Chocolate Dips, 1 oz	150	7	20
White Creme Dips, 1 oz	140	6	21

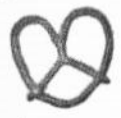
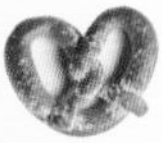

Pretzels ~ Brands

	C	F	Cb
Flipz: Milk Choc, 8 pieces, 1 oz	140	5	21
White Fudge, 7 pcs, 1 oz	140	5	21
Rold Gold *(Frito-Lay):*			
Braided Twists,			
Honey Wheat (8), 1 oz	110	1	23
Pretzel Thins, Orig. (9), 1 oz	110	1	23
Rods, Original (3), 1 oz	110	1	22
Tiny Twists, Original, (18), 1 oz	110	0	23
Sticks, Original, 1 oz	100	0	23
Snackwell's Pretzels, Minis:			
Fudge Dipped, 1 pack	100	4	16
Yogurt Dipped, 1 pack	100	5	16
Snyder's of Hanover:			
Butter Snaps, (24), 1 oz	120	1	25
Gluten Free, Sticks (32), 1 oz	120	3	24
Mini Pretzels,(20), 1 oz	110	0	25
Sticks, (26), 1 oz	110	1	23
Special K, Salted Choc. Coated, 1 oz	100	3	18
SuperPretzel:			
6 Count Soft, Original (1), 2.3 oz	160	0	34
Bites, (3), 2 oz	160	4.5	21
Softstix, (2), 1.76 oz	130	3.5	21
Utz:			
Sourdough Pretzels: Extra Dark, 1 oz	110	1	21
Hard (1)	90	0	18

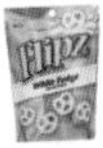

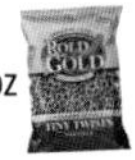
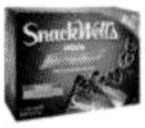
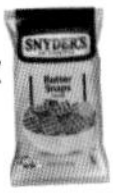

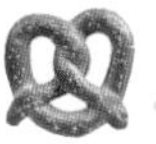

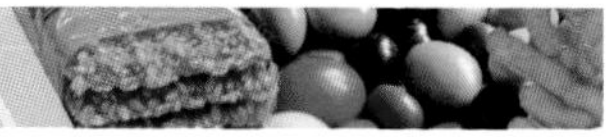

Snacks

Note: Actual weight of packaged snacks is usually 5-10% more than label Net Wt. For accuracy, weigh snack and allow extra calories, fat and carbs for any extra weight.

Snacks	C	F	Cb
Apple Chips *(Seneca),* av., 1 oz	140	7	20
Bagel Crisps *(N.Y. Style)*, 6 crisps, 1 oz	130	6	17
Baguette Chips, 1 oz	130	5	19
Banana Chips *(T.Joe's)*, 13 chips, 1 oz	160	11	13
Beef Jerky *(Jack Link's),* av., 1 oz	80	1	6
Beef Sticks:			
Slim Jim, Giant, Smoked, 1 oz	130	10	5
Jack Link's, Original (1), 1.5 oz	190	16	3
Beet Chips *(Rhythm)*, Sea Salt, 1oz	130	4	20
Trader Joes, 1.3 oz	140	0.5	29
BodyKey *(Amway)*:			
Zesty Protein Snack, 1 oz	120	3.5	15
Bugles, Orig.; Nacho Cheese, 1 oz	150	6.5	18
Cheese Balls *(Utz)*, 1 oz serving	150	9	16
Cheese Bites *(Tr. Joes)*, 1 oz	170	12	0.5
Cheese Nips *(Nabisco)*, (29), 1 oz	150	6	19
Cheese Puffs, average, 1 oz	160	10	15
Cheetos: 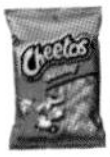			
Crunchy: Av. all flavors, 1 oz	165	10	15
4 oz package	640	40	60
Baked!; Fantastix, av., 1 oz	130	5	19
Simply Puffs, Wh. Cheddar, 1 oz	160	9	16
Cheez-It *(Sunshine)*:			
Snack Mix: Classic, ½ cup, 1 oz	140	5	20
Double Cheese, ½ cup, 0.9 ozz	120	5	17
Sweet & Salty, ½ cup, 1oz	140	5	21
Chester's: Fries, Flamin' Hot, 1 oz	150	8	17
Puffcorn, Cheese, 1 oz	160	11	13
Chex Mix *(General Mills)*:			
Muddy Buddies, Mint Choc, 0.9 oz	120	3.5	21
Traditional, 1 oz	130	3.5	23
Chicharrones ~ *See Pork Skins*			
Crackers *(Tr. Joes)*, Mini Edaname (28)	120	2	21
Churro Bites *(Great Value)*, Cinn., 1 oz	100	5	12
Combos, Crackers, av., ⅓ cup, 1 oz	140	6	18
Cool Cuts, Carrot & Ranch, 2.3 oz	60	5	6
Corn Chips ~ *See Page 149* 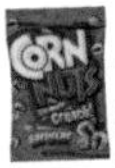			
Corn Nuts: Av all flav., 1 oz	130	4.5	20
1.7 oz bag	210	8	34
Corn Puffs, Buttery C'rml, 1 oz	130	4.5	22
Edamame,			
Seapoint Farms, Dry Roasted, 1 oz	130	5	9
Fritos,			
Corn Chips, Orig.; Flamin' Hot, 1 oz	160	10	16

Snacks (Cont)

Snacks (Cont)	C	F	Cb
Fruit Snacks ~ *See Page 102 & 151*			
Funyuns, Onion Flavored, 1 oz 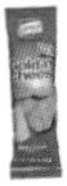	140	6	19
Goldfish, Crackers, av., 1 oz	140	5	20
Gold-n-Chees *(Lance)*:			
Snack Crackers, 1 oz	140	6	18
Gripz *(Sunshine)*, Mighty Tiny (1)	120	6	15
Flamin Hot Peanuts *(Munchies)*, 1 oz	170	15	5
Kale Chips *(Rhythm):* 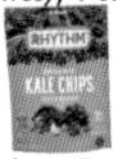			
Kool Rancch, 1 oz	130	9	6
Zesty Nacho, 1 oz	130	9	8
Lance ~ *See Sandwich Crackers Page 151*			
Munchies *(Frito-Lay)*,			
Snack Mix, all flavors, 1 oz	140	7	18
Munchos *(Fritolay)*, all flavors, 1 oz	160	10	16
Newtons: 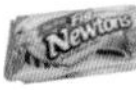			
Single Serve: 2 oz pkg	200	4	42
Fat-Free, 2 oz package	180	0	46
Nutella, w/ Breadsticks/Pretzels (1)	270	14	35
Nutter Butter, Sandwich Cookies: 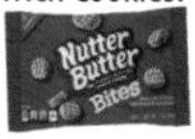			
2 Cookies	120	5	17
Bites, 1 pack	130	5	20
Wafers (5), 1.2 oz	160	9	19
Oreo Cookies, all Creme Fillings: 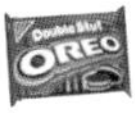			
Double Stuf (2), 1 oz	145	7	21
Mini: 1 Pack, 1 oz	135	5.5	20
Snak-Sak (9), 1 oz	140	6	21
Oriental Mix Rice Snacks, 1 oz	125	3.5	21
Peanut Butter Nuggets, (10), 1 oz	140	6	15
Pepitas, dried or roasted, 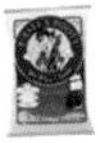			
¼ cup, 1 oz	155	14	3
Pirate's Booty: 1 oz	140	6	18
Aged White Cheddar, 4 oz	560	24	72
Veggie, 4 oz bag 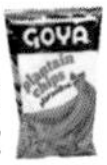	560	28	72
Pita Chips *(Stacy's)*, (10), 1 oz	130	5	9
Plaintain Chips *(Goya)*, 1 oz	150	8	19
PopChips Ridges, av., 1 oz	130	5	19
PopCorners, Kettle, 1 oz	125	3.5	20
Popcorn ~ *See Page 148*			
Pork Cracklins, 1 oz 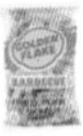	160	12	0
Pork Skins/Rinds: 1 oz	160	10	0
Baken-ets, Traditional, 0.5 oz	80	5	0
Mission, Chiccarones, 4 oz package	640	40	0
Potato Chips ~ *See Page 149*			
Potato Skins Chips *(TGI Friday)*,			
all flavors, 16 chips, 1 oz	140	8	16
Puffed Wheat, 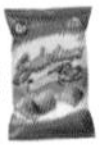			
Sabritones, Chili & Lime, 1 oz	140	8	16
Pretzels ~ *See Page 149*			

Snacks (Cont)

	C	F	Cb
Rice Cakes:			
Lundberg: Honey Nut (1)	80	0.5	19
Thin Stackers, Brown Rice (4), 1 oz	110	1	4
Quaker:			
100% Whole Grain, lightly salted (1)	35	0	7
Chocolate (1)	60	1	12
Rice Chips,			
Lundberg, average, 1 oz	135	6	18
Sandwich Crackers:			
Austin, Cheese Sandwich Crackers:			
w/ Cheddar, 1.4 oz	190	9	24
w/ Peanut Butter, 1.3 oz	190	9	24
Cheese Crackers, with PB, 0.8 oz	130	6	15
Lance: Nekot Lemon Creme, 1pkg	240	11	35
Toasty, PB, 1 pkg	180	9	21
Toast Chee, PB, 1.5 oz	220	10	25
Ritz Bits: Cheese (13), 1 oz Pkg	160	9	19
P'nut Butter:,1.5 oz pkg	220	13	24
Sesame Sticks, Salted,			
SunRidge Farm, 1 oz	170	11	14
Smart Puffs,			
Pirates Booty, 1 oz	140	7	17
Soybeans in Pods,			
AFC, ½ Cup, 3.2 oz	90	5	3
Soy Crisps, average, 1 oz	120	3	17
Soy Nuts: Dry Roasted, ¼ cup, 1 oz	130	6	9
Choc-Coated, 1 oz	140	7	13
Sun Chips,			
Fritolay, average, 1 oz	140	6	19
Takis: Crunchy Fajitas, 1 oz	140	8	17
4 oz package	560	32	68
Tings *(Robert's)*, 2 oz bag	300	16	36
Toasted Chips (*Ritz***)**, av. all, 1 oz	130	5.5	20
Tortilla Chips, White,			
Garden of Eatin, Touch of Lime, 1 oz	130	7	17
Trail Mix (Nuts/Seeds/Dried Fruit):			
Regular, 3 Tbsp, 1 oz	140	9	13
Tropical, 3 Tbsp, 1 oz	130	7	16
Turkey Jerky: Teriyaki, 1 oz	80	1	8
Trader Joe's, Original, 1 oz	60	0.5	6
Veggie Crisps,			
Snyder's, 1 oz	150	8	19
Wheat Thins *(Nabisco)*, av. all, 1 oz	135	5	21
Woats, Oatsnack, av., ¼ cup, 1 oz	120	5	17
Yogurt Pretzels *(Larissa)*, 5 pces, 1 oz	150	8	20
Yogurt Raisins, Vanilla,			
Sun-Maid, 1 oz	120	4.5	20

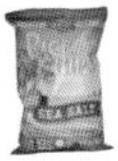
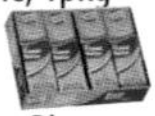
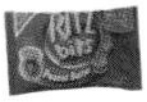
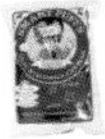
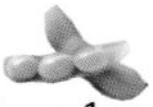
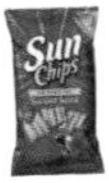

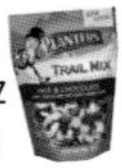

Fruit Snacks

	C	F	Cb
Betty Crocker: Fruit Gushers, 0.9 oz	80	1	18
Fruit by the Foot, 1 roll, 0.8 oz	80	1	17
Fruit Roll Ups, 1 roll, 0.5 oz	50	1	11
Sunkist:			
Fruit Lover's Trail Mix:			
Pineapple Coconut Blend, 1 oz	120	5	18
Strawberry Banana, 1 oz	110	4	19

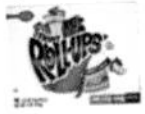

Fruit Snack Cups ~ See Page 102

Vending Machines

	C	F	Cb
Bugles, Nacho Cheese, 1 oz	150	9	18
Cheese Balls *(Utz)*, 1 oz	150	9	16
Cheetos, Crunchy, av., 1 oz	165	10	15
Cheeze-It, Classic Snack Mix, 1 oz	140	5	20
Chester's, Flamin' Hot Fries, 1 oz	150	8	17
Choc Chip Cookies:			
Chips Ahoy, 2 oz pkg	280	14	38
Famous Amos, 1.2 oz pouch	170	8	23
Grandma's, (1), 1.4 oz	200	10	25
Chocolate Bars:			
Hershey's, Milk Choc.,1.5 oz	220	13	26
Kit Kat, 1.5 oz	210	11	28
Snickers, 1.7 oz bar	250	12	32
Donut, plain cake, 1.4 oz	160	9	18
Doritos, av. all flavors, 1 oz	145	8	18
Fritos, Corn Chips, Orig., 2.75 oz	440	28	44
Fruit Pie,			
Hostess, Apple, 4.5 oz	430	17	67
Granola/Cereal Bars, av., 1 oz	140	3	26
M & M's:			
Milk Chocolate, 2 oz	280	10	40
Peanuts, 2 oz	280	14	34
Oreo Cookies, (3), 1.2 oz	160	7	25
Peanut Butter Cups,			
Reese's, 1.5 oz	210	12	24
Popcorn, plain, 1 oz	160	10	16
PopChips Ridges, 1 oz	130	5	19
Pork Skins, 1.5 oz	240	15	0
Potato Chips: 1 oz	150	10	15
Baked! *(Ruffles)*, Orig.,1 oz	120	3	22
Potato Skins Chips *(TGI Friday's)*,			
all flavors, 1 oz	140	8	16
Pretzels *(Snyder's)*, Olde Tyme, 1 oz	120	1	24
Raisins, 0.5 oz package	45	0	11
Rice Krispies Treat, Original, 0.78 oz	90	2	17
Skittles, Original,1 oz	110	1	26
Starburst, Fruit Chews, Orig., 1 oz	120	2.5	24
Tortilla Chips, 1 oz	140	7	18

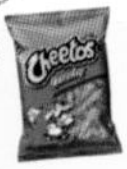
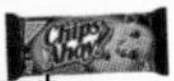
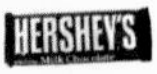

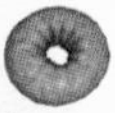
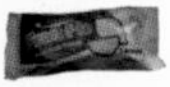
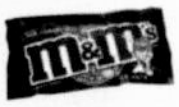
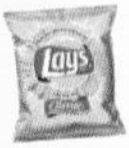

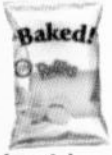

Updated Nutrition Data ~ www.CalorieKing.com
Persons with Diabetes ~ See Disclaimer (Page 22)

S Soups

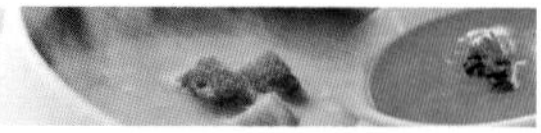

Homemade & Restaurant

Restaurant & Take-Out: *Average All Preparations: Per 8 fl.oz*	C	F	Cb
Bean Medley	**200**	3	34
Beef Consomme	**30**	0	2
Borscht, with Sour Cream	**130**	8	14
Bouillabaisse	**400**	15	10
Chicken & Corn	**290**	14	20
Chicken & Wild Rice	**80**	4	9
Chicken Consomme	**50**	0	2
Chicken Curry	**180**	8	18
Chicken Jambalaya	**160**	7	8
Chicken Noodle	**80**	2	12
With Chicken	**160**	4	12
Chicken Soup	**80**	2	6
Chili with Beans	**250**	12	25
Clam Chowder	**240**	15	17
Corn & Crab	**120**	3	18
Corn Chowder	**150**	8	16
Cream of Broccoli	**200**	12	20
Cream of Potato	**150**	6.5	17
Cream of Mushroom	**200**	13	15
Fish Chowder	**220**	15	6
French Onion	**420**	15	25
Gazpacho	**50**	0	5
Lentil Soup	**250**	9	28
Lobster Bisque	**320**	15	10
Matzo Ball, with 1 large ball	**180**	7	24
Minestrone	**125**	2.5	20
Mulligatawny	**300**	15	8
Pea & Ham	**240**	10	25
Potato & Bacon	**170**	7	19
Pumpkin, Creamy	**210**	10	26
Shark Fin Soup	**100**	4	8
Spicy Shrimp Soup, 1 bowl	**160**	7	10
Split Pea Soup	**180**	2.5	30
Vegetable (Fat Free)	**75**	0	18
Vegetable Beef	**80**	2	10
Vichyssoise	**200**	9	15
Watercress	**90**	4	13

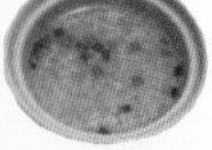
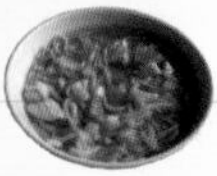
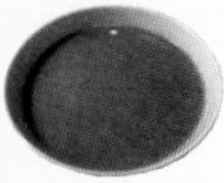
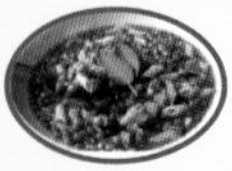
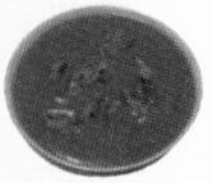
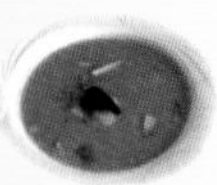

Other Soups ~ *See International & Fast-Foods Sections (Arby's, Au Bon Pain, Boston Market, Dunkin' Donuts, Denny's, Schlotzsky's, Sizzler, Souplantation,Sweet Tomatoes, Zoup!)*

Homemade Soups: *Calculate calories, fat and carbohydrates from recipe ingredients.*

Bouillon Cubes & Powders

Bouillon Cubes: *Average all types*	C	F	Cb
Regular, 1 cube	**5**	0	1
Extra Large, 1 cube	**20**	1	1
Powders, average, 1 tsp	**10**	0	1
Herb-Ox:			
Instant Broth & Seasoning,			
Beef, 1 envelope, 0.14 oz	**5**	0	1
Chicken, 1 envelope, 0.14 oz	**5**	0	1

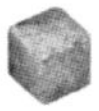
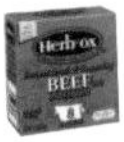

Soup ~ Brands

Amy's:

Heat & Serve (Organic): *Per 1 Cup,*			
Alphabet	**110**	2	21
Black Bean Vegetable	**140**	1.5	26
Chunky Vegetable	**70**	1.5	11
Carrot Ginger	**200**	13	18
Cream of M'shrm, $^3/_4$ cup	**150**	9	13
Lentil Vegetable	**160**	4	24
Rustic Italian Vegetable	**250**	9	35
Southwestern Vegetable	**140**	5	20
Split Pea	**110**	1	19
Thai Coconut	**210**	14	15
Thai Curry Sweet Pot. Lentil	**280**	20	20
Tuscan Bean & Rice	**170**	4.5	28

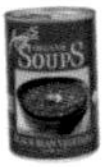

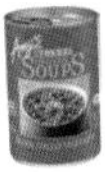

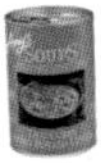

Campbell's:

Chunky: *Per Cup, Unless Indicated*			
Baked Potato w/ Ched. & Bacon Bits	**190**	9	22
Baked Potato with Steak & Cheese	**190**	9	21
Beef with Country Vegetables	**110**	1.5	16
Buffalo-Style Chicken Soup	**150**	7	15
Chicken Corn Chowder	**190**	9	20
Chipotle Chkn & Corn Chowder	**180**	8	20
Classic Chicken Noodle	**120**	3	14
Creamy Chkn & Dumplings	**170**	9	14
Grilled Chicken & Sausage Gumbo	**140**	3.5	21
Hearty: Bean & Ham, Smoked	**150**	1.5	27
Jambalaya Chkn, Ssg & Ham	**140**	4	20
Manhattan Clam Chowder	**100**	2.5	15
Old Fashioned Vegetable	**110**	2	16

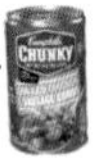

Campbell's (Cont):

Condensed Soup: *Per ½ Cup*

	C	F	Cb
Beef Broth	15	0	1
Beef Consume	20	0	1
Beef with Veggie & Barley	100	1	18
Broccoli Cheese	100	5	11
Cheddar Cheese	90	4	14
Chicken Gumbo	70	2	12
Cream of: Asparagus	100	7	8
Celery	100	7	8
Mushroom with Roasted Garlic	90	5	9
Onion	120	7	12
French Onion	70	1.5	13
Golden Mushroom	80	3.5	10
Mega Noodle	60	2	8
Old Fashioned Tom. Rice	120	1.5	25
Tomato	90	0	20
25% Less Sodium,			
Cream of Mushroom	100	7	8
98% Fat Free:			
Broccoli Cheese	80	2.5	11
Cream of: Celery	60	2.5	9
Chicken	60	2	8
Mushroom	60	2	9

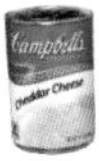

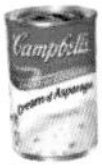

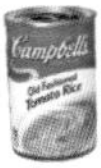

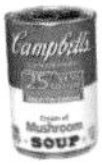

Healthy Request: *Per ½ cup, Unless Indicated*

	C	F	Cb
Beef with Country Vegetables	110	1.5	17
Cheddar Cheese	60	1	12
Chicken Corn Chowder	140	3	22
Chicken Noodle	110	3	13
Golden Mushroom	70	2.5	10
Old Fashioned Vegetable Beef	110	2	17

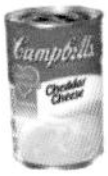

Homestyle: *Per Cup*

	C	F	Cb
Chicken Noodle	60	2	8
Chkn w/ Whole Grain Pasta	70	1.5	10
Harvest Tomato with Basil	110	1	23
Mexican-Style Chkn Tortilla	130	2	20
New England Clam Chowder	170	10	15
Savory Chicken with Brown Rice	110	2.5	16

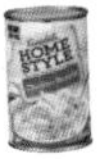

Soup on the Go: *Per Container*

	C	F	Cb
Cheesy Chicken Tortilla	100	4	13
Cheesy Potato w/Bacon Flav.	130	6	16
Classic Tomato	140	0.5	32
Creamy Tomato	230	10	30
Creamy Tomato Parmesan Bisque	230	8	35

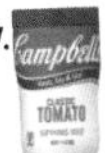

Campbell's (Cont):

Slow Kettle Style: *Per Container*

	C	F	Cb
Baked Potato with Smoked Bacon	440	32	32
Creamy Broccoli Cheddar Bisque	370	28	23
Mediterranean Vegetable	180	2	34
Rstd Red Pepper & Gouda Bisque	320	20	30
Tomato & Sweet Basil Bisque	550	33	56
Vegetarian Black Bean	340	3	61

Health Valley Organics: *Per Cup*

	C	F	Cb
40% Less Sodium:			
Chicken Noodle	80	2	11
Vegetable	90	0	18
Creamed:			
Cream of Chicken	120	3	17
Cream of Mushroom	90	1.5	16
No Salt Added:			
Chicken & Rice	100	1.5	19
Chicken Noodle	80	2	11
Lentil	150	1.5	27
Minestrone	100	2	18
Split Pea	160	2.5	26
Tomato	110	2	22
Vegetable	90	2	15

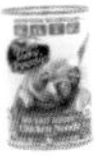
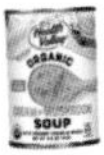

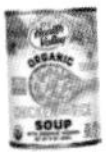

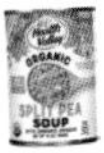

Healthy Choice:

Canned: *Per Cup*

	C	F	Cb
Chicken & Dumplings	150	3	22
Chicken Noodle	90	2	12
Chicken with Rice	110	3	15
Country Vegetable	100	0.5	21
Vegetable Beef	120	1	21

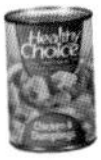

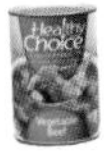

Imagine:

Broths, Organic: *Per Cup*

	C	F	Cb
Beef	20	1	2
Free Range Chicken	20	1	2
Vegetable, unsalted	20	0	4
Vegetarian, No-Chicken	15	0	2

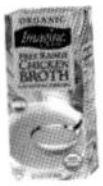

Chunky Style, Organic: *Per Cup*

	C	F	Cb
Italian Style Wedding	150	5	20
Italian Vegetables & Beans	130	2	25
Loaded Baked Potato	120	5	18
Moroccan Chickpea & Carrot	100	1	1
Tomato Bisque	80	3	15
White Bean & Kale	110	1	21

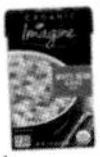

Continued Nex Page...

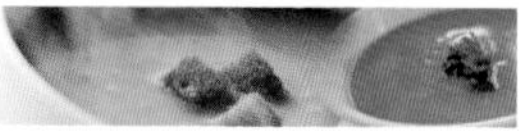

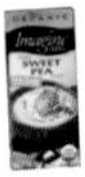
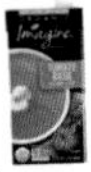

Imagine (Cont):	C	F	Cb
Creamy: *Per 8 fl.oz Cup*			
Butternut Squash	100	2	20
Broccoli	70	1	14
Garden Tomato, Light Sodium	80	1	16
Potato Leek	90	3	14
Portobello Mushroom	80	3	12
Tomato; Tomato Basil, av.	85	1	16

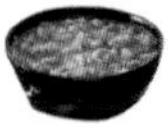
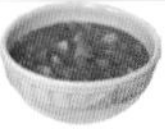
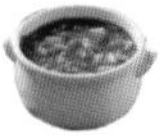

Kettle Cuisine: *Per 8 fl.oz Cup*	C	F	Cb
Albondigas Meatball Soup	150	7	17
Beef, Barley & Vegetable	110	3	13
Broccoli Cheddar	320	24	16
Buffalo Chicken	240	15	14
Carrot Ginger	110	4	18
Chicken Tortilla	120	3	15
Chipotle Sweet Potato	150	6	22
Classic Gazpacho	60	1	10
Cream of Crab	290	22	16
Hot Honey & Butternut Squash	140	4	26
Lobster Bisque	250	18	18
Manhattan Clam Chowder	120	3	16
Minestrone	80	2	14
North Atlantic Haddock Chowder	260	17	14
Organic, Split Pea	80	1	13
Portuguese Kale with Linguica	170	7	23

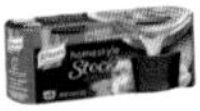

Knorr:	C	F	Cb
Cubes: *Per ½ Cube, 1 Cup, Prepared*			
Beef; Chicken; Vegetable, average	12	1	0.5
Homestyle Stock: *Per 1 Tsp*			
Beef	10	0.5	1
Chicken	10	1	0.5

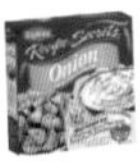

Lipton:	C	F	Cb
Cup-a-Soup: *Per Envelope, 6 fl.oz Prepared*			
Chicken Noodle, White Meat	50	1	8
Cream of Chicken Flavor	70	1.5	12
Recipe Secrets:			
Onion, 1 Tbsp	20	0	4
Onion Mushroom, 1⅔ T.	35	0	7
Savory Herb w/ Garlic, 1 T.	30	0	6

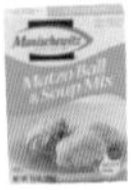

Manischewitz:	C	F	Cb
Dry Soup Mix:			
Matzo Ball, 0.5 oz	40	0	8
Tetra Pack: *Per 1 cup*			
Chicken Broth	15	0.5	1

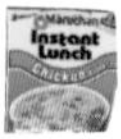

Maruchan:	C	F	Cb
Instant Lunch, average all flavors, 1 pkg	290	12	38
Ramen, all flavors, 1 pkg, 3 oz	380	14	52

Nissin:	C	F	Cb
Soup'd Up Cup Noodles: *Per Package*			
Roasted Chicken Flavor, 2.57 oz	330	12	45
Savory Shrimp Flavor, 2.57 oz	330	13	45
Souper Meal, Beef, 1.45 oz pkg	550	22	753

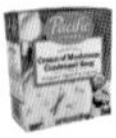
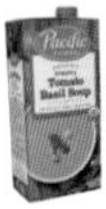
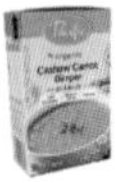

Pacific Foods:	C	F	Cb
Condensed: *Per Container*			
Cream of Chicken	190	6	23
Cream of Mushroom	190	8	27
Creamy: *Per 1 Cup*			
Golden Cauliflower	120	6	13
Moroccan Sweet Potato	130	5	19
Tomato Basil	90	2	13
Hearty Organic: *Per 1 Cup*			
Butternut Squash Bisque	120	3	22
Cashew Carrot Ginger Bisque	140	5	22
Coconut Curry	200	9	28
Rosemary Potato Chowder	170	8	22

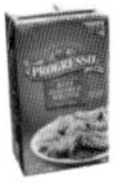
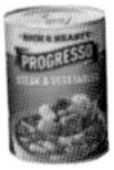
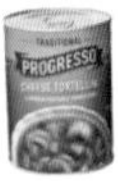
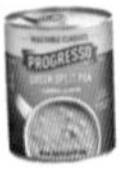
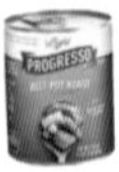

Progresso: *Per Cup*	C	F	Cb
Broths: Beef	15	0	1
Classic Chicken	5	0	0
Vegetable	5	0	1
Rich & Hearty:			
Beef Pot Roast w/ Country Vegetables	110	1.5	16
Chicken & Homestyle Noodles	110	2.5	14
Chkn Pot Pie w Dumplings	130	4	17
Lasagna Style w Ital Ssc	170	7	20
Minestrone w/ Italian Ssg	150	5	17
New England Clam Chowder	170	7	23
Steak & Vegetables	100	1.5	16
Traditional: *Per 1 Cup*			
Cheese Tortellini Garden Vegetable	100	1	20
Chickarina	110	4	12
Chicken & Rotini	90	1.5	13
Italian-Style Wedding	120	4	15
Manhattan Clam Chowder	100	2	17
Potato, Broccoli & Cheese	210	13	19
Vegetable Classic: *Per 1 Cup*			
Creamy Mushroom	130	9	12
Green Split Pea w/ Bacon	150	1.5	29
Minestrone	110	2	20
Tuscan-Style White Bean	130	1.5	23
Light: *Per 1 cup*			
Beef Pot Roast	70	1	9
Broccoli Cheese	120	6	11
Chicken Noodle	60	0.5	9
Vegetable	70	0	15

Swanson:	C	F	Cb
Broth: *Per 8 fl.oz Cup*			
Beef, unsalted	15	0	1
Chicken/Chicken unsalted	10	0	1
Organic Chicken	15	0	0.5
Vegetable	10	0	2
Stock: Beef	15	0	1
Chicken	20	0	1
Vegetable	15	0.5	2
Tabatchnick:			
Frozen:			
Dairy: *Per 7.5 oz Pouch*			
Corn Chowder	130	4.5	21
Cream of Mushroom	100	5	11
New England Potato	140	4.5	21
Gluten Free: *Per 7.5 oz Pouch*			
Balsamic Tomato & Rice	100	1.5	20
New England Potato	140	4.5	21
Old Fashioned Potato	100	1.5	21
Southwest Bean	220	5	36
Split Pea	180	0.5	33
Tuskany Lentil	160	0	29
Wilderness Wild Rice	90	0.5	19
Low Sodium: *Per 7 .5oz Pouch*			
Barley & Mushroom	80	0.5	17
Split Pea	110	1.5	20
Vegetable	110	1.5	20
Meat: *Per 7.5 oz Pouch*			
Chkn Broth with Noodles & Dumplings	120	4	16
Chkn Broth NY Style w/ Noodles & Veg.	70	1.5	12
Frenchman's Onion	60	1.5	11
Pareve: *Per 7.5 oz Pouch*			
Barley & Mushroom	80	0.5	17
Black Bean	220	2.5	38
Cabbage	90	0.5	21
Minestrone	110	1.5	19
Vegetarian Chili	200	3.5	32
Yankee Bean	180	1.5	32
Thai Kitchen:			
Rice Noodle Soup Bowls: *Per Bowl*			
Hot and Sour Rice Noodle	250	4	51
Lemongrass & Chili	250	3.5	52
Roasted Garlic	250	3	52
Spring Onion	260	4.5	50
Thai Ginger	260	3	52

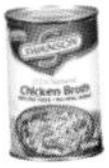
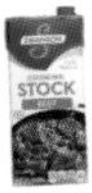

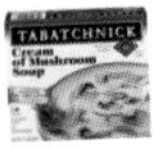

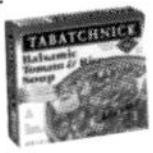

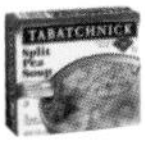

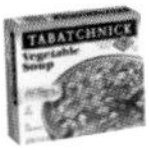

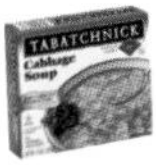

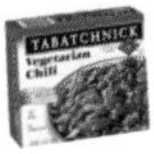

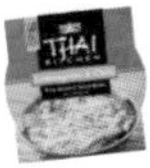

Trader Joe's:	C	F	Cb
28 fl.oz Cans: *Per Cup*			
Chunky, Low Fat:			
Lentil with Vegetables	140	3	21
Minestrone	110	2.5	19
14.5 oz Cans: *Per Cup*			
Organic: Black Bean	140	1.5	26
Lentil Vegetable	160	4	24
Split Pea	100	0	19
10.75 oz Can,			
Low Sodium, Minestrone	200	4	37
15 oz Can,			
Low Fat, Chicken Noodle, 1 cup	90	1	14
32 fl oz. Cartons: *Per Cup*			
Butternut Squash	90	2	16
Carrot & Ginger	80	1	17
Creamy Corn & Rstd Pepper	110	2	23
Latin Style Black Bean	70	1	12
Sweet Potato Bisque	130	1	28
Organic: Butternut Squash	70	0	17
Tomato & Rstd Red Pepper	100	3.5	15
Low Sodium, Creamy Tomato	90	3.5	15
17.6 fl.oz Cartons: *Per Cup*			
Beef, Barley with Veggies	100	0.5	16
Chicken Noodle with Veggies	100	1	16
Ramen Soups: *Per 43g Container*			
Chicken	180	4	29
Miso	180	3	31
Whole Foods: *Per Cup*			
365 Organic:			
Caribbean Black Bean	170	0	35
Chicken Noodle	70	0	10
Lentil	100	0	18
Minestrone	140	1.5	23
Sthwestern Black Bean	120	1	23
Vegetable Medley	70	0	16
Condensed,			
Cream of Mushroom, ½ cup	60	1.5	10
Wolfgang Puck: *Per Cup*			
Organic:			
Chicken with White & Wild Rice	130	4	18
Classic Minestrone	120	2.5	20
Creamy Butternut Squash	140	11	10
Old Fashioned Potato	170	10	20
Thick Hearty Lentil Vegetable	160	1	29
Tomato with Basil	150	6	21
Tortilla	160	3.5	27
Vegetable	130	5	19

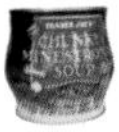
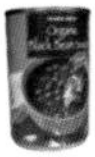
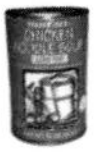
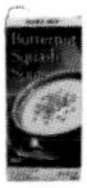
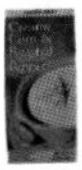
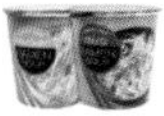
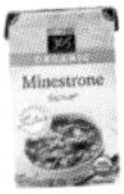

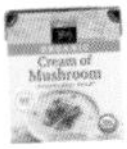

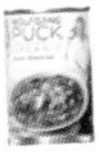

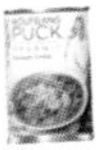

Soybean Products

	C	F	Cb
Cheeses (Soy) ~ *See Page 78*			
Miso Soy Bean Paste:			
Cold Mountain: Light Yellow, 1 tsp	10	0	1
Mellow Red, 1 tsp	15	0	3
Red, 1 tsp	10	0	1
Miso Soup (dry mix):			
1 Tbsp., dry mix	35	1	5
1 cup, prepared	35	1	5
Natto, ½ cup, 3 oz	160	7	14
Okara (Tofu fiber residue), ½ c., 2 oz	47	1	8
Tempeh: 1 piece, 3 oz	180	8	12
Fried, 3 oz	250	14	14
Seitan *(Westsoy)*, Strips, 3 oz	120	2	4
Soybean Protein *(TVP)*, 1 oz	95	0	8
Soy Bean Paste, 1 tsp	10	0	2
Soy Beans ~ *See Page 160*			
Soy Drinks ~ *See Page 49*			

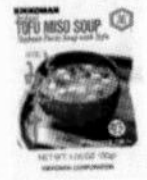

Tofu ~ Brands

	C	F	Cb
Azumaya Tofu:			
Extra Firm; Firm, av., 3 oz	70	4	2
Firm (Silken), 3.2 oz	50	2.5	2
House Foods: *Per 3 oz*			
Premium: Firm	70	4	2
Extra Firm	80	4.5	2
Grilled, Super Firm	80	4.5	3
Medium Firm	60	3	2
Soft (Silken)	60	3	2
Super Firm, cubed	80	4.5	2
Organic Tofu: Firm	70	4	2
Extra Firm	70	3.5	2
Grilled, Super Firm	70	3.5	3
Mori-Nu Tofu: *Per 3 oz*			
Extra Firm	45	1.5	1
Firm Silken	50	2	1
Lite	30	1	0
Organic, Silken	45	2	1
Soft	45	2	1
Nasoya: *Per 3 oz*			
Organic: Extra Firm	80	4	3
Firm	70	3.5	2
Silken	45	2	1
Organic Tofubaked: *Per 3.5 oz*			
Sesame Ginger	150	8	5
Teriyaki	140	7	6
Organic Toss'ables,			
Garlic & Herb, 3 oz	150	8	5

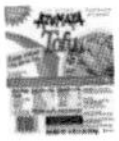
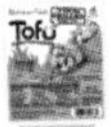

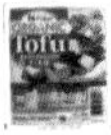
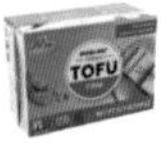

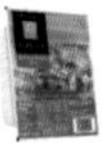
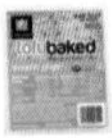

Supplements

	C	F	Cb
Aloe Vera Juice, undiluted, 2 fl.oz	5	0	1
Flakes, 1 heaping Tbsp, 0.3 oz	30	0.5	4
Powder, 1 heaping Tbsp, 0.5 oz	50	0.5	6
Tablets, 2 tabs	4	0	0.5
Calcium Chews: *CVS*, 1 chew	20	0	3
Trader Joe's, Chocolate, 1 chew	20	1	3
Cod Liver Oil, 1 Tbsp	125	13	0
Fiber Choice, 2 tabs	15	0	4
Fiber,			
Fibersure, 1 heaping tsp	25	0	6
Fish Oil Capsules, (1), av.	10	1	0
Flax Oil:			
Capsules (2)	10	1	0
Barlean's, softgels (3)	110	11	0
Garlic Tablets/Capsules, each	3	0	0
Glowelle:			
Beauty Drink, 8 fl.oz	100	0	24
Powder Stick (1)	50	0	12
Lecithin Granules, 1 Tbsp	55	4	0.5
Metamucil, Powder:			
Orange (Smooth Texture),			
1 rounded Tbsp	45	0	12
Sugar-Free, 1 rounded tsp	20	0	5
Pink Lemonade, Sugar-Free,			
1 rounded tsp	20	0	5
Capsules: Heart & Digestive (6)	10	0	3
Strong Bones (5)	10	0	3
Meta, Fiber Wafers (2)	100	4.5	16
Protein, Powders, av., 1 oz	100	0.5	0
Seaweed: Dried, 1 oz	85	0.5	22
Soaked, drained, 1 oz	15	0.5	3
Spirulina, 1 tablet	2	0	0.5
Vitamins/Minerals: Tabs/Caps (1)	2	0	0
Vitamin E Capsules, each	5	0.5	0
Viactiv Chews, Choc. (1)	20	0.5	4

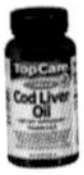

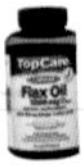

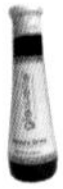
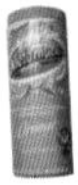
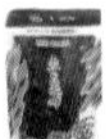
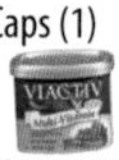

Cough & Pharmaceutical

	C	F	Cb
Antacids: Av., 1 tablet	4	0	1
Liquid, 1 Tbsp	6	0	1
Antacid Sodium Counts ~ *See Page 280*			
Cough/Cold Syrups:			
Regular: With sugar, 1 Tbsp	35	0	9
With alcohol, 1 Tbsp	46	0	9
Diabetic Tussin, Sugar Free, 1 T.	0	0	0
Cough Drops/Lozenges ~ *See Page 75*			
Sudafed, Syrup 1 tsp	14	0	3
Tylenol, Liquid: Child, 1 tsp	17	0	4
Extra Strength, 1 tsp	11	0	3

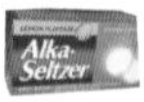

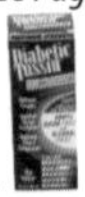

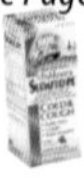

Sugar

	C	F	Cb
White Sugar, granulated:			
1 level teaspoon, 4g	15	0	4
1 heaping teaspoon, 6g	25	0	6
1 Tablespoon, 12g	50	0	12
1 ounce, 1 oz	110	0	28
1 cup, 7 oz	775	0	200
1 lb (16 oz)	1760	0	454
Single Portion Packages:			
1 stick	15	0	4
1 packet	15	0	4
1 cube	10	0	2.5
Brown Sugar: 1 Tbsp	50	0	13
1 ounce, 1 oz	110	0	28
1 cup, not packed, 5 oz	550	0	140
1 cup, packed, 7.8 oz	835	0	216
Powdered Sugar:			
Sifted, 1 cup, 3.5 oz	390	0	100
Unsifted, 1 cup, 4¼ oz	470	0	120
Coconut Palm Sugar, 1 tsp, 4g	15	0	4
Dextrose, 1 tsp	12	0	3
Fructose, powder, 1 tsp	12	0	3
Glucose Powder, 1 oz	110	0	27
Glucose Tablets, (1)	20	0	5
Palm Sugar, 3 Tbsp	45	0	11
Piloncillo, (Brown Sugar), 3oz	325	0	81
Turbinado Sugar, 2 Tbsp, 1 oz	110	0	27

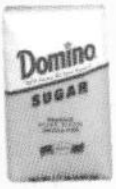

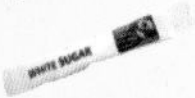
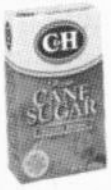

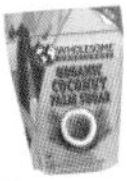

Sugar Substitutes

	C	F	Cb
Agave, 1 Tbsp, 0.7 oz	60	0	16
DiabetiSweet, 1 teaspoon	9	0	4.5
Note: Carb figure includes 4.5 g sugar alcohol			
Domino, Light, ½ tsp	5	0	2
Equal: Tablet (2)	0	0	0
Granular, 1 tsp	0	0	0
Packet (1)	0	0	0
Next, 1 packet	0	0	0
Nectresse, 1 packet	0	0	0
NutraSweet, 1 tsp	0	0	0
Splenda, Granulated No Calorie Sweetener:			
1 tsp	0	0	0
1 cup	95	0	24
Packets, all flavors	0	0	0
Sugar Blend,Orig/Brown, ½ cup	385	0	96
Stevia, single serving	0	0	0
Sugar Twin, 1 packet	0	0	0
Sweet 'N Low, 1 packet	0	0	0
Truvia, 1 packet	0	0	0
Walgreens, Wal-Sweet, 1 packet	0	0	0
Whey Low, 1 tsp	4	0	1

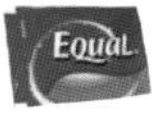

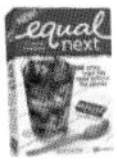

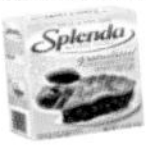

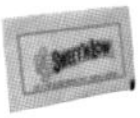

Syrups, Molasses, Agave

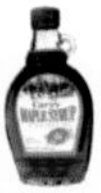

Syrups, Plain: *Average All Brands (Corn/Rice/Maple/Pancake/Sundae/Waffle) Includes Aunt Jemima, Cary's, Karo, Hershey's, Hungry Jack, IHOP, Log Cabin, Mrs Butterworth's*

	C	F	Cb
Regular/Dark/Light Color:			
1 Tbsp, 0.5 fl.oz	55	0	14
¼ cup (4 Tbsp)	220	0	55
Single Portion, 1.5 oz pkg	170	0	42
Lite, 1Tbsp, 1 oz	25	0	6
Sugar-Free: 2 Tbsp, 1 oz	18	0	5
Maple Grove, Cozy Cottage, 2 Tbsp	10	0	3
IHOP, 4 Tbsp, 2 oz	20	0	7
Fruit Syrups, *(IHOP)*, ¼ cup, 2 oz	200	0	52
Honey Cream Syrup, ¼ cup, 2 oz	220	0	55
Molasses: Dark/Light: 1 T, 0.7 oz	60	0	15
1 cup, 12 oz	975	0.5	252
Blackstrap, 1 Tbsp, 0.8 oz	47	0	13
Agave Nectar, av. all flavors,			
1 Tablespoon, 0.8 oz	60	0	15

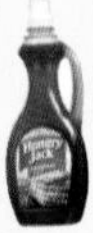
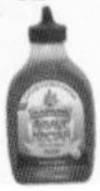

Flavored Syrups/Ice Cream Toppings

	C	F	Cb
Hershey's: *Per 2 Tbsp*			
Double Chocolate,	200	0	50
Choc.; Strawb; Caramel, av.	95	0	25
Sugar Free	10	0	6
Smuckers: *Per 2 Tbsp*			
Magic Shell, average all flavors	215	16	16
Spoonables: Hot Caramel/Fudge, av	140	3.5	27
Sugar Free: Caramel; Hot Fudge	90	0.5	24
Strawberry	30	0	10
Note: Carb figures include 9g-17g sugar alcohol			
Sundae Syrups: Regular, av. all flavors	105	0	25
Sugar Free, average all flavors	95	0.5	24
Note: Carb figures includes 15g-16g sugar alcohol			

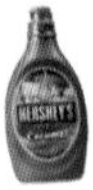

Honey, Jam, Preserves

Average all Brands

	C	F	Cb
Honey: 1 tsp, 0.23 oz	20	0	5.5
1 Tbsp, 0.7 oz	60	0	17
1 oz	85	0	24
½ cup, 6 oz	515	0	145
Single Portion, 0.5 oz package	45	0	12
Jams/Jellies/Marmalade/Preserves:			
Regular: 1 tsp, 0.3 oz	20	0	5
1 Tbsp, 0.8 oz	55	0	14
1 ounce, 1 oz	80	0	20
Single Portion, 0.5 oz pkg	40	0	11
Apple/Fruit Butters, 1 T., 0.6 oz	20	0	6
Fruit Spreads: Regular, 1 tsp	15	0	4
Low Sugar, 1 tsp	8	0	2
Jelly: Regular, average, 1 tsp	18	0	4.5
Imitation, Low Calorie, 1 tsp	4	0	1

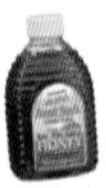
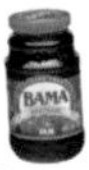

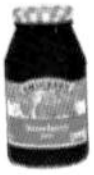

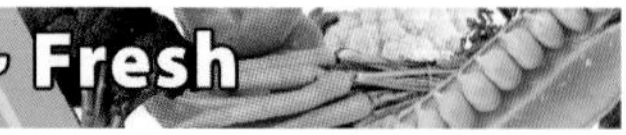

Vegetables

Vegetables	C	F	Cb
Alfalfa Sprouts, ½ cup, 0.5 oz	5	0	0.5
Artichokes, Globe/French:			
1 medium, 4.5 oz	60	0	13
1 large, 5.7 oz	75	0	17
Artichoke Heart, plain, 2 pieces	15	0	3
Asparagus, raw/frozen:			
Cuts & Tips, ½ cup, 4.3 oz	20	0	3
Spears, 3 medium	10	0	2
Bamboo Shoots, cooked, ½ cup, 2 oz	7	0	1
Beans, Green/Snap/String:			
10 beans (4" long), 2 oz	20	0	4
Pieces, ½ cup, 3 oz	30	0	7
Dried Beans (Kidney, Brown, Lima, Navy, Pinto, White):			
Raw: 2 Tbsp, 1 oz	95	0.5	18
1 cup, 7 oz	665	3	126
Cooked: 1 oz	35	0	7
½ cup, 3 oz	105	0	21
Bean Sprouts, average, ½ cup, 2 oz	15	0	3.5
Beets (Beetroot):			
Raw, 1 beet (2" diam.), 4 oz	35	0	8
Cooked, 1 cup, slices, 3 oz	35	0	8
Canned ~ *See Page 161*			
Beet Greens, cooked, ½ cup, 2.5 oz	20	0	4
Bell Pepper ~ *See Peppers*			
Bitter Melon/Gourd, 1 cup, 1.5 oz	15	0	1.5
Blackeye Peas, cooked, ½ cup, 3 oz	100	0.5	18
Bok Choy (Chinese Chard), cooked, 3 oz	10	0	1.5
Breadfruit, ¼ small fruit, 3 oz	100	0	26
Broadbeans (Fava Beans):			
Green, raw, (in pod): 4 pods (3.5 oz with shells, 1.2 oz beans)	30	0	6
1 cup beans, without shell, 4.5 oz	110	1	22
Mature Seeds: Raw, 1 cup, 5.3 oz	510	2.5	87
Cooked, ½ cup, 3 oz	95	0	17
Broccoflower, ⅕ head, 3.5 oz	35	0	7
Broccoli: Raw, chopped, 1 cup, 3 oz	30	0	6
3 Florets, 2.5 oz	25	0	5
1 Spear (5" long), 1.oz	10	0	2
1 Whole: Medium, 14 oz	135	1.5	26
Large, 21 oz	205	2	40
1 Head (no stalk), 11 oz	105	1	21
1 Stalk, small (5" long), 5.3 oz	50	0.5	10
Brocco Sprouts, ½ cup, 1 oz	15	0	2
Brussels Sprouts:			
Cooked, ½ cup, 2.8 oz	30	0.5	6
2 Sprouts, 1.5 oz	15	0	3
Butterbeans, cooked, ½ cup, 3 oz	90	0	16
Cabbage, average other flavors:			
Raw: 1 leaf, large, 1 oz	5	0	2
Shredded, 1 cup, 2.5 oz	15	0	4
½ large head (7" diam), 22 oz	150	1	35
Cooked, shredded, ½ cup, 2.5 oz	15	0.5	3.5

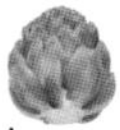
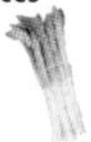
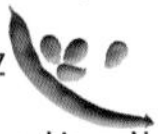
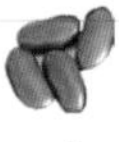
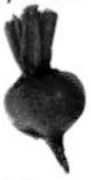
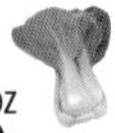
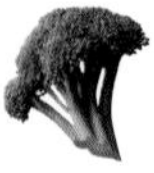
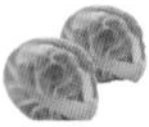
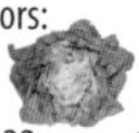

Vegetables (Cont)

Vegetables (Cont)	C	F	Cb
Cactus Leaf (Nopales):			
1 leaf, 4.5 oz	20	0	4
1 cup (slices), 3 oz	15	0	3
Carrots, regular thick variety:			
1 small, 4 oz	45	0	11
1 medium, 6 oz	70	0	16
1 large, 8 oz	95	0	22
Chopped, 1 cup, 4.5 oz	50	0	12
Grated, 1 cup, 4 oz	45	0	11
Slices, 1 cup, 4.5 oz	50	0	12
Sticks (4"), 4-5, 1.5 oz	20	0	4
Long thin variety, 1 medium, 2.2 oz	25	0	6
Baby: Snack size, 3 medium, 1 oz	10	0	2.5
Snack Pack, 3 oz	30	0	7
Cassava, raw, 1 cup, 2.5 oz	330	0.5	78
Cauliflower, raw:			
Pieces, 1 cup, 3.5 oz	25	0	5
½ medium head, 10 oz	70	0	15
Cooked, 3 florets, 2 oz	10	0	2
Celeriac, ½ cup, raw, 2.8 oz	35	0	7
Celery: 1 large stalk, 11", 2.2 oz	10	0	2
4 Strips, thin sticks, 0.5 oz	5	0	1
Chopped, 1 cup, 3.5 oz	15	0	3
Chard (Swiss), ½ cup, cooked, 3 oz	20	0	3.5
Chayote Squash:			
1 medium, 7 oz	40	0	9
Pieces, 1 cup, 4.5 oz	25	0	6
Chickpeas, (Garbanzo Beans):			
Dry, 1 cup, 7 oz	730	12	121
Cooked, 1 cup, 5.8 oz	270	4	45
Chicory Greens, 1 cup, 1 oz	7	0	1.5
Chili Peppers ~ *See Peppers*			
Chinese Long Bean, slices, 1 cup, 3.2 oz	45	0	8
Chives, chopped, 1 Tbsp	1	0	0
Choy Sum, 3 oz	15	0	3
Cilantro, (Coriander), 1 cup	5	0	0.5
Collards, cooked, ½ cup, 3 oz	25	0	5
Corn, Yellow/White:			
Raw: Kernels, ½ cup, 3 oz	80	0.5	19
Ear (5"x 1¾"), 5.5 oz	155	1	37
Cooked: Kernels, ½ cup, 3 oz	77	0.5	18
Cob, small, 2.3 oz	60	0.5	14
Ear, large, 5.5 oz	120	1	28
Cress, garden, raw, 1 cup, 1.8 oz	15	0	3
Cucumber, average other flavors:			
Slices, ½ cup, 2 oz	10	0	2
Green, 1 medium (9"), 11 oz	45	0	11
Persian, 1 medium (8"), 6 oz	25	0	5
Daikon Radish, ½ cup, slices, 2 oz	9	0	2
Dandelion Greens, raw, ½ cup, 1 oz	10	0	2.5
Edamame, (Immature green soybeans):			
Shelled, ½ cup, 2.6 oz	110	5	8
With shells, 10 pods, 1.3 oz	30	1	3

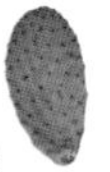
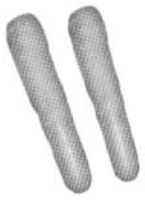
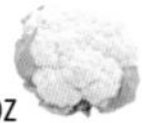
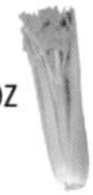
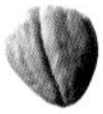
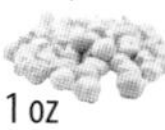
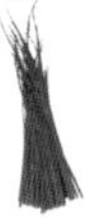
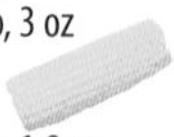
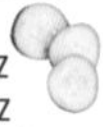
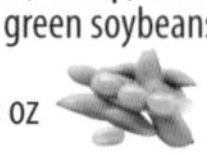

Vegetables (Cont)	C	F	Cb
Eggplant, raw: 4 oz	30	0	7
½ cup, 1" pieces, 1.5 oz	10	0	2
1 slice, fried, 1 oz	75	4	10
Endive, Belgian/French: Raw,			
1 medium head (6"), 2.5 oz	12	0	3
Fennel, 1 cup, sliced, 3 oz	25	0	7
Gai Choy Cabbage, cooked, 1 cup, 6 oz	20	0	3
Gai Lan, (Chinese Kale), cooked, 1 cup	35	0.5	7
Garbanzo Beans ~ *See Chick Peas*			
Garlic, 1 clove	4	0	1
Ginger: ¼ cup slices, 1 oz	20	0	5
Crystallized (sugared), 7 pieces, 1.5 oz	130	0	35
Horseradish, raw, 1 pod, 0.5 oz	5	0	1
Jerusalem Artichoke, raw, ½ cup	55	0	13
Jicama, raw, sliced, ½ cup, 2.3 oz	25	0	6
Kale, 1 cup, chopped, 2.5 oz	35	0.5	7
Kalettes, 1 cup, 2 oz	30	0	4
Kohlrabi, cooked, ½ cup, 1.8 oz	17	0	5
Leek, cooked, 1 whole, 4.5 oz	40	0	9
Lentils, green/brown: Dry, 1 oz	100	0.5	17
1 cup, 6.8 oz	675	3	115
Cooked, ½ cup, 3.5 oz	115	0.5	20
Lettuce: 1 cup, chopped/shredded, 2 oz	7	0	1
Butterhead, 2 leaves, 0.5 oz	2	0	0.5
Cos/Romaine, shredded, 1 cup	10	0	2
Iceberg: 1 outer leaf, 0.5 oz	2	0	0.5
1 medium head, 16 oz	75	1	16
Lima Beans, baby, cooked, ½ cup, 3 oz	105	0	20
Lotus Root, cooked, 10 slices, 3 oz	60	0	14
Mung Bean Sprouts, ½ cup, 2 oz	15	0	3
Mushrooms, average all varieties:			
Raw, diced/siced, 1 cup, 3 oz	20	0	3
Pieces, 1 cup, 1.3 oz	8	0	1
Fried/Sauteed, 6 oz	220	16	10
Grilled, pieces, ½ cup, 2.5 oz	20	0.5	4
Shitake, dried, 1 oz package	90	0	22
Mustard Greens, raw, ½ cup, 1 oz	7	0	2
Okra: Raw, 8 pods, 4 oz	30	0	7
Cooked, ½ cup, 2.8 oz	20	0	4
Onions, Raw: 1 small, 2.5 oz	30	0	7
1 medium, 4 oz	50	0	11
1 large, 5.5 oz	65	0	15
1 jumbo, 16 oz	190	0.5	46
Chopped: ½ cup, 3 oz	35	0	8
1 Tbsp, 0.4 oz	5	0	1
Slices: 1 cup, 4 oz	50	0	12
1 medium slice (⅛"), 0.5 oz	5	0	1
1 large slice (¼"), 1.3 oz	15	0	4
Flakes, dried ¼ cup, 0.5 oz	50	0	12
Rings, breaded & fried, 2 rings	80	5	9
Scallions, ½ cup, 2 oz	15	0	3
Spring, chopped, ½ cup, 2 oz	15	0	3

Vegetables (Cont)	C	F	Cb
Parsley, chopped, ½ cup, 1 oz	10	0	2
Parsnip: 1 medium, 4 oz	85	0	20
Cooked, slices, ½ cup, 2.8 oz	55	0	13
Peas: Green, raw, ¼ cup, 1.5 oz	30	0	5
With pods, 0.5 lb	70	0	13
Snow Peas, 10 pods, 1.2 oz	15	0	3
Split: Dry, hulled, 1 oz	100	0.5	17
Cooked, 1 cup, 7 oz	230	1	42
Peppers:			
Sweet, 1 medium, 4.2 oz	30	0	7
Bell: 1 medium, 4.2 oz	30	0	7
raw, chopped, ½ cup, 2.5 oz	20	0	5
2 rings (5" diam. x ¼" thick)	3	0	1
Chili: Green/Red, 1.5 oz	20	0	5
Habanero, 1 only, 0.3 oz	10	0	2
Pigeon Peas, cooked, ½ cup, 3 oz	95	1	17
Pimientos, 3 medium, 3.5 oz	25	0	5
Poi, ½ cup, 4.2 oz	135	0	33
Potatoes:			
Raw (with skin):			
1 baby, 2 oz	45	0	10
1 small, 6 oz	135	0	30
1 medium, 8 oz	180	0	40
1 large, 12 oz	270	0	60
1 extra large, 16 oz	360	0	80
Baked, (no added fat), 1 medium:			
Plain: With skin, 7 oz (cooked wt)	185	0	42
Without skin, 5.5 oz (cooked wt)	145	0	34
With Skin/Toppings:			
With 2 tsp fat	255	8	42
With Grated Cheese, 1 oz	300	9	42
With Plain Yogurt, 2 Tbsp	220	2	45
With Sour Crm & Chives, 2 Tbsp	240	5	43
Mashed:			
With milk plus fat, ½ cup, 4 oz	120	4.5	18
KFC Style without gravy, 4 oz	90	3	15
Loaded (fat/cream/cheese/bacon):			
Side serving, 6 oz	180	9	22
Large serving, 12 oz	360	18	44
Roasted, with oil:			
Whole, 1 small, 3 oz	140	5	20
Diced, 1 cup, 5 oz	180	8	30
Potato Skins, baked w/ cheese topping,			
½ whole, 4 oz	240	13	22
French Fries: Small serving, 2.6 oz	250	13	30
Medium serving, 4 oz	380	20	47
Frozen, uncooked, 18 fries, 4 oz	165	5.5	28
Oven-heated, 18 fries, 4 oz	165	5.5	28
Take-Out, 1 cup, 5 oz	440	25	60
Au Gratin, ½ cup, 4.3 oz	160	9	14
Scalloped, 8.5 oz	220	9	26

Persons with Diabetes ~ See Disclaimer (Page 22)

Vegetables (Cont)

	C	F	Cb
Pumpkin:			
Raw, 1" cubes, 1 cup, 4 oz	30	0	7
Cooked:			
Baked, without fat, 4 oz	90	7	9
Mashed: 1 scoop, 2 oz	10	0	2
1/2 cup, 4.3 oz	25	0	6
Pumpkin Flowers, 1 cup, 1.2 oz	5	0	1
Purslane: Cooked, 1/2 cup, 2 oz	10	0	2
Raw, 1" cubes, 1 cup, 1.5 oz	5	0	1.5
Radicchio: 2 leaves, 0.5 oz	5	0	1
Shredded, 1 cup, 1.5 oz	20	0	4
Radishes: 1 small	0	0	0
10 medium/5 large, 1.6 oz	5	0	1
Slices, 1/2 cup, 2 oz	10	0	2
Rhubarb, raw, 1/2 cup, 2 oz	15	0	3
Rutabaga, cubes, cooked, 1/2 cup, 3 oz	30	0	7
Salsify, cooked, slices, 1/2 cup, 2.5 oz	50	0	11
Sauerkraut, 1/2 cup, 2.5 oz	15	0	3
Seaweed: Dried, 1 oz	5	0	2
Soaked, drained, 1 oz	15	0	4
Nori/Laver, dried, 6 sheets, 0.5 oz	35	0	5
Shallots, chopped, 1 Tbsp, 0.5 oz	5	0	1
Sorrel, raw, 1/2 cup, 4 oz	20	0	4
Soybeans: Dry, 1/2 cup, 3.3 oz	390	18	28
Mature, dry, 1 oz	120	5.5	9
Cooked, 1/2 cup, 3 oz	150	7.5	8
Soy Products/Tofu/Tempeh ~ *See Page 156*			
Spinach: Cooked, 1/2 cup, 3 oz	20	0	4
Creamed, average, 1/2 cup, 4.5 oz	190	15	8
Raw: 3 leaves,1 cup, 1 oz	7	0	1
1 Bunch, 12 oz	80	1.5	12
Squash:			
Summer: Raw, 1/2 cup, 2.5 oz	10	0	2
Cooked, slices, 1/2 cup, 3 oz	15	0	3
Winter, cooked:			
Acorn: Cubes, 1/2 cup, 3.5 oz	35	0	9
1/2 medium (10 oz raw weight)	115	0	30
Butternut: Cubes, 1/2 cup, 3.5 oz	40	0	10
1/4 medium (9 oz raw weight)	115	0	30
Spaghetti, 1/2 cup, 1.8 oz	15	0	3
Succotash, cooked, 1/2 cup, 3.3 oz	110	1	23
Sweetcorn ~ *See Corn*			
Sweet Potatoes:			
Cooked with skin (w/o fat), 1 medium, 4 oz	105	0	24
Without skin, mashed, 1/2 cup, 5.5 oz	125	0	29
Fries (Alexia, Julienne syle), approximately 12 pieces, 3 oz	140	5	24

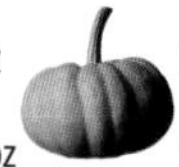
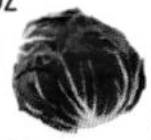
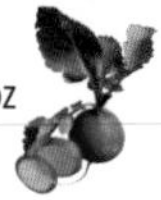
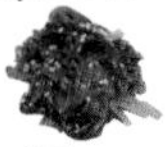
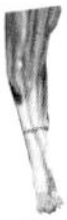
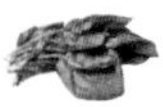
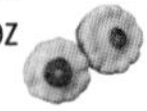
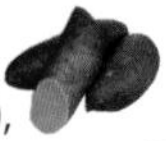

Vegetables (Cont)

	C	F	Cb
Swiss Chard, cooked, chopped,1 c., 6 oz	35	0	7
Taro, cooked, 1/2 cup, 2.3 oz	95	0	23
Tomatoes: 1 small (2 1/4" diam.), 3 oz	15	0	3
1 medium (2 3/4" diameter), 5 oz	25	0	5
1 large (3 1/2" diameter), 8 oz	40	0.5	9
1 extra lge (4" diam.), 12 oz	60	0.5	14
Chopped, 1 cup, 6.5 oz	35	0.5	7
Tomatillo: 1 medium, 1.2 oz	10	0	2
1lb quantity for recipe	135	4.5	27
Turnip: Cooked, 1/2 cup, 2.8 oz	15	0	4
Greens, cooked, 1/2 cup, 2.5 oz	15	0	3
Water Chestnuts: 5-6 nuts, 1 oz	56	0.5	13
Raw, slices, 1/2 cup, 2.3 oz	60	0	15
Canned, 1 oz	15	0	3
Watercress, 10 sprigs, 1 oz	3	0	0.5
Yams: Cooked, steamed, 1/2 cup, 2.5 oz	80	0	19
Baked:			
1 medium (6") 8 oz	265	0.5	63
1 large (9") 12 oz	400	0.5	94
Yardlong Bean, 1 pod, 0.5 oz	5	0	1
Yucca Root, raw, 1/2 cup, 3.5 oz	165	0	39
Zucchini: Raw, 1 medium, 7 oz	30	0.5	7
1 large, 12 oz	60	1	12
Cooked, slices, 1/2 cup, 3 oz	15	0	4

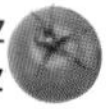
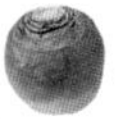
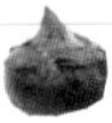
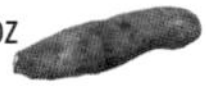
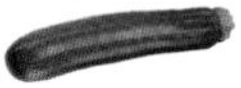

Frozen Vegetables

	C	F	Cb
Birds Eye:			
Flavor Full:			
Buffalo Cauliflower, 3.3 oz	50	2	7
Ranch: Broccoli, 3 oz	50	1.5	5
Cauliflower, 3.3 oz	50	2	6
Salt & Vinegar Potatoes, 3.9 oz	150	4	25
Steakhouse Green Beans, 3 oz	60	2.5	6
Teriyaki Broccoli, 3 oz	50	1.5	7
Steamfresh:			
Asparagus Spears (6)	20	0	3
Chopped Kale, 3.1 oz	25	0	4
Cut Green Beans, 3 oz	30	0	5
Mixtures: Brocc. Cauliflower, 3 oz	25	0	4
Brocc, Cauliflower, Carrots,	30	0	5
Italian Blend, 2.7 oz	30	0	5
Roasted Red Potato Blend, 2.7 oz	50	0	11
Power Blends: Barley Kale, 10 oz	240	3.5	40
Black Rice & Edamame, 10 oz	290	4.5	48
Chickpea & Spinach, 10 oz	320	7	51
Quinoa & Spinach, 10 oz	310	5	57

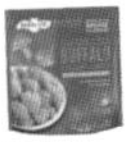
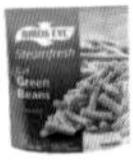

Frozen Vegetables (Cont)

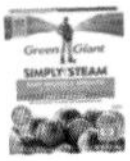

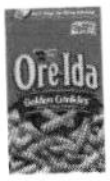

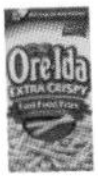

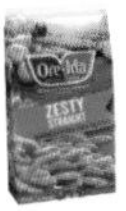

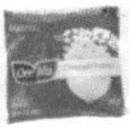

Item	C	F	Cb
Green Giant:			
Grilled, Zucchini, 3.17 oz	40	0.5	7
Mashed Cauliflower: Original, 4.2 oz	80	5	7
Cheddar & Bacon, 4.2 oz	90	6	6
Garlic & Herb., 4.2 oz	80	4.5	8
Marinated Veggies: *Per ⅓ Package*			
Eggplant, Peppers & Zucchini, 4.33 oz	70	3	7
Mushrooms, 3.3 oz	80	7	4
Riced Veggies: *Per ¼ Cup, 1.76 oz*			
Chickpea, Cauliflower	180	2.5	32
Red Lentils, Green Pea, Chickpea	180	1.5	32
Roasted Veggies:			
Brussels Sprouts, 3 oz	30	0	6
Corn, 3 oz	120	1.5	25
Simply Steam: *Prepared*			
Baby Bruss. Sprouts & Butter Sce, ½ c.	50	1.5	8
Baby Lima Beans, 1/2 cup	80	0	14
Chopped Spinach, ⅓ cup	20	0	3
Garden Vegetable Medley, ½ cup	70	0.5	14
Riced Cauliflower & Cheese Sce, ½ c.	70	3	10
Sugar Snap Peas, ½ cup	40	0	9
Sweet Peas, ½ cup	60	0	12
Ore-Ida: *Per 3 oz Unless Indicated*			
Fries:			
Classic: Golden Crinkles	90	4.5	12
Golden Fries	90	4	13
Steak Fries	80	3	13
Extra Crispy:			
Fast Food Fries	130	7	16
Golden Crinkles	130	7	16
Seasoned Crinkles	150	6	22
Flavored:			
Country Style French Fries	90	4	13
Garlic & Bl. Pepper Steakhouse Fries	150	8	16
Zesty Curly Fries	150	9	17
Zesty Straight Fries	140	8	16
Hash Browns:			
Golden Patties (1)	120	8	10
Potatoes O'Brien	50	0	12
Shredded Hash Brown Potatoes	60	0	13
Mashed Potatoes: Bites (8)	170	10	17
Homestyle Steam 'n' Mash, 3.35 oz	60	0	15
Onion:			
Gourmet Rings, 2.7 oz	185	9	24
Onion Ringers, 2.85 oz	180	10	21
Sweet Potato Straight Fries	150	7	19
Tater Tots, Reg., Crispy Crowns, av.	135	9	12

Updated Nutrition Data ~ www.CalorieKing.com
Persons with Diabetes ~ See Disclaimer (Page 22)

Canned/Bottled

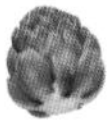

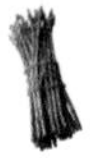

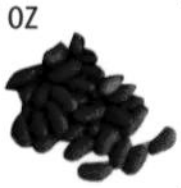

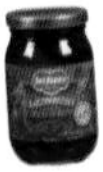

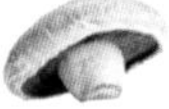

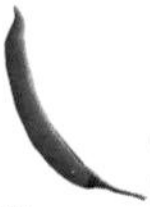

Item	C	F	Cb
Solids & Liquid			
Artichoke Hearts:			
Fancifoods: Plain, 1 oz (1)	8	0	1
Marinated, ¼ bottle, 1 oz	25	1.5	2
Asparagus: Drained, 3 spears	10	0	1.5
Pieces, ½ cup, 4.3 oz	25	0.5	3
Bamboo Shoots, 1 cup, 4.5 oz	25	0	4
Bean Salad, ½ cup, 4.4 oz	90	0	20
Beans: Baked, ½ cup, 4.5 oz	120	0.5	27
Butter, ½ cup, 4.5 oz	90	0	16
Green, ½ cup, 2.5 oz	15	0	3
Italian, ½ cup, 4.5 oz	30	0	6
Kidney, ½ cup 3.5 oz	105	0.5	19
Lima, ½ cup, 4.5 oz	80	0	15
Pinto, ½ cup, 4.5 oz	105	1	18
Beets: Sliced, ½ cup, 3 oz	25	0	6
Crinkle/Pickled, ½ cup	80	0	20
Carrots: Sliced, ½ cup, 2.5 oz	20	0	4
Del Monte, Honey Glazed, ½ cup	75	0	18
Corn: Kernels, ½ cup, 4.5 oz	80	0.5	18
Creamed style, ½ cup, 4.5 oz	90	0.5	23
Garbanzo/Chick Peas, ½ c, 4.2 oz	145	1.5	27
Hearts of Palm, (1), 1.2 oz	7	0	1
Mushrooms: ½ cup, 2.5 oz	20	0	4
In Butter Sauce, 2 oz	20	1	2
Onions: Cocktail (1)	0	0	0
Pickled, 1 medium, 0.5 oz	10	0	2
Peas, ½ cup, 3 oz	60	0.5	10
Peppers: Hot Chili, Jalapeno (1), 1 oz	5	0	1
Red/Green, 1 oz	5	0	1
Sweet, undrained, 2.5 oz	13	0	3
Jalapeno, with liquid, ½ cup chopped	20	0.5	3
Fried, drained, 2 Tbsp, 1 oz	60	5	3
Salsa, average all varieties, 2 Tbsp	10	0	2
Sauerkraut, drained, 1 cup, 5 oz	25	0	6
Spinach, ½ cup, 3.5 oz	25	0.5	3.5
Succotash: Cream Style, ½ cup	100	0.5	23
w/ whole kernels, undrained, ½ cup	80	0.5	18
Sweetcorn ~ *See Corn*			
Sweet Potato, ½ cup, 3.5 oz	90	0	24
Tomatoes, Sundried: Nat., 5-6 pieces	20	0	5
In Oil, drained, 6 pieces, 0.5 oz	40	2.5	4
Tomato Products ~ *See Page 144*			
Vegetables, mixed, ½ cup, 4 oz	45	0	8
Yams: In Light Syrup, ½ cup, 4 oz	105	0	25
Candied, ½ cup, 5 oz	170	0	46
Zucchini, in Tomato Sauce, ½ cup, 4 oz	30	0	8

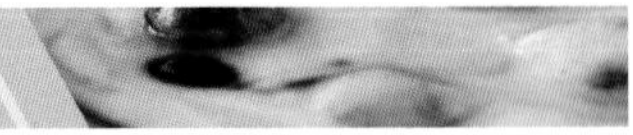

Quick Guide

	C	F	Cb
Yogurt: *Average All Brands: Per 8 oz Container*			
Plain Yogurt: Whole	140	8	10
Low-Fat	145	3.5	16
Fat-Free	125	0.5	17
Fruit Flavored: Whole	225	8	32
Low-Fat	230	3	43
Fat-Free, regular	215	0.5	43
Fat-Free, no sugar added	80	0	15
Yogurt Parfait/Deli Cups:			
With Fruit Pieces: (2/3 Yogurt + 1/3 Fruit)			
Small, 8 oz cup	140	3	20
Large, 12 oz cup	210	4.5	30
With Fruit + Granola:			
Small, 8 oz cup (+ 0.75 oz Granola)	235	7	30
Large, 12 oz cup (+ 1.3 oz Granola)	400	13	58

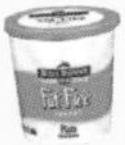

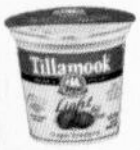

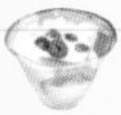

Yogurt ~ Brands

	C	F	Cb
Activia:			
Dairy Free, all flavors	120	4	18
Probiotic Yogurts: *Per 4 oz Container*			
60 Calorie, all flavors	60	0	10
Greek: Vanilla	140	0	23
Other Flavors	120	0	17
Less Sugar, all flavors	130	4.5	11
Lacatose Free, Strawberry	90	2	15
With Fiber, Strawberry	90	0	22
With Fruit, average all flavors	85	1.5	15
With Fruit On The Bottom, all	90	2	15
Axelrod:			
32 oz Ctn: Regular Plain, 8 oz	160	8	15
Fat Free, Plain, 8 oz	130	0	19
6 oz Containers:			
Low Fat, Fruit flavors, av.	180	1.5	36
NonFat Vanilla	90	0	17
Brown Cow:			
Cream Top: *Per 5.3 oz Ctn*			
Whole Milk: Plain	130	7	11
Cherry Vanilla; Choc	160	5	26
Coffee; Vanilla	150	6	19
Average Other Flavors	155	6	23

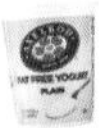

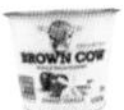

	C	F	Cb
Cabot: *Per 8 oz Serving*			
Greek Style:			
Whole Milk, Plain	230	16	9
Lowfat (2%): Plain	130	3.5	8
Strawberry; Vanilla Bean	180	2.5	26
Triple Cream, Vanilla Bean	260	13	26
Nonfat, Plain	80	0	13
Chobani Greek Yogurt: *Per 5.3 oz Unless Indicated*			
Blended: Coconut	140	4.5	15
Mixed Berry	140	2.5	17
Coconut Based: Plain, slightly swt	130	8	16
Average Other flavors	140	7	20
Creamy Blended, average	150	4.5	17
Flip: Almond Coco Loco	230	10	23
Coffee Brownie Bliss	180	4	25
Fruit On The Bottom:			
Apricot; Mango; Strawb Banana, av,	130	2.5	16
Strawberry/Blueberry	110	0	16
Gimmies, average all flavors, 4 oz	145	4	20
Less Sugar, all flavors, 5.3 oz	120	2.5	11
Nut Butter, average all flavors, 5.3 oz	165	7	15
Plain, 32 oz Ctn:: Lowfat, 8 oz	130	3.5	7
Nonfat, 8 oz	90	0	6
Whole Milk, 8 oz	170	9	7
Dannon:			
Activia ~ *See Activia*			
Creamy, Strawberry, 4 oz	70	0	14
Fruit On The Bottom, all flavors, 5.3 oz	130	1.5	25
Lowfat: Plain, 6 oz	100	2.5	12
Coffee; Vanilla, 6 oz	140	2	24
Plain, 32 oz Ctn: Lowat, 8 oz	110	2.5	12
Nonfat, 8 oz	80	0	13
Whole Milk, 8 oz	110	6	7
Fage Greek Yogurt:			
Best Self: Plain, 5.3 oz	110	3	5
Blueberry, 5.3 oz	120	2.5	14
Strawberry, 5.3 oz	110	2.5	12
Vanilla, 5.3 oz	100	2.5	11
Total: Plain 5% Milk Fat, 7 oz	190	10	6
Plain, 2% Milk Fat, 7 oz	140	4	6
Plain, 0% Milk Fat, 6oz	90	0	5
Total Split Cups: *Per 5.3 oz*			
5% Milk Fat: Fruit Flav., av.	150	6	13
Honey	210	6	28
2% Milk Fat: Fruit Flavors	120	2.5	13
Honey	180	2.5	28
Tru Blend: *Per 5.3 oz*			
Fruit Flavors	110	2.5	10
Vanilla; Coconut	110	2.5	9

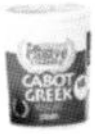

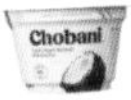

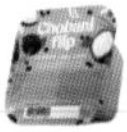

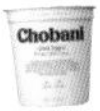

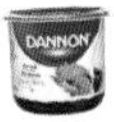

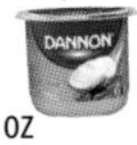

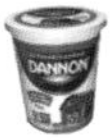

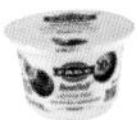

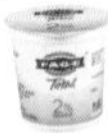

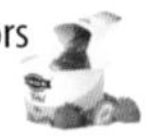

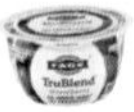

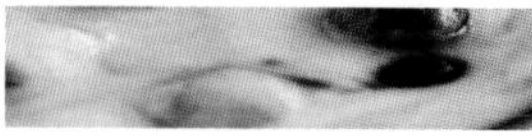

Yogurt Brands (Cont)

Great Value *(Walmart)*:

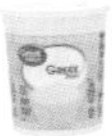
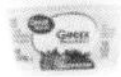
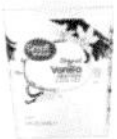

	C	F	Cb
Greek, Fat Free,			
32 oz Ctn, Plain, 6 oz	90	0	7
Greek Non Fat Light: *Per 5.3 oz Ctn*			
Banana Cream; Peach; Vanilla	80	0	9
Strawberry	80	0	9
Original Lowfat:			
5.3 oz, Blueberry	120	1	23
6 oz, Strawberry; Peach	130	1.5	26
32 oz, Vanilla, 6 oz	130	1.5	26

Kemps:

	C	F	Cb
5 lb Containers:			
Lowfat: Plain, Sweeetened, 6 oz	120	2	15
Nonfat: Raspberry, 6 oz	130	0	27
Strawberry; Blueberry, 6 oz	120	0	26
Vanilla, 6 oz	130	0	28
Kroger, CarbMaster, all flavors, 6 oz	70	1.5	5

La Yogurt: *Per 6 oz Container*

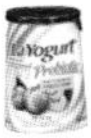

	C	F	Cb
Low Fat: Orig., Fruit Flavors, av.	155	1.5	30
Rich & Creamy, Fruit Flav., av.	180	1.5	33

LALA:

	C	F	Cb
Blended Yogurt: Plain, 6 oz	110	1.5	14
Fruit Flavors, average, 6 oz	155	1	29

Lucerne:

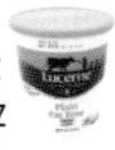

	C	F	Cb
Greek Nonfat, Plain, 8 oz	130	0	14
Low-Fat, Blueberry Flav., 6 oz	140	2	26
Light Nonfat, Blueberry, 6 oz	100	0	18
Nonfat, Vanilla Flavored, 8 oz	190	0	32

Mountain High: *Per 8 oz*

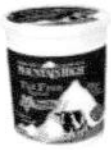
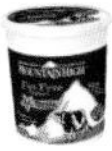

	C	F	Cb
32 oz Containers:			
Whole Milk Original: Plain	170	7	15
Strawberry; Vanilla, av.	200	7	27
Lowfat: Plain	130	2.5	16
Vanilla	170	2.5	28
Fat Free: Plain	110	0	16
Vanilla	160	0	28

Nancy's:

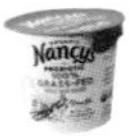
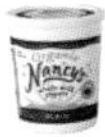

	C	F	Cb
Natural:			
Whole Milk, Honey, 8 oz	170	8	17
Low fat: Fruit Flavors, 5.3 oz	120	2	18
Nonfat, Vanilla, 6 oz	90	0	15
Organic:			
Greek: Plain, 6 oz	160	6	7
Honey, 6 oz	180	6	12
Lowfat, Plain, 8 oz	150	3	16
Nonfat: Plain, 8 oz	120	0	17
Vanilla, 6 oz	90	0	15
Whole Milk: Plain, 8 oz	180	8	16
Fruit Flavors, 5.3 oz	140	4.5	19

Oikos *(Dannon)*: *Per 5.3 oz Single Sve*

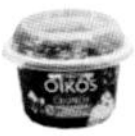
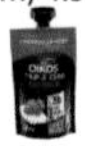

	C	F	Cb
Protein Crunch:			
Vanilla with Blueberries	160	1	21
Other Flavors	150	2	17
Nonfat, Plain	80	0	6
Triple Zero Greek: Av all flavors	110	0	12
Go Pack: Strawberries & Crm, 4.5 oz	80	0	13
Fruit Flavors, 4.5 oz	80	0	11
Whole Milk, av. all flav.	160	4	20

O Organics *(Vons)*:

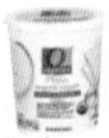

	C	F	Cb
Greek, Nonfat Strained, Vanilla, 6 oz	130	0	15
Whole Milk: Plain, 6 oz	130	6	11
Vanilla, 6 oz	160	6	22

Siggi's:

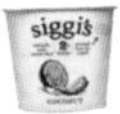

	C	F	Cb
Skyr: *Per 5.3 oz Unless Indicated*			
0%: Plain	90	0	6
Fruit Flavors	110	0	13
2%: Coconut	160	5	14
Fruit Flavors, average	140	3	14
4%: Fruit flavors, 4.4 oz	130	4.5	11
Fruit, no added sugar, av., 4.4 oz	95	2	8
Plant Based, Fruit Flavors, average	180	10	12
With Almond Butter, average, 5 oz	255	14	14

Silk: *Per 5.3 oz Containers*

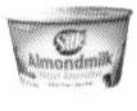
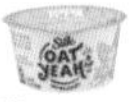
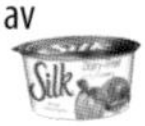

	C	F	Cb
Almond Yogurt: Plain	170	13	10
Fruit flavors, average	180	11	18
Vanilla	190	11	19
Oat Yeah, Vanilla	80	0	17
Soy Yogurt: Fruit flavors, av	125	3.5	19
Vanilla	140	3.5	21

So Delicious:

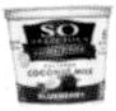
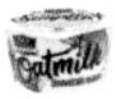

	C	F	Cb
Coconut Milk: *Per 5.3 oz*			
Blueberry	140	4	24
Chocolate	140	4.5	24
Salted Caramel Cluster	190	7	30
Vanilla	130	4	22
Oatmilk, av, all flavors, 5.3 oz	75	0	16

Stonyfield Organic:

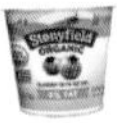
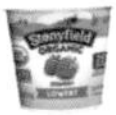
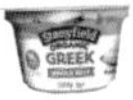

	C	F	Cb
Dairy Free (Soy):			
Fruit Flav., 5.3 oz	150	2.5	26
Vanilla	130	2.5	20
0% Fat Fruit On The Bottom:			
Blueberry On The Bottom, 5.3 oz	100	0	18
Chocolate Underground, 5.3 oz	110	0	22
Low Fat: Plain, 6 oz	90	1.5	11
Strawberry, 5.3 oz	100	1.5	16
Vanilla, 6 oz	110	0	20
Whole Milk: Strawb.; Van., av., 5.3 oz	140	5	18
32 oz Ctn: Plain, 6 oz	120	7	9
Vanilla, 6 oz	150	6	20
Greek: Plain, 6 oz	150	6	7
Vanilla Bean, 6 oz	170	5	18

Yogurt Brands (Cont)

	C	F	Cb
Trader Joe's:			
Organic: Greek, Nonfat, Plain	80	0	6
Whole Milk, Strawb., 5.3 oz 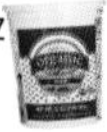	150	5	17
Lowfat, av. all flavors, 6 oz	150	2.5	26
Nonfat, plain, 6 oz	80	0	6
Greek, Lowfat (2%):			
Almond Butter coconut, 5.3 oz	170	6	16
Plain, 1 cup, 8 oz 	120	0	7
Greek, Whole Milk:			
5.3 oz Cups, av. all flavors	180	6	18
16 oz Ctn: Plain, 1 cup, 8 oz	280	22	12
Icelandic Style: 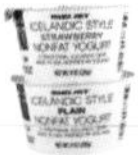			
Non Fat: Plain, 8 oz	130	0	10
Strawberry, 8 oz	190	0	26
Low Fat:			
Vanilla with Almonds, 4.6 oz 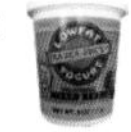	160	7	20
Prestirred, Strawberry, 8 oz	220	3	40
European Style:			
Organic, Plain: Whole Milk, 1 cup, 8 oz	170	7	14
Nonfat, 1 up, 8 oz 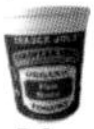	120	0	17
Voskos:			
Greek:			
2x Protein (0%), Exotic Fig, 5.3 oz	160	0	28
Real Fruit: Fruit Flavors, av., 6 oz	140	0	19
Coconut Cream, 6 oz 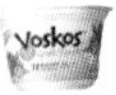	160	0	22
16 oz Tubs: Orig. Plain, 8 oz	280	20	15
Nonfat Vanilla, 8 oz	200	0	30
Wallaby Organic:			
Lowfat Greek, Plain, 5.3 oz 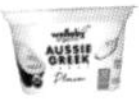	100	2	7
Nonfat, Plain, 5.3 oz	90	0	7
Whole Milk: Fruit Flavors, av., 5.3 oz			
Aussie Smooth,			
Fruit Flav., av., 5.3 oz 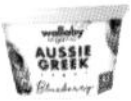	145	4	21
Wegmans:			
Fruit On The Bottom, Lowfat:			
Blueberry; Cherry Vanilla, 6 oz	160	2	29
Average other Fruit Flavors, 6 oz	175	2	34
Greek Non-Fat: Plain, 5.3 oz	80	0	5
Fruit flavors, av., 5.3 oz 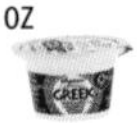	125	0	18
Vanilla, 5.3 oz	100	0	11
Whole Foods (365 Orgainic):			
Whole Milk: Plain, 8 oz	170	9	13
Unsweetened, 6 oz 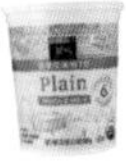	120	6	9
Blueberry, 5.3 oz	150	4.5	15
Vanilla, 5.3 oz	140	5	18
Low-Fat, European Style, 6 oz	110	2	13
Greek Nonfat, 6 oz	100	0	7
YoCrunch: *Per 4 oz Container*			
Lowfat Vanilla Yogurt: 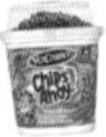			
Chips Ahoy; Twix, av.	185	4	32
M&M's; Oreo, av.	125	3	22

Yogurt Brands (Cont)

	C	F	Cb
Yoplait: 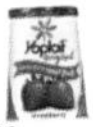			
Single Serve Cups: *Per 6 oz*			
Original, all Flavors, average	150	2	29
Lactose Free, av. all flavors, 6 oz	150	2	26
Light, 6 oz cup, average all flavors	90	0	17
FruitSide, all flavors, 5.3 oz	160	4	25
Greek 100 Protein, av. all flav., 5.3 oz	100	0	11
Go-Gurt: Tube, 2 oz	50	0.5	10
Dunkers, all flavors, 2.2 oz tray	120	2	22
Simply, all flavors, 2 oz 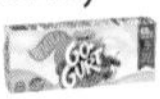	45	0.5	8
Just 3, av. all flavors, 5 oz	175	9	19
Lactose Free, av. all flavors, 6 oz	150	2	27
Light, av. all flavors, 6 oz 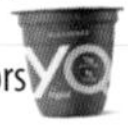	90	0	18
Starburst, average all flavors	160	1.5	29
Whips!:			
Regular: Coconut Crème, 4 oz	160	4	24
Chocolate, 4 oz 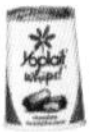	160	4	25
Sea Salt Caramel, 4 oz	170	4	27
Average other flav., 4 oz	140	2.5	25

Yogurt Drinks & Probiotics

	C	F	Cb
Dannon:			
Activia Probiotics: 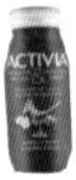			
Dailies, all flavors, 3.15 fl.oz	70	1.5	11
Drinks, av. all flavors, 7 fl oz	160	35	25
Smoothies, av. all flavors, 7 fl.oz	135	4	18
DanActive Dailies, all flav., 3.1 fl.oz	75	1	13
Danimals Smoothies: All flavors, 3.1 fl.oz	50	0	11
Pouches, all flavors, 3.5 oz	80	1	13
Organic, all flavors, 3.1 fl.oz 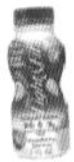	45	0	8
Wild, all flavors, 7 fl.oz	90	1	17
Glen Oaks, all flavors, 6 fl.oz	150	2.5	27
Lifeway:			
Kefir: *Per 8 fl.oz*			
Organic Whole Milk: Plain	160	8	12
Other Flavors	190	8	20
Organic Lowfat: Plain 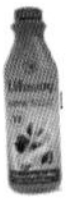	110	2	12
Other flavors	140	2	20
Plantiful: Plain	90	1	9
Other Flavors	110	1	14
Probugs, 3.5 fl.oz	80	3	11
Stonyfield:			
Smoothies: Low Fat, av., 6 oz 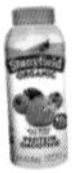	110	1.5	17
10 oz bottle, average	180	3	29
Daily Probiotics, all flav., 3.1 fl.oz	60	1	11
Yakult: Regular, 2.7 fl.oz bottle	50	0	12
Light, 2.7 fl.oz	25	0	6

Cafeteria-Style Foods

Cafeteria-Style Foods	C	F	Cb
Average All Preparations:			
Beef Stroganoff, 5 oz	**195**	13	7
Beef Stroganoff, with 4 oz noodles	**350**	14	36
Chicken Lasagna, 1 piece	**300**	11	32
Chicken Chop Suey, with 4 oz rice	**245**	4	37
Deep Dish Burrito, 7 oz	**265**	13	20
Ground Beef Casserole, 2 scps, 6 oz	**245**	13	17
Italian Meat Sce, for Spaghetti, 5 oz	**150**	9	9
with 5 oz Spaghetti	**350**	10	49
Lasagna, 1 piece	**275**	11	25
Meatloaf, 3 oz	**205**	13	4
Ranch Beans, 2 scoops, 6 oz	**350**	11	45
Red Beans & Rice, 7 oz	**280**	9	37
Scalloped Potato/Ham, 2 scoops, 6 oz	**160**	6	20
Stuffed Shells in Sauce, (1)	**105**	3	17
Swedish Meatballs, (3)	**205**	12	9
Sweet & Sour Pork/Rice, 9 oz	**240**	3	40
Swiss Steak, w/ Mushroom Gravy, 6 oz	**280**	11	4
Tator Tot Casserole, 2 scoops, 6 oz	**260**	15	20
Tenderloin Tips/Mshrm Gravy: 5 oz	**210**	13	3
With 5 oz noodles	**395**	15	38
Tuna Noodle Casserole, 2 scoops, 6 oz	**180**	6	17
Turkey Tetrazzini, 2 scoops, 6 oz	**195**	7	17
Vegetable Lasagna, 1 piece	**250**	13	21

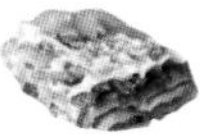

Croissants

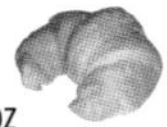

Croissants	C	F	Cb
Unfilled, medium 1.5 oz	**180**	10	21
Filled: With Ham (2 oz), garnish	**280**	14	24
With Ham (2 oz), Cheese (2 oz)	**470**	30	20
With Chick (2 oz) Cheese (2 oz)	**470**	30	20
With Turkey/Ham/Cheese (2 oz ea.)	**580**	36	20
Au Bon Pain: Ham & Cheese	**390**	21	35
Spinach & Cheese	**290**	17	28

7-Eleven ~ *See Page 236*

Bagels

Bagels	C	F	Cb
Plain: Large, 4 oz (without filling)	**320**	2	65
With 2 oz Cream Cheese	**500**	27	54
With 2 oz Lox (Smoked Salmon)	**400**	4	65

Also see Bagels Section ~ *Page 56*
Fast-Foods Restaurants ~ *Page 175*
Au Bon Pain ~ *Page 178*
Brueggerʼs ~ *Page 185*
Einstein Bros Bagels ~ *Page 199*

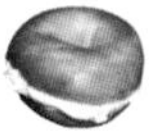

Sandwiches

Sandwiches	C	F	Cb
No Spreads Unless Indicated:			
Includes 2 Slices Bread ~ 3 oz			
BLT, (5 strips Bacon, 2 Tbsp Mayo)	**600**	40	46
Breaded Chicken & Garnish	**540**	28	46
Chicken Salad, with Mayo., 5 oz	**580**	30	49
Chopped Liver, Egg Mayonnaise	**630**	25	44
Corned Beef with Mustard, 5 oz	**560**	28	44
Egg Salad, with Mayonnaise	**570**	29	49
Egg Salad Club, with Bacon & Mayo,	**780**	53	49
Grilled Cheese, (3 oz)	**540**	30	44
Ham, (4 oz), Cheese (4 oz), & Mayo.	**910**	56	44
Lobster Salad, (4 oz), w/ Mayo.	**530**	25	45
Overstuffed Tuna Salad, (7 oz)	**870**	39	75
Philly Cheese Steak Sandwich	**550**	23	42
Reuben, (6 oz Beef/Pastrami, 2 oz Cheese, 2 Tbsp Dressing)	**920**	60	28
Roast Beef, (4 oz), with Mustard	**460**	12	45
Roast Pork, (4 oz), with Apple Sauce	**500**	16	55
Shrimp Salad Club, w/ Bacon & Mayo	**800**	57	48
Sloppy Joe with Sauce, (7 oz)	**600**	30	45
Steak Sandwich, (5 oz cooked)	**680**	32	41
Triple Cheese Melt, (4 oz)	**720**	45	46
Tuna Salad, (5 oz), with Mayonnaise	**610**	30	49
Turkey Breast, (5 oz), w/ Mayo.	**460**	18	44
Turkey Breast, (5 oz,) with Mustard	**360**	7	44
Turkey Club, with Bacon & Mayo.	**830**	38	31
Vegetarian, with Avocado & Cheese	**820**	49	72

7-Eleven ~ *Page 236*
Schlotzskyʼs ~ *Page 237*
Subway ~ *Page 245*

Wraps & Roll-Ups

Wraps & Roll-Ups	C	F	Cb
Average All Types			
Meat/Chicken/Fish/Veggie:			
Small, approximately 9 oz	**500**	25	48
Regular, approximately 15 oz	**830**	40	80
Large, approximately 22 oz	**1400**	70	134

Fast-Foods Restaurants ~ *Page 175*
Au Bon Pain ~ *Page 178*
Sonic Drive-In ~ *Page 241*
Subway ~ *Page 245*
WAWA ~ *Page 254*

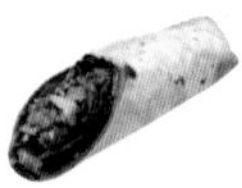

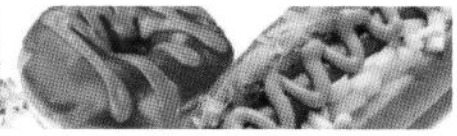

Fair & Carnival Foods

Food	C	F	Cb
Barbeque Chicken/Meats:			
Chicken, ½ chicken, 15 oz	740	24	34
Grilled Chicken Pita, with dressing	680	19	82
Teriyaki Chicken, on stick, w/ dress.	250	6	4
Pork Ribs, 18 oz	1360	68	21
Turkey Leg: Regular, 19 oz	1135	54	0
Caveman (2lb Turkey Leg, with 1lb Bacon)	2360	177	3
Bacon: Fried, on-a-stick, with syrup	230	16	5
Choc-covered Bacon, 4.5 oz dish	640	43	30
Beef Stew over Rice, 2 cups	440	14	61
Butter Balls, deep fried, 4 Balls	460	38	24
Cheese Curds, Breaded & fried, *Culver's*, 6.7 oz	670	38	54
Corn Dogs: Regular, 4 oz	250	14	23
Jumbo, 6 oz	375	21	36
Pretzel-Wrapped Dog	300	16	30
Papa Pup, on-a-stick	400	24	32
Pronto Pup, on-a-stick	170	9	16
Corn On The Cob, 8" (1), 16 oz	200	1	42
Finger Foods:			
Artichoke, fried, 9 pieces	250	14	24
Chicken Nuggets, (6)	340	17	26
Chicken Strips, (4), 4.5 oz	445	21	33
Onion Rings, 3 rings	310	13	40
Onion Flower	1320	72	140
Shrimp, Fried, 10-12 pieces, 5 oz	555	30	36
Spam, deep-fried in batter, 2 pieces	330	24	18
Gator:			
Big Gator, Nuggets/Hushpuppies	550	31	54
Stick Gator, 1 sausage	250	20	4
Greek:			
Baklava, 2" square	245	13	32
Falafel, 11.6 oz	660	27	85
Greek Salad, 14 oz	520	48	17
Gyro, 7.5", 12 oz	680	40	55
Spanakopita, 8 oz	200	7.5	23
Hamburgers:			
⅓ Pound Burger, 7.5 oz	670	41	26
Cheeseburger, 6 oz	550	36	25
Hot Dogs: *With Bun*			
Regular: No extras	215	14	28
With Chili, 6 oz	450	32	32
With Chili & Cheese, 7.3 oz	500	36	31
⅓ Pound Hot Dog	550	41	31
Foot Long Hot Dog	470	26	41
Jumbo, Bratwurst/Kielbasa, average	800	60	28

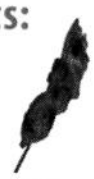
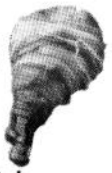
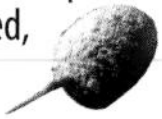
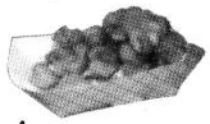

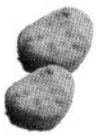
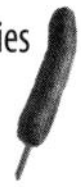
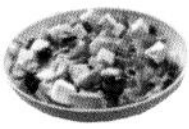
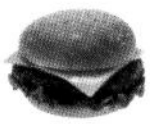
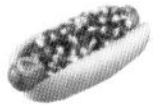
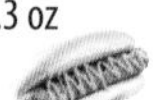

Fair & Carnival Foods (Cont)

Food	C	F	Cb
Mexican:			
Burrito, with Bean/Beef, 17 oz	1100	41	104
Carne Asada, 14.5 oz	820	44	58
Cheese Quesadilla, 1.8 oz	480	27	40
Chicken Taco, 3.3 oz	210	12	16
Fish Taco, 5 oz	270	13	31
Jalapeno Pepper, choc-covered (3)	270	15	31
Nachos with Cheese, 9" plate	860	59	70
Tamale, 3.5 oz	180	8	21
Taquito, 5 oz	370	17	43
Pizza:			
Pizza Bread, Pepperoni, ½ loaf, 12 oz	1115	32	151
Pizza on-a-stick, 1 piece	535	28	55
Personal Pizza: *Per 7"*			
Cheese	670	24	80
Pepperoni	795	35	80
Ham & Pineapple	800	31	87
Potatoes & Fries:			
Australian Battered Potatoes	1290	66	155
Baked Potato, 14 oz	435	0.5	100
Fries: French, 7 oz	560	24	79
Cheese Fries, 10 oz	645	38	62
Chili Fries, 10 oz	700	36	83
Curly Fries, 7 oz	620	30	78
Jamaican Jerk Fries, 7 oz	640	34	77
Sweet Potato, baked, 14 oz	405	0.5	97
Tornado, on-a-stick	210	15	18
Salads/Sides:			
Chili, 1 cup	280	11	24
Cole Slaw, 5 oz	350	21	37
Pickle, whole (6")	30	0	8
Potato Salad, 5 oz	290	15	35
Sandwiches: *7½" Roll*			
Ham, 11 oz	645	39	47
Hot Pastrami, 9 oz	760	17	62
Roast Beef, 11 oz	620	36	46
Philadelphia Cheese Steak, 13 oz	680	36	49
Turkey, 11 oz	665	24	65
Drinks:			
Icee, 16 fl.oz	235	0	59
Shakes, average, 16 fl.oz	690	33	85
Slushies: Horchata, 16 fl.oz	280	8	50
Lemonade, 18 fl.oz	210	0	52
Orange Julius, 20 fl.oz	490	10	96
Strawberry Julius, 20 fl.oz	430	0	98
Soft Frozen Lemonade, 12 fl.oz	300	0	78
Smoothies, Berry Flavors, 16 fl.oz	350	1	80

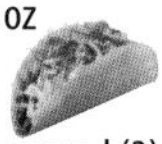
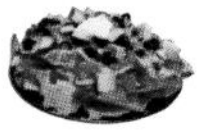
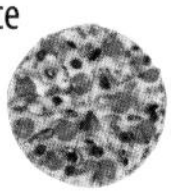
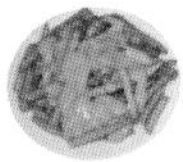
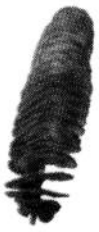
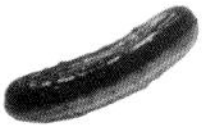
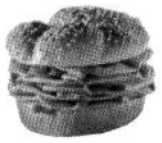
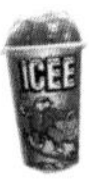

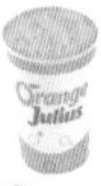

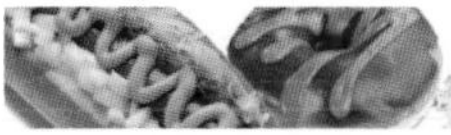

Fair & Carnival Foods (Cont)

Cakes, Pastries:	C	F	Cb
Funnel Cake, Plain (1) 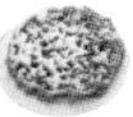	760	44	80
Toppings:			
Apple Cinnamon, 2 oz	85	3	16
Cinnamon & Sugar, 2 tsp	40	0	10
Strawberry & Cream, 2 oz	70	0	16
Cheesecake on-a-stick, 6 oz	655	47	56
Churro, (1), 9", 1.6 oz	170	8	22
Cream Puff, 4.3 oz 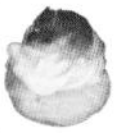	500	43	22
Fried Twinkie, (1)	420	34	45
Puff-on-a-Stick, (4), 8.6 oz	995	86	44
Strawberry Crepe, 4.3 oz	280	14	36
Twinkie Dog, (Sundae) 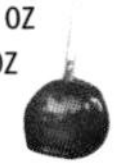	500	14	89
Candied Apple, 7 oz	330	0	80
Cookies: 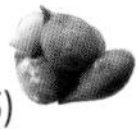			
Sweet Martha, (1), 0.8 oz	90	4	14
Deep Fried: Oreos, tray (5)	890	48	108
Cookie Dough on stick, 3 pieces	670	32	89
Cotton Candy: 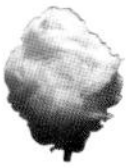			
Small, 1 oz	110	0	27
Large, 2.3 oz	250	0	62
Family Size, 5.5 oz	610	0	151
Dirt Dessert, 1 cup, 9.3 oz	405	12	69
Donuts, Jumbo Twist, (1), 7.5 oz	905	49	109
Fried Dough/FryBread:			
Plain: 7", 3.7 oz 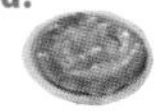	390	19	47
9", $4^3/_4$ oz	510	25	61
Toppings: Cinnamon Sugar, 2 tsp	40	0	10
Butterscotch; Caramel, 2 Tbsp	115	0	29
Hot Fudge, average, 2 Tbsp	110	4	22
Cheese Powder, 2 tsp	70	3	2
Honey, 1 Tbsp, 0.8 oz	65	0	17
Fudge, 1.5 oz	200	11	25
Ice Cream & Frozen Treats:			
Deep-fried Klondike Bar, w/ syrup	430	16	18
Dippin' Dots Ice Cream, 6 oz cup	380	20	46
Frozen Banana, choc. coated, 5 oz	240	4	53
Frozen Yogurt, in sugar cone, 14 oz	475	2	94
Ice Cream: Small, sugar cone, 10 oz	775	42	83
Large, sugar cone, 14 oz	935	54	96
Sherbet, 8 oz	270	4	59
Snow Cone, with 3 oz syrup	270	0	68
Strawberry, Choc. Dipped, 1 piece	125	7	15
Popcorn: 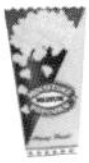			
Plain: Small, 3 oz	450	24	48
Large, 6 oz	900	48	96
Kettle Corn: Small, 5 oz	600	15	110
Large, 10 oz	1200	30	220
Pretzels, Soft, 4.5 oz 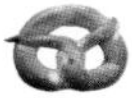	340	2	70
S'more, on stick	275	16	27

Stadium Foods

Burgers:	C	F	Cb
Bacon Burger, 8.3 oz 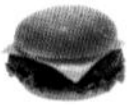	470	25	34
Cheeseburger, 8.3 oz	450	23	33
Hamburger, 7.8 oz	400	19	33
French Fries, 6.4 oz	470	34	39
Fruit Cup, 6 oz	80	0	20
Hot Dogs: 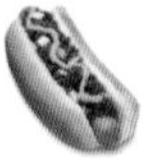			
Chili Dog, 7.7 oz	520	29	45
Hot Dog, 6.4 oz	465	21	50
Jumbo Dog, 6 oz	440	25	38
Kraut Dog with Sauerkraut, 7.8 oz	490	27	41
Individual Pan Pizza (6"): *Per Pizza*			
BBQ Chicken 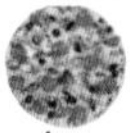	630	24	71
Cheese	630	27	71
Pepperoni	660	30	70
Nachos, 40 chips, with 4 oz cheese	1100	59	132
Sandwiches:			
Chicken: With Bacon, 8.3 oz	530	31	41
With Cheese, 8.3 oz	510	29	40
Without Cheese, 7.7 oz	460	25	40
Polish Sausage Sandwich, 7 oz	565	33	46
Snacks: 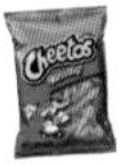			
Brownie, 2.5" x 4.5"	360	18	44
Cheese Sauce, 1.3 oz	100	8	4
Cheetos, 2.8 oz package	440	28	42
Chocolate Chip Cookie, 2.3 oz	280	12	40
Churro, (1), 10", 2 oz	210	10	26
Doritos, Nacho, 2.8 oz package	390	20	48
King Size Candy: 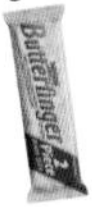			
Butterfinger, 3.8 oz	480	18	75
Nestle Crunch, 2.8 oz	390	21	85
Lay's, Chips, 2.8 oz package	440	28	42
Peanuts, in shell, 8 oz	930	80	24
Popcorn: Small (9 cup size) 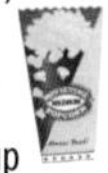	575	35	56
Large (15 cup size)	950	58	93
Pretzel, Soft, Reg., 5.5 oz	490	3.5	101
Red Vines, 5 oz box	500	0	117
Snow Cone: With 3 oz syrup	270	0	68
With 6 oz syrup	540	0	136
Beverages: 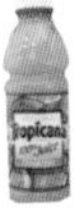			
Orange Juice, 12 fl.oz	180	0	2
Beer:			
Heineken, 16 fl.oz	200	0	16
Miller: Draft, 16 fl.oz	195	0	17
Lite, 16 fl.oz	125	16	4
Jack Daniels, Punch, 12 fl.oz 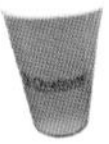	235	0	34
Wine, White, 9 fl.oz	190	0	6
Soda, (with $^1/_2$ ice), average: 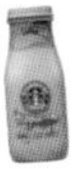			
20 fl.oz	160	0	40
32 fl.oz	260	0	65
Starbuck's, Coffee, Frappuccino, 9.5 fl.oz	200	3	37

Updated Nutrition Data ~ www.CalorieKing.com
Persons with Diabetes ~ See Disclaimer (Page 22)

Asian & Chinese Dishes

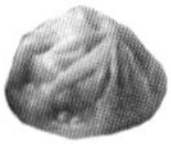
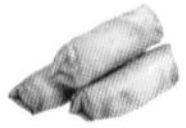
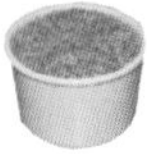
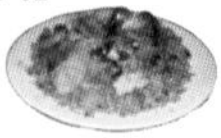
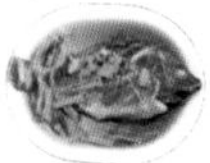

	C	F	Cb
Appetizers:			
Crab Cake, 2.3 oz	125	10	1
Dumplings: *Per Dumpling*			
Pork: Steamed	80	4.5	5
Fried	90	6	5
Vegetable, steamed	35	1	5
Egg Rolls, Mini, 3 rolls	100	3	11
Spring Roll:			
Small, 1.5 oz	85	4	9
Medium, 3 oz	170	8	17
Large, 5 oz	290	15	29
Wonton, 1 only	75	4	5
Soup: Egg Flower, bowl 12 oz	90	2	16
Hot & Sour Soup, bowl 12 oz	110	3.5	14
Rice: Plain,1 cup, 6.5 oz	320	2	66
2 Cups, 13 oz	640	4	132
Fried: 1 cup, 5 oz	365	11	55
Large dish, 16 oz	950	28	67
Noodles, Chinese Egg, cooked, 1 cup	200	4	37
Entrees & Mains: *Per Serving*			
Almond Chicken, 6 oz	270	10	21
BBQ Pork, 5.5oz	440	23	15
Beef in Black Bean Sauce, 8.5 oz	390	17	17
Broccoli Beef, 6 oz	370	21	13
Chicken & Broccoli, 5.5 oz	160	8	10
Chicken Skewers, 3 oz	210	9	18
Chop Suey:			
Chicken, 5 oz	140	9	2
Pork, 5 oz	170	12	3
Chow Mein, Beef/Chicken, 8 oz	390	12	59
Crab Puff/Rangoon, 1 dumpling	190	11	13
Crispy Fried Chicken, 8 oz	485	33	12
Egg Drop Soup: With Noodles, 1 cup	110	3	16
Without Noodles, 1 cup	60	3	4
Egg Foo Yung with Sauce, 1 cup	270	15	16
Kung Pao Chicken, 5.5 oz	240	15	12
Lemon Chicken, 5 oz	525	21	57
Lo Mein, stir-fried, 8 oz	705	42	49
Omelet, Chicken/Shrimp, 16 oz	990	82	10
Orange Chicken, 5.5 oz	500	27	42
Steamed Whole Fish, ½ Sockeye Salmon	646	36	23
Sweet & Sour:			
Fish, 20 oz	1160	58	106
Pork, 5.5 oz	400	23	35
Vegetable Combo, with oil, 6 oz	367	5	66
Vegetables, Steamed, without oil, 6 oz	135	1	29
Sauces: Mandarin Sauce 1.5 oz	70	0	17
Potsticker Sauce, 1.5 oz	35	0	8
Bubble Tea, average, 12 fl oz	280	0.5	68
Fortune Cookie, each	32	0.5	7

Cajun & Creole

	C	F	Cb
Alligator, cooked, 4 oz	160	2	0
Baked Herb Chicken, 1 serving	850	53	2
Bouillabaisse	400	15	10
Cajun Fried Turkey, 1 serving	630	25	0
Cocktail Sauce, 2 Tbsp	30	0	6
Couche-Couche, ½ cup	80	0	17
Crawfish Bisque, 1 serving	500	10	10
Crawfish, cooked, 2 oz	45	0.5	0
Creole Jambalaya, 1 serving	550	30	15
Frog Legs, steamed (2)	45	0	0
Guinea Fowl, flesh, 4 oz, cooked	160	4	0
Hogshead Cheese, ¼ cup	80	5.5	0
Jambalaya, Shrimp & Crabmeat	520	14	12
Red Beans & Rice, 1 serving	400	17	52
Roasted Quail, with Bacon, on Toast	550	25	15
Remoulade Sauce, 2 Tbsp, 1 oz	110	11	2
Shrimp Creole, 1 serving	450	20	10
Stuffed Smothered Steak, with 1 cup Rice	890	50	50
Turtle, cooked, 3 oz	120	3	0

Canadian Foods

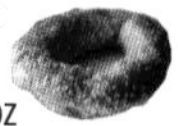
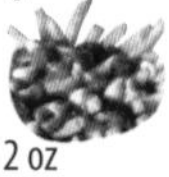
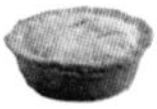

	C	F	Cb
Bagels, Montreal-Style:			
Plain, 100g/3.5 oz	300	2	60
Poppyseed, 100g/3.5 oz	310	4	58
Sesame, 100g/3.5 oz	320	6	56
Bannock: Plain 33g/1.2 oz	120	3	20
With currants/raisins, 85g/3 oz	215	9	32
Meals:			
Baked Beans in Maple Syrup, 1 cup, 250g/8.8 oz	320	1	62
Donnairs (*Pizza Delight*):			
Famous, regular, 250g/8.8 oz	510	21	60
Super, regular, 310g/11 oz	685	34	62
Poutine:			
A&W, 330g/12 oz	610	33	58
Boston Pizza, regular, 400g/14 oz	610	30	67
Burger King, Classic, 330g/11.6 oz	680	36	72
Harvey's, 240g/8.5 oz	730	41	63
McDonald's, 1 serving	510	29	44
Swiss Chalet, Chalet -Style, 340g/12 oz	150	12	195
Shish Taouk:			
Chicken: 1 skewer, 200g/7 oz	270	25	9
Wrap, 455g/16 oz	1150	12	195
Tassot:			
Beef, 283g/10 oz	430	28	12
Goat, 100g/3.5 oz	360	36	9
Toutiere, 170g/6oz	600	42	35

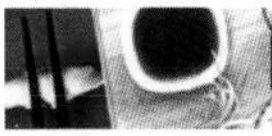

Restaurant & International Foods

Canadian (Cont)

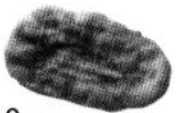
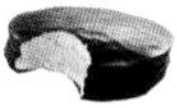

	C	F	Cb
Pastries:			
Beaver Tails:			
Cheese & Garlic, 80g/2.8 oz	390	30	28
Cinnamon & Sugar, 80g/2.8 oz	315	13	30
Butter Tart, mini, 1 tart	120	3	16
May West,			
Original, 54g/1.9 oz	240	11	34
Nanaimo Bar, 56g/2 oz	270	16	30
Snacks: Maple Syrup Taffy, 40g/1.4 oz	130	0	33
Potato Chips: Dill Pickle Flav., 40g	160	10	15
Ketchup Flavor, 50g/1.8 oz	260	16	26

French Foods

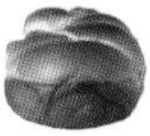
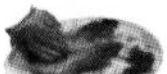
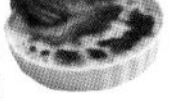

	C	F	Cb
Blanquette d' Agneau, (Lamb Stew)	800	30	17
Brioche, 1 cake	280	14	34
Bouillabaisse	400	15	10
Coq au Vin, leg/thigh	700	28	31
Coquilles St. Jacques	320	13	36
Crème Brulée, 1 serving	460	40	21
Baguette, 3 slices, 2.2 oz	150	1	35
Creme Caramel, (Caramel Custard)	260	10	38
Crepe Suzette, 1x6" crepe with sauce	220	10	13
Duck a l'Orange, 1/4 duck, 22 oz	970	44	19
Escargot, (Snails), in garlic butter (6)	200	10	4
Frog Legs, fried, 4 medium pairs	400	20	10
Lamb Noisettes, fried, 2 chops	500	40	1
Potage Creme Crecy, (Carrot Soup)	360	18	14
Salade Nicoise, (Tuna/Olives/Vegs)	450	13	14
Veal Cordon Bleu, (Veal/Ham)	650	25	18
Vichyssoise, (Potato /Leek Soup), 1 c.	200	9	15

Baguette & French Stick ~ *Page 54*

German Foods

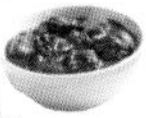
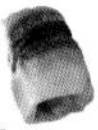
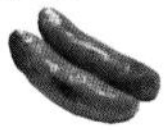

	C	F	Cb
Beef: Goulash with Veggies	520	20	46
Weiner Schnitzel, 1 medium	750	35	38
Chicken: Fried, Viennese-style	530	20	28
Livers with Apple/Onion, 6 oz	460	28	10
Herring, pickled: Rollmops, 4 oz	260	16	3
With Sour Cream, 4 oz	310	20	3
Pork, Sauerbraten (Pot Roast)	650	35	15
Sausage: Bratwurst, grilled, 6 oz	450	37	2
Hot Sausage Curry	300	7	6
Cakes:			
Black Forest, 1 slice	380	16	30
Bavarian Bread Dumpling, 3 small	330	10	28
Kugelhupf Cake, 1 large slice, 4 oz	400	23	40
Torte: Linzer (Almond/Raspb. Jam)	430	18	58
Sacher (Chocolate/Apricot Jam)	260	12	23

Greek Foods

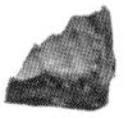

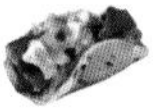
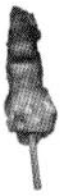
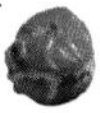

	C	F	Cb
Baklava Pastry: Small	240	13	32
Large, 3.8 oz	400	21	45
Calamari, deep fried, 1 cup	300	13	17
Chicken Kebob Plate	345	13	8
Dolmades, 2 rolls, 6 oz	200	5	13
Galactobureko, 1 only			
(Filo, Custard, Pastry in Syrup)	360	15	48
Greek Chicken Salad	400	18	9
Gyros: 6" Pita, 8 oz	475	32	35
7 1/2" Pita, 12 oz	680	40	55
Hummus & Pita, 4 oz	260	12	30
Kataifi, (Filo, Nut, Pastry in Syrup)	350	11	56
Moussaka: Small serving, 8 oz	350	22	22
Large serving, 16 oz	700	44	44
Soup, Avgolemono (Egg & Lemon			
with Chicken & Rice), 1 cup	85	6	5
Souvlaki, (Lamb), each, 2 oz	120	6	1
Stuffed Tomatoes, (2)	250	12	17
Taramosalata, 1 T., 0.5 oz	40	3	2
Tyropita, (Filo/Egg/Cheese Pastry)	350	26	31

Hawaiian

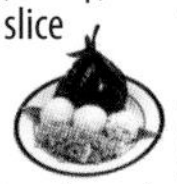
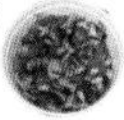
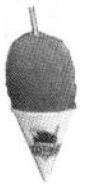

	C	F	Cb
Ahi Tuna, grilled w/o fat, 6 oz fillet	220	2	0
Chicken Long Rice, 1 cup, 7 oz	240	14	12
Gyoza, 1 only	55	2	6
Haupia, (Coconut Pudd.), 1 pce, (4"x 2 1/2")	120	6	17
Hawaiian Sweet Bread, 1/2" slice, 2 oz	180	4.5	29
Kalua: Chicken, 4 oz	280	16	0
Pork, 4 oz	350	24	0
Kim Chee, (pickled cabbage), 1/2 cup, 4 oz	20	0	5
Kulolo, (Taro Pudding), 1 slice	125	5	19
Lau Lau:			
Chicken (1), 7 oz	280	21	3
Pork (1), 7 oz	320	26	5
Loco Moco, (rice/burger/egg/gravy)	650	27	63
Lomi Salmon, 1/4 cup, 4 oz	20	1	2
Malasadas, (Donut), 2 oz	240	13	26
Manapua, (Char Siu Pork Bun), 2.3 oz	180	8	25
Poi ,(mashed cooked taro), 1 cup., 8.5 oz	270	0.5	65
Poke, average all types, 3 oz	90	1	0
Portuguese Sausage, 2 oz	180	15	2
Potato Salad, 1/2 cup, 5 oz	170	10	17
Shave Ice, *(Matsumoto)*, all flavors:			
With Ice Cream, 1 large	300	4	64
With Beans, 1 large	290	0	72
Spam Musubi:			
With Regular Spam	265	11	34
(4 oz rice+1.3 oz Spam/7-Eleven Hawaii)			
Homemade, w/ Lite Spam (50% less fat)	220	5	34
Taro Pancake Mix, 1/3 cup (makes 2)	140	2	26

Restaurant & International Foods

Hawaiian (Cont)

	C	F	Cb
Plate Lunches:			
Chicken Katsu, (9 oz:) With Rice	**1110**	48	108
+ Macaroni Salad, 3/4 cup	**1360**	68	123
or Tossed Salad + 2 T. French Dress.	**1240**	61	111
Hamburger, (5 oz): With Rice	**710**	24	81
Gravy + Macaroni Salad	**1135**	49	112
Mahi Mahi, (7 oz): With Rice	**650**	12	90
+ Macaroni Salad + Tartar Sce	**1150**	58	109
or Macaroni Salad, w/o Tartar ce	**935**	34	108
or Tossed Salad + 3 Tbsp Fr. Dress.	**815**	27	96
or Tossed Salad, without dressing	**670**	12	93
Teri Beef, (5 oz): With 2 scoops Rice	**790**	23	94
+ Macaroni Salad, 3/4 cup	**1095**	47	113
or Tossed Salad, without dressing	**800**	23	95

Indian & Pakistani

Per Serving, Meat dishes allow 4 oz meat/serving

	C	F	Cb
Aloo Samosa, each	**155**	12	12
Alu Gosht Kari, (Meat/Potato Curry)	**600**	40	23
Chicken Korma	**500**	35	6
Chicken Pilaf	**700**	53	50
Chicken Tikka	**260**	16	2
Chicken Vindaloo	**400**	20	8
Chapati/Roti, 7" diameter, 1 piece	**60**	0.5	11
Dahl, (Lentil Puree):			
1 cup, without oil	**230**	1	37
1 Tbsp Tadka (oil topping)	**120**	13	0
Dhakla, (Lentil Dish), 1" square, 1 oz	**105**	5	13
Dhansak, ½ cup	**105**	3.5	11
Gosht Kari	**460**	25	17
Lamb Pilaf	**520**	35	40
Lassi, (Sweet or Mango), 1 cup, 8 oz	**160**	4	24
Masala Gosht, (Beef/Tomato/Gravy)	**400**	25	18
Mulligatawney Soup	**300**	15	8
Murgh Tikka, 1 cup	**300**	4	7
Naan Flatbread, 2 oz	**160**	3.5	29
Pappadum, 1 large/2 small	**50**	3	5
Pesrattu, (Lentil Crepe), 9", 2.6 oz	**130**	5	15
Pork Vindaloo Curry, without Rice	**620**	47	3
Rajmah, 1 cup	**225**	5	35
Rogan Josh,			
without Rice/Potatoes	**500**	30	3
Shahi Korma, (Braised Lamb)	**430**	28	3
Tandoori Chicken:			
Breast	**260**	13	5
Leg/Thigh portion	**300**	17	6

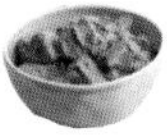
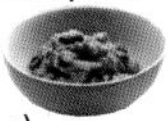
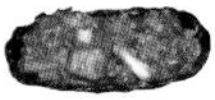
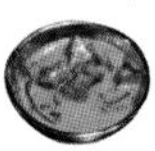
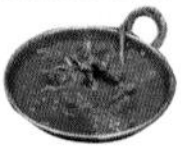
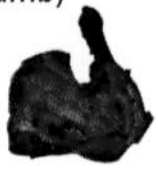

Italian Dishes

	C	F	Cb
Entrees:			
Baked Ziti: Small	**370**	27	32
Regular	**575**	42	49
Breadstick, 2 oz piece	**120**	2.5	25
Broccoli Fettucine Alfredo, regular	**815**	23	125
Bruschetta, 2 slices	**380**	17	53
Calzones, av. all varieties	**840**	34	101
Cannelloni, 1 tube, 6 oz	**280**	15	18
Cheese Breadstick, 2.4 oz piece	**180**	8	20
Cheese Ravioli, with sauce	**495**	17	65
Chicken Alfredo	**775**	29	82
Chicken Parmigiana, 11 oz	**520**	22	16
Chicken Scallopine, dinner	**1110**	71	68
Eggplant Parmigiana	**900**	39	78
Fettucine Alfredo: Lunch, 9 oz	**885**	65	63
Dinner, 15 oz	**1475**	108	104
Linquine & Seafood, dinner	**1130**	71	79
Manicotti Formaggio	**800**	38	57
Meat Lasagne:			
Small, 10 oz	**440**	23	39
Large, 16 oz	**700**	36	60
Meat Ravioli	**725**	22	102
Minestrone Soup, 1 bowl	**110**	2	18
Penne Rustica: Lunch	**1300**	71	76
Dinner	**1540**	80	101
Ravioli, over-stuffed, average	**990**	67	57
Panini Sandwich:			
Chicken, 16 oz	**900**	38	81
Meats, average, 18 oz	**940**	39	81
Vegetarian, 15 oz	**750**	31	83

Pizza, Ready-To-Eat ~ *See Page 135*

	C	F	Cb
Spaghetti & Meatballs:			
With Tomato Sauce: Kids	**500**	20	58
Medium/Lunch	**1080**	63	89
Large/Dinner	**1430**	81	119
With Meat Sauce: Kids	**550**	25	56
Medium/Lunch	**1300**	79	84
Large/Dinner	**1700**	103	110
Veal Marsala, dinner	**1320**	66	132
Veal Parmigiana, dinner	**1270**	65	116
Vegetable Primavera	**610**	8	116
Salad,			
Caprese , 11 oz	**445**	34	10
Desserts:			
Gelato: Vanilla (Milk Base), 1/2 cup	**200**	15	18
Choc. Hazelnut (Milk), 1/2 cup	**370**	29	26
Water Base, 1/2 cup	**100**	0	25
Lemon Ice,	**180**	0	45
Tiramisu, 1 piece, 5 oz	**400**	29	30

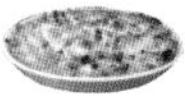
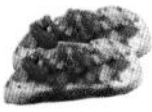
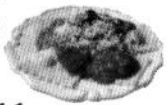
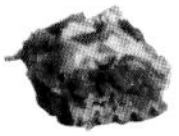
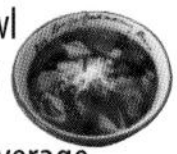
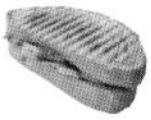
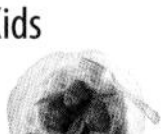
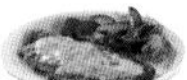
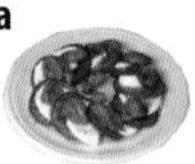
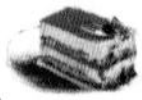

Further listings ~ *See Fast-Foods Section*

Japanese

	C	F	Cb
Sashimi: (Sliced Raw Seafood/Beef)			
Ika (Squid), 4 oz	**105**	2	0
Hamachi (Yellowtail), 4 oz	**165**	6	0
Maguro (Yellowfin Tuna), 4 oz	**120**	1	0
Niku (Beef), 5 oz	**200**	10	0
Saba (Mackerel), 4 oz	**160**	7	0
Suzuki (Sea Bass), 4 oz	**110**	0.5	0
Tako (Octopus), 4 oz	**95**	1	0
Sushi Rice: Cooked, 1 Tbsp	**25**	0	5
1 cup, 5.3 oz	**380**	3	82
Sushi (Maki) Rolls: *Per Piece*			
Average all types (California Rolls; Cream Cheese with Crab; Eel; Salmon; Shrimp; Tuna; Yellowtail; Vegetable)			
Small (1.2" diam. x 1.2" high), 0.8 oz	**25**	0.5	3.5
Medium (1 3/4" diam. x 1 3/4" high), 1.6 oz	**50**	1	7
Large (2 1/4" diam. x 7/8" high), 2 oz	**60**	1.5	9
Sushi Packs: *Per Pack*			
Average all types: 6 large pieces	**370**	5	55
9 medium pieces	**360**	6	60
12 small pieces	**265**	3	45
Futomaki (thick roll), 6 pieces	**380**	5	72
Hand Roll (Cone), 4 oz	**120**	2	18
Inari (rice filled soybean pocket), 4 pces	**420**	9	73
Sushi-Nigiri, (fish on rice), average all varieties, 1 piece	**70**	0.5	12
Sushi Plate, Assorted: 6 pieces	**420**	3	36
Combination (Sushi & Sushi Rolls) 2 Sushi + 6 small & 3 medium rolls	**400**	7	72
Dipping Sauces: Average, 2 Tbsp	**30**	0	7
Ginger Vinegar Dressing, 2 Tbsp	**20**	0	5
Edamame: (young green soybeans):			
Boiled beans (no pods), 4 oz	**160**	7	12
Steamed (in pods), 4 oz	**60**	3	5
Katsu-don, Pork with Rice	**1100**	39	141
Miso Soup, with Tofu pieces, 1 cup	**85**	3	11
Sake Wine, (16% alcohol), 3 fl.oz	**115**	0	7
Seaweed Salad, 1.5 oz	**20**	2	0
Sukiyaki, (Beef/Tofu/Veggies), 8 oz	**400**	24	32
Tempura:			
3 large shrimp & veggies	**320**	18	25
1 shrimp only	**60**	4	3
Teppan Yaki, (Steak, Seafood & Veggies), 10 oz serving	**470**	30	15
Teriyaki: Beef, 4 oz	**350**	25	4
Chicken, 4 oz	**260**	9	7
Salmon, medium, 6 oz	**270**	8	3
Yakatori, 1 skewer, 2.5 oz	**140**	5	1

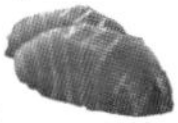
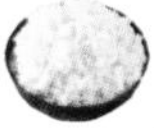
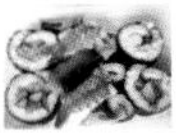
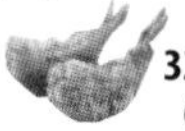
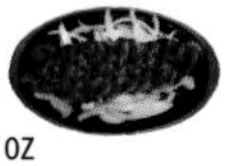

Kosher/Deli Foods

	C	F	Cb
Bagel/Bialy, 1 small, 2 oz	**160**	2	32
Beiglach, (Cheese Knish)	**350**	17	35
Blintzes: Average, 1 only	**120**	1	25
With Sour Cream & Preserves	**370**	10	30
Borscht, (Without Sour Cream): 1 cup	**85**	3	14
Diet/Reduced Calorie, 1 cup	**30**	1	7
Cabbage Rolls, (meat/rice), 5 oz	**170**	6	21
Chicken Broth: 1 cup	**80**	8	0
With vegetables	**100**	8	5
With noodles	**150**	9	16
Lowfat, plain, 1 cup	**25**	1	0
Cholent, 1 medium serving, 1 cup	**350**	16	48
Chopped Liver: 1 serving, 3 oz	**110**	6	5
With Egg Salad, 1/4 cup	**100**	7	3
Farfel, dry, 1/2 cup	**90**	0.5	21
Gefilte Fish Balls:			
Regular, 2 oz	**55**	2	4
With Jelled Broth	**80**	2	6
Cocktail size, 1 oz	**30**	1	2
Sweet: Medium, 2 oz	**65**	2	4
With Jelled Broth	**95**	2	9
Hallah, (Yeast Bread), 1 slice, 1 oz	**85**	2	14
Herring: Smoked, 2 oz	**120**	8	0
In Sour Cream, 2 oz	**150**	10	0
Kasha, cooked, 1/2 cup	**100**	0.5	20
Kipfel, (Vanilla/Almdond Cookie), 1 pce	**60**	2	7
Knaidlach ~ *See Matzo Balls*			
Knish: Kasha/Potato, 1 only	**130**	4	22
Cheese, 1 only	**350**	17	35
Kreplach, beef, 1 piece	**40**	1	6
Kugel, potato/noodle, 1 serving	**300**	20	25
Latkes, (Potato Pancake): 2 oz	**200**	11	22
3 Latkes w/ Sour Cran Apple Sauce	**750**	25	95
Lochshen: Plain, 1 cup	**130**	2	26
Pudding, 1 cup	**380**	13	48
Lox, (Smoked Salmon), 2 oz	**65**	2	0
Mandelbrot, (Almond Bread), 1 slice, 1/4" thick	**45**	2	5
Matzo, 1 oz board	**110**	0.5	21
Matzo Balls: 2 small, or 1 large, 2"	**90**	3	12
Extra large ball, 3"	**180**	6	24
Matzo Ball Soup:			
Cup w/ 2 small or 1 large ball	**150**	5	27
Bowl w/ Chkn & Noodles	**325**	13	34
Jerry's Deli, large bowl	**560**	17	56
NY Cheesecake, 4 oz	**350**	24	26
Pierogi, potato/cheese, 1 piece	**90**	4	11
Reuben S'wich, w/ 1/2 lb Corned Beef	**920**	60	28
Schmaltz, (Rend'd Chicken Fat), 1 T.	**90**	10	0

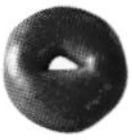
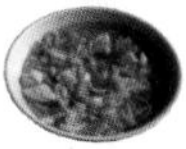
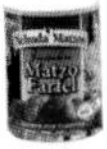

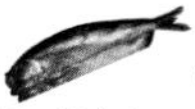
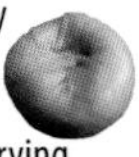
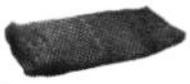
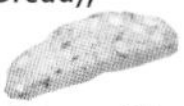
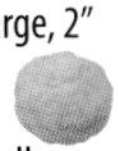
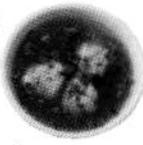

Restaurant & International Foods

Korean Food

	C	F	Cb
Bibimbab, (Veg. & Beef on Rice), 1 cup	**565**	15	89
Bulgogi, (Barbeque Beef), 3.5 oz	**325**	12	15
Galbi (Short Ribs), 16 oz	**975**	61	16
Gujeolpan, (Pancake with Meat & Vegetables), 1 cup with 1 pancake	**340**	11	39
Japchae, (Noodle w/ Veggies & Meat), 1¼ cups	**365**	19	34
Sides:			
Kimchee, (Cabbage Relish), ½ cup	**30**	0	6
Namool, (Assorted Vegetables), 1 cup	**125**	6.5	9
Soups: *Per Serving*			
Muguk, (Radish & Chive Soup), 6 oz	**105**	7	6
Samgyetang, (Ginseng Chkn Soup):			
Without Chicken Skin, 1 cup	**520**	11	60
With Chicken Skin, 1 cup	**725**	35	60
Yuk Gae Jang, (Spicy Beef Soup), 1¼ cups	**180**	13	5

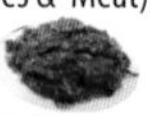
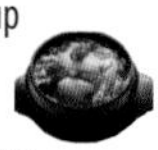

Lebanese/Middle East

	C	F	Cb
Baba Ghannouj, 2 Tbsp, 1 oz	**70**	6	2
Baklava, (Pastry, Nuts, Syrup), 1 pastry, 1¾ oz	**245**	18	18
Cabbage Rolls, (Cabb. Leaf, Meat, Rice), 1 roll, 3 oz,	**100**	3	12
Cous Cous, (Semolina, Milk, Fruit, Nuts), 1 cup	**400**	21	43
Falafel, (Chick Pea Fritter), Fried, 1 medium, 1 oz	**60**	4	4
Hummus, ¼ cup, 2.2 oz	**105**	3	5
Fried Kibbi, (Wheat, Meat Pinenuts), 1 piece, 3 oz	**180**	8	15
Kafta, (Ground Lamb, Ssge on Skewer), 1 skewer, 1.5 ozoz	**85**	5	2
Kibbeh Naye, (raw Lamb, Bulgur & Spice) 1 cup, 9 oz	**450**	18	28
Lebanese Omelet, 1 serving, 4 oz (Egg, Spinach, Pinenuts, Onion)	**200**	12	13
Pilaf, (Rice, Onion, Raisins, Apr., Spice) 1 cup	**400**	11	60
Shawourma, (Spit-Roast Beef), 4 oz serving	**280**	15	2
Shish Kabob, 1 stick, 2.5 oz	**130**	7	2
Spinach Pie, 1 piece, 3.5 oz	**290**	21	20
Sweet Almond Sanbusak, (Pastry, Almonds, Spices), 1 piece	**200**	15	11
Tabouli, 1 serving, 4 oz	**125**	7	13
Tahini Sauce, average, 1 Tbsp	**90**	8	2

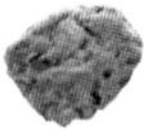
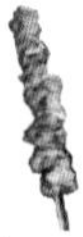

Mexican Food

	C	F	Cb
Burritos *(Taco Bell):* Bean	**370**	10	56
Supreme Beef	**420**	16	53
Chili, plain, ¼ cup	**90**	6	8
Chili con Carne: With Beans, 1 cup	**310**	17	15
Without Beans, 1 cup	**370**	28	10
Chimichangas, Beef, 5 oz	**400**	19	43
Chorizo Sausage, 2 oz	**265**	23	0
Churro, (1), 1.5 oz	**150**	8	18
Corn Chips, ½ cup, 1 oz	**160**	10	17
Enchilada, average	**330**	10	49
Fajitas, Chicken	**200**	7	20
Guacamole, average, 2 Tbsp, 1 oz	**45**	4	2
Horchata: *(Don Jose)*, 1 cup, 8 fl.oz	**140**	4	25
Cacique, 1 pint bottle, 16 fl.oz	**320**	7	62
Margarita, with 1.5 oz Tequila	**160**	0	6
Masa, (Pre-mixed for Tamales), 1 oz	**80**	5	9
Menudo:			
With Hominy, 1 cup	**240**	9	19
Without Hominy, 1 cup	**170**	9	2
Nachos: With cheese, peppers, 1 portion, 6-8 nachos, 7 oz	**600**	33	60
With cheese, beans, beef, peppers, 1 portion, 6-8 nachos, 9 oz	**570**	31	56
Del Taco: Regular, 4 oz	**300**	19	30
Macho Nachos, 17 oz	**1000**	56	94
Taco Bell, BellGrande®, 10.8 oz	**780**	40	84
Nopal Cactus Salad, 1 cup	**130**	9	11
Papas Fritas, (1), 6 oz	**325**	18	40
Piloncillo, (Brown Sugar):			
1 Tbsp, 0.5 oz	**50**	0	13
Cone, small, 3", 3 oz	**325**	0	81
Quesadilla, Cheese	**490**	28	39
Queso Fresco, ¼ cup	**80**	4.5	8
Refried Beans, ¾ cup, 6 oz	**160**	3	26
Rice Pudding, (Arroz Con Leche), 4 oz	**140**	3	24
Soup, Black Bean, 1 bowl	**200**	3	34
Tacos *(Taco Bell):*			
Crunchy: Regular	**170**	10	12
Supreme	**200**	12	15
Soft: Crispy Potato	**270**	13	31
Grilled Steak	**250**	14	19
Taco Salad with Salsa	**840**	52	85
Taco Sauce, average, ¼ cup	**15**	0	3
Taco Shell, regular	**50**	2	8
Tamales, Beef/Chicken, av. 4.5 oz	**250**	11	27
Taquitos, Beef & Cheese, 4.5 oz	**330**	15	36
Tostada (*Taco Bell*)	**250**	10	29
Tortilla, Corn, 6" diameter	**70**	1	14
Tortilla Chips, 1 oz	**150**	8	18
Soup, Black Bean, 1 bowl	**200**	3	34

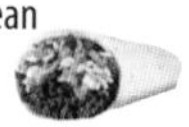
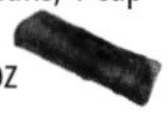
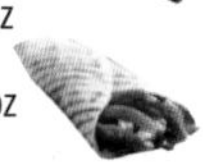
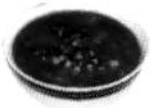
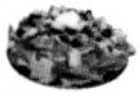
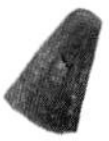
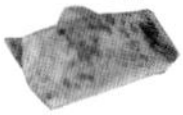
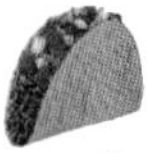
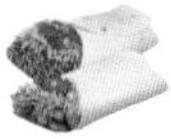
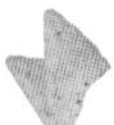

Extra Food Listings ~ See Fast Food Section
(Examples: Del Taco, Taco Bell, Taco Cabana, Taco Time)

Mexican (Cont)

Food	C	F	Cb
Breads:			
Bolillos, 1 roll, 3.5 oz	240	4	42
Mexican Cornbread, 4″ square	210	11	19
Pan de Leche, 1 roll, 1.3 oz	110	2.5	20
Telera, 2 oz	150	1.5	19
Cakes· Cookies· Pastries Pan Dulce:			
Banderilla, 1 piece	140	10	8
Bigotes, 7″	570	22	44
Capirotada, (Bread Pudding), 10 oz	810	38	107
Cinnamon Cookies, 2	125	8	13
Concha, av. all varieties:			
Small (3″ diameter), 2.5 oz	250	8	38
Medium (4″ diameter), 3.5 oz	350	11	53
Large (5″ diameter), 5.5 oz	550	18	84
Cream Puff, with Custard, 4.3 oz	255	14	25
Cuernos, (Horns), 3 oz	340	17	41
Donut, large, 4″, 3.5 oz	440	21	58
Elotes, 3.5 oz	450	24	51
Empanadas, average all varieties:			
Medium, 3 oz	300	14	42
Large, 4 oz	400	19	56
Fiesta Cookie, (1), 2.3 oz	280	8	47
Galletas Mixtas:			
Small, 1 oz	100	2.5	16
Medium, 2 oz	200	5	32
Large, 3 oz	300	7.5	48
Guayaba, 3.3 oz	360	14	53
Jelly Roll, (1), 3.3 oz	240	4	46
Mantecadites, 4.5 oz	670	42	64
Mini Cupcake, (1),1.8 oz	180	8	25
Muffins/Nino Enbuelto, large, 6 oz	465	11	48
Nuez, 3.3 oz	380	17	52
Ojo de Buey, 4 oz	360	15	55
Orejas, 1 medium, 3 oz	310	15	38
Pan Dulce, 1 bun	330	10	45
Panquecitos, 2.5 oz	260	11	36
Piedras, 4 oz	470	15	76
Polvorones: Small, 1.5 oz	180	9	24
1 large, 3 oz	370	18	48
Pound Cakes, mini, 3.5 oz	380	16	52
Puerquitos, 3.5 oz	350	12	55
Rebanadas, 3.5 oz	390	18	51
Roles De Canela, (Cinn. Roll), 4.5 oz	490	15	81
Roscas, 1 piece, 2.8 oz	360	18	44
Semitas *(Bimbo)*, 1 piece, 2.2 oz	210	6	33
Sopapillas, (flaky pastry puffs): 1 piece	100	7	10
With Honey & Cream	200	14	18
Strawberry Crema Roll, 2.5 oz slice	240	5	45

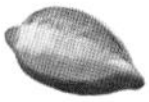
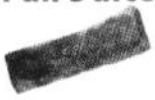
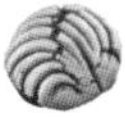
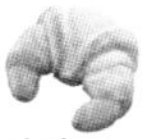
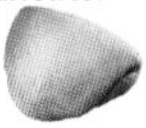
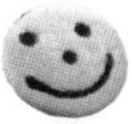
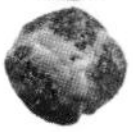
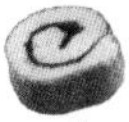
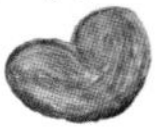
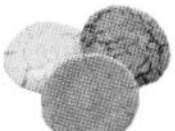
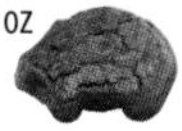

Extra Food Listings ~ *See CalorieKing.com*

Polish

Food	C	F	Cb
Cabbage Rolls, w/ Sour Cream, 2 small	220	10	30
Chicken Casserole, w/ Mshrms, 1 cup	520	27	5
Kielbasa, (Sausages, Onions, fried), 2 large	350	28	2
Meatballs, in sour cream, 3 x 1½″ balls	300	16	11
Pierogi, Fruit/Vegetables, 3″ ball	80	2	15
Pork Goulash, (Pork/Vegetable Stew)	550	21	38
Pot Roast, with Vegetables	630	21	28

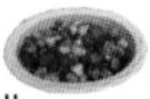

Soul Foods

Food	C	F	Cb
Breakfast Sausage, fried, 2 patties	250	17	0
Brunswick Stew, 1 cup, 8.5 oz	320	14	19
Cornbread, homemade, 3 oz	200	7.5	28
Fatback, 0.5 oz	110	11	0
Ham Hock, pickled, 3 oz	200	12	0
Hog Maw, 1 oz	70	4.5	0
Hominy, cooked, ¾ cup	110	0.5	25
Hush Puppies, 5 pieces	260	12	35
Kale, cooked, ½ cup	20	0.5	4
Opossum, roasted, without bone, 3 oz	190	9	0
Oxtail, cooked, without bone, 2 oz	85	4.5	0
Pig's Ear, ¼ ear	50	3	0
Pig's Foot, ½ foot	70	4.5	0
Pig's Tail, ⅓ tail	115	10	0
Poke Salad, cooked, ½ cup	16	0.5	3
Pork Brains, braised, 3 oz	115	8	0
Pork Chitterlings, simmered, 3 oz	260	25	0
Pork Cracklings, 0.5 oz	80	6	0
Pork Neck Bones, cooked, no bone, 2 oz	100	4.5	0
Pork Skin, 1 cup	70	4.5	0
Pork Tongue, ⅓ tongue	75	5.5	0
Sousemeat, 1 oz	60	4.5	0
Succotash, ½ cup	80	1	17
Sweet Potato Pie, ⅛ of 9″ pie	250	12	34
Tripe, 2 oz	55	2	0
Vienna Sausage:			
2 small, 1 oz	90	8	1
1 small, 0.5 oz	45	4	0.5

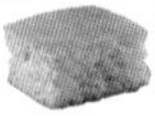
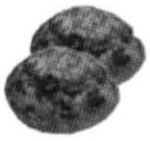
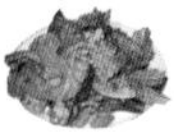
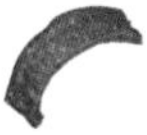
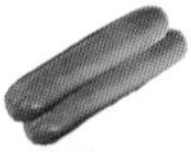

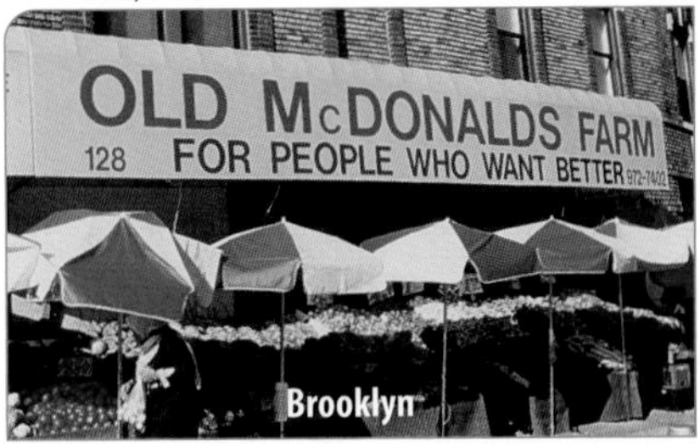

Brooklyn

Restaurant & International Foods

Spanish

	C	F	Cb
Arroz Abanda, (Fish with Rice)	340	8	31
Arroz Con Pollo, (Rice/Chkn Salad)	500	23	50
Clams Marinara, 8 clams	330	16	22
Cochifrito, (Lamb with Lemon/Garlic)	650	25	5
Cochinillo Asado, (Rst Suckling Pig), 2 slices	300	15	3
Cocido Madrileno, (Madrid-Style Boiled Dinner)	450	27	18
Flan de Leche, (Caramel Custard)	325	9	52
Fritadera de Ternera, (Sauteed Veal)	450	27	2
Gazpacho, 1 bowl	60	0	15
Mole Poblano, ½ cup	205	14	16
Paella a la Valenciana, (Chicken & Shellfish Rice)	900	42	70
Pollo a la Espanola, (Chicken)	475	30	4
Ternera al Jerez, (Veal with Sherry)	660	29	6
Zarzuela, (Fish & Shellfish Medley)	530	27	40

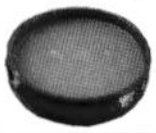

Thai Foods

	C	F	Cb
Appetizers: Satay Pork, 1 oz	100	4	2
Spring Roll, 1.3 oz	110	6	13
Soups, Tom Yam (Hot & Sour): Spicy Shrimp/Seafood:			
1 cup	100	4	6
1 bowl	160	7	10
Vegetarian, 1 cup	50	0	11
Curries: Chicken with Ginger, 1 cup	390	34	4
Thick Red Curry with Beef, 1 cup	600	50	7
Thai Chicken Curry, 1 cup	340	23	4
Massaman Curry, 1 cup	680	57	8
Green Curry with Pork, 1 cup	480	44	5
Pad Thai, large serving, 18 oz	990	38	125
Fish: Steamed with Spicy Thai Sce	450	8	46
Crispy Fried, 5 oz	290	15	9
Spicy Chicken, stir-fry	450	22	14
Spicy Garlic Tofu, stir-fry	340	18	18
Sticky Thai Rice: Plain 1 cup, 6 oz	170	0.5	36
With Coconut & Sesame Seeds, 1 cup	880	28	120
Stir-fried Rice Noodles, 1 cup 5.5 oz	270	9	40
Stir-fried Vegetables, 1 cup	100	3	18
Salads: Green Papaya Salad	160	0	40
Spicy Prawn, 9 shrimp	170	3	15
Thai Beef Salad, 1 serving	260	9	15
Thai Chicken, 1 serving	330	9	17
Thai Noodle, 1 serving	410	13	45
Satay Chicken & Peanut Sauce, 1 satay stick	390	24	20
Sauce, Peanut Satay, ½ cup, 4 oz	160	10	13

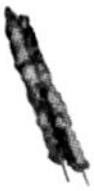
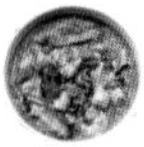
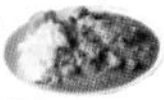
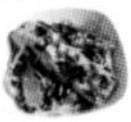
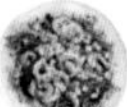
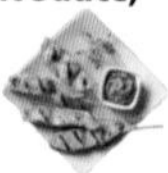

Vietnamese

	C	F	Cb
Banh Cuon, (Steam Rice w/ Pork), 1 roll	105	7	8
Bo Nuong, (Beef Satay), 2 sticks	265	9	4
Bo Xao Dau Phong, (Ginger Beef with Onion, Fish Sce)	750	30	10
Ca Chien Gung, (Whole Snapper/Ginger)	600	16	6
Canh Chay, (Vegetable/Tofu Soup)	80	3	13
Cari Chicken, 1 cup	475	29	16
Cari Chicken, with Rice Noodle, 1 cup curry & 1 cup noodles	660	29	60
Cari Chicken, with Steamed Rice, 1 cup curry & 1 cup rice	650	29	55
Cuu Xao Lan, (Curried Lamb and Veggies in Coconut)	900	40	80
Ga Chien, (Crisp Chick + Plum Sauce)	900	40	105
Ga Nuong, (Chicken Satay + Sauce)	240	10	4
Ga Xao Rau, (Marinated Chicken Braised with Vegetables)	800	26	100
Gio Lua, (Lean Pork Pie), ⅛ of pie	245	12	0
Goi Cuon, (Cold Spring Rolls), 1 roll	60	1	7
Rau Cai Xao Chay, (Stir Fried Veggies)	400	15	65
Thit Bo Vien, (Beef Balls), 6 balls	225	14	2
Thit Heo Goi Baup Cai, (Spicy Cabb. Rolls with Pork), 1 roll	200	7	11
Soup: *Per Bowl, ½ Cup*			
Bun Bo Hue, (Hot & Spicy Soup):			
Without Pork Feet	340	9	35
With Pork Feet	830	45	35
Chicken & Rice Noodle Soup	400	3	55
Pho Bo, (Beef Noodle Soup)	410	7	59
Pho Ga, (Chicken Noodle Soup)	460	6	58
Pho Tai, (Rare Beef & Noodle Soup)	440	7	73
Salad, Goi Du Du, (Green Papaya), ½ cup	155	3	29
Sauce, Nuoc Cham (Hot Sauce)	5	0	1

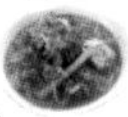
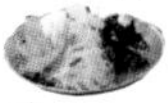

Gourmet & Miscellaneous

	C	F	Cb
Ants Eggs/Larvae, 1 Tbsp	20	0	0
Ants, chocolate coated, 3 Tbsp	140	7	2
Bee Maggots, canned, 3 Tbsp	65	2	0
Caviar, black/red, 1 Tbsp	40	3	0
Caterpillars, canned, 2 oz	60	2	0
Frog Legs, fried, 1 pair (large)	125	7	0
Haggis, boiled, 4 oz	350	24	22
Locusts, roasted, 1 oz	35	1	0
Silkworms, raw, 1 oz	60	2	0
Snails in garlic butter, 6 large	200	10	4
Snake, roasted, 4 oz	160	6	0

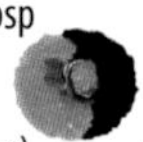
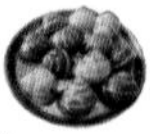

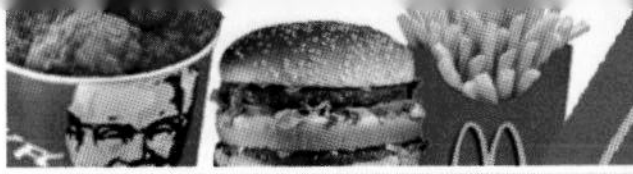

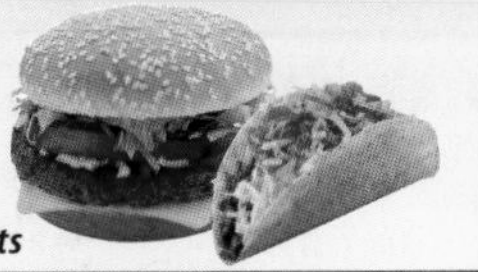

Nutritional data is based on U.S. outlets

For More Restaurants & Full Nutritional Data ~ See CalorieKing.com

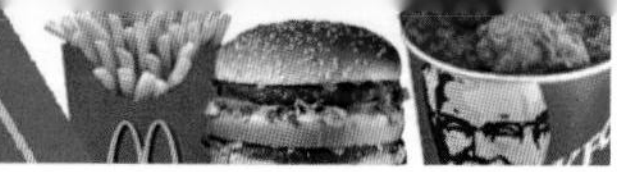

A&W® (Nov '20)

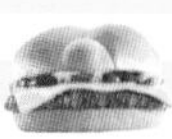
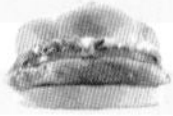
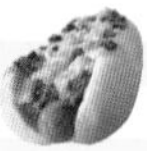
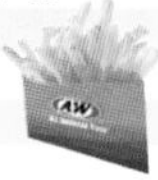
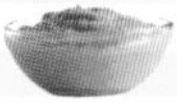
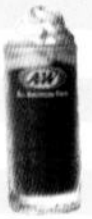
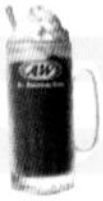

Burgers:	C	F	Cb
Original Bacon Cheeseburger:			
Single	460	23	40
Double	650	36	41
Cheeseburger	400	16	42
Double Cheeseburger	590	29	42
Hamburger	350	11	41
Papa Burger: Single	450	22	42
Double	640	35	42
Sandwiches: Crispy Chicken	480	20	51
Fish	440	21	61
Grilled: Chicken	410	12	38
Chicken Club	470	17	39
Hand-Breaded: Chicken	475	13	51
Chicken Club	490	20	42
Chicken Tenders, breaded, 3 pcs	260	9	5
Corn Dog Nuggets, 10 pieces	540	26	40
Hot Dogs: Plain	310	18	28
Coney	320	19	26
Coney Cheese Dog	360	22	29
Footlong Hotdog	610	34	52
Fries: Chili Cheese Fries, 7 oz	410	18	51
French Fries:			
Small/Kids, 2.5 oz	210	8	29
Regular, 4 oz	310	13	45
Large, 5.5 oz	430	17	61
Onion Rings, 5.1 oz	280	4	53
Dipping Sauces: *Per 1 oz Cup*			
BBQ	40	0	10
Buttermilk Ranch	130	14	1
Honey Mustard	45	0	10
Spicy Papas	130	12	6
A&W Root Beer Float:			
16 oz Cup	300	5	64
20 oz Cup	330	5	71
32 oz Cup	590	11	124
Diet Root Beer, 16 oz	160	5	24
Cones: Choc./Vanilla, reg., 5.5 oz	270	8	42
Root Beer, regular, 5.5 oz	260	8	41
Freeze:			
A&W Root Beer: 16 oz	380	9	68
20 oz	520	12	92
Diet Root Beer, 16 oz	270	9	41
Polar Swirls: M&M, 12 oz	810	29	123
Oreo, 12 oz	660	17	100
Reese's Peanut Butter Cup, 12 oz	690	29	95
Shakes: Chocolate/Vanilla, av., 16 oz	540	17	87
Strawberry, 16 oz	520	17	81
Sundaes: Caramel, regular	380	11	65
Chocolate, regular	360	11	61
Hot Fudge/Hot Caramel, reg., av.	385	13	63

Applebees® (Nov '20)

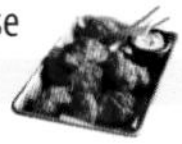
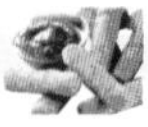
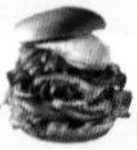
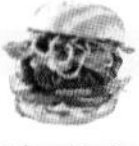
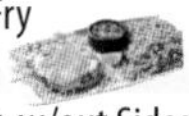
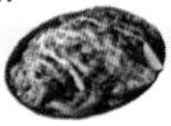
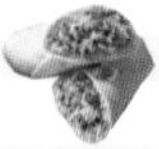
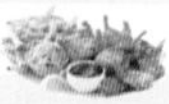

Appetizers: *As Served*	C	F	Cb
Boneless Wings, plain	640	32	47
Dressings: Bleu Cheese	210	22	2
Ranch	160	16	2
Sauces: Honey BBQ	220	0	54
Sweet Asian Chili	250	2	55
Brew Pub Pretzels & Beer Chse Dip	1190	47	153
Chipotle Lime Chicken Quesadillas	940	61	58
Chips & Salsa	630	29	83
Crunchy Onion Rings	1250	56	173
Mozzarella Sticks	850	43	79
Neighborhood Nachos, Chicken	1770	110	114
Spinach & Artichoke Dip	980	60	88
Burgers: *With Fries*			
Brunch	1640	100	118
Classic	1180	68	99
Classic Bacon Cheeseburger	1400	85	102
Quesadilla	1670	109	100
Whisky Bacon	1680	102	126
Chicken: *With Menu Set Sides Unless Indicated*			
Bourbon Street Chicken & Shrimp	740	36	43
Chicken Tenders Plate	1130	63	104
Chicken Wonton Stir Fry	750	19	92
Fiesta Lime Chicken	1190	63	96
Grilled Chicken Breast, w/out Sides	190	3	0
Sweet & Savory Grilled Chicken	560	24	41
Fajitas: Loaded Chicken	1560	76	129
Loaded Shrimp	1400	74	129
Loaded Sirloin Steak	1630	88	129
Sandwiches & More: *With Menu Set Sides*			
BBQ Brisket Tacos	1620	88	165
Chicken Fajita Rollup	1470	83	120
Clubhouse Grille S'wch	1460	79	133
The Prime Rib Dipper	1410	75	125
Pasta: *As Served, with Breadstick*			
Broccoli Blackened Shrimp Alfredo	1360	80	105
Broccoli Grilled Chicken Alfredo	1470	82	103
Three Cheese Chicken Penne	1370	75	98
Seafood: *Without Sides*			
Blackened Cajun Grilled Salmon	240	9	5
Double Crunch Shrimp	630	23	78
Shrimp Wonton Stir Fry	640	17	93

Updated Nutrition Data ~ www.CalorieKing.com
Persons with Diabetes ~ See Disclaimer (Page 22)

Applebees® cont... (Nov '20)

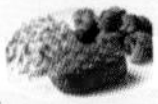
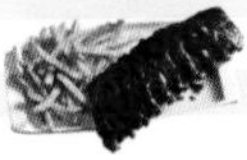
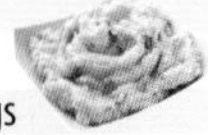
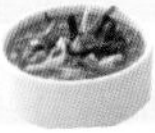
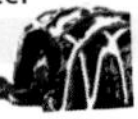

Steaks & Ribs: W/out Sauce, Sides, or Steak Toppings	C	F	Cb
6 oz TopSirloin	200	7	0.5
8 oz USDA Sirloin	270	10	0.5
Bourbon Street Steak	420	25	3
Double Glazed Baby Back Ribs:			
Full Rack	860	64	0.5
Half Rack	430	32	0
Riblets: Plate	480	30	4
Platter	760	49	6
Shrimp & Parmesan Sirloin, 8 oz	560	34	6
Ribs Sauce:			
Honey BBQ/Texas Style BBQ, av:			
Full Rack	155	1	36
Half Rack	75	0.5	18
Ribs Toppers: Grilled Onions	45	2.5	5
Crispy Onion Tanglers	170	12	14
Sauteed Garlic Mushrooms	170	15	6
Shrimp 'n Parm Toppers	290	24	5
Salads: Per Regular, with Dressing, without Bread			
Caesar with Grilled Chicken	940	60	49
Crispy Chicken Tender	1060	73	63
Oriental Grilled Chicken	1280	83	89
Strawberry Balsamic Chicken	690	43	34
Tuscan Garden Shrimp	570	39	29
Fries & Sides: Baked Potato, plain	210	5	38
Loaded	530	35	42
Caesar Side Salad, with Dressing	210	18	10
Cole Slaw	130	8	16
Classic Fries	430	20	57
Crunchy Onion Rings	510	28	60
Four-Cheese Mac & Cheese	420	22	35
Garlic Mashed Potatoes	250	11	32
Garlic Mashed Potatoes, loaded	430	27	35
Garlicky Green Beans	160	13	10
House Salad without dressing	120	6	12
Steamed Broccoli	100	7	6
Soup: Chicken Tortilla	190	9	18
Clam Chowder, regular	330	23	18
French Onion	340	20	22
Loaded Potato	520	45	17
Portsmith Clam Chowder	210	10	24
Tomato Basil	230	14	20
Desserts: Blue Ribbon Brownie	1400	61	196
Chocolate Chip Cookie Sundae	1290	62	173
Hot Fudge Sundae Shooter	340	18	44
Sizzlin' Crml Apple Blondie	1240	50	190
Triple Choc. Meltdown	1000	54	118

Arby's® (Nov '20)

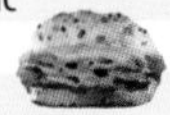
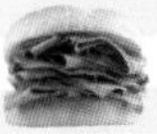
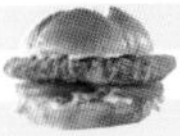
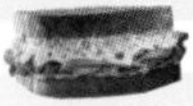
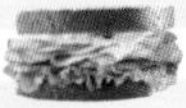
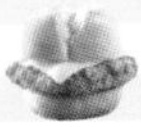
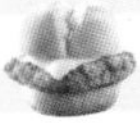
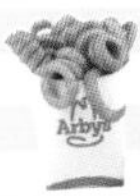
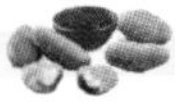
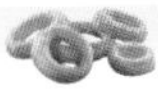

Sandwiches:	C	F	Cb
Beef 'n Cheddar: Classic	450	20	45
Double	630	32	48
½ Pound	740	39	48
Roast Beef: Classic	360	14	37
Double	510	24	38
½ Pound	610	30	38
Buttermilk Chicken:			
Buffalo Chicken	500	23	49
Chicken Bacon & Swiss	610	30	51
Chicken Cordon Bleu	660	34	49
Crispy Chicken	510	25	48
Signature: Loaded Italian	680	40	49
Reuben	680	31	62
Roast Beef Gyro	550	29	48
Smokehouse Brisket	600	35	42
Turkey Gyro	470	20	48
Turkey:			
Grand Turkey Club	480	23	38
Roast Turkey & Swiss	710	28	79
Roast Turkey, Ranch & Bacon	800	34	79
Wraps: Roast Turkey & Swiss	520	27	39
Roast Turkey, Ranch & Bacon	620	34	39
Sliders: Buffalo Chicken	290	13	31
Chicken Tender 'n Cheese	290	12	30
Ham 'n Cheese	230	9	22
Jalapeno Roast Beef 'n Cheese	240	11	21
Pizza	300	17	22
Roast Beef 'n Cheese	240	11	21
Turkey 'n Cheese	200	7	21
Chicken Tenders: 3 pieces	360	17	28
5 pieces	600	28	47
Dipping Sauces: Buffalo, 1 oz	10	1	2
Honey Mustard, 1 oz	140	13	5
Ranch, 1 oz	100	11	2
Curly Fries: Small, 4.5 oz	410	22	49
Medium, 6 oz	550	29	65
Large, 7 oz	650	35	77
Loaded Curly Fries, 8 oz	670	44	57
Sides: Without Sauce			
Jalapeno Bites:			
5 pieces	290	17	31
8 pieces	470	27	50
Mozzarella Sticks: 4 pieces	440	23	37
6 pieces	650	35	56
Potato Cakes: 3 pcs	370	21	35
4 pieces	490	28	46
Onion Rings, 5 rings	420	21	52

continued next page...

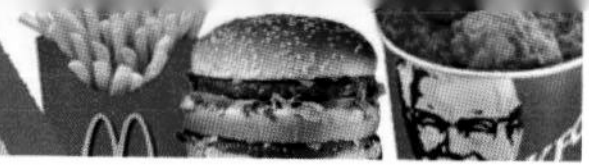

Arby's® cont... (Nov '20)

Item	C	F	Cb
***Salads:** Without Dressing*			
Chopped Farmhouse:			
Crispy Chicken	430	24	26
Roast Turkey	240	13	9
Chopped Side Salad	70	5	4
***Dressings:** Per 1.5 oz Packet*			
Balsamic Vinaigrette	130	12	4
Buttermilk Ranch	210	22	2
Dijon Honey Mustard	180	16	8
Light Italian	20	1	2
Kids Menu: Chicken Tenders (2)	240	11	19
Chicken Tender 'N Cheese Slider	290	12	30
Curly Fries	250	13	29
Ham 'n Cheese Slider	230	9	22
Roast Beef 'n Cheese Slider	240	11	21
***Breakfast:** Per Serving*			
Biscuits: Bacon, Egg & Cheese	480	29	38
Ham, Egg & Cheese	470	25	39
Sausage, Egg & Cheese	640	45	39
Croissants: Bacon, Egg & Cheese	440	27	29
Ham, Egg & Cheese	420	23	30
Sausage, Egg & Cheese	590	44	30
Sourdoughs:			
Bacon, Egg & Cheese	490	23	46
Ham, Egg & Cheese	470	19	47
Sausage, Egg & Cheese	640	39	47
Wraps: Bacon, Egg & Cheese	500	27	42
Ham, Egg & Cheese	440	22	42
Sausage, Egg & Cheese	630	41	42
Sauces: Arby's, 0.5 oz	15	0	3
Bronco Berry, 1 oz	60	0	15
Cheddar Cheese, 1.5 oz	50	3.5	4
Horsey, 0.5 oz	60	5	3
Marinara, 1 oz	20	0	4
Spicy Three Pepper, 0.5 oz	25	1	3
Tangy BBQ, 1 oz	40	0	9
Desserts:			
Apple Turnover	430	18	65
Cherry Turnover	390	13	65
Salted Caramel & Chocolate Cookie	430	18	63
Triple Chocolate Cookie	450	21	60
Iced Tea, Unsweetened, small cup	5	0	1
Juice, Capri Sun Fruit Juice, 6.5 oz	80	0	21
***Shakes:** Per Medium*			
Jamocha; Ultimate Choc.	755	23	125
Vanilla	630	23	95

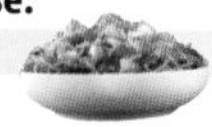
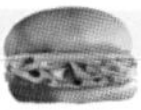
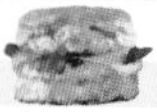
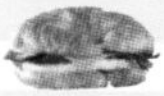
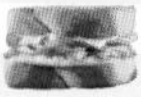
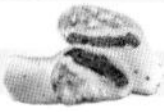
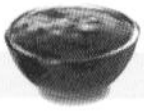
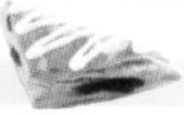

Atlanta Bread Co® (Nov '20)

Item	C	F	Cb
Breakfast Bagel Sandwiches:			
Egg & Cheese	525	17	69
Egg, Cheese & Ham	505	13	69
Egg, Cheese & Turkey Sausage	500	14	68
Side, Breakfast Potatoes	170	9	20
Paninis: Chicken Pesto	735	30	76
Cuban	845	41	75
Steakhouse	725	33	68
Sandwiches: Chicken Salad	745	42	57
Grilled Caprese	700	36	64
Roast Beef	475	16	52
Roasted Turkey	510	16	58
Tuna Salad	720	38	60
***Salads:** Per Full Size, with Dressing, without Bread*			
Balsamic Blue	605	44	40
Caesar	790	55	60
Chopstix Chicken	855	46	80
Cobb	730	17	32
Greek	700	51	40
Sides, Black Beans & Corn	190	9	24

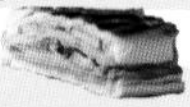
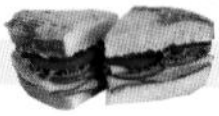
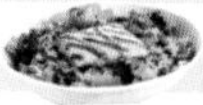

Au Bon Pain® (Nov '20)

Item	C	F	Cb
***Bagels:** Per Bagel*			
Ancient Grain, 3.8 oz	290	4	53
Asiago Cheese, 4 oz	310	5	54
Cinnamon Raisin, 3.7 oz	270	1	57
Everything, 3.6 oz	270	1.5	54
Plain, 3.5 oz	260	0.5	53
Sesame Seed Bagel, 3.6 oz	280	2	54
Whole Wheat Skinny , 1.6 oz	90	1	21
Breakfast Sandwiches:			
2 Eggs on a Bagel	400	11	54
with Bacon	450	15	55
with Bacon & Cheese	480	20	51
Egg Whites On Skinny Wheat Bagel:			
Cheddar	210	7	22
Cheddar & Avocado	360	23	25
Smoked Salmon Wasabi,			
on Skinny Wheat Bagel	400	10	59
Classic Oatmeal, 12 oz	260	5	47
Fruit Cup, large, 12 oz	140	0.5	36
Yogurt Parfait:			
Blueb. Yog. & Wild Blueb. 10.2 oz	370	9	65
Greek Van. Yog. & Wild Blueb., 10.2 oz	320	8	44
***Sandwiches:** Per Whole Sandwich*			
Cafe: Extra Bacon BLT	500	24	52
Prime Roast Beef	630	25	69
Tuna Salad	460	11	53
Signature: 2 Tomato Caprese	570	28	59
Toasted Chicken & Avocado	730	34	68

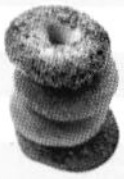
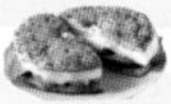
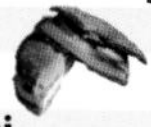
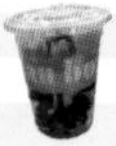
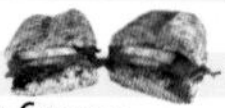

Updated Nutrition Data ~ www.CalorieKing.com
Persons with Diabetes ~ See Disclaimer (Page 22)

Au Bon Pain® cont... (Nov '20)

	C	F	Cb
Harvest Hot Bowls:			
Mayan Chicken	**550**	10	84
Mediterranean Chicken	**700**	27	76
Roasted Vegetarian	**640**	32	75
Teriyaki Steak	**650**	11	98
Soups: *Per 12 fl.oz*			
Baked Stuffed Potato	**390**	24	34
Broccoli Cheddar	**340**	24	20
Chicken Noodle	**120**	2.5	15
Clam Chowder	**350**	20	32
Corn & Green Chili Bisque	**270**	16	26
Harvest Pumpkin	**230**	13	24
Lemon Orzo Chicken	**230**	12	20
Roasted Eggplant	**190**	6	25
Wild Mushroom bizque	**190**	9	23
Salads: *Without Dressing*			
Chicken Caesar Asiago	**290**	9	21
Chicken Cobb, w/ Avocado	**460**	25	17
Harvest Turkey	**370**	14	30
Vegetarian Deluxe	**260**	13	26
Dressings: Bals. Vinaigrette, 1.5 oz	**80**	7	5
Caesar, 1.5 oz	**190**	19	3
Ranch, 1.5 oz	**180**	19	4
Cake, Cookies, Croissants, Danish, Dessert:			
Cake, Iced Lemon Pound, 4.5 oz	**470**	21	66
Cinnamon Swirl Roll, 5.2 oz	**530**	25	73
Cookies:			
Chocolate Chip, 2.8 oz	**370**	18	54
Oatmeal Raisin, 2.2 oz	**290**	11	46
Croissants: Almond, 4 oz	**500**	31	47
Apple & Cinnamon, 3.4 oz	**220**	8	35
Chocolate, 4 oz	**470**	25	55
Plain, 2.4 oz	**280**	16	28
Danish, Sweet Cheese, 4.4 oz	**410**	20	50
Muffins:			
Banana Walnut, 4.9 oz	**580**	31	66
Blueberry, 4.9 oz	**480**	25	59
Chocolate Chip, 4.7 oz	**580**	30	73
Raisin Bran, 4.7 oz	**430**	12	75
Palmier, 2.6 oz	**380**	20	46
Beverages:			
Caffe Latte, 16 fl.oz	**140**	7	12
Caramel Macchiato, 16 fl.oz	**270**	8	41
Hot Chocolate, 16 fl.oz	**350**	12	51
Raspberry Iced Tea, 24 fl.oz	**180**	0	50
Strawb. Banana Smoothie, 16 fl.oz	**290**	0	68

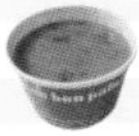
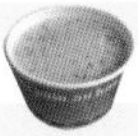
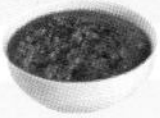
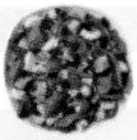
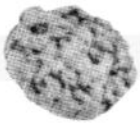
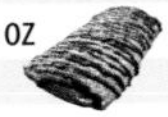
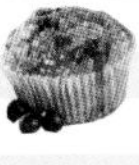
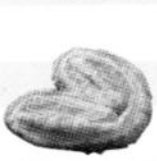

For Complete Items ~ See CalorieKing.com

Auntie Anne's® (Nov '20)

	C	F	Cb
Pretzels: *With Butter*			
Cinnamon Sugar	**470**	12	84
Jalapeno	**330**	5	63
Original	**340**	5	65
Pepperoni	**480**	16	65
Roasted Garlic & Parm.	**380**	8	68
Sour Cream & Onion	**380**	8	68
Sweet Almond	**390**	6	74
Dipping Sauces:			
Caramel, 1.7 oz	**170**	2	37
Cheese, 1.4 oz	**90**	8	2
Hot Salsa, 1.4 oz	**90**	8	2
Light Cream Cheese, 1.25 oz	**80**	6	1
Marinara, 2 oz	**45**	1	7
Melted Cheese, 2 oz	**150**	12	6
Sweet Glaze, 1.7 oz	**150**	0	39
Sweet Mustard, 1.5 oz	**90**	3	14
Pretzel Dogs: Original	**360**	20	33
Cheese with Butter	**370**	20	33
Jalapeno & Cheese	**370**	20	34
Mini Pretzel Dogs w/ Butter (10)	**630**	35	56
Pretzel Nuggets, Orig., w/ Butter, 16 oz	**390**	5	75
Beverages, Frozen Lemonade Mixer, Blue Raspberry; Strawb., 16 fl.oz	**235**	0	58

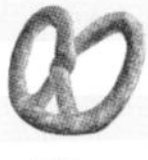
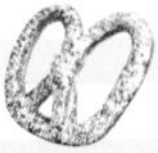
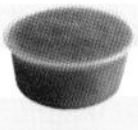
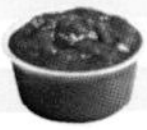
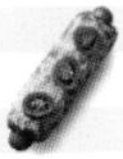

Back Yard Burgers® (Nov '20)

	C	F	Cb
Black Angus Burgers: *On Brioche Bun*			
Back Yard: *Without Cheese*			
Classic Burger	**760**	47	49
Double Classic	**1210**	84	49
Black Jack Burger	**940**	65	49
Black & Bleu Burger	**940**	65	46
Chipotle Burger	**1000**	67	56
Mushroom Swiss Burger	**850**	56	44
Chicken Sandwiches: *On Brioche Bun*			
Blackened Chicken w/out cheese	**620**	27	51
Black Jack Chicken Club	**710**	37	47
Grilled Chicken, w/out cheese	**460**	11	46
Hawaiian Chicken, w/out cheese	**530**	11	64
Specialties:			
Breaded Chicken Tender Basket, w/o Toppings, Chse, Sce or Bread	**540**	36	27
Veggie Burger, without cheese	**430**	10	68
Turkey Burgers: *On Brioche Bun*			
Classic, without cheese	**540**	28	42
Club	**660**	38	43
Wild	**610**	33	44

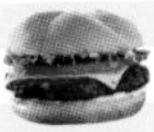
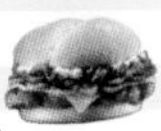
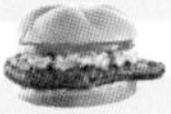

continued next page ...

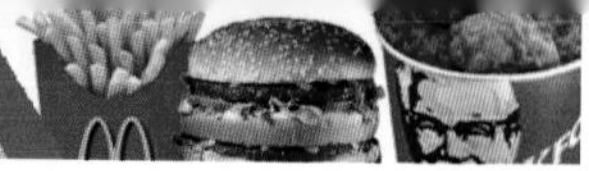

Back Yard Burgers® cont... (Nov '20)

Fries:	C	F	Cb
Chili Cheese Fries, seasoned, reg.	790	59	52
Seasoned Fries: Regular, 4.5 oz	480	36	38
Large, 6 oz	640	47	50
Sweet Potato Fries, regular, 6 oz	450	29	40
Waffle Fries: Reg., 6 oz	820	56	66
Large, 8 oz	1100	75	88
Sides: Back Yard Chili	310	18	15
Creamy Coleslaw	200	16	15
Loaded Baked Potato	420	21	45
Panko Onion Rings, regular, 4 oz	340	13	47
Salads: *Without Dressing*			
Back Yard Salad: w. Grilled Chicken	350	10	21
with Blackened Chicken	450	21	22
Cranberry Pecan Grilled Chicken	660	30	52
Side Salad	140	6	14
Dressings:			
Bleu Cheese	220	24	1
Caesar	260	26	4
Gorgonzola Vinaigrette	170	15	6
Honey Mustard	200	20	7
Ranch, Homestyle	150	16	1
Dessert/Cobblers: Apple/Cherry	390	16	58
Apple/Cherry Cobbler A La Mode	540	24	78
Ice Cream, A La Carte	150	8	20
Milk Shakes: *With Whole Milk & Whipped Topping*			
Chocolate: Vanilla, av.	745	35	98
Chocolate Oreo	850	40	115
Peanut Butter	830	51	79

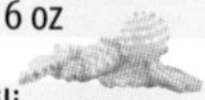
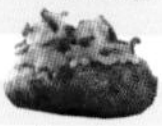
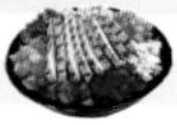
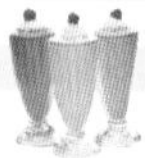

Baja Fresh® (Nov '20)

Baja Bowls: *With Black Beans*	C	F	Cb
Carnitas	680	18	92
Chicken	700	22	82
Shrimp	660	20	83
Steak	690	22	82
Veggie	540	14	90
Burritos: *With Standard Components*			
Baja: with Carnitas	800	41	63
with Chicken	820	45	53
with Steak	810	45	53
Mexicano: *With Black Beans*			
Chicken	800	27	94
Roasted Veggie	640	19	102
Steak	790	27	94
Ultimo: Carnitas	950	45	88
Chicken	970	50	78
Steak	960	50	78
Nachos: *Regular Size, with Black Beans*			
Chicken	1960	105	162
Shrimp	1920	104	164
Steak	1950	105	162

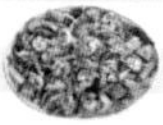
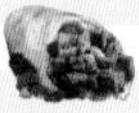
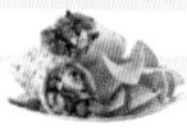
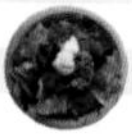

Baja Fresh® cont... (Nov '20)

Fajitas: *With Black Beans*	C	F	Cb
Chicken: with Corn Tortilla	1050	38	119
with Flour Tortilla	1240	44	144
Shrimp: with Corn Tortilla	980	35	120
with Flour Tortilla	1170	41	145
Steak: with Corn Tortilla	1040	38	119
with Flour Tortilla	1230	44	144
Wahoo: with Corn Tortilla	980	35	119
with Flour Tortilla	1170	40	144
Tacos: *With Standard Toppings*			
Americano, Soft Taco: Carnitas	220	9	21
Chicken	230	11	19
Baja, meat/fish varieties, average	160	6	17
Wahoo Crispy Taco	265	16	25
Salads: *Without Dressing*			
Baja Ensalada:			
with Chicken	260	11	18
with Shrimp	325	14	20
with Steak	255	11	18
Tostada:			
Chicken	880	52	60
Shrimp	890	53	62
Steak	875	52	60
Sides: Guacamole, 8 oz	310	27	19
Queso, 8 oz	470	37	13
Rice & Black Beans, 17 oz	550	11	90
Rice & Pinto Beans, 17 oz	570	11	95
Tortilla Chips, 5 oz	710	28	99

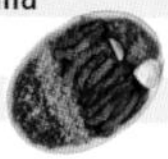
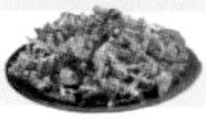
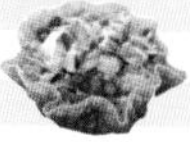
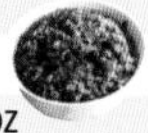

For Complete Nutritional Data ~ see CalorieKing.com

Baskin Robbins® (Nov '20)

Cones:	C	F	Cb
Cake	25	0	5
Fresh-Baked Waffle	160	3.5	29
Sugar	45	0.5	9
Ice Creams: *Per 4 oz Scoop*			
Classic Flavors: Baseball Nut	260	14	29
Cherries Jubilee	240	11	31
Chocolate Chip	250	16	23
Chocolate	240	14	26
Jamoca Almond Fudge	260	15	27
Lemon Custard	240	13	26
Made with Snickers Bars	270	14	32
Mint Chocolate Chip	250	16	23
Nutty Coconut	290	19	24
Old Fash. Butter Pecan	260	18	20
Oreo Cookies 'n Cream	260	15	28
Peanut Butter 'n Chocolate	300	20	25

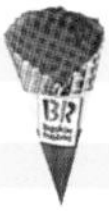
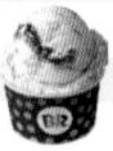
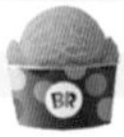
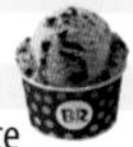

Updated Nutrition Data ~ www.CalorieKing.com
Persons with Diabetes ~ See Disclaimer (Page 22)

Baskin Robbins® cont... (Nov '20)

Ice Creams (Cont): Per 4 oz Scoop

	C	F	Cb
Classic Flavors Cont:			
Pistachio Almond	270	19	21
Pralines 'n Cream	270	14	31
Quarterback Crunch	300	17	33
Reese's P'nut Butter Cup	280	17	27
Rocky Road	290	15	35
Rum Raisin	250	11	33
Strawberry Cheesecake	250	13	29
Vanilla	240	16	21
Very Berry Strawberry	200	11	24
No Sugar Added Reduced Fat:			
Caramel Turtle Truffle	200	8	38
Key Lime Pie	230	11	37
Non Dairy/Vegan,			
Choc. Chip Cookie Dough	270	14	36
Wild 'n Reckless Sherbet	130	2	26
***Bakery:** Per 1.3 oz Cookie*			
Brownie	240	9	36
Dark Chocolate Chunk Cookie	170	6	26
Double Fudge Cookie	160	6	25
Peanut Butter Chocolate Cookie	170	8	23
White Chunk Macadamia Cookie	180	9	24
Ice Cream Quarts: *Per ⅔Cup, 3.46 oz*			
Chocolate/ Mint Chocolate Chip	210	13	20
Jamoca Almond Fudge	230	14	25
Old Fashioned Butter Pecan	230	16	18
Vanilla	210	14	18
Very Berry Strawberry	180	9	21
Sundaes:			
Banana Royale	690	28	103
Choc. Chip Cookie Dough	1130	48	164
Made with Snickers	1110	43	165
Oreo Layered	920	44	122
Reese's Peanut Butter Cup	1250	85	106
***Beverages:** Per Medium, 24 fl.oz*			
Blasts: Caramel Cappuccino	790	25	130
Mocha Cappuccino	590	22	97
Oreo Cookies 'n Cream	730	31	105
Turtle	820	23	148
Milkshakes: Chocolate Chip	1030	54	118
Mint Chocolate Chip	1030	55	117
Smoothie: Mango Banana	600	1	145
Strawberry Banana	520	1	126

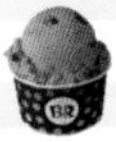
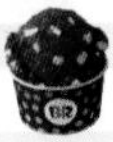
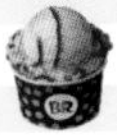
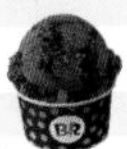
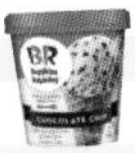

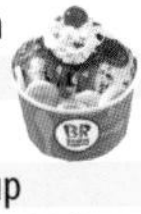
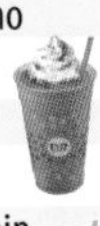
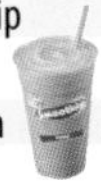

Big Apple Bagels® (Nov '20)

Bagels:	C	F	Cb
Asiago Melt; Swiss Melt	370	6	65
Cinnamon Sugar	370	2	78
Fruit Varieties, average	330	3	66
Plain or Salt	320	2	64
***Cream Cheese:** Per 1.5 oz*			
Chedd. & Bacon; Walnut Raisin, av	140	13	4
Plain/Scallion, average	135	12	2
Plain, Lite	100	9	2
Strawberry	130	11	5
Tomato-Basil	140	13	3
***Muffins:** With Whole Egg*			
Mini: Blueberry; Lemon Poppyseed	90	4.5	12
Cinnamon Swirl Cheesecake	90	5	9
Large:			
Blueberry	590	28	78
Choc. Cheesecake, 6 oz	650	38	70
***Breakfast Sandwiches:** French Toast with Egg:*			
on BAB Bagel	1020	55	107
On MFM Bagel	1060	55	117
Salads:			
Caesar, with Caesar Dressing	450	34	19
Chicken Club, with Ranch Dressing	760	59	18
Mediterranean Bread Salad, with Balsamic Vinaigrette	740	41	63
***Beverages:** Per Medium, 16 fl.oz*			
Hot Chocolate	440	12	71
Mocha; White Chocolate Latte, av.	380	8	67
Vanilla Creme Latte	310	7	50

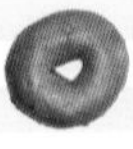
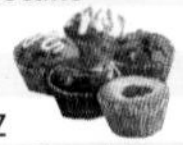
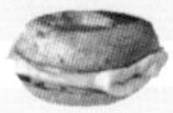

Biggby Coffee® (Nov '20)

***Hot Drinks:** Per Tall, 16 fl.oz, without Whipped Cream*	C	F	Cb
Caffe au Lait: with 2% Milk	100	4	9
with Nonfat Milk	65	0	9
with Soy	90	3	11
Caffe Latte: with 2% Milk	175	7.5	16
with Nonfat Milk	115	0	16
with Soy	160	5	19
Cappuccino: with 2% Milk	105	4.5	10
with Nonfat Milk	70	0	10
with Soy	95	3	11
Chai Latte: with 2% Milk	315	7.5	51
with Nonfat Milk	255	0	51
Dark Hot Chocolate: w/ 2% Milk	320	9	50
with Non-Fat Milk	260	1.5	50
***Frozen Creme Freeze:** Per 20 fl.oz, with 2% Milk, Whipped Cream & Sugar, without Reduced Calorie*			
Avalanche Latte	640	19	108
Banana Chip	750	20	135
Coconut Creme	640	19	110
Mellow Mochanut	645	19	109

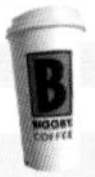
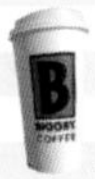
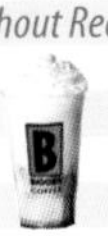

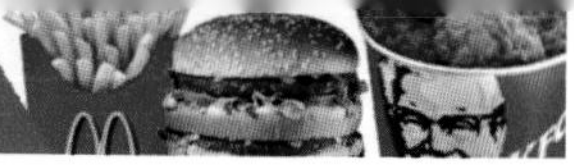

BJ's Restaurant® (Nov '20)

Shareable Appetizers: Full Order	C	F	Cb
Ahi Poke	**320**	10	24
BJ's Original Wings	**820**	63	8
Chicken Lettuce Wraps	**490**	19	46
Mozzarella Sticks	**810**	39	76
Root Beer Glazed Ribs	**560**	17	85
Sliders	**800**	30	81
Spinach Stuffed Mushrooms	**290**	20	17
***Burgers:** With French Fries*			
Bacon Cheeseburger	**1350**	80	98
Bacon Guacamole Deluxe	**1420**	85	102
Classic Burger	**1180**	66	97
Crispy Jalapeno Burger	**1430**	87	105
Mushroom Swiss Burger	**1600**	105	102
Brunch: Avocado Toast	**410**	20	47
Buttermilk Pancakes, short stack	**910**	31	143
Calif. Scramble, w/ sourdough	**1210**	69	90
Enlightened Veggie Omelette w/ Fruit	**250**	8	23
***Enlightened Entrees:** Includes Menu Set Sides*			
Cherry Chipotle Glazed Salmon	**580**	26	40
Lemon Thyme Chicken	**630**	19	52
Mediterranean: Chicken Pita Tacos	**720**	24	80
Spiced Chicken	**750**	50	21
Seared Ahi Salad	**570**	31	42
Turkey Burger	**850**	45	72
***Pasta:** Includes Garlic Knot*			
Deep Dish Ziti	**1400**	91	99
Grilled Chicken Alfredo	**1460**	71	129
Italiano Veggie Penne	**700**	28	91
Jumbo Spaghetti & Meatballs	**1600**	82	161
Shrimp Scampi	**1660**	100	130
***Deep Dish Pizza:** Per Slice, ⅛ Med. Pizza*			
BBQ/Buffalo Chicken, average	**310**	10	35
Classic Combo; Pepperoni Extreme, av.	**335**	17	32
Gourmet Five Meet	**360**	18	33
Sweet Pig; Vegetarian, average	**265**	10	34
***Tavern Crust Pizza:** Per Slice (1/12 Pizza)*			
Brewhouse; Italian Market, average	**115**	6	9
Garlic Chicken Pesto	**100**	5	9
Spicy Pig; Old Country Tomato, average	**80**	4	9
***Sandwiches:** With French Fries*			
Brewhouse Philly	**1490**	90	108
California Chicken Club	**1310**	69	91
Slow Roasted Turkey Club	**1560**	99	104
***Ribs & Steaks:** Without Sides*			
Baby Back Pork Ribs, half rack, with Peppered BBQ Sauce	**710**	34	74
Classic Rib-Eye	**1080**	67	5
Dble Bone In Pork Chop	**760**	44	32
Prime Rib Dinner	**1310**	106	6
Soups: Chicken Tortilla, Bowl	**280**	12	30
Clam Chowder: Bowl with Crackers	**510**	31	37
Sourdough Loaf with Crackers	**1470**	42	219

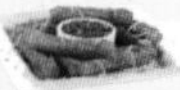
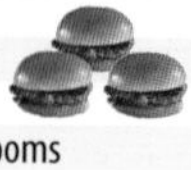
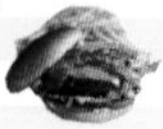
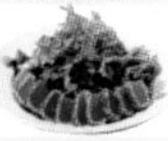
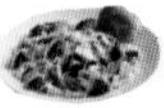
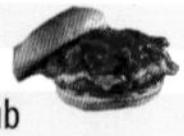
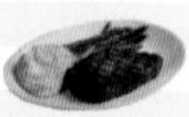

BJ's Restaurant® cont...(Nov '20)

Salads: With Dressing & Toppings	C	F	Cb
BBQ Chicken Chopped Salad	**930**	47	64
Caesar Salad	**810**	64	44
Derby-Style Chicken Cobb Salad	**940**	69	20
Honey-Crisp Chicken Salad	**1370**	103	75
Tri-Tip Wedge Salad	**1300**	91	68
Sides: Broccoli	**40**	0	6
Classic Baked Potato	**590**	28	70
French Fries	**350**	19	40
Honey Sriracha Brussels Sprouts	**160**	4	23
Rice Pilaf	**230**	6	39
White Cheddar Mashed Potatoes	**330**	18	33
Desserts: Baked Beignet	**640**	25	93
Monkey Bread Pizookie	**1380**	67	182
Salted Caramel Pizookie	**1380**	56	204
Soda Floats, Black Cherry/Or. Crm	**535**	19	83

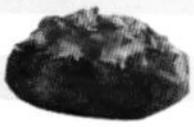

Blimpie® (Nov '20)

Cold Deli Subs: *Per Regular, 6" White Sub, with Standard Menu Board Toppings*	C	F	Cb
Blimpie Best; Turkey & Prov., av.	**465**	16	54
Club; Ham & Swiss	**430**	14	54
Roast Beef & Provolone	**460**	14	53
Tuna	**480**	22	48
Wraps, average	**580**	30	52
***Hot Deli Subs:** Per Regular White Sub with Standard Menu Board Toppings Unless Indicated*			
BLT	**510**	27	48
Meatball Parmigiana	**740**	38	59
Philly Cheesesteak	**570**	28	49
***Salads:** Regular, without Dressing*			
Buffalo Chicken; Grilled Chicken, av.	**185**	9	7
Garden	**40**	0	8
Macaroni	**290**	21	22
Potato	**190**	10	24
Ultimate Club	**310**	16	11
***Dressings:** Per 1.5 oz*			
Blue Cheese; B'mlk Ranch, average	**254**	26	3
Creamy Ital.; Pepp. Ranch, average	**240**	25	2
Thousand Island; Creamy Caesar, av.	**205**	21	4
Soup: Chicken Noodle	**210**	4	29
Cream of Broccoli with Cheese	**190**	11	15
Crm of Potato w/ Bacon	**190**	9	24
New Eng. Clam Chowder	**170**	3	28
Vegetable Beef with Barley	**100**	3	14
Breakfast:			
Biscuits: Bacon, Egg & Cheese	**410**	22	37
Sausage, Egg & Cheese	**560**	36	37
Bluffin, Egg & Cheese	**240**	8	29
Burritos: Ham, Egg & Cheese	**570**	27	51
Sausage, Egg & Cheese	**710**	43	50
Sandwich, Grilled Bacon	**520**	23	49

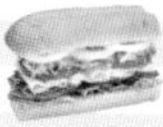
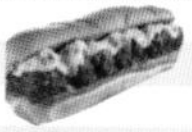
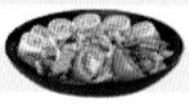
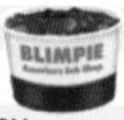

Persons with Diabetes ~ See Disclaimer (Page 22)

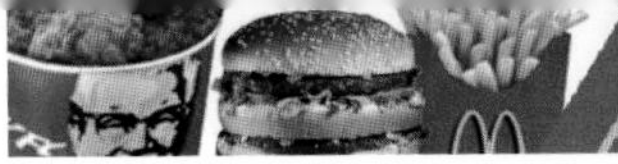

Bob Evans® (Nov '20)

Burgers: With Fries

	C	F	Cb
Big Farm Burgers:			
Double Bacon Cheeseburger	**1100**	61	81
Double Steakhouse	**1350**	78	88
Sandwiches: *With Fries*			
Farmhouse Chicken	**890**	50	87
Slow Roasted:			
Pot Roast	**1130**	57	104
Turkey Bacon Melt	**970**	46	92
Dinners: *With Menu Set Sides*			
Chicken 'n Noodle Deep Dish	**620**	33	54
Down-Home Country Fried Steak	**730**	45	58
Fork Tender Pot Roast	**950**	62	62
Smaller Portion	**620**	44	37
Heartland Chicken Pot Pie	**1430**	87	106
Herb Rubbed Turkey & Dressing	**820**	40	81
Smaller Portion	**650**	32	67
Wildfire Meatloaf	**740**	51	40
Dinners: *Without Sides*			
Great Alaska Cod with Tartar Sauce	**640**	39	39
Grilled Chicken Breast (2)	**370**	9	0
Homestyle:			
Boneless Fried Chicken Breast (2)	**570**	30	41
Fried Chicken Tenders	**640**	36	46
Golden Fried Shrump w/ Cocktail Sauce	**350**	2.5	65
USDA Choice Sirloin with Toppings	**750**	54	17
Sides: Baked Potato	**330**	12	51
Bread & Celery Dressing	**340**	15	42
Broccoli, with Butter	**110**	10	5
Carrots	**90**	4.5	13
Coleslaw	**200**	14	19
Corn	**170**	10	20
French Fries	**330**	14	47
Green Beans with Ham	**30**	1.5	4
Hash Browns	**220**	12	28
Homefries	**250**	17	24
Mac & Cheese	**250**	12	25
Mashed Potatoes: w/ Chicken Gravy	**210**	14	19
with Country Gravy	**170**	10	17
Salads: *Regular Size, with dressing*			
Cranberry Pecan Chicken	**870**	51	55
Wildfire: without Chicken	**470**	26	50
with Grilled Chicken	**560**	28	50
with Homestyle Chicken	**590**	33	64

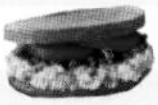
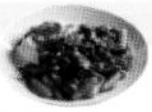
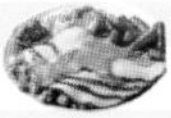
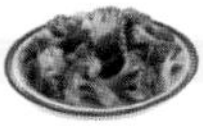
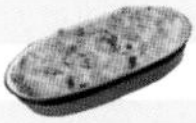
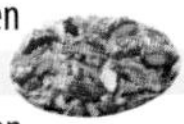

Bob Evans® cont... (Nov '20)

	C	F	Cb
Soups: *Per Bowl, with 2 Saltine Crackers*			
Cheddar Baked Potato	**390**	21	32
Chicken N Noodles	**290**	15	26
Hearty Beef Vegetable	**230**	5	36
Kid's: *With Menu Set Items*			
Chicken & Noodles	**150**	7	14
Cheeseburger with Fries	**760**	36	84
Grilled Cheese & Tomato Basil Soup	**430**	22	43
Grilled Chicken	**360**	6	52
Grilled Cheese Triangles	**330**	15	40
Mac & Cheese	**280**	12	31
Turkey Lurkey	**410**	23	34
Breakfast: *With Menu Set Items, without Added Sides Unless Indicated*			
Brioche French Toast, w/ butter & syrup	**830**	25	134
Cntry Fried Steak & Gravy	**540**	33	38
Everything Breakfast	**1130**	73	63
Goat Cheese Veg. Omelet	**850**	54	12
Ham Biscuit Benedict	**440**	23	43
Hotcakes: *With Menu Set Toppings*			
Buttermilk (4)	**1150**	28	209
Cinnamon Supreme (4)	**1070**	26	190
Doule Blueberry Hotcakes (4)	**1090**	23	203
Double Chocolate (4)	**1120**	27	199
Multigrain (4)	**1200**	31	214
Pot Roast Hash	**580**	39	28
Sunshine Skillet	**760**	59	27
Western Omelet, without sides	**650**	50	11
Breakfast Sides:			
Eggs: Egg White	**60**	0	0.5
Freshly Cracked	**200**	16	0.5
Scrambled	**160**	11	1
Homefries	**250**	17	24
Grits with butter	**240**	21	13
Hardwood Smoked Bacon	**190**	14	0.5
Hashbrowns	**200**	12	28
Hickory-Smoked Ham	**100**	2.5	2
Sausage Links (3)	**190**	16	0
Sausage Patties (2)	**320**	26	2
Turkey Sausage Links (2)	**140**	7	2
Dessert: Cherry Pie, plain, slice	**490**	24	66
Coconut Cream Pie, 1 slice	**600**	38	64
Chocolate Peanut Butter Pie, 1 slice	**680**	41	74
Double-Crust Apple Pie, 1 slice	**530**	24	77

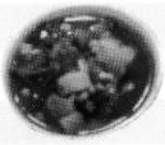
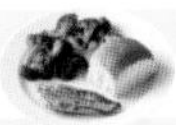
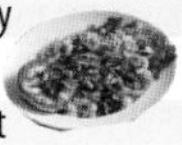
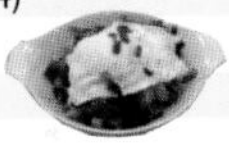
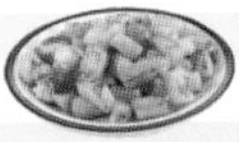
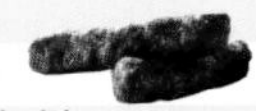

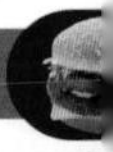

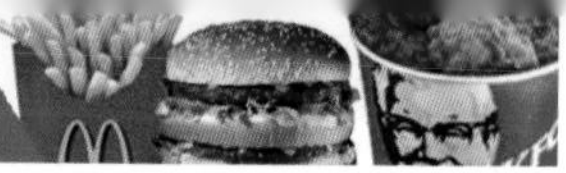

Bojangles® (Nov '20)

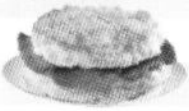
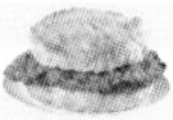

Biscuit:	C	F	Cb
Plain	310	15	37
Bacon, Egg & Cheese	470	27	39
Cajun Filet	570	27	57
Country Ham	380	20	38
Gravy Biscuit	430	21	49
Sausage	470	28	38
Sausage & Egg	550	34	38
Southern Filet	550	27	54
Steak	620	40	48
Biscuit Add Ons: American Cheese	40	3.5	1
Egg	80	6	0
Chicken: Breast (1)	540	29	24
Leg (1)	190	13	8
Thigh (1)	240	10	14
Wing (1)	150	8	8
Homestyle Tenders, 4 pieces	490	24	39
Supremes, 4 pieces	500	25	33
Sandwiches:			
Cajun Filet: Regular	670	40	55
Club	750	46	56
Grilled Chicken: Regular	570	33	36
Club	650	40	37
Fixins': Per Individual Size, Unless Indicated			
Bo-Tato Rounds, medium	390	24	40
Cole Slaw	170	11	20
Green Beans	20	0	5
Macaroni & Cheese	280	18	21
Mashed Potatoes 'N Cajun Gravy	120	3	18
Seasoned Fries: Small	360	21	39
Medium	450	26	49
Picnic	670	38	73
Salads: Without Dressing or Croutons			
Chicken Supreme	490	28	28
Garden	120	9	3
Grilled Chicken	270	14	4
Sweets: Bo-Berry Biscuit (1)	370	17	49
Cinnamon Twist (1)	380	24	8
Sweet Potato Pie	350	20	41

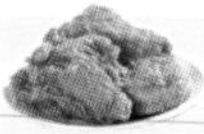
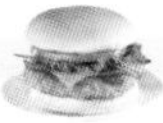
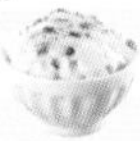
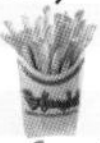
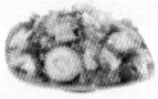
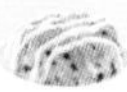

Boston Market® (Nov '20)

Sandwiches: Per Whole Sandwich	C	F	Cb
Avocado Club on Ciabatta Roll	1110	66	75
Chkn Salad Carver on Multigr. Roll	870	51	63
Rstd Turkey Carver on Ciabatta Roll	970	55	73
Sthwest Chkn Carver on Ciabatta Roll	1110	65	76
Individual Meals: Without Sides or Corn Bread			
Meatloaf, regular	470	33	17
Roasted Garlic & Herb Half Chkn	650	35	13
Rotisserie Half Chicken	500	24	1
Rotisserie Prime Rib	630	47	0
Sesame Half Chicken	630	30	18
Turkey Pot Pie	710	38	64

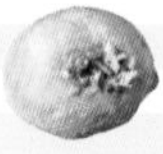

Boston Market® cont...(Nov '20)

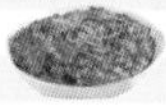

Salad Bowls: With Dressing	C	F	Cb
Chicken Caesar	770	51	49
Southwest Cobb	760	53	43
Sides: Corn Bread	240	17	11
Creamed Spinach, medium	240	17	11
Fresh Steamed Veggies, medium	60	3.5	7
Fresh Vegetable Stuffing	220	10	28
Garlic Dill New Potatoes, medium	100	2	20
Macaroni & Cheese, medium	310	10	41
Mashed Potatoes, medium	270	11	37
Sweet Corn, medium	160	7	20
Swt Pot. Casserole, med.	460	12	87
Soup, Chicken Noodle	240	9	20
Kid's: Without Sides or Corn Bread			
Chicken: Dark, 1 thigh, 1 drumstick	230	13	0.5
White, 1 breast, 1 wing	270	11	0
Meatloaf	240	16	9
Turkey	80	2.5	0
Sauce: Cranberry Walnut Relish	140	2	31
Gravy, Beef/Au Jus/Chicken	10	0	2
Horseradish	60	3	6
Zesty BBQ	40	0	10
Desserts: Apple Pie, 1 slice	560	32	66
Chocolate Brownie (1)	340	14	53
Chocolate Cake, 1 slice	570	33	66
Chocolate Chunk Cookie (1)	370	18	53

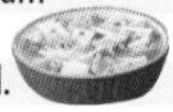
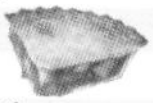

For Complete Nutritional Data ~ see CalorieKing.com

Boston Pizza® Canada (Nov '20)

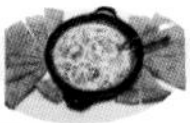

Starters:	C	F	Cb
Nonna's Meatballs	1280	67	116
Poutine	880	28	128
Spinach & Artichoke Dip	1260	58	137
Burgers: Black Bean Veggie	510	19	74
Boston Brute	800	24	108
Most Valuable Burger	1040	77	49
Vegan	460	16	73
Pastas: Full Order, without Garlic Toast			
Boston's Lasagna	790	23	107
Chicken & Mushroom Fettuccini	1250	56	142
Seven Cheese Ravioli	710	31	70
Pizza: Per 8" Individual Pizza			
Original Crust: Boston Royal	820	28	97
Deluxe	720	24	92
Hawaiian	660	16	100
Pepperoni	710	25	89
Vegetarian	620	15	94
Thin Crust Pizzas: *Per Slice of 13" Medium Pizza*			
Fiesta Chicken, 2.86 oz	200	11	18
Pesto Caprese	230	13	18
Pizza Bella, 2.3 oz	150	6	17

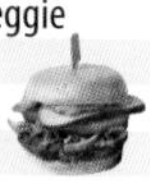
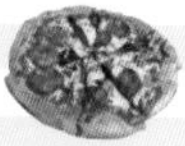
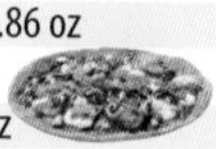

Boston Pizza® Canada cont... (Jn '21)

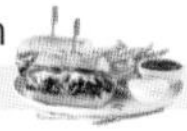
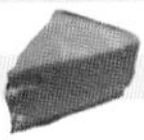

Sandwiches: Without Sides	C	F	Cb
Grilled Chicken Clubhouse	1040	44	98
Kick'n Memphis Chicken	1210	75	86
Montreal Smoked Meat	910	59	40
Wrap, Thai Chicken	820	33	87
Salads: Full Order with Set Dressing			
Crispy Chicken Pecan	950	72	50
Pineapple, Beet & Goat Cheese	390	24	36
Thai Chicken	720	24	86
Desssert:			
NY Cheesecake	580	37	54
The Panookie, with Ice Cream	940	45	125

For Complete Nutritional Data ~ see CalorieKing.com

Braum's® ~ *see CalorieKing.com*

Bruegger's® (Nov '20)

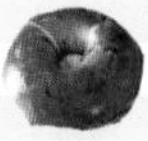
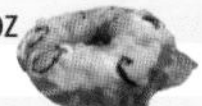
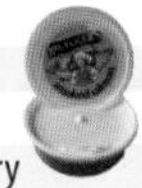
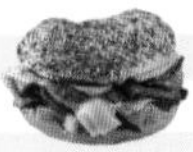

Bagels:	C	F	Cb
Blueberry, 4.1 oz	310	2	63
Cinnamon Sugar, 4.1 oz	320	2	63
Everything, 4.1 oz	310	2.5	62
Five Cheese, 4.1 oz	350	9	53
Jalapeno Cheddar, 5.5 oz	440	9	75
Plain, 4.1 oz	300	2	60
Rosemary Olive Oil, 4.1 oz	330	6	59
Cream Cheese: Per 1.5 oz			
Bacon Scallion; Jalapeno, average	140	12	6
Honey Walnut	150	12	8
Light Herb Garlic/Plain	100	6	4
Plain; Garden Veggie	130	11	6
Smoked Salmon; Strawberry	150	13	3
Breakfast Bagel S'wiches: With Standard Toppings			
Egg, Cheese & Bacon	520	20	63
Egg, Cheese & Ham	500	15	64
Egg, Cheese & Turkey Sausage	530	19	62
Egg, Cheese & Sausage	610	30	62
Deli Sandwiches: Plain Bagel With Standard Toppings			
BLT	530	23	64
Garden Veggie	360	2	72
Ham	410	7	64
Tuna Salad	550	21	65
Signature & Bagel Sandwiches: With Stndrd Toppings			
Herby Turkey on Sesame Bagel	570	15	75
Hot Pastrami on Everything Bagel	590	19	66
Hot Tuna on Ciabatta	500	24	51
Leon. da Veggie on Asiago Parm. Bagel	490	14	70
Sm. Salmon Egg Salad on Pumpnkl Bgl	570	21	64
Turkey Chipotle Club on Evrythng Bagel	810	45	66

Bruegger's® cont... (Nov '20)

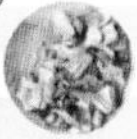

Salads: Without Dressing	C	F	Cb
Chicken Caesar	200	8	14
Garden with Chicken	270	14	22
Mixed Green Base	20	0	4
Dressings: Balsamic Vinaig., 1 oz	60	6	3
Caesar, 1 oz	80	7	2
Sides, Twice Baked Hashbrowns	170	11	12
Soup: Chicken & Wild Rice, 8 oz	230	16	14
Chicken Spaetzle, 8 oz	140	3.5	14
Dessert: Blueberry Muffin, Main St.	290	7	54
Marshmallow Chew, 2.7 oz	290	7	54

For Complete Menu & Data ~ see CalorieKing.com

Burgerville® (Nov '20)

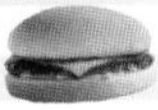
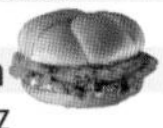
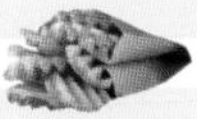
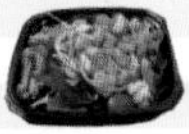
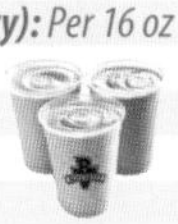
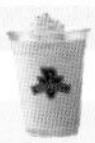

Burgers: With Standard Ingredients	C	F	Cb
Colossal on Non Seeded Bun	540	28	40
½ lb Colossal On Non Seeded Bun	790	46	40
Double Cheeseburger on Plain Bun	490	28	31
Original: Hamburger on Plain Bun	340	17	31
Cheeseburger on Plain Bun	380	21	31
Northwest Cheeseburger on Non Seeded Bun	590	33	38
Pepper Bacon Cheeseburger on Non Seeded Bun	660	39	37
Number 6 Burger on Brioche Bun	620	37	30
Vegetarian on Non Seeded Bun	700	43	60
Chicken Tenders, (3), with Fries	770	43	71
Sandwiches: Without Cheese			
Best Coast Chkn on Non Seeded Bun	430	16	36
Crispy Chkn, on Non Seeded Bun	610	32	61
Halibut Fish on Plain Bun	460	27	40
Turkey on Non Seeded Bun	450	18	40
French Fries: Small, 2.8 oz	220	11	28
Regular, 5 oz	400	19	50
Large, 6.5 oz	510	25	65
Waffly Fries, regular	280	14	34
Salads: Full Size, without Dressing			
Blue Cheese Crumbles	220	14	15
Grilled Chicken Breast	200	8	16
Smoked Salmon	190	9	15
Dressing: Balsamic Vinaigrette	180	18	5
Blue Cheese	180	18	2
Ranch	190	20	2
Bliss Shakes (Non Dairy): Per 16 oz w/out Wh. Cream			
Chocolate	840	31	143
Mint Patty	940	38	148
Oregon Strawberry	640	27	97
Sweet Cream	610	28	89
Ice Cream Milkshakes: Per 16 oz with Whipped Cream			
Chocolate Hazelnut	1080	72	98
Portland Cold Brew	910	55	89
Sweet Cream	930	57	92

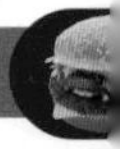

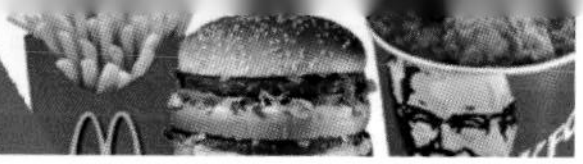

Burger King® (Nov '20)

Whopper Sandwiches:	C	F	Cb
Whopper: Regular	660	40	49
with Cheese	740	46	50
Double Whopper	900	58	49
with Cheese	980	64	50
Bacon & Cheese	790	51	50
Impossible Whopper, with Mayo	630	34	58
Triple Whopper	1130	75	49
with cheese	1220	82	50
Whopper Jr	310	18	27
Flame Grilled Burgers:			
Bacon Cheeseburger	320	16	27
Bacon Double Cheeseburger	420	24	27
Bacon King Sandwich	1150	79	49
Big King XL	1005	63	56
Cheddar Bacon King Sandwich	1190	33	50
Cheeseburger	280	13	27
Double Cheeseburger	390	21	27
Hamburger	240	10	26
Quarter Pound King	580	29	49
Double	900	54	50
Stacker King: Single	700	42	48
Double	1050	68	49
Chicken Sandwiches:			
Original	660	40	48
Crispy Chicken: Regular	670	41	54
Bacon & Cheese	800	52	55
BBQ Bacon	790	49	60
Spicy	700	42	57
Spicy Crispy Chkn Jr.	390	21	37
Crispy Taco	170	9	19
Chicken Nuggets: 4 pieces	170	11	11
6 pieces	260	16	16
Chicken Fries, 9 pieces, w/out sauce	280	17	20
Dipping Sauces: BBQ	40	0	11
Buffalo	80	8	2
Ranch; Zesty Onion Ring, av.	145	15	2
Big Fish S'wich	510	28	51
French Fries: Small, 4.3 oz	320	13	49
Medium, 5.8 oz	380	16	58
Large, 7 oz	430	18	66
Onion Rings: Small	320	16	41
Medium	410	21	53
Large	500	25	64
Salads: Without Dressing			
Club, Crispy Chicken	540	33	31
Garden, Crispy Chicken	440	25	31
Garden, Side Salad	60	4	3
Salad Dressings: Gldn Italian, 1.5 oz	160	17	4
Lite Honey Bals. Vinaigrette, 1.5 oz	120	8	14
Ranch, 1.5 oz	260	28	2

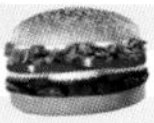
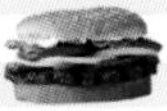
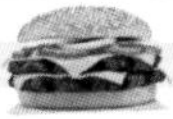
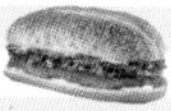
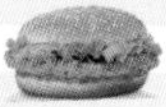
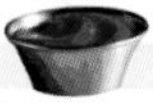
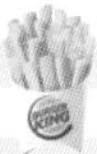
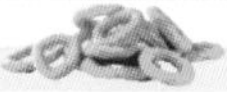
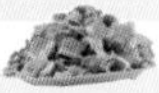

Burger King® cont... (Nov '20)

Breakfast:	C	F	Cb
Biscuits: Bacon, Egg & Cheese	400	26	29
Ham, Egg & Cheese	400	24	29
Sausage	420	28	28
Sausage, Egg & Cheese	530	38	29
BK Ultimate Breakfast Platter	930	44	110
Burrito: Egg-Normous	780	42	68
Breakfast Burrito Jr.	370	23	27
Croissan'wich:			
Bacon, Egg & Cheese	370	21	30
Egg & Cheese	340	18	29
Fully Loaded	610	40	31
Ham, Egg & Cheese	370	19	30
Double Croissan'wich:			
with Sausage	710	52	31
with Ham & Sausage	580	38	31
with Sausage & Bacon	580	40	31
Sausage, Egg & Cheese	510	32	30
French Toast Stick:			
3 pieces	230	11	29
5 pieces	380	18	49
Hash Browns: Small, 3 oz	250	16	24
Medium, 6 oz	500	33	48
Large, 8 oz	670	44	65
Oatmeal, Kid's	170	3	32
Pancakes & Sausage Platter	610	31	72
Desserts:			
Chocolate Chip Cookie	160	8	24
Pies: Dutch Apple	340	14	51
Hershey's Sundae	310	19	32
Sundaes: Caramel	240	5	42
Chocolate Hershey's	260	5	49
Vanilla Soft Serve: Cone	190	4.5	32
Cup	170	4.5	28
Shakes: Chocolate Oreo	740	22	121
Oreo	720	20	118
Strawberry	640	15	113
Vanilla	580	15	98
Smoothie, Strawb. Ban.,16 fl.oz	310	1	71
Beverages: Frappes, all, 16 fl.oz	400	10	68
Orange Juice, 10 fl.oz	140	0	33
Frozen Coke/Fanta	130	0	35
Iced Coffee: Mocha, 16 fl.oz	150	8	19
Vanilla, 16 fl.oz	200	10	27
Sweet Tea, 20 fl.oz	120	0	35

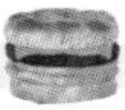
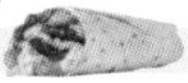
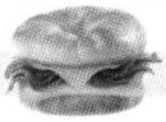
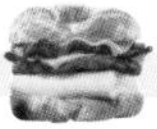
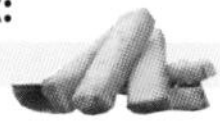
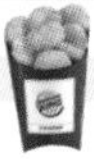
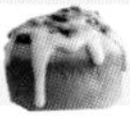
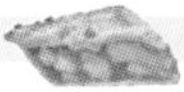
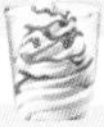
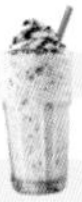
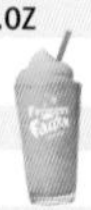

Updated Nutrition Data ~ www.CalorieKing.com
Persons with Diabetes ~ See Disclaimer (Page 22)

Captain D's Seafood® (Nov '20)

	C	F	Cb
From The Grill: *Without Sides, Rice, Hushpuppies or Breadstick*			
Blackened Tilapia	210	7	1
Grilled Wild Salmon	230	10	2
Grilled Whitefish & Shrimp Skewer	280	11	3
Lemon Pepper Whitefish Fillet	180	8	1
Shrimp Skewers (2)	200	6	2
Variety Meals: *W/out Sides Or Hush Puppies*			
Deluxe Seafood Platter	1100	75	67
Fish & Shrimp	810	56	45
Supreme Sampler	1180	79	68
The Captain Sandwich	1130	74	82
White Fish, Shrimp & Crab	940	64	52
Salads: *Without Dressing or Breadstick*			
Grilled Tilapia	310	13	9
Southern Style Breaded Chicken	290	17	20
Add-Ons:			
Baked Potato, plain, (1)	210	0	48
Loaded	400	15	49
Coleslaw, 1 order	180	13	15
French Fries, 1 serving	330	22	28
Hushpuppy (1)	80	4	9
Jalapeno Poppers	510	36	40
Dessert, Chocolate Cake, 1 order	300	11	49

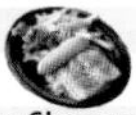
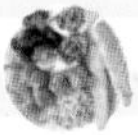
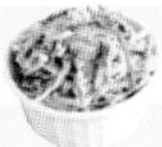

Caribou Coffee® (Nov '20)

With Standard Recipe Ingredients.

	C	F	Cb
Hot Beverages:			
Chai Tea, 16 fl.oz	310	7	48
Chocolate, 16 fl.oz	450	22	49
Crafted Press Coffee: Small, 12 fl.oz	90	6	7
Medium, 16 fl.oz	160	9	12
Large, 20 fl.oz	190	11	17
Macchiato: Small, 12 fl.oz	15	0.5	1
Medium, 16 fl.oz	20	1	1
Large, 20 fl.oz	20	1	1
Cold Beverages: *Per Medium 20 fl.oz, without Whipped Cream*			
Smoothies:			
Mango Orange Key Lime	420	0	106
Strawberry Banana	360	0	87
Coolers:			
Berry White Mocha	770	24	126
Caramel High Rise	720	27	113
Mint Condition	790	27	121

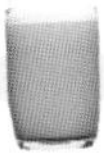
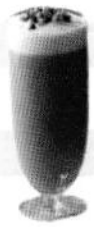
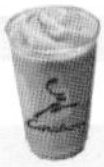
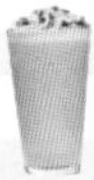

For Complete Menu ~ See Calorieking.com

Carl's Jr.® (Nov '20)

California menu only. Please check instore for further nutritional information.

	C	F	Cb
Charbroiled Burgers:			
Beyond Famous Star with Cheese	710	40	61
Famous Star with Cheese	670	37	57
Super Star with Cheese	920	56	59
The Big Carl	920	58	56
Western Bacon Cheeseburger	750	35	75
Double	1010	55	76
⅓ lb Thickburgers: Original $6	780	48	56
Guacamole Bacon	950	67	50
Lettuce Wrapped	420	33	8
Chicken Sandwiches:			
Bacon Swiss Crispy Chicken Fillet	770	41	58
Big Chicken Fillet	650	33	55
Charbroiled:			
BBQ Chicken	390	7	50
Chicken Club	580	28	46
Santa Fe Chicken	560	27	46
Chicken Tenders, hand breaded, 5 pieces, without sauce	440	21	21
Low Carb Options, Chicken Club	370	24	8
Trim It: Charbr. BBQ Chicken S'wich	390	8	51
Famous Star	430	18	46
Veg It, Guacamole Thickburger	670	46	56
Breakfast:			
Bacon & Egg Burrito	570	35	32
Bacon, Egg & Cheese Biscuit	480	29	38
Breakfast Burger, Single	730	43	47
Loaded Breakfast Burrito	760	48	46
Monster Biscuit	820	59	39
Sausage, Egg & Cheese Biscuit	610	42	38
Steak & Egg Burrito	630	36	37
Hash Rounds: Small, 3.8 oz	350	23	32
Medium, 4.2 oz	390	26	36
Large, 6 oz	560	37	52
Fries: CrissCut Fries, 5 oz	450	29	42
Natural Cut: Small, 3.5 oz	300	15	39
Medium, 6 oz	430	21	55
Large, 6.5oz	460	22	59
Fried Zucchini, 5 oz	330	18	36
Onion Rings, 4.5 oz	530	28	61
Salads: *Without Dressing*			
Charbroiled Chicken	280	9	19
Garden, side	140	7	15
Dressings: *Per 2 oz Package*			
House	220	22	3
Low-Fat Balsamic	35	1.5	5
Dessert: Choc. Chip Cookies (2)	330	17	43
Chocolate Cake, 3 oz	290	11	46
Strawb. Swirl Cheesecake, 3.5 oz	320	17	35
Shakes: *With Ice Cream*			
Oreo Cookie	710	39	79
Vanilla; Chocolate; Strawberry, av.	695	35	85

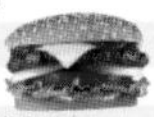
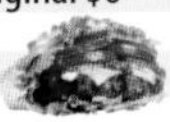
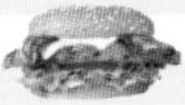
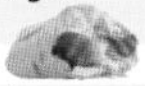
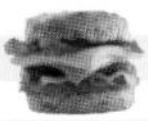
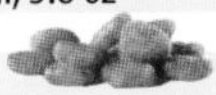
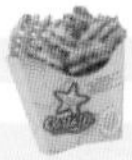
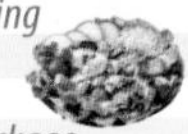

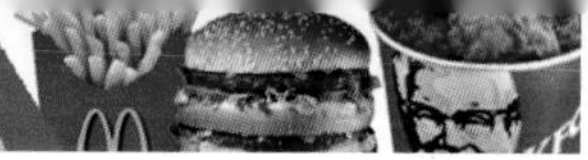

Carvel® (Nov '20)

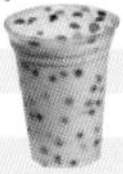
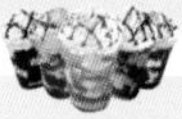
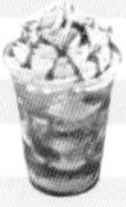
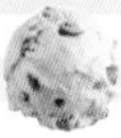
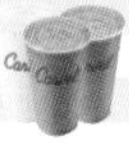

	C	F	Cb
Carvelanche:			
M&M'S: Small, 12 oz	650	32	73
Regular, 16 oz	850	43	97
Large, 24 oz	1320	66	152
Classic Sundaes: *Per Small, 12 oz*			
Hot Caramel	620	27	79
Hot Fudge	620	32	72
Strawberry	530	26	61
Sundae Dashers: *Per Regular, 16 oz*			
Banana's Foster	1050	33	171
Fudge Brownie	1250	62	166
Mint Chocolate Chip	1080	56	144
Peanut Butter Cup	1850	110	174
Strawberry Shortcake	880	37	125
Ice Cream Scoops: *Per Medium*			
Butter Pecan	750	51	57
Chocolate	520	27	59
Mint Chcolate Chip	670	35	78
Peanut Butter Treasure	680	41	73
Thick Shakes: *Per 16 oz*			
Chocolate; Vanilla, av.	650	27	90
Strawberry	590	27	73

Charley's Philly Steaks® (Nov '20)

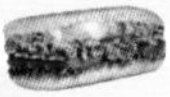
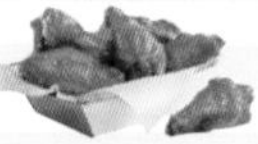
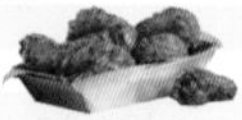
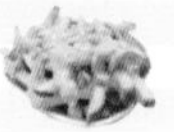
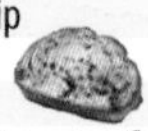

	C	F	Cb
Philly Cheessesteaks: *Per Regular*			
Bacon 3 Cheesesteak	720	31	56
Chicken Buffalo/Teriyaki, average	620	18	61
Chicken California	690	28	52
Jalapeno Cheesesteak	640	24	57
Pepperoni Cheesesteak	780	37	55
Philly Cheesesteak	640	24	58
Chicken: *Per Piece*			
Boneless: Plain/Buffalo/Habanero	110	7	6
Garlic Parmesan	160	12	8
Nashville Hot	180	14	9
Thai Chili	150	7	16
Classic: Plain	120	9	0
Angry Ghost	140	10	3
Buffalo/Cajun Rub/Smokin Habanero	130	9	1
Nashville Hot	190	16	2
Thai Chili/Cajun Rub	130	10	1
Tenders, Plain	190	13	11
Fries:			
Original	400	22	46
Gourmet: Cheese & Bacon	690	42	63
Cheese	550	31	62
Ultimate	790	54	61
Sides:			
Baked Beans, regular	180	0	41
Celery Sticks w/ Ranch Dip	210	21	3
Coleslaw regular	190	16	11
Texas Toast, 1 piece	170	6	26

For Complete Menu & Data ~ see CalorieKing.com

Cheesecake Factory® (Nov '20)

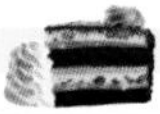
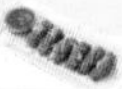
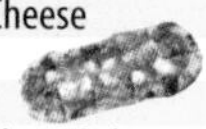
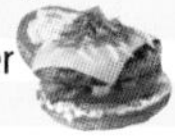
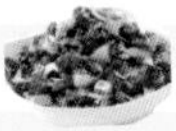
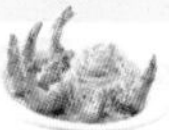
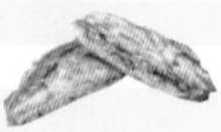
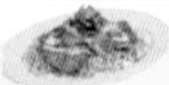
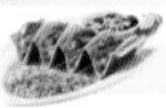
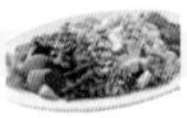

	C	F	Cb
Cheesecake: *Per Slice*			
Original	830	59	63
Godiva Chocolate	1400	105	110
Reese's P.B. Chocolate Cake	1530	94	157
White Chocolate Raspberry Truffle	1220	89	92
Appetizers: Avocado Egg Rolls	930	48	111
Buffalo Blasts	1670	93	129
Chicken Pot Stickers	420	14	42
Fried Macaroni & Cheese	1310	147	70
Thai Lettuce Wraps w/ Satay. Chkn	850	27	105
Spicy Ahi Tempura Roll	770	51	44
Small Plates & Snacks: As Served			
Beets & Avocado Salad	290	12	40
Chicken Samosas	480	28	29
Crispy Fried Cheese	1080	97	50
Korean Fried Cauliflower	1150	71	113
Stuffed Mushrooms	510	42	19
Flatbread Pizza: Cheese	1000	50	86
Margherita	760	30	85
Pepperoni	1110	61	87
Glamburgers: *Without Sides*			
American Cheeseburger	1400	93	79
Bacon-Bacon Cheeseburger	1590	108	76
Classic Burger	1340	87	69
Macaroni Cheeseburger	1340	85	81
Mushroom Burger	1470	102	72
Veggie Burger	1160	57	136
Glamburger Sides: French Fries	530	23	76
Green Salad	130	12	6
Sweet Potato Fries	510	20	63
Fish & Seafood:			
Fish & Chips	1860	121	133
Shrimp Scampi	1350	77	123
Seared Ahi Tuna	1090	54	107
Pasta: Carbonara	2070	143	141
Fettuccine Alfredo with Chicken	2310	155	145
Louisiana Chicken Pasta	2120	125	168
Sandwiches: Club	1210	60	111
Cuban	1190	71	64
Sthwst Chicken	1040	57	80
Specialties: Baja Chicken Tacos	1250	53	123
Cajun Chicken "Littles"	2130	110	177
Chicken Bellagio	1790	100	135
Chicken Madeira	1180	66	70
Crispy Chicken Costoletta	1760	116	102
Factory Burrito Grande	2150	129	160
Grilled Fish Tacos	1030	42	121
Grilled Steak Tacos	1030	42	121
White Chicken Chili	590	16	33
Super Salads: *Includes Dressing*			
California Guacamole	890	66	69
Vegan Cobb	1080	89	58
Wellness	810	68	44

Updated Nutrition Data ~ www.CalorieKing.com
Persons with Diabetes ~ See Disclaimer (Page 22)

Chick-fil-A® (Nov '20)

	C	F	Cb
Breakfast:			
Bagel, Chicken, Egg & Cheese	500	20	50
Biscuits: Plain, buttered	290	15	37
Bacon, Egg & Cheese	420	23	38
Chicken	460	23	45
Egg White Chicken Grill	290	8	29
Sausage, Egg & Cheese	630	43	38
Bowl, Hash Brown Scramble	470	30	19
Burrito, Hash Brown Scramble	700	40	51
Chick-n-Minis, 4 pieces	360	13	41
Hash Browns, 2.7 oz	270	18	23
Parfait, Greek Yogurt, fruit topping	280	8	37
Sandwiches: Without Sauce			
Chick-fil-A: Chicken	440	17	41
Deluxe	500	22	44
Grilled Chicken	320	6	41
Grilled Chicken Club	460	17	41
Spicy Deluxe	550	25	47
Breaded Chick-n-Strips, 3 count	310	14	16
Grilled Nuggets: 6 count	80	2	1
8 Count	100	2	1
Salads: Without Dressing			
Cobb: with Chick-n Strips	600	31	37
with Grilled Nuggets	400	20	22
with Spicy Grilled Filet (cold)	390	19	22
Market: with Nuggets	470	22	35
without Chicken	210	11	24
Spicy Southwest: with Nuggets	600	28	47
with Spicy Grilled Filet (cold)	450	19	39
Dressings: Creamy Salsa	290	31	2
Fat Free Honey Mustard	90	0	23
Garlic Herb Ranch	280	29	2
Light Italian	25	1	3
Sauces: BBQ/Honey Roasted	45	0	11
Chick-fil-A	140	13	6
Honey Mustard Sauce	45	0	11
Sweet & Spicy Sriracha Sauce	45	0	10
Sides: Fruit Cup, medium	60	0	15
Chicken Noodle Soup, cup	120	3	16
Side Salad, with toppings	160	10	13
Mac & Cheese, small	270	17	17
Waffle Potato Fries	220	13	25
Dessert: Chocolate Chunk Cookie	350	16	49
Frosted Coffee, large	300	7	53
Milkshakes: Chocolate, large	670	21	109
Cookies & Cream, large	710	26	107
Vanilla, large	580	21	86

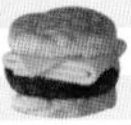
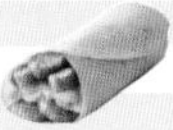
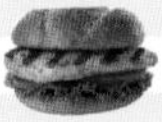
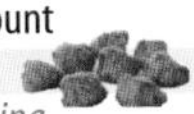
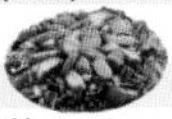
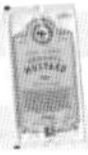
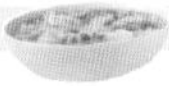
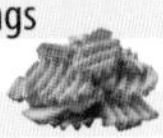

Chili's® (Nov '20)

	C	F	Cb
Appetizers: As Served			
Awesome Blossom Petals	760	50	70
Classic Nachos: Beef	1580	103	54
Chicken	1360	86	56
Southwestern Eggrolls	800	41	82
Texas Cheese Fries, full order	1860	127	97
Triple Dipper: *Serving for One*			
Big Mouth Bites	780	54	40
Original Chicken Crispers	510	34	23
Baby Back Ribs: Full Rack, without Sides			
Dry Rub	1480	107	30
Original BBQ	1430	106	21
Honey Chipotle BBQ	1520	106	47
House BBQ	1440	107	21
Burgers: Without Side Fries			
Just Bacon Beef	1030	71	43
Oldtimer, with Cheese	860	55	42
Southern Smokehouse Beef	1260	83	68
Crispers & More: As Served, with Set Sides			
Cajun Pasta with Grilled Chicken	1180	53	110
Orig. Tempura, with Honey Mustard	1320	67	120
Fresh Mex: As Served			
Bacon Ranch Chicken Quesadilla	1680	125	70
Chicken Enchiladas	1140	53	104
Chipotle Chicken Bowl	1030	51	80
Ranchero Chicken Tacos	1050	47	99
Guiltless Grill: As Served			
Ancho Salmon	630	30	42
Grilled Chicken Salad	440	23	23
Mango Chile Chicken	510	20	50
Margarita Grilled Chicken	650	17	68
Sirloin (6 oz), with Grilled Avocado	330	16	13
Sandwiches: Without Fries			
Bacon Avocado Chicken	1170	61	75
Buffalo Chicken Ranch	960	51	81
CA Turkey Club	1030	59	78
Steaks: Without Sides			
Classic Ribeye	630	40	0
Classic Sirloin, 6 oz	260	13	1
Country-Fried Steak, with gravy	590	35	30
Sides: Asparagus	35	1	5
Black Beans	120	1	20
Coleslaw	250	19	14
Loaded Mashed Potatoes	350	20	33
Mexican Rice	160	4.5	27
Roasted Street Corn	390	28	31
Steamed Broccoli	40	0	8
Salads: As Served			
Boneless Buffalo Chicken	1020	64	60
Caribbean with Seared Shrimp	600	26	80
Quesadilla Explosion	1410	94	82
Sweet Stuff: Per Slice			
Cheesecake	720	43	74
Molten Chocolate Cake	1170	59	155

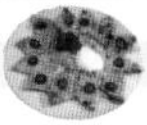
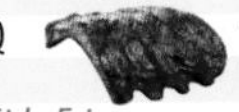
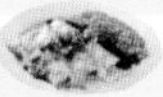
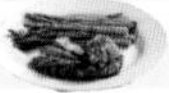
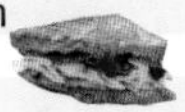
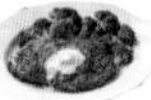
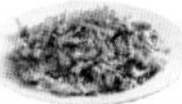
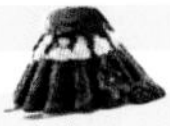

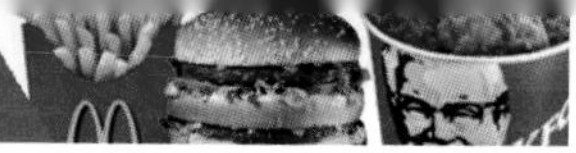

Chipotle® (Nov '20)

Tortillas:	C	F	Cb
Burrito Size Flour Tortillas (1)	320	9	50
Tacos: Crispy Corn Tortilla (3)	200	9	29
Soft Flour Tortillas (3)	250	8	40
Meal Components:			
Barbacoa, 4 oz	170	7	2
Black/Pinto Beans, average, 4 oz	130	1.5	22
Cilantro Brown or White Rice, 4 oz	210	5	38
Carnitas, 4 oz	210	12	0
Chicken, 4 oz	180	7	0
Fajita Vegetables, 2.5 oz	20	0	5
Guacamole, 3.5 oz	230	22	8
Lettuce Blend	15	0	3
Monterey Jack, 1 oz	110	8	1
Sofritas, 4 oz	150	10	9
Steak, 4 oz	150	6	1
Condiments:			
Queso, 2 oz	120	8	4
Salsa: Chili Corn, 3.5 oz	80	1.5	16
Green Tomatillo, 2 oz	15	0	4
Red Tomatillo, 2 oz	15	0	4
Sour Cream, 2 oz	110	9	2
Extras, Chips, 4 oz	540	25	73

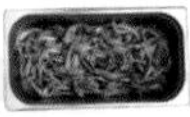

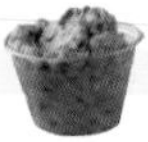

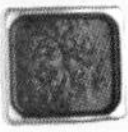

Chuck E. Cheese® (Nov '20)

Appetizers:	C	F	Cb
Cheesy Breadsticks (1)	140	6	15
French Fries, 8 oz	420	13	67
Parmesan Breadstick (1)	200	7	29
Sub Sandwiches: Per Half Sub Without Fries			
Chicken Bacon Ranch	290	13	24
Ham & Cheese	280	13	25
Italian	290	14	24
Specialty Pizzas: Per Slice, 1/10 Medium Pizza			
BBQ Chicken	170	6	22
Cali Alfredo; Meat Combo	200	9	18
Supreme	190	9	19
Veggie	160	6	19
Traditional Wings: Per 12 oz Wings with 2 oz Sauce			
Small: with BBQ or Sweet Chili Sauce	680	33	43
with Buffalo Sauce	600	37	16
Desserts: Choc. Chip Cookie, 1/8 slice	200	9	28
Churros (4)	550	10	111

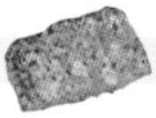

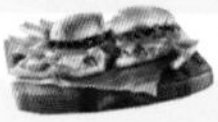

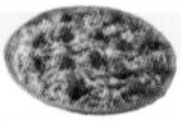

Church's Chicken® (Nov '20)

Chicken: Per Piece	C	F	Cb
Original: Breast, 1 piece	250	14	9
Leg, 1 piece	150	8	6
Thigh, 1 piece	360	27	12
Wing, 1 piece	290	18	8
Spicy: Breast, 1 piece	280	17	12
Leg, 1 piece	160	9	9
Thigh, 1 piece	380	25	21
Wing, 1 piece	350	20	19
Tender Strips, average, 1 piece	110	5	6.5
Sides: Per Regular Serving			
Baked Macaroni & Cheese, 4.7 oz	210	12	19
Cole Slaw, 4.2 oz	170	11	16
French Fries, 2.6 oz	210	9	29
Honey Butter Biscuit, 2.2 oz	230	15	25
Jalapeno Cheese Bombers (4)	220	11	24
Mashed Potatoes & Gravy, 4.5 oz	110	1	24
Okra, 3.4 oz	260	15	30
Sauces: Honey BBQ, pkt	45	0	11
Creamy Jalapeno, pkt	120	13	2
Honey Mustard/Ranch, av., pkt	140	14	3
Dessert, Apple Pie	270	13	37

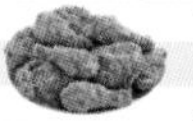

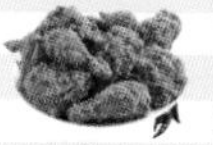

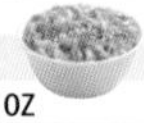

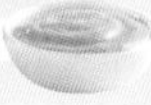

Cici's Pizza® (Nov '20)

Pizza:	C	F	Cb
Regular Crust: *Per Slice, 1/10 of Large 14" Pizza*			
Alfredo; Zesty Ham & Cheddar, av.	170	6	22
Pepperoni	200	8	23
Deep Dish: *Per Slice, 1/6 Pizza*			
Average all varieties	165	6	21
Flatbread: Chicken Bacon Club	150	7	14
Honey BBQ Chicken	140	6.5	19
Stuffed Crust, Cheese; Pepperoni	190	7.5	21
Boneless Wings: BBQ (5)	350	10	40
Buffalo (5), average	325	11	27
Garlic Parmesan (5)	400	25	30
Sides: Chicken & Pasta Soup, 8 oz	90	2.5	13
Garlic Cheesy Bread, 2 slices	70	3	9
Pasta	270	4	50
Sauce, Alfredo	90	8	3
Dessert: Brownie	140	6	21
Apple/Barvarian Pizza, 1 slice	130	3	24

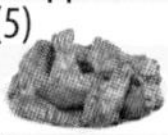

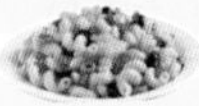

Cinnabon® (Nov '20)

	C	F	Cb
Cinnabon Classic Roll (1)	880	37	127
MiniBon Roll (1), 3.4 oz	350	15	51
Cheese Roll Paninis:			
Grilled Cheese	480	26	41
Black Forest Ham	590	25	48
Smoked Turkey Club	520	25	48
Chillata: Per 16 fl.oz			
Double Chocolate Mocha	360	13	59
Oreo Cookies & Cream	700	25	112
Strawberries & Cream	540	18	89

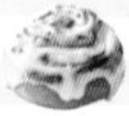

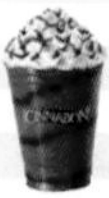

Updated Nutrition Data ~ www.CalorieKing.com
Persons with Diabetes ~ See Disclaimer (Page 22)

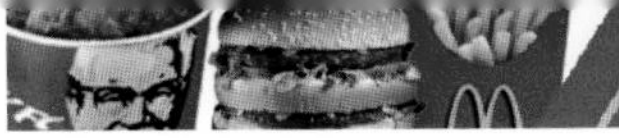

Claim Jumper® (Nov '20)

Appetizers: As Served	C	F	Cb
Beef Sliders with Cheese	740	35	67
Chips & Salsa	540	10	90
Spinach & Artichoke Dip, share	1735	64	233
***Burgers:** Without Sides*			
Bacon & Mac	950	48	89
Classic Hamburger	750	40	60
Impossible Burger	1230	75	91
Widow Maker Burger	1565	89	126
***Meals:** As Per Menu Description*			
Classics: Country Fried Steak	1175	50	116
Fish & Chips	1115	37	148
Meatloaf & Mashed Potatoes	1180	73	83
Combo Plates: Steak & Shrimp	770	52	17
Surf & Turf	1050	51	66
The Tri-Tip Prospector	765	42	9
Pasta: Black Tie Pasta	1895	97	161
Shrimp Fresca	2005	143	110
Seafood: Blackened Salmon	405	26	3
Coconut Shrimp	1305	36	202
Grilled Shrimp	550	22	53
Wood Fired Pizza, Classic Crust:			
BBQ Chicken, whole pizza	1960	80	230
Sausage & Pepperoni, whole pizza	2010	100	190
Sides: Baked Potato with Butter	635	27	82
Brussels Sprouts	190	14	11
Charbroiled Asparagus	235	19	7
Chili French Fries	580	35	44
Loaded French Fries	550	35	39
Mac & Cheese	460	25	40
Mashed Potatoes	270	16	28
Roasted Veggies	55	3	6
Sweets: Chocolate Motherlode Cake	3415	158	459
Raspberry Cream Cheese Pie	1570	97	147

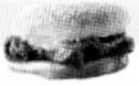
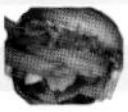
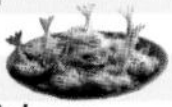
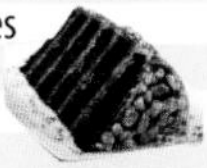

Cold Stone Creamery® (Nov '20)

Ice Cream:	C	F	Cb
Amaretto: Like it	340	21	36
Love it	550	33	57
Gotta have it	820	49	85
Chocolate: Like it	330	20	34
Love it	520	31	54
Gotta have it	780	47	81
Sorbet:			
Strawberry Mango Banana:			
Like it, 5 oz	210	0	54
Love it, 8 oz	340	0	87
Gotta have it, 12 oz	510	0	130
***Shakes:** Per 20 oz With Whipped Topping*			
Cake Batter 'n Shake	1440	76	176
Oh Fudge; Very Vanilla, average	1320	76	148
Savory Strawberry	1200	71	133
Sundaes: Banana Split Decision	650	37	77
Who You Callin' Shortcake	560	31	68

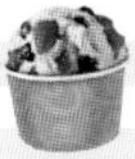
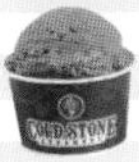

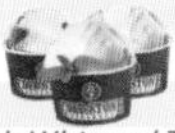

Costco Food Court® (Sept '19)

(Approximate Figures Only)	C	F	Cb
Baked Potato, with Chicken Chili	840	24	120
French Fries, 11 oz	870	45	106
Hot Dogs: Hebrew National	550	34	42
KS	570	33	46
Sinai	540	30	48
***Pizza:** Per Slice*			
Cheese Pizza, 9.8 oz	700	28	70
Combo Pizza, 10.7 oz	680	29	72
Pepperoni Pizza, 8.9 oz	620	24	68
Chicken Bake, 12.75 oz	770	25	78
Wrap, Turkey, 14.4 oz	810	38	65
Salad, Chicken Caesar, w/ Dressing	650	40	34
Sandwiches: Hebrew Sausage	540	32	44
Italian Sausage	700	42	46
KS Polish/Sinai Sausage, av.	570	33	47
Desserts: California Churro	410	18	51
Ice Cream Bar	870	65	60
J&J Churro	470	22	61
Yogurt, 12 oz	390	0	82
Smoothies: Fruit, 16 fl. oz	290	0	72
Strawberry Banana, 16 fl.oz	300	0	74
Sundae, Berry, 12.3 oz	410	0	87
Beverages: Hot Latte, 9.6 fl.oz	190	5	24
Hot Mocha, 11.3 fl.oz	310	9	45

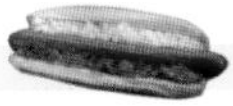
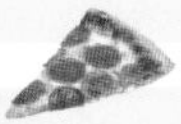
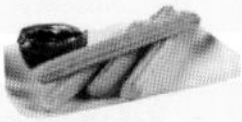

Cousins Subs® (Nov '20)

Subs: Per 7.5", Standard Toppings	C	F	Cb
Grilled To Order:			
Chkn Bacon Cheddar	610	23	53
Chicken Cheese Steak	560	18	52
Double Steak Cheese Steak	800	31	56
Classics:			
Club, with Mayo	670	32	53
Italian Special, with Oil	830	48	52
Tuna with Mayo	650	36	51
Deli Fresh:			
Ham & Provolone, with Mayo	630	32	51
Roast Beef & Cheddar, with Mayo	740	37	52
Turkey Breast with Mayo	550	25	53
Cheese Curds: Regular, 4 oz	550	47	10
Large, 8 oz	1110	94	20
French Fries: Regular, 3 oz	260	14	31
Large, 5.9 oz	520	27	62
***Soup:** Per Cup*			
Beef Steak, with Noodles	105	3.5	12
Cheddar Cauliflower	110	5	13
Chicken Noodle	110	3	16
Cream of Potato	170	8	21
New England Clam Chowder	150	2.5	25

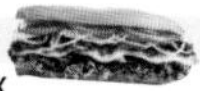
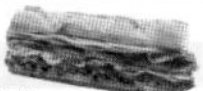
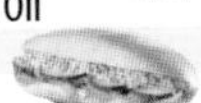
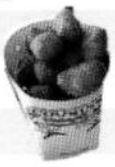
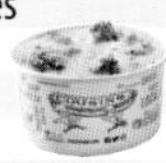

For Complete Nutritional Data ~ see CalorieKing.com

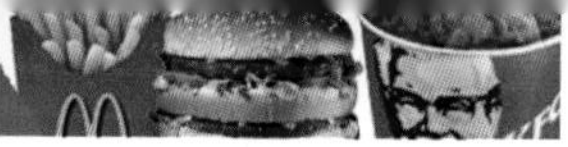

Culver's® (Nov '20)

ButterBurgers:	C	F	Cb
Original: Single	390	17	38
Double	560	30	38
Triple	730	43	38
Cheddar:			
Single	470	24	38
Double	720	44	38
Culver's Bacon Deluxe:			
Single	610	38	40
Double	850	57	41
Culver's Deluxe:			
Single	570	34	41
Double	810	53	42
Mushroom & Swiss, Single	500	26	40
Sourdough Melt, Single	490	25	42
Sandwiches:			
Beef Pot Roast	410	13	40
Crispy Chicken	460	14	56
Grilled Reuben Melt	660	37	43
North Atl. Cod Filet	600	33	49
Pork Tenderloin	630	25	72
Sides: Chili Cheddar Fries	690	32	80
Coleslaw, regular	200	16	15
Crinkle Cut Fries, reg.	360	14	53
Mashed Potatoes & Gravy, regular	130	1	25
Onion Rings, regular	400	22	44
Steamed Broccoli	40	0	7
Wisconsin Cheese Curds, reg., 5.3 oz	510	25	51
Dinners: With Dinner Role, Butter & Menu Set Sauce			
Butterfly Jumbo Shrimp, 6 pieces	530	22	63
North Atlantic Cod, Fried, 2 pieces	920	68	42
Soup:			
Broccoli Cheese	220	12	17
Chicken Noodle	100	2	15
Potato with Bacon	240	10	28
Salads: Without Dressing			
Chicken Cashew with Gilled Chicken	450	24	13
Cranberry Bacon Bleu, with Grilled Chicken	360	14	14
Garden Fresco with Grilled Chicken	350	13	15
Side Salad	50	2	4
Kid's Meals:			
Corn Dog	240	14	23
Chicken Tenders, Breaded, 2 pieces	270	12	21
Grilled Cheese Sourdough Sandwich	360	16	39
Dressings: Chunky Bleu Cheese	310	33	2
French	190	13	19
Honey Mustard	130	6	20
Ranch	180	19	2
Raspberry Vinaigrette	45	0	11

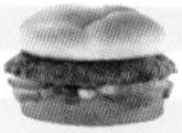
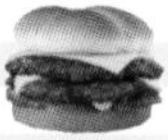
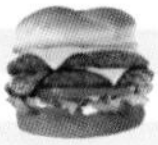
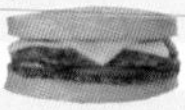
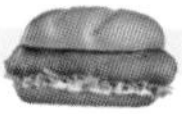

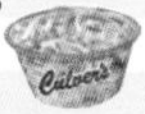
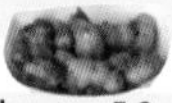
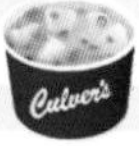

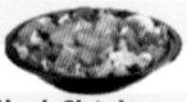
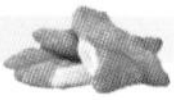
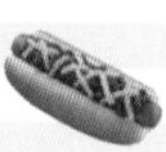

Culver's® cont... (Nov '20)

Concrete Mixers: No Toppings	C	F	Cb
Chocolate & M&M's, reg.	980	46	124
Cookie Dough, regular	1010	56	113
Sundaes: Per 2 Scoops			
Banana Split	1090	61	122
Caramel Cashew	1000	52	121
Turtle	1040	61	111
Beverages: Chocolate Malt, reg.	850	38	114
Chocolate Shake, reg.	820	38	108
Strawberry Malt, reg.	760	38	92
Strawberry Shake, reg.	730	38	86

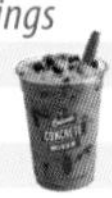
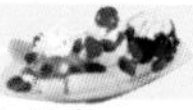
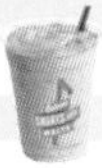

D'Angelo® (Nov '20)

Deli Sandwiches: Per Medium	C	F	Cb
Italian Sub Bread	310	3.5	57
Add Chicken Salad	700	62	3
Add Ham & Cheese	310	24	6
Add Tuna Salad	640	64	3
Wraps: Per Medium			
Tortilla Wrap Only	250	6	42
Add Buffalo Chicken	520	38	13
Add Chicken Caesar	600	41	20
Add Greek	390	31	17
Fresh Entree Salads: With Dressing, without Pokket			
Entree: Caesar	490	39	24
Greek	520	45	19
Grilled Topped:			
Chicken Cobb	810	59	25
Steak Cobb	880	65	25
Steak Greek	780	62	20
Soup: Per Bowl			
Beef Stew	330	12	34
Broccoli & Cheddar	370	28	18
Main Lobster Bisque	540	43	24
New England Clam Chowder	480	27	46

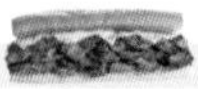
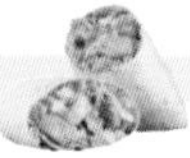
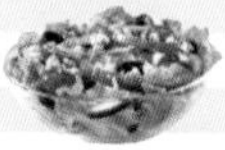
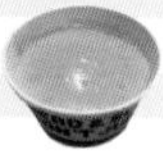

For Complete Menu & Data ~ see CalorieKing.com

Dairy Queen® (Nov '20)

Burgers:	C	F	Cb
Deluxe Cheeseburger	660	25	86
½ lb Cheese	800	49	44
½ lb Flame Thrower	980	70	40
⅓ Double with Cheese	560	31	36
Hot Dogs:			
Cheese Dog	390	24	27
Classic Hot Dog	330	19	25
Chili Cheese Dog	420	26	28

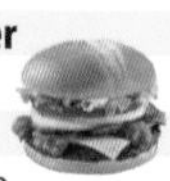

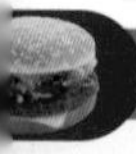

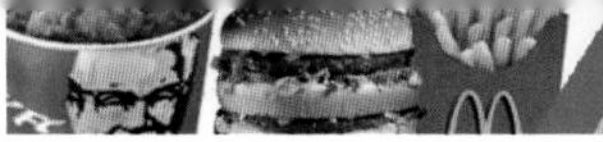

Dairy Queen® cont... (Nov '20)

Sandwiches:	C	F	Cb
Chicken Bacon Ranch	500	20	46
Crispy Chicken	550	28	49
Grilled Chicken	390	15	34
Turkey BLT	580	28	45
Salads: *Without Dressing*			
Chicken BLT:			
Crispy Chicken	400	21	28
Grilled Chicken	280	11	12
Strips, 3 pieces	360	18	28
Side Salad	25	0	5
French Fries: Regular, 4 oz	290	13	39
Large	470	21	63
Sides: Cheese Curds, Regular	500	34	26
Large	1000	67	52
Onion Ring: Regular	360	16	48
Large	540	24	71
Pretzel Sticks with Zesty Queso	330	9	52
Desserts: *Per Medium*			
Blizzard Treats: Butterfinger	730	26	107
Choco Brownie Xtreme	810	36	111
Choc. Chip Cookie Dough	1030	41	151
Heath	860	37	119
M&M's	800	27	124
Oreo Cheesecake	1220	58	159
Reese's P'nut Butter Cup	750	31	102
Snickers	800	28	120
Turtle Pecan Cluster	900	48	105
Cupcakes: Blue Striped Swirl	440	18	64
Swirl with Bright Quins	450	18	63
Curl On Top Treats:			
Fudge Stuffed Cookie	640	33	80
Peanut Buster Parfait	710	31	95
Triple Chocolate Brownie	540	24	75
Dipped Cone, Chocolate	460	22	58
DQ Sundaes: Caramel	420	12	75
Hot Fudge	430	16	68
Strawberry	320	11	54
Moo Latte: Caramel	570	17	96
Mocha	580	22	88
Vanilla	530	16	90
Shakes: Caramel	750	25	115
Chocolate	710	23	110
Strawberry	620	23	87
Vanilla	660	23	97
Treatzza Pizza: Heath	190	9	26
Reese's Peanut Butter Cup	200	10	24

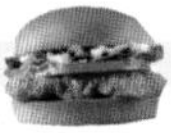
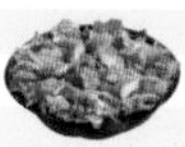
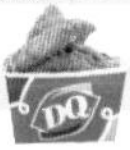

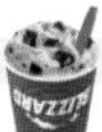
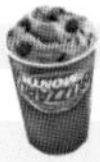
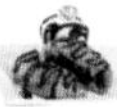
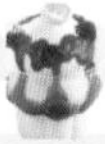
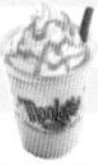
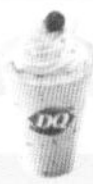

Daphne's Greek Cafe® (Nov '20)

Califonia Menu Only. Check Instore for Latest Information

Starters:	C	F	Cb
Fire Feta & Warm Pita	340	17	39
Hummus & Warm Pita	320	12	47
Classic Pita Sandwiches: *Without Tzatziki Sauce*			
with Chicken	410	16	41
with Crispy Shrimp	410	17	48
with Falafel	640	17	96
with Gyro	680	45	49
Plates: *Without Pita or Tzatziki Sauce*			
Cali-Greek Bowls:			
with Crispy Shrimp	930	38	117
with Falafel	1160	39	165
with Gr. Chicken	930	37	109
with Grilled Shrimp	1060	46	91
Mediterranean Veggie	1300	56	161
Surf & Turf	690	25	85
Classic Greek Salads: *W/ Dressing, w/o Pita & Sauce*			
Crispy Shrimp	440	31	25
Falafel	670	31	74
Grilled Chicken	440	30	18
Add, Pita & Tzatziki	130	3	21
Sides: Cucumber-Tomato Salad	120	11	5
Fire Roasted Vegetables	70	3	12
French Fries	440	22	55
Greek Salad, small	140	12	7
Lemon Chicken Soup	280	12	37
Moroccan Carrot Salad	180	13	15
Pita Chips	220	6	36
Pita Bread	190	3	36
Seasoned Rice	360	8	68
Tabouli	220	15	20
Dessert, Traditional Baklava	250	9	36

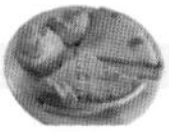
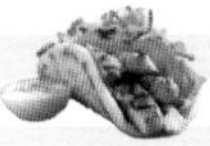
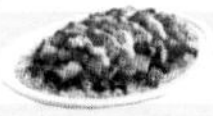
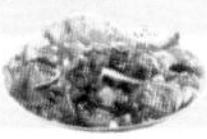
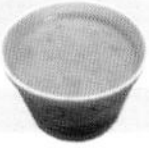
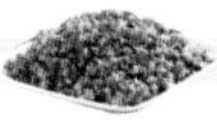

Davanni's® (Nov '20)

Hot Hoagies: *Per Half, with 6" White Bun & Standard Toppings*	C	F	Cb
Assorted	490	30	39
Cheese	500	31	39
Chicken & Bacon, w/ Honey Mustard	505	22	46
Chicken Parmigiana	445	16	40
Club	495	27	40
Pastrami	470	27	40
Roast Beef	470	25	39
Southwestern Chicken	535	26	43
Tuna Melt	645	44	42
Turkey Bacon Chipotle	565	33	39
Pasta: *As Served, with Garlic Toast*			
Chicken Florentine, half portion	610	28	56
Lasagna, half portion	625	43	37

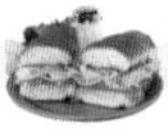
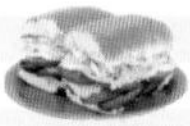
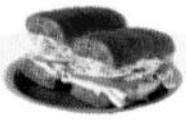

continued next page...

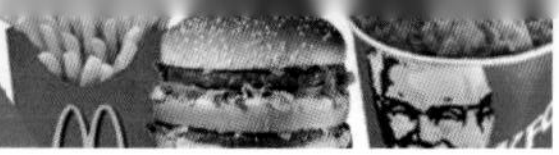

Davanni's® cont... (Nov '20)

Pizzas: Per ⅛ of Med. Pizza with Red Sauce	C	F	Cb
Five Meat: Thin Crust	255	13	19
Traditional Crust	305	13	30
Gluten Free Crust	215	12	16
Veggie: Thin Crust	220	10	19
Traditional Crust	275	10	30
Works: Thin Crust	265	14	19
Traditional Crust	315	15	30

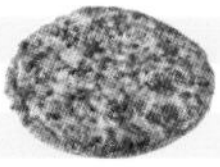

Del Taco® (Nov '20)

Breakfast:	C	F	Cb
Burritos: Breakfast	430	21	38
Bacon	640	36	38
Chorizo/Steak, average	510	26	39
Hash Brown Sticks, 5 pieces	230	17	18
Tacos: Bacon	230	14	15
Chorizo	240	15	16
Carne Asada	240	13	16
Egg & Cheese	190	11	15
Burgers: Without Fries			
Bacon Double Del Cheeseburger	740	51	35
Del Cheeseburger	470	28	34
Double Del Chseburger	690	47	35
Burritos:			
Bean & Cheese, red	470	10	69
Beyond Burrito	550	21	60
Classic Grilled Chicken	530	33	40
Del Beef	500	24	40
Del Combo	470	17	54
Epic: Beyond Cali	860	44	82
Carne Asada	740	25	88
Cali Steak & Guacamole	800	39	80
Grilled Chicken Avocado	830	36	88
Macho Combo	950	37	100
Queso Loaded Nachos: Per Regular			
Beef; Carne Asada, average	570	30	52
Chicken	550	28	52
Quesadillas: Mini Bacon	170	9	14
Cheddar	460	26	31
Chicken/Cheddar or Spicy Jack, av.	550	31	35
Tacos:			
Beer Battered Fish	230	12	26
Beyond: Avocado Taco	260	14	22
Taco	300	19	15
Chicken Al Carbon	150	4.5	19
Del Taco: Crunchy Beef	310	20	14
Soft Beef	300	18	17
Grilled Chicken	210	12	16

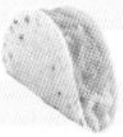

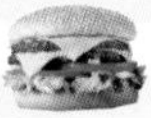

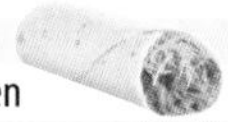

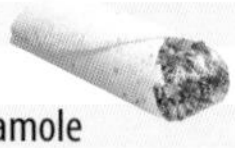

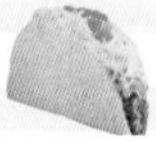

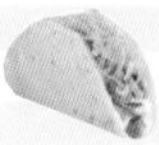

Del Taco® cont... (Nov '20)

Salads: Without Dressing	C	F	Cb
Chicken, Bacon Avocado	550	40	27
Mexican Chopped Chicken	510	23	39
Signature Taco	550	29	38
Sides:			
Bean & Cheese Cup, 7.8 oz	320	3.5	52
Potato Poppers: 4 pieces	240	14	20
6 pieces	360	21	30
Desserts:			
Caramel Cheesecake Bites (2)	460	28	43
Chocolate Chip Cookie (1)	200	10	27
Premium Shakes: Per Regular			
Chocolate	560	11	105
Strawberry or Vanilla	520	10	95

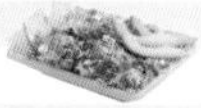

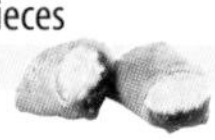

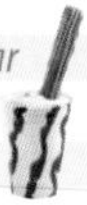

Denny's® (Nov '20)

Breakfast:	C	F	Cb
Favorites: *W/ith Scrambled Eggs, Hash Browns*			
Country Fried Steak with Muffin	950	60	61
Moons Over My Hammy, no Muffin	950	60	57
T'Bone Steak with Muffin	1090	69	38
Omelettes: *With Hash Browns & English Muffin*			
My Hammy & Cheese	930	60	41
Philly Cheese Steak	1040	71	46
Wild West	910	60	45
Pancakes: *With Bacon, Scrambled Eggs & Hash Browns*			
Blueberry Pancakes Breakfast	950	48	97
Cinnamon Roll Breakfast	1500	64	205
Skillets:			
Crazy Spicy Sizzlin, without bread	1040	70	44
Santa Fe, with Sunny Side Up Eggs	910	69	35
Slams: *With Cheesy Scrambled Eggs & Bacon Strips*			
All American with 2 B'Milk P'cakes	1150	66	81
French Toast	1120	73	67
Lumberjack with 2 B'Milk Pancakes, & English Muffin	1140	60	103
Sides: Bacon Strips (2)	100	8	1
1 Egg: Over Easy/Medium/Hard	125	11	0
Scrambled	110	9	1
Scrambled with cheese	160	14	1
English Muffin without Margarine	130	1	25
Grilled Ham, slice	90	11	1
Hash Browns:			
Regular	340	24	30
Cheddar Cheese	420	30	30
Everything	480	33	39

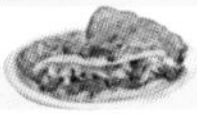

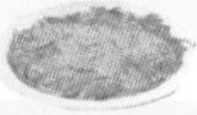

Updated Nutrition Data ~ www.CalorieKing.com
Persons with Diabetes ~ See Disclaimer (Page 22)

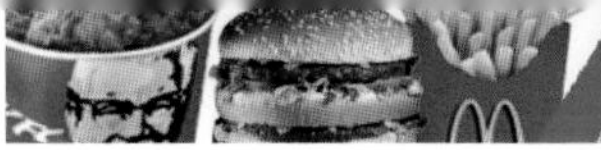

Denny's® cont... (Nov '20)

Breakfast Sides (Cont):	C	F	Cb
Pancakes: Buttermilk (2)	**450**	11	77
Hearty 9-grain (2)	**410**	11	68
Sausages: 4 links	**300**	30	4
Hearty Sausage	**350**	31	5
Toast: Wheat, with Margarine , 2 sl.	**230**	11	29
White, with Margarine, 2 slices	**240**	10	31
Appetizers:			
Beer Battered Onion Rings	**400**	27	35
Chips & Queso	**670**	39	69
Prem. Chkn Tenders			
without sauce	**680**	40	38
Zesty Nachos	**1650**	105	135
Lunch Burgers & Sandwiches: *On Brioche Bun, without Sides*			
Burgers: Bourbon Bacon	**910**	51	64
Double Cheeseburger:			
with Cheddar Cheese	**1140**	68	50
with Swiss Cheese	**1200**	70	52
Sandwiches: BBQ Chicken	**520**	18	69
Buffalo Chicken	**520**	26	50
Club	**830**	39	74
Honey Buttermilk Chicken	**530**	24	58
Prime Rib Mega Philly Cheese Melt	**910**	52	62
The Super Bird	**600**	28	43
Dinners: *Without Sides or Sauces*			
Bourbon Chicken Sizzlin Skillet	**880**	39	69
Premium Chicken Tenders	**730**	39	55
Seafood & Steak: *With Garlic Bread, without Sides or Toppings*			
Classic Battered Fish Fillets	**1010**	68	65
Sirloin Steak, 8 oz	**530**	25	27
T-Bone Steak, 13 oz	**680**	38	25
Lunch/Dinner Sides:			
Beer Battered Onion Rings	**400**	27	35
Broccoli, 3 oz	**25**	0	4
Garden Salad, without dressing	**170**	9	16
House Salad, w/out meat or drssng	**190**	9	19
Sauteed Zucchini & Squash	**70**	6	3
Seasoned Fries	**490**	26	57
Seasonal Fruit	**110**	0	27
Southwest Creamed Corn	**240**	18	13
Sweet Petite Corn	**210**	13	20
Wavy-Cut Fries	**400**	22	46
Whole Grain Rice	**240**	2.5	48

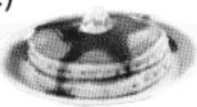
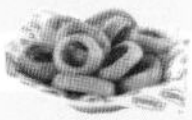
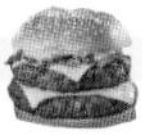
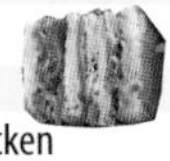
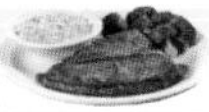
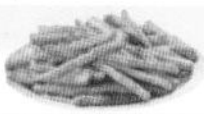
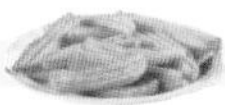

Denny's® cont... (Nov '20)

55 & Over: *Without Extras*	C	F	Cb
B'fast, Scrambled Eggs & Cheddar	**1010**	58	80
Club Sandwich with Wavy Cut Fries	**1090**	58	97
Grilled Cheese Sandwich	**440**	25	39
Loaded Veggie Omelette Fit Fare	**440**	9	64
Salads: *Without Dressing*			
House Salad:			
without Meat, 10 oz	**190**	9	19
with Chicken Tenders (3)	**600**	33	42
with Prime Rib, 12.5 oz	**320**	17	22
with Wild Alaska Salmon, 17 oz	**500**	28	21
Condiments: Pico de Gallo, 2 oz	**15**	0	3
Sour Cream, 1 oz	**45**	4	1
Tomato Sauce, 1.5 oz	**25**	1	3
Whipped Margarine, 0.5 oz	**40**	4.5	0
Dressings: *Per 1.5oz*			
Balsamic Vinaigrette	**130**	4	24
Blue Cheese	**160**	16	2
Honey Mustard	**180**	15	12
Mayo	**100**	11	0
Light Italian	**30**	0	8
Ranch	**200**	21	1
Thousand Island	**160**	16	7
Sauces: *Per 1.5 oz*			
BBQ	**80**	0	20
Bourbon	**110**	0	26
Buffalo	**110**	12	1
Den	**220**	22	4
Mango Habanero	**110**	0	27
Desserts: *As Served*			
Caramel Apple Pie Crisp, 13 oz	**760**	26	126
Chocolate Lava Cake	**700**	34	85
New York Style Cheesecake, plain	**500**	34	42
Beverages:			
Hot Chocolate, 8 oz	**190**	3	37
Iced Tea, sweetened, 12 oz	**160**	0	40
Lemonade Iced Tea, 12 oz	**80**	0	21
Mango Lemonade, 15 oz	**210**	0	57
Strawb. Lemonade, 12 oz	**210**	0	55
Milk Shakes: Chocolate, 16 oz	**870**	43	111
Vanilla, 16 oz	**800**	43	97
Smoothie: Groovy Mango, 15 oz	**340**	0	86
Strawberry Banana Bliss, 15 oz	**330**	0.5	82

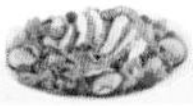
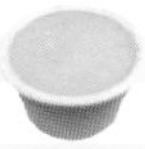
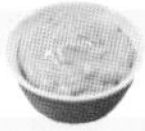
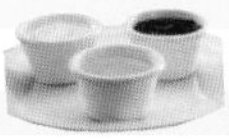
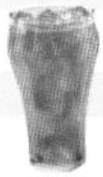

For Complete Nutritional Data ~ see CalorieKing.com

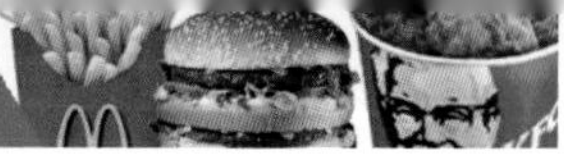

Dippin' Dots® (Nov '20)

Flavored Ices,	C	F	Cb
Medium, all flavors, 5.53 oz	190	0	48
Dot Shakes: Banana Split	350	14	42
Brownie Sundae/Brownie Batter	390	15	49
Cookie Dough;Choc Strawb;Strawb, av.	355	15	43
Strawberry Cheesecake	300	5	50
Vanilla	300	10	22
Dot Sundaes: All Shook Up	310	16	38
Brownie Batter Cup; C'rml Toffee, av.	370	18	48
Nut Caramel Crunch	350	15	49
Split Decision	300	14	39
Ice Cream: Banana Split, medium	310	16	36
Brownie/ Batter; Crmel Sundae, med.	380	19	48

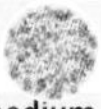

Donatos Pizza® (Nov '20)

Pizzas: Per Slice	C	F	Cb
Hand Tossed Signature Pizzas: *Per Slice of 14" Pizza*			
Chicken Spinach Mozzarella	340	15	31
Founder's Favorite	330	14	33
Mariachi Beef	310	12	34
Mariachi Chicken	310	12	34
Serious Meat, Ground Beef	340	15	33
The Works	320	14	34
Thick Crust Signature Pizzas: *Per Slice of 14" Pizza*			
Chicken Spinach Mozzarella	160	7	15
Double Bacon Pepperoni	200	10	16
Founders Favorite	170	8	16
Margherita	160	8	14
Serious Meat, Ground Beef	190	9	17
The Works	170	8	17
Oven Baked Subs:			
Big Don with Marinara Sauce	600	25	63
Chicken Bacon Cheddar	770	37	62
Fresh Vegy	490	19	63
Ham & Smoked Prov.	560	21	62
Hot Chicken	840	42	73
Meatball	850	38	80
Salad: Entree Size, with Menu Set Dressing			
Chicken Caprese	400	25	17
Italian Chef	500	42	12
Side: Caprese	220	18	11
Italian	330	31	7
Wings: Per 6 pieces, without Dipping Sauce			
Boneless Chkn: Mild/Hot Sce, av.	415	23	26
BBQ Sauce	400	17	39
Sweet Thai Chili	470	18	53
Dessert: Cinnamon Bread, ¼ bread	280	10	44
Fudge Brownie (1)	360	21	39
Salty Caramel Apple Pie, 2 pieces	330	10	53
Triple Chocolate Chunk Cookie (1)	320	23	22

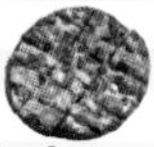

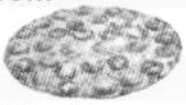

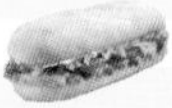

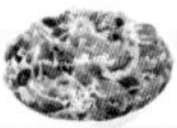

For Complete Nutritional Data ~ see CalorieKing.com

Domino's® (Nov '20)

With Regular Cheese Base	C	F	Cb
12" Hand Tossed: *Per Slice, ⅛ Pizza, with BBQ Sauce Unless Indicated*			
Bacon, Beef, & Sausage	290	15	26
Beef, Green Peppers, Onions, & Mshrm	220	9	25
Black Olives, Green Peppers, Onions, Mshrm &Tomatoes, Marinara Sauce	190	7	25
Ham & Pineapple, no sauce	190	7	23
Pepperoni, no sauce	200	9	22
Pepperoni & Sausage, no Sauce	230	12	22
Sausage	240	11	25
Sausage, Beef & Pepperoni	270	14	26
14" Brooklyn: *Per Slice, ⅙ Pizza, with BBQ Sce Unless Indicated*			
Beef, Green Pepp., Onions & Mshrm	300	13	32
Black Olives, Green Peppers, Onions, Mushrooms, Tomatoes	280	11	32
Ham & Pineapple, no sauce	290	11	33
Pepperoni, no sauce	290	15	24
Pepperoni & Sausage, no sauce	340	20	24
Sausage	350	19	30
14" Thin Crust: *Per Slice, ⅛ Pizza, with BBQ Sauce Unless Indicated*			
Bacon, Beef & Sausage	270	17	20
Beef, Green Pepp., Onions & Mshrm	210	11	21
Black Olives, Green Peppers, Onions, Mushrooms & Tomatoes	1200	10	21
Ham & Pineapple, no sauce	190	9	17
Pepperoni, no sauce	210	12	15
Pepperoni & Sausage, no sauce	250	16	15
Sausage	260	15	20
12" Specialty Handmade Pan: *Per Slice, ⅛ Pizza*			
Cali Chicken Bacon Ranch	380	22	29
Deluxe	320	17	29
Memphis BBQ Chicken	340	17	33
Spinach & Feta	310	17	29
12" Specialty Hand-Tossed: *Per Slice, ⅛ Pizza*			
Buffalo Chicken	260	12	24
Deluxe	220	10	24
ExtravaganZZa	280	14	25
MeatZZa	270	13	24
Ultimate Pepperoni	260	14	24
14" Specialty Thin Crust: *Per Slice, ⅛ Pizza*			
Buffalo Chicken	270	16	17
Cali Chicken Bacon Ranch	330	22	17
Honolulu Hawaiian	260	14	19
Memphis BBQ Chicken	270	15	21
Wisconsin 6 Cheese	260	15	18

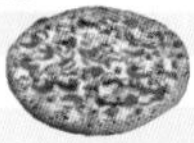

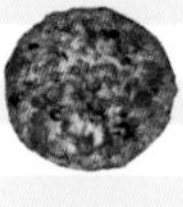

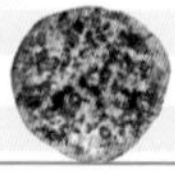

Updated Nutrition Data ~ www.CalorieKing.com
Persons with Diabetes ~ See Disclaimer (Page 22)

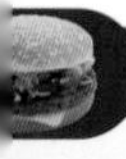

Domino's® cont... (Nov '20)

Chicken Wings: Without Sauce	C	F	Cb
Barbecue, 4 wings	**270**	16	18
Hot, 4 wings	**230**	16	8
Chicken Dipping Cups: BBQ, 1.25 oz	**60**	0	14
Blue Cheese, 1.25 oz	**200**	21	2
Kicker Hot, 1.25 oz	**40**	3.5	1
Ranch, 1.5 oz	**160**	17	1
Sweet Mango Habanero, 1.25 oz	**70**	0	17
BreadBowl Pasta: *Per ½ Bowl*			
Chicken Alfredo, 10.5 oz	**690**	25	92
Chicken Carbonara, 11.6 oz	**730**	28	93
Italian Sausage Marinara, 11.85 oz	**740**	28	96
Pasta Primavera, 11 oz	**660**	23	92
Oven Baked Sandwiches: *Per Sandwich*			
Buffalo Chicken with Blue Cheese	**840**	42	74
Chicken Bacon Ranch	**880**	44	70
Chicken Parmesan	**760**	30	72
Italian	**820**	40	70
Mediterranean Veggie	**700**	30	76
Philly Cheese Steak	**720**	30	74
Sweet & Spicy Chicken Habanero	**800**	32	84
Pasta In Dish: Chkn Alfredo, 11.5 oz	**600**	29	60
Chicken Carbonara, 13 oz	**690**	34	63
Italian Sausage Marinara, 13.5 oz	**700**	36	68
Pasta Primavera, 11.9 oz	**530**	26	62
Salads: *Without Dressing*			
Chicken Caesar	**220**	8	14
Classic Garden	**80**	4	8
Ken's Salad Dressings: *Per 1.5 oz Package*			
Caesar Dressing	**210**	23	2
Italian	**160**	17	4
Light Balsamic Dressing	**90**	9	5
Ranch Dressing	**200**	21	2
Bread Side Items:			
Garlic Bread Twists, 2 pcs	**220**	11	27
Jalap. Bacon Stuffed Cheesy Bread (1)	**170**	8	17
Parmesan Bread Bites, 4 pieces	**220**	10	27
Spin. & Fetta Stuffed Cheesy Bread, 1 piece	**160**	7	17
Stuffed Cheesy Bread, 1 piece	**150**	7	17
Bread Dipping Sauces: *Per Container*			
Garlic, 1 oz cup	**250**	28	0
Marinara, 2 oz cup	**30**	0	6
Dessert: Choc. Lava Crunch Cake, 3 oz	**350**	19	46
Cinnamon Bread Twists, 2 pcs	**250**	12	31
Marbled Cookie Brownie, 1.5 oz	**190**	9	25
Sweet Icing, Dipping Cup, 2.25 oz	**230**	4	52

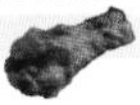
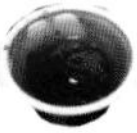
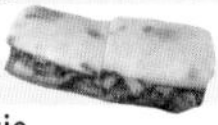
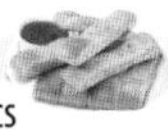

Dunkin'® (Nov '20)

Bagels: Per Bagel	C	F	Cb
Plain	**300**	1	64
Cinnamon Raisin	**320**	1	67
Everything	**340**	3	67
Multigrain	**380**	8	63
Sesame Seed	**350**	5	64
White Cheddar Twist	**390**	8	64
Donuts: Apple 'n Spice	**230**	10	31
Apple Crumb	**290**	11	44
Bavarian Kreme	**240**	11	31
Bismark	**480**	22	63
Boston Kreme	**270**	11	39
Butternut	**430**	21	57
Chocolate Butternut	**440**	23	55
Chocolate Frosted Cake	**360**	20	41
Chocolate Headlight	**310**	14	41
Coconut; Coffee Roll, average	**400**	20	49
Double Chocolate	**370**	22	40
French Cruller	**230**	14	21
Glazed	**240**	11	33
Glazed Chocolate	**360**	22	39
Glazed Jelly	**280**	10	44
Jelly	**250**	10	36
Lemon	**230**	10	31
Maple Frosted	**260**	11	35
Maple Vanilla Creme	**330**	15	45
Old Fashioned	**310**	19	30
Peanut	**470**	27	50
Powdered	**330**	20	34
Strawberry Frosted	**260**	11	35
Sugared	**210**	11	24
Toasted Coconut	**430**	22	52
Vanilla Creme	**300**	15	37
Muffins: Blueberry	**460**	15	77
Chocolate Chip	**550**	21	85
Coffee Cake	**590**	24	88
Corn	**460**	16	73
Munchkins: Cinnamon	**60**	3.5	6
Glazed	**60**	3	7
Glazed Chocolate	**60**	3.5	8
Jelly	**60**	3	8
Old Fashioned	**60**	3.5	6
Powdered	**60**	3.5	6
Other Bakery Items:			
English Muffin	**190**	2	35
Plain Croissant	**340**	19	37
Sandwiches:			
Bacon, Egg & Cheese Croissont	**560**	36	41
Ham, Egg & Cheese Croissant	**530**	32	40
Ssg, Egg & Cheese English Muffin	**560**	35	40
Turkey Sausage English Muffin	**460**	22	39

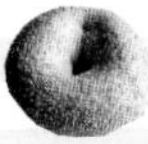
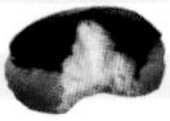
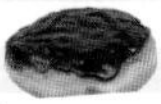
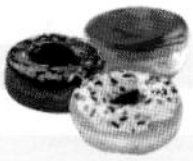
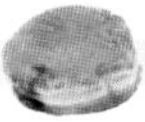
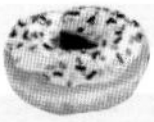
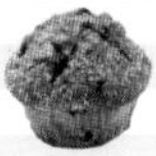
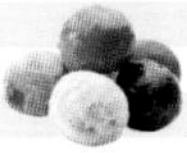
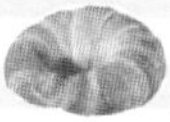

continued next page...

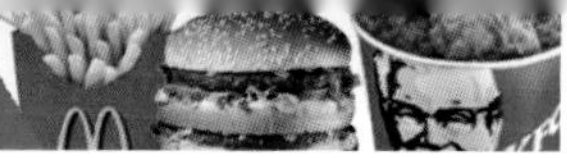

Dunkin'® cont... (Nov '20)

Breakfast:

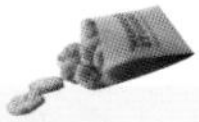

	C	F	Cb
Hash Browns,			
6 pieces	130	6	12
Multigrain Oatmeal, with			
Br. Sugar & Dried Fruit Topping	300	2.5	65
Sandwiches:			
Plain Bagels:			
Bacon, Egg & Cheese	520	18	67
Egg & Cheese	460	13	66
Ham, Egg & Cheese	490	14	67
Sausage, Egg & Cheese	680	34	68
Big N' Toasted, with Toast	600	36	41
Biscuit, Chicken	460	22	46
Croissants: Bacon, Egg & Cheese	560	36	41
Egg & Cheese	500	31	40
Ham, Egg & Cheese	530	32	40
Sausage, Egg & Cheese	720	52	42
English Muffins:			
Bacon, Egg & Cheese	400	19	39
Ham, Egg & Cheese	340	15	38
Sausage, Egg & Cheese	560	35	40
Sandwich, Beyond Sausage	510	26	40
Wake-Up Wraps:			
Bacon, Egg & Cheese	220	13	15
Beyond Sausage	280	18	15
Egg & Cheese	180	10	14
Ham, Egg & Cheese	190	11	15
Turkey Sausage	240	15	15
Veggie Egg White	150	7	15
Hot Beverages: *Per Medium Size*			
Chocolate: Original	330	10	59
Salted Caramel	310	10	52
Dunkaccino	350	15	52
Cold Beverages: *Per Medium, 24 fl.oz*			
Coolatta: Blue Raspberry	350	0	84
Strawberry	350	0	86
Vanilla Bean	590	4.5	129
Iced Latte: *Per Medium, 24 fl.oz, with Whole Milk, without Sugar*			
Butter Pecan Swirl	330	9	52
Caramel Craze Signature	410	14	61
Cocoa Mocha	400	14	60
French Vanilla Swirl	330	9	52
Mocha Swirl	330	10	52
Iced Macchiato: *Per Medium, 24 fl.oz, with Whole Milk, without Sugar*			
Caramel Swirl	290	6	49
French Vanilla Swirl	280	6	49
Hazelnut Swirl	280	6	49
Mocha Swirl	280	7	48

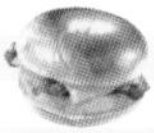
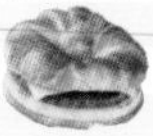
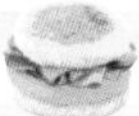
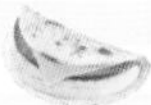
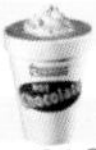
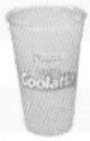
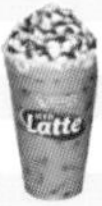

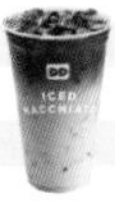

Eat 'N Park® (Nov '20)

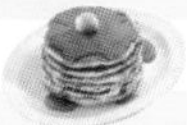
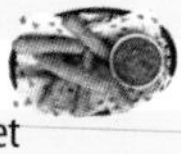
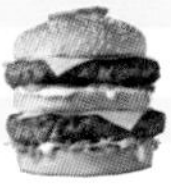
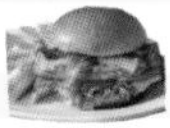
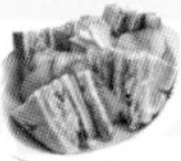
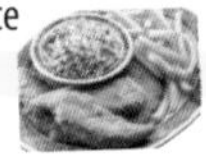

	C	F	Cb
Breakfast: *Without Extras*			
Home Made French Toast,			
with Maple Syrup & Sugar, 2 slices	300	10	38
Omelettes: Ham & Cheese	660	47	6
Mushroom & Swiss	490	25	5
Pancakes,			
Buttermilk (2)	320	2.5	65
Scramblers:			
Philly Steak & Egg	620	24	59
All-American with Sausage	740	42	58
Appetizers:			
Fried Cheese Sticks	590	35	41
Fresh Potato Chip Basket	620	40	63
Burgers: *Without Sides*			
Black Angus:			
Bacon Cheeseburger	810	51	37
Cheeseburger	760	47	40
Mushroom & Onion	790	48	41
Superburgers: Black Angus	1100	71	39
Original	670	42	37
Sandwiches: *Without Sides*			
Chargrilled Chicken	470	16	41
Classic Grilled Cheese	720	37	70
Crispy Buff. Chicken Wrap with Ranch	970	54	68
Grilled Chicken Club	810	49	39
Philly Cheesesteak	800	42	50
Shredded Pot Roast	540	31	28
Turkey Club	850	46	48
Whale of a Cod Fish	930	35	96
Dinners: *Without Sides*			
Baked Chicken Parmigiana:			
with Marinara Sauce	920	41	84
with Meat Sauce	1030	50	75
Baked Cod, 2 fillets	410	24	6
Chicken Bruschetta, 2 pieces	890	51	35
Fried Chicken, 4 pieces	1650	97	79
Grilled Chicken & Broccoli Alfredo	880	44	67
Nantucket Cod & Stuffing, 2 pieces	740	56	20
Pasta Noodles w/ Marinara Sauce	680	8	130
Rosemary Chicken, 2 pieces	470	17	9
Whale of a Cod	620	30	39

Updated Nutrition Data ~ www.CalorieKing.com
Persons with Diabetes ~ See Disclaimer (Page 22)

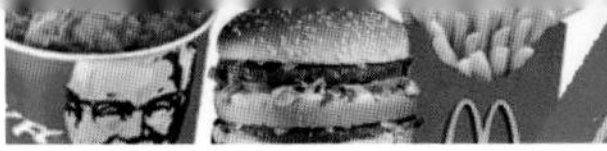

Eat 'N Park® cont... (Nov '20)

Salads: With Fries, w/out Dressing	C	F	Cb
Crispy Buffalo Chicken	390	23	31
Grilled Buffalo Chicken	570	28	31
Eat'n Park, with Rib Eye	730	44	31
Sides: Broccoli	40	0	8
Carrots	40	1	9
Coleslaw	120	8	12
French fries	350	17	47
Mac'n Cheese	450	22	44
Mashed Potatoes	110	6	13
Onion Rings	170	9	20
Soup Bowls: Chicken Noodle	270	8	34
Clam Chowder	420	18	48
Cream of Broccoli	300	12	39
Cream of Potato	310	14	39
Desserts: Per Slice, without Whipped Cream			
Pies: Apple Pie	390	14	65
Bananas Foster Creme Pie	560	29	74
Blackberry Pie	430	14	72
Coconut Cream Pie	470	23	59
Dutch Apple Pie	410	16	65
Lemon Meringue Pie	250	10	35
Oreo Creme Pie	970	47	128

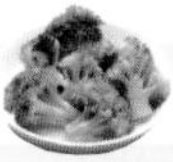
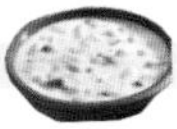
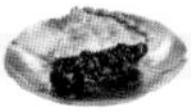

Edo Japan® (Nov '20)

Bento Box: Without Teriyaki Sauce	C	F	Cb
Beef Yakisoba, 20.3 oz	840	29	102
Chicken Yakisoba, 20.5 oz	790	24	102
Sizzling Shrimp, 22 oz	790	15	122
Sukiyaki Beef, 20.3 oz	880	27	120
Teriyaki: Without Teriyaki Sauce			
Beef & Shrimp, 17 oz	660	18	82
Sukiyaki Beef, 14.8 oz	580	15	80
Soup: Per Bowl			
Beef Udon	720	25	82
Chicken Udon	670	19	82
Maki Sushi: Per 6 Pieces			
California Roll, 7.6 oz	430	17	61
Spicy Tuna Roll, 6.5 oz	300	2.5	54
Nigiri Sushi: Per 1 Piece			
Ebi	70	0.5	12
Smoked Salmon	70	0.5	12
Sushi Platters: Easi with Sukiyaki	790	19	131
Easi with Beef & Edamame, 15 pcs	695	22	97
Easi, Spicy, 15 pieces	830	22	134
Enjoi	650	12	111
Kami	660	14	105

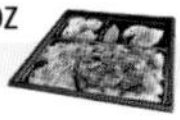
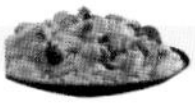
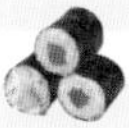
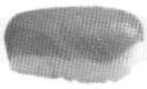
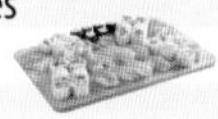

Einstein Bros® (Nov '20)

Bagels:	C	F	Cb
Bagels: Ancient Grain	280	5	49
Asiago Cheese	300	4	54
Blueberry	290	1	59
Chocolate Chip	300	4	58
Cinnamon Sugar	300	4	54
Everything	280	2	56
Garlic	280	2	57
Green Chili	390	12	54
Honey Whole Wheat	260	3	49
Onion	270	2	55
Poppyseed	290	2.5	56
Power Protein	350	6	64
Sesame	290	3	56
Six-Cheese	370	10	53
Spinach Florentine	370	12	53
Lunch Sandwiches: On Menu Set Bagels/Rolls			
Albacore Tuna Salad	590	28	57
Avocado Veg Out	420	15	68
Ham & Swiss	560	23	60
Nova Lox	480	17	60
Tasty Turkey	510	15	64
Hot Sandwiches:			
Cheese Bagel Pizza	440	14	58
Pepperoni Bagel Pizza	530	23	59
Cream Cheese: Per 1.2 oz Schmear			
Reduced Fat:			
Garlic Herb/Garden Veggie	110	9	5
Honey Almond; Strawberry, av.	120	8	10
Plain	120	12	2
Onion and Chive	120	10	4
Smoked Salmon	110	10	4
Breakfast:			
Applewood Bacon Cheddar	450	15	57
Bagelrito	930	41	104
Chorizo & Pepper Jack	610	31	56
Farmhouse	680	32	64
French Toast Chicken	840	37	92
Turkey Sausage & Cheddar	480	15	58
Side, Twice Baked Hash Brown	170	11	11
Sweets: Blueberry Muffin, 4 oz	420	20	57
Chocolate Chip Cookie	460	23	60
Chocolate Croissant	310	17	33

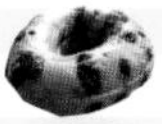
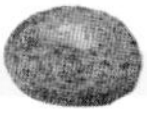
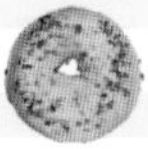
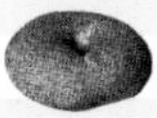
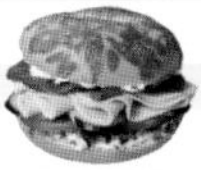
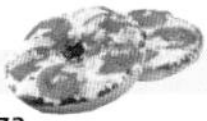
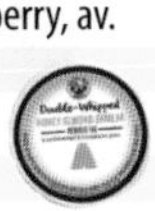
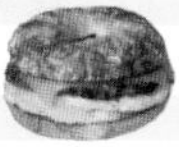

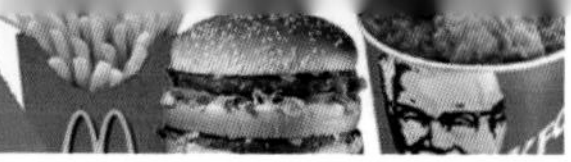

El Pollo Loco® (Nov '20)

	C	F	Cb
Bowl:			
Original Chicken	**520**	8	80
Double Chicken	**840**	28	87
Grand Avocado Chicken	**760**	27	89
Burritos:			
Chicken Avocado	**870**	47	69
Chipotle Chicken Avocado	**880**	40	84
Original BRC	**410**	11	61
Fire-Grilled Combos:			
Chicken Tacos Al Carbon	**430**	13	51
Chicken Nachos	**840**	48	68
Classic Chicken Burrito	**510**	15	65
Extras:			
Chicken Tortilla Soup: Small	**210**	9	17
Large	**440**	19	36
Chips & Chunky Guacamole, 13.5 oz	**1010**	67	98
Tostada Salads: *With Shell, without Dressing*			
Classic	**820**	42	76
Double Chicken	**980**	50	80
Under 500 Calories: *Without Dressing*			
Chicken Black Bean Bowl	**450**	11	57
Chicken Avocado Tortilla Wrap	**460**	19	46
Double Chicken Avocado Salad	**350**	15	15
Dressings: Citrus Vinaig., 1.5 oz	**70**	4	9
Creamy Cilantro: 1.3 oz	**140**	15	0.5
Light Creamy Cilantro, 1.5 oz	**110**	8	9
Ranch, 1.5 oz	**220**	24	2
Sides: Black Beans: Small	**140**	1	25
Large	**370**	2.5	65
Cole Slaw, 4 oz	**130**	10	9
Loco Side Salad, small	**170**	15	8
Macaroni & Cheese: Small	**310**	19	24
Large	**770**	48	60
Mashed Potatoes & Gravy: Small	**105**	1	20
Large	**340**	4.5	69
Pinto Beans, small	**150**	2.5	24
Spanish Rice: Small	**160**	1.5	32
Large	**380**	4	76
Tapatio Fries, 4.1 oz	**230**	12	29
Condiments: Pico de Gallo, 1.5 oz	**10**	0	2
Salsa: Avocado, 1.5 oz	**30**	2.5	2
House; Roja, 1.5 oz	**10**	0	2
Sour Cream, 1.3 oz	**80**	7	1
Dessert, Two Cinnamon Churros	**320**	22	30

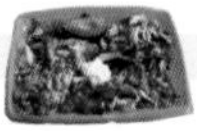
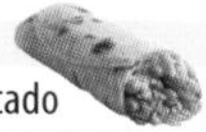
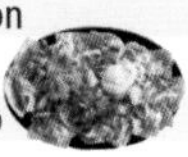
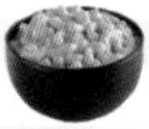
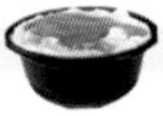
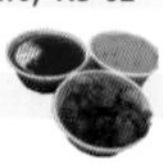

Fatburger® (Nov '20)

	C	F	Cb
Burgers: *Without Extras*			
Fatburger: Baby Fat	**400**	21	37
Original	**590**	31	46
Kingburger	**850**	41	69
Impossible Burger	**525**	13	54
Thousand Island	**770**	47	46
Turkeyburger	**480**	21	50
Veggieburger	**510**	20	60
Hot Dogs: *Without Extras*			
Chili Cheese	**330**	15	27
Regular Hot Dog	**510**	20	60
Sandwiches: *Without Extras*			
Bacon & Egg	**350**	16	37
Chicken: Crispy	**560**	27	53
Grilled	**430**	14	42
Sausage & Egg	**780**	53	47
Spicy Chicken	**520**	21	58
Fries: Fat Fries	**380**	18	47
with Chili & Cheese	**590**	33	53
Skinny Fries	**390**	15	58
with Chili Cheese	**600**	30	64
Salad: Buffalo Chicken	**640**	32	16
Cajun Chicken	**200**	12	8
Wings & Tenders: Bone In Wing (1)	**60**	3.5	2
Boneless Wing (1)	**50**	2.5	2
Chicken Tenders (4)	**670**	34	31
Add-Ons: American Cheese	**70**	5	1
Cheddar Cheese, 1 slice	**110**	9	1
Mayonnaise, 1 serving	**90**	10	1
Relish, 1 serving	**20**	0	5
Vegan Cheese	**60**	4.5	5
Sides: Chili Cup	**200**	11	10
with Cheese & Onions	**320**	20	12
Onion Rings	**540**	29	64
Shakes: Chocolate	**910**	45	115
Maui Banana	**940**	44	126
Strawberry	**880**	44	111
Vegan Strawberry/Vanilla	**355**	12	69

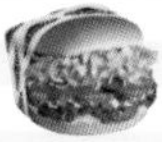
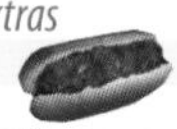
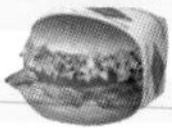
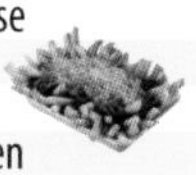
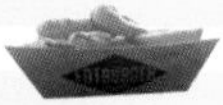
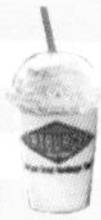

For Complete Nutritional Data ~ see CalorieKing.com

Fazoli's® (Nov '20)

	C	F	Cb
Oven-Baked Pasta: *Per Serving*			
Baked Lasagna	**630**	25	69
Chicken Broccoli Penne	**860**	38	74
Chicken Parmigiano	**840**	25	114
Penne with Creamy Basil Chicken	**900**	45	70
Spicy Sausage Penne	**770**	38	76
Classic Pastas:			
Chicken Fettuccine Alfredo	**870**	28	106
Fettuccine Alfredo	**690**	22	104
Spagh. with Marinara	**510**	3.5	108
Spaghetti with Meatballs	**740**	21	113

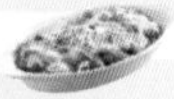

Updated Nutrition Data ~ www.CalorieKing.com
Persons with Diabetes ~ See Disclaimer (Page 22)

Fazoli's® cont... (Nov '20)

Samplers: Per Serving	C	F	Cb
Classic	820	25	120
Oven Baked	930	35	116
Ultimate	1050	30	163
Signature Pasta:			
Chicken Carbonara	940	33	110
Three Cheese Tortellini Alfredo	890	35	78
Submarinos:			
Meatball da Vinci	920	56	65
Primo Italiano	840	45	60
Salads:			
Caesar Side, without dressing	80	3	9
Chicken Bacon Caesar, with dressing	740	51	26

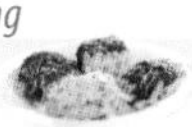
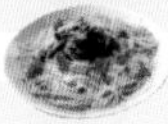
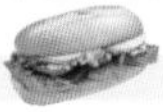

For Complete Nutritional Data ~ see CalorieKing.com

Firehouse Subs® (Nov '20)

Cold Sub,	C	F	Cb
Tuna on White Sub, medium	910	57	61
Hot Subs: *Per Medium White Sub, Standard Toppings and Dressings*			
Cajun Chicken	710	34	54
Club on a Sub	770	40	63
Engineer	690	35	60
Italian	940	58	65
Meatball	840	50	61
Steak & Cheese	830	51	53
Sides, Chili, Bowl	300	15	22
Under 500 Calorie Salads:			
Firehouse Chopped: *Without Dressing*			
with Grilled Chicken	380	10	14
with Ham	310	10	27
with Turkey	220	7	15
Italian, w/ Gr. Chicken, w/o dressing	410	22	13

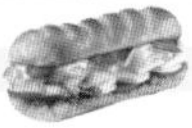
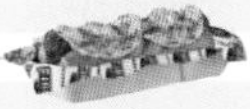
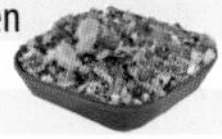

Five Guys® (Nov '20)

Burgers: *Without Toppings or Sauce*	C	F	Cb
Bacon Burger	920	50	39
Bacon Cheeseburger	1060	62	40
Cheeseburger	980	55	40
Hamburger	840	43	39
Little Burgers: Bacon Burger	620	33	39
Bacon Cheeseburger	690	39	40
Hamburger	540	26	39
Hot Dogs: Bacon	600	42	40
Bacon Cheese	670	48	41
Cheese	590	41	41
Sandwiches: BLT	600	34	42
Cheese Veggie	420	21	61
Grilled Cheese	470	26	41
Veggie	280	15	60

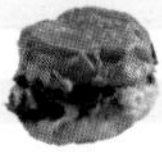
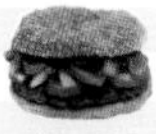
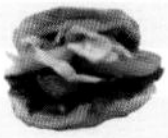

Five Guys® cont... (Nov '20)

Burger Sauces:	C	F	Cb
A.1 Original	15	0	3
BBQ Sauce	50	0	15
Ketchup	30	0	5
Mayo	110	11	0
Fries: Little, 8 oz	530	23	72
Regular, 14.5 oz	955	41	131
Large, 20 oz	1315	57	181

Flame Broiler® (Nov '20)

Bowls: *Regular Single Protein with White Rice, without Toppings or Sauce*	C	F	Cb
Beef	660	10	103
Chicken, white meat	590	6	82
Chicken & Veggie	510	14	49
Tofu	550	9	88
Plates: *Regular Single Portion with White Rice, without Toppings or Sauce*			
Beef	850	15	126
Angus Rib	1000	35	107
Tofu	700	14	106

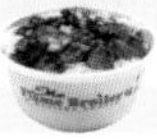
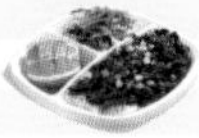

Freshens® (Nov '20)

Smoothies: *100% Juice*	C	F	Cb
Blended Fruit Classics: *Per 20 fl.oz*			
Bangin' Berry	330	0	80
Caribbean Craze	300	0	73
Jamaican Jammer	330	0	70
Peach On The Beach	330	2.5	75
Peanut Butter Protein	480	12	69
Tropical Therapy	530	4	81
Vegan PowerUp	320	0	71
Wild Strawberry	300	0	76
Crepes: Buffalo Chicken	410	22	25
Chicken Caesar	600	44	25
Chipotle Ranch Turkey Melt	520	31	25
Denver, with Bacon	520	29	27
Honey Mustard Chkn	460	22	36
Pesto Chicken	490	29	27
Southwest Chicken	580	33	36
Rice Bowls: Buffalo Chicken	600	23	70
Florence	550	11	73
KC BBQ	610	11	97
Mexican	710	29	83
Power Protein	700	28	75
Spicy Korean	520	8	90
Salads: Buffalo Chkn	480	27	29
Gr. Chicken Caesar	520	37	26
Roadhouse BBQ Chkn	420	17	42
Strawberry & Kale	490	15	56

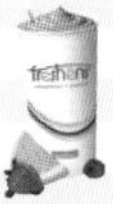
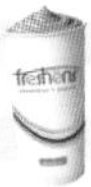
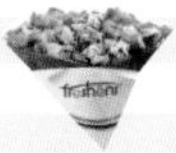
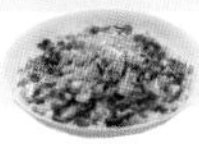
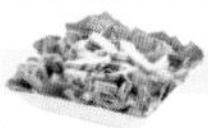

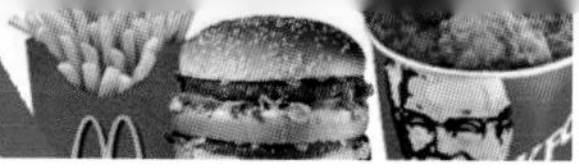

Godfather's Pizza® (Nov '20)

Golden Crust Pizza: Per Slice	C	F	Cb
Cheese: Medium, ⅛ pizza	**210**	8	26
Large, 1/10 pizza	**240**	10	28
Combo: Medium, ⅛ pizza	**280**	13	28
Large, 1/10 pizza	**310**	15	30
Super Combo:			
Medium, ⅛ pizza	**310**	16	28
Large, 1/10 pizza	**360**	18	31
Mozza-Loaded:			
All Meat Combo: Med., ⅛ pizza	**340**	18	29
Large, 1/10 pizza	**380**	20	31
Original Crust Pizza:			
BLT: Small, ⅙ pizza	**300**	14	30
Medium, ⅛ pizza	**320**	15	33
Jumbo, 1/12 pizza	**440**	21	43
Buffalo Chicken: Small, ⅙ pizza	**250**	9	30
Medium, ⅛ pizza	**270**	9	33
Jumbo, 1/12 pizza	**380**	14	43
Taco Pie: Small, ⅙ pizza	**300**	12	33
Medium, ⅛ pizza	**340**	14	36
Jumbo, 1/12 pizza	**460**	20	47
Thin Crust Pizza:			
BBQ Chicken: Medium, ⅛ pizza	**200**	8	20
Large, 1/10 pizza	**240**	10	24
Pepperoni: Medium, ⅛ pizza	**200**	11	15
Large, 1/10 pizza	**230**	13	18
The Don: Medium, ⅛ pizza	**250**	14	16
Large, 1/10 pizza	**290**	17	19
Sides: Baked Beans, 4 oz	**120**	1	25
Biscuit, 1 oz	**90**	3.5	13
Cheesy Potatoes, 4 oz	**300**	19	30
Coleslaw, 4 oz	**210**	17	12
Gravy, 2 oz	**30**	1	4
Mashed Potatoes, 4 oz	**100**	3	17
Mixed Vegetables, 4 oz	**90**	0	18
Potato Wedges, 4 oz	**180**	7	26

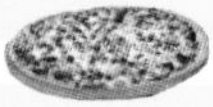
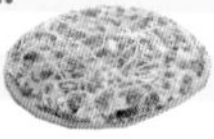
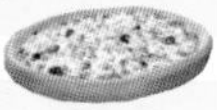
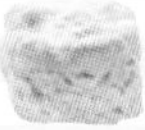

Gold Star Chili® (Nov '20)

Burgers: Per Single	C	F	Cb
Bacon Cheeseburger	**870**	58	46
Chili Burger	**680**	39	50
Hamburger	**560**	33	44
Coneys: Cheese, plain	**300**	18	21
Plain	**210**	11	21
Mustard & Onion	**230**	11	23
Ways, Orignminal Chili:			
Regular: 2-Way	**410**	12	56
3-Way	**760**	41	56
5-Way	**850**	41	74
Super, 5-Way	**1160**	53	111
Chili Bowls, Original:			
Plain, 8 oz	**200**	11	12
Beans & Onions, 8 oz	**290**	12	30

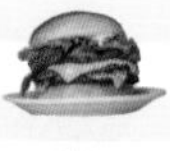
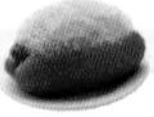
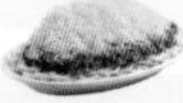
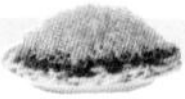

Gold Star Chili® cont...(Nov '20)

Double Deckers: With White Bread	C	F	Cb
Ham & Bacon	**1080**	80	46
Ham & Turkey	**760**	46	46
Turkey & Bacon	**1070**	78	46
Salads: Full Salad, without Dressing			
BBQ Chicken	**490**	24	36
Harvest Chicken	**340**	16	25
Fries: French, regular	**460**	19	67
Cheese	**810**	48	68
Chili Cheese	**840**	51	64
Garlic Parmesan	**870**	62	71
Vegetarian Chili	**540**	24	71

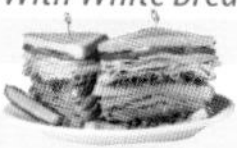
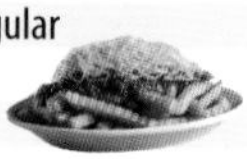

Golden Corral® (Nov '20)

Breakfast:	C	F	Cb
Corned Beef Hash, ½ cup	**230**	15	14
Hash Brown Casserole, ½ cup	**100**	3.5	14
Sausage & Egg Burrito	**320**	19	22
Scrambled Eggs, ½ cup	**180**	14	2
Hot Buffet: Without Sides			
Beef: Pot Roast, 1/2 cup	**130**	7	8
Roast, flat, 3 oz	**180**	10	1
Smoked Beef Short Ribs, 3 oz	**340**	27	0
Steak, Smothered Chopped, 5.9 oz	**290**	18	4
Chicken: Buffalo Chicken S'wich	**210**	10	20
Fried Chicken, 3 oz	**240**	15	6
Orange Chicken, 6 oz	**390**	15	40
Smoked White Meat Chicken, 3 oz	**150**	6	0
Fish: Baked, 3 oz	**150**	8	1
Fried Catfish, 3 oz	**180**	10	12
Pork: Baby Back Ribs, 3 oz	**190**	13	3
Sweet & Sour, 6 oz	**220**	11	18
Sides: BBQ Baked Beans, ½ cup	**160**	1	35
Creamed Spinach, ½ cup	**170**	12	10
Fries, Seasoned Wedges (10)	**190**	12	21
Fried Okra (10)	**110**	7	10
Mac & Cheese, ½ c.	**180**	10	19
Mshd Potatoes,½ c.	**160**	8	20
Rice Pilaf, ½ cup	**130**	4.5	18
Salad Buffet: Per ½ Cup Unless Indicated			
Caesar, without dressing, 1 cup	**110**	8	8
Chicken	**250**	22	3
Coleslaw	**110**	9	6
Potato	**150**	5	26
Seafood	**140**	10	9
Spinach, 1 cup	**15**	0	2
Tuna	**190**	12	4
Dressings: Balsamic Vinaig., 2 Tbsp	**20**	0	5
Caesar, 2 Tbsp	**150**	15	2
Ranch, 2 Tbsp	**110**	12	2

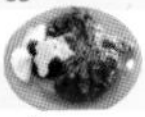
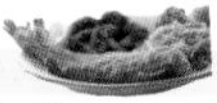
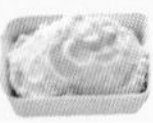
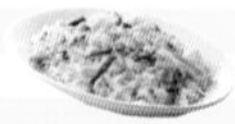

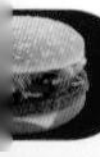

Updated Nutrition Data ~ www.CalorieKing.com
Persons with Diabetes ~ See Disclaimer (Page 22)

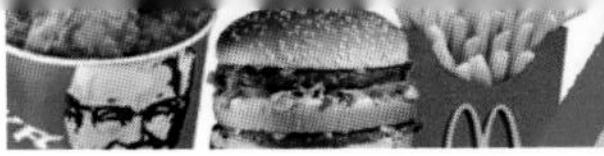

Great American Bagel Co® (Nov '20)

Bagels:	C	F	Cb
Asiago Cheese	520	16	72
Cheddar Herb	390	8	66
Cinnamon Raisin	380	3.5	76
Jalapeno Cheddar	370	7	63
Plain	360	4	71
Spinach Tomazzo	640	20	86
Tomazzo	520	13	77
Paninis: On Regular Baguette			
Chicken Pesto	770	35	70
Ham & Swiss	600	26	58
Philly Beef	920	40	92
Turkey Club	680	29	67
Sandwiches: Asiago Omelet	720	29	80
BLT	550	17	72
Chicken Parmigiana	740	22	81
Ham	460	9	71
Roast Beef	465	9	71
Turkey	435	5	72
Cream Cheese Filling: Per 1 oz			
Plain	100	10	1
Strawberry; Vegetable, average	90	8	4
Pastries:			
Cookies: Chocolate Chunk, 4 oz	110	3.5	19
Oatmeal Raisin, 4 oz	120	5	18
Muffins: Banana Nut, 4.25 oz	430	18	61
Blueberry, 4.25 oz	430	16	64

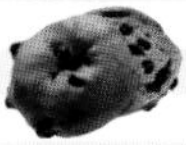

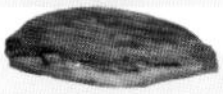

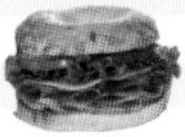

Green Burrito® (Nov '20)

Burritos:	C	F	Cb
Bean, Rice & Cheese	730	26	93
Green: Chicken	930	38	96
Steak	940	38	96
Grilled, Beef; Chicken; Steak, av.	840	33	89
Specialties:			
Quesadillas: Cheese	640	34	53
Chicken	780	40	56
Steak	790	39	56
Rice, Bean & Chips Platter	340	10	51
Taco Salad, Chicken; Steak	875	53	60
Taquitos: Chicken, 3 pieces	410	28	34
Chicken, 5 pieces	640	43	56
Tacos:			
Crunchy Beef	210	12	16
Soft Chicken	250	12	18
Sides: Chips, 2 oz	300	17	35
Cilantro Lime Rice, 3.4 oz	90	5	21
Guacamole, 2.7 oz	100	8	5
Pinto Beans, 3.7 oz	90	1.5	13

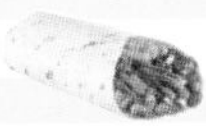

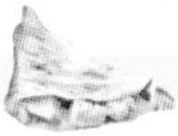

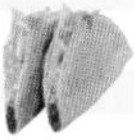

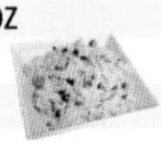

(The) Great Steak® (Nov '20)

Breakfast Sandwiches:	C	F	Cb
Bacon, Egg & Cheese	550	31	38
Sausage, Egg & Cheese	660	42	38
Steak, Egg & Chse	540	27	38
Burgers:			
Bacon Cheeseburger	1050	72	45
Cheeseburger	840	54	45
Hamburger	730	46	44
Philly Cheeseburger	780	48	44
Sandwiches: Regular Sie			
Bacon Cheddar Cheesesteak	590	23	55
Buffalo Chicken Philly	750	38	61
Chicagoland Cheesesteak	610	24	59
Chicken Bacon Ranch	820	44	60
Great Steak Cheesesteak	790	45	55
Ham Delight	780	44	64
Original Philly Cheesesteak	510	17	55
Pastrami Philly	800	46	57
Reuben Philly	710	37	56
Super Steak Cheesesteak	800	45	57
Turkey Philly	750	42	57
Ultimate Chicken Philly	800	44	60
Veggie Delight	490	19	61
Wisconsin Inside-Out	530	26	50
Baked Potatoes:			
Bacon & Cheese	440	23	36
Broccoli & Cheese	250	6	45
The Great Potato: Chicken	460	19	49
Ham	450	19	52
Steak	470	20	46
Turkey	430	17	48
The King	540	32	38
Fries:			
Bacon Ranch: Regular	650	42	51
Large	1520	91	139
Great Fry: Kids	270	13	36
Regular	370	18	48
Large	930	40	132
King Fry, regular	480	27	52
Salads: Without Dressing			
Great Salad: Chicken	370	22	16
Ham	360	22	19
Steak	390	23	17
Turkey	350	20	19
Salad Dressings: Mayo, reg., 1 oz	200	22	0
Ranch, 1 oz	150	16	2
Thousand Island, 1 oz	130	12	4
Sauce: BBQ, 1 oz	50	0	12
Buffalo, 1 oz	10	0	1
Honey Mustard, 1 oz	40	1	7
Teriyaki, 1 oz	20	0	3

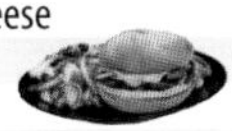

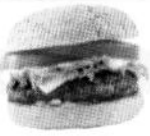

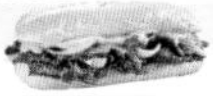

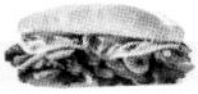

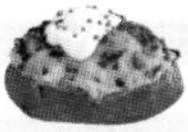

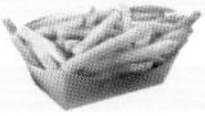

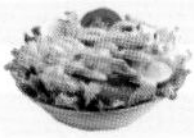

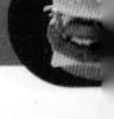

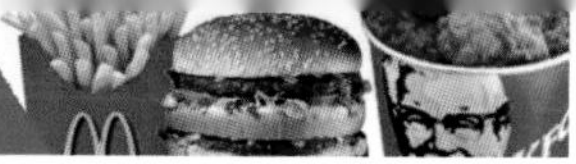

Haagen-Dazs® (Nov '20)

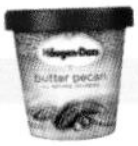
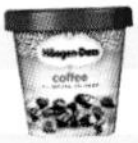
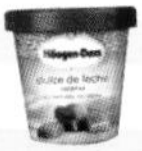
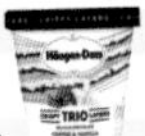

Classic Flavors: Per ⅔ Cup	C	F	Cb
Banana Peanut Butter Chip	**440**	30	33
Bourbon Praline Pecan	**380**	21	42
Bourbon Van. Bean Truffle	**340**	20	36
Butter Pecan	**370**	28	26
Caramel Cone	**400**	25	38
Cherry Vanilla	**290**	18	29
Chocolate	**260**	17	22
Chocolate Chocolate Chip	**380**	24	34
Chocolate Peanut Butter	**450**	29	36
Coffee; Cookies & Cream, av.	**310**	21	27
Cold Brew Espresso Chip Heaven	**220**	9	27
Double Belgian Chocolate Chip	**330**	21	30
Dulce de Leche	**350**	20	36
Green Tea	**310**	21	25
Honey Salted Caramel Almond	**350**	22	33
Irish Cream Brownie	**360**	21	37
Mango	**330**	17	40
Mint Chip	**360**	23	33
PB Chocolate Fudge	**380**	19	47
Pineapple Coconut; Rose & Crm. av.	**300**	17	33
Pistachio	**280**	19	22
Rocky Road; Rum Tres Leches, av.	**365**	21	38
Rum Raisin; Vanilla, average	**310**	20	27
Sea Salt Caramel Truffle	**300**	17	32
Strawberry	**240**	15	22
Vanilla Choc. Chip/Swiss Alm., av.	**370**	24	32
Whisky Hazelnut Latte	**380**	25	32
Light: Chocolate Sea Salt Heaven	**230**	8	30
PB Chip Heaven	**230**	10	26
Strawberry Waffle Cone Heaven	**210**	6	33
Non Dairy: Per ⅔ cup			
Amaretto Black Cherry Almond Toffee	**320**	12	49
Chocolate Salted Fudge Truffle	**270**	11	40
Peanut Butter Chocolate Fudge	**380**	19	47
Trio Crispy Layers: Per ⅔ cup			
Coconut Caramel Chocolate	**370**	24	34
Coffee Vanilla Chocolate	**360**	25	29
Lemon Raspberry White Chocolate	**360**	22	36
Salted Caramel Chocolate	**300**	20	26
Triple Chocolate Trio	**290**	19	26
Van. Blackberry Chocolate	**280**	19	24

Ice Cream Bars/Cones ~ See Page 109

Hardee's® (Nov '20)

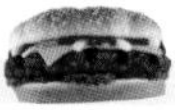
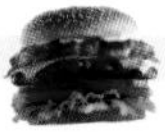
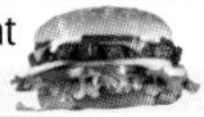
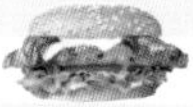
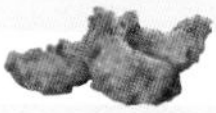
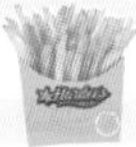
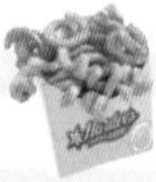

Burgers:	C	F	Cb
Charbroiled Slider: Double, 5 oz	**340**	20	20
Single, 3.5 oz	**220**	11	20
Cheeseburgers: Big	**540**	23	56
Classic Double	**610**	40	38
Thickburgers: Original, ⅓ lb	**780**	48	56
Bacon Cheese, ⅓ lb	**850**	54	54
Frisco, ⅓ lb	**840**	55	46
Monster, ⅔ lb	**1300**	90	53
Mushroom 'N' Swiss, ⅓ lb	**680**	38	53
Original Beyond Meat	**780**	46	61
Sandwiches:			
Beef: Monster Roast Beef	**870**	33	52
Roast Beef	**380**	11	50
Big Hot Ham 'N' Cheese	**530**	20	51
Chicken: Big Chicken Fillet, 11 oz	**710**	36	64
Charbroiled: BBQ Chicken, 7.8 oz	**350**	6	46
Chicken Club	**560**	28	38
Spicy Chicken	**440**	23	44
Chicken Tenders: Without Sauce			
Hand Breaded:			
3 pieces, 4.5 oz	**260**	13	13
5 pieces, 7.5 oz	**440**	21	21
Chili Dog, Jumbo	**390**	26	23
Natural Cut Fries:			
Kid's, 3 oz	**240**	12	31
Small, 3.7 oz	**300**	15	47
Medium, 5.9 oz	**490**	24	63
Large, 6.5 oz	**530**	26	69
Sides:			
Beer Battered Onion Rings	**410**	24	45
Dipping Sauce: B'milk Ranch, 1 oz	**100**	10	2
Honey Mustard	**120**	12	4
Sweet & Bold BBQ, 0.9 oz	**50**	0	13
Crispy Curls:			
Small, 4.1 oz	**360**	18	46
Medium, 5.36 oz	**470**	23	60
Large, 6.5 oz	**570**	28	72
All Star Meals: Per Set Menu, without Dipping Sauce			
Double Cheeseburger & Hot Dog	**1160**	64	111
Hand Breaded Chicken Tender	**690**	34	68

Updated Nutrition Data ~ www.CalorieKing.com
Persons with Diabetes ~ See Disclaimer (Page 22)

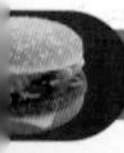

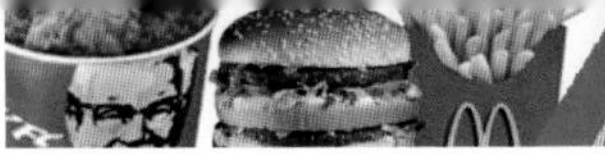

Hardee's® cont... (Nov '20)

Better For You Options:	C	F	Cb
Low Carb It: ⅓ lb Thickburger	470	36	9
Charbroiled Chicken Club S'wich	340	22	13
Trim It: ¼ lb Little Thickburger	220	15	6
Big Hot Ham Sandwich	290	6	31
Charbroiled BBQ Chicken Sandwich	190	3.5	24
Veg It: Egg & Cheese Biscuit	410	23	38
Thickburger, hold the Patty	550	33	56
Breakfast:			
Breakfast Burrito, Loaded	580	30	46
Made From Scratch Biscuits:			
Bacon, Egg & Cheese	610	38	46
Beyond Sausage	530	29	47
Biscuit 'N' Gravy	620	39	57
Chicken	650	41	53
Country Ham	500	30	44
Country Fried Steak	640	42	52
Loaded Omelet	620	39	48
Monster	880	61	48
Pork Chop 'N' Gravy	590	33	49
Sausage	620	43	44
Sausage and Egg	690	48	46
Smoked Sausage, Egg & Cheese	790	57	48
Platter, with Bacon	760	45	51
Sandwich, Frisco Breakfast	450	19	45
Sunrise Croissant	450	28	30
Breakfast Sides:			
Hash Rounds: Small, 2.9 oz	260	15	23
Medium, 4.2 oz	370	22	33
Large, 5.8 oz	510	30	45
Desserts:			
Apple Turnover, w/out Cinnamon Sugar	270	13	35
Chocolate Chip Cookies (2), 2 oz	290	15	35
Ice Cream Shakes: Per 14 oz			
Hand Scooped: Chocolate	710	33	87
Strawberry	710	33	87
Vanilla	710	33	87

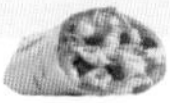
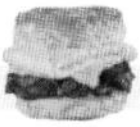
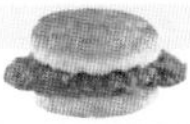
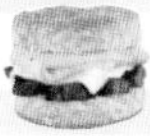
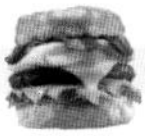
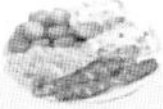
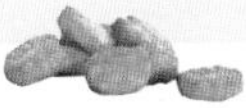
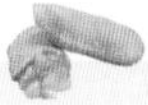
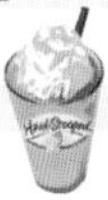

Hissho Sushi® (Nov '20)

Natural Food Store Menu Items	C	F	Cb
Maki Sushi Rolls: Per Package			
Blazing California, 13 oz	440	16	66
California, 11.5 oz	330	7	60
Dazzling Dragon, 13 oz	510	22	52
Krispy Krab, 9.8 oz	410	19	53
Living Color, 10.6 oz	340	11	40
Philadelphia, 11.4 oz	470	20	62
Rising Sun, 13.4 oz	680	40	50
Salmon Lover, 12.4 oz	600	34	41
Spicy Pepper, 8.9 oz	250	9	40
Spicy Salmon, 12 oz	420	15	53
Spicy Tuna, 12 oz	390	9	53
Tempura Shrimp, 12.87 oz	520	23	70
TNT, 10.3 oz	440	19	42
Veggie, 12 oz	320	7	60
Veggie TNT, 10.3 oz	220	4.5	43
Wasabi Crunch, 9.45 oz	290	9	43

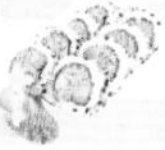
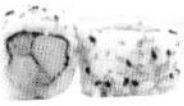
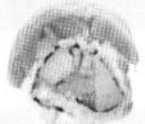
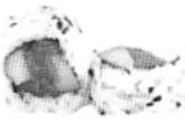
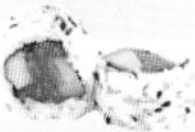

Hot Dog on a Stick® (Nov '20)

Menu Items:	C	F	Cb
On A Stick: American Cheese	260	16	20
Beef Hot Dog	330	21	25
Pepper Jack Cheese	260	15	22
Turkey Hot Dog	240	5	27
Veggie Dog	200	6	26
Fish & Zucchini Platter	470	15	53
Fish Platter with Tartar Sauce	320	14	27
Zucchini Platter with Ranch Sauce	420	23	45
French Fries: Small, 7.2 oz	500	29	57
Regular, 14.4 oz	1000	59	113
Funnel Cake Sticks:			
with Chocolate Sauce, 3.4 oz	300	6	48
with Powdered Sugar, 2.6 oz	210	5	26
with Raspberry Sauce, 3.4 oz	270	5	40
Beverages: Per Regular Size, 16 fl.oz			
Lemonade: Original	150	0	38
Cherry	210	0	52
Lime	230	0	57

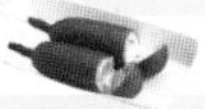
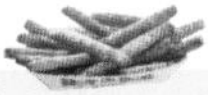
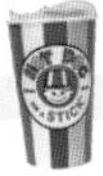

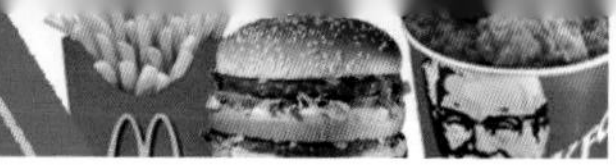

Hungry Howie's Pizza® (Nov '20)

Counts may vary in Florida.

	C	F	Cb
Specialty Pizza: *12" Pizza, Per ⅛ Slice*			
BBQ Chicken	230	8	29
Buffalo Chicken	210	8	24
Works	250	11	26
Veggie	200	6	28
Subs: *Per ½ of Large Sub, with Set Menu Toppings*			
Ham & Cheese	630	25	62
Italian	620	27	62
Steak & Cheese	650	29	62
Turkey Club	860	47	59
Veggie	750	36	73
Salads: *Regular Size, without Dressing*			
Antipasto	400	26	14
Chef; Chicken Asiago av,	240	11	14
Chicken Caesar	220	8	15
Garden	120	2.5	21
Greek	250	11	21
Spicy Chicken	510	29	31
Dressings: *Per 1 oz*			
Caesar	180	18	2
Creamy Italian	120	12	2
Greek	110	11	2
Ranch	140	14	1
Thousand Island	140	14	4

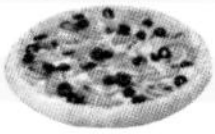
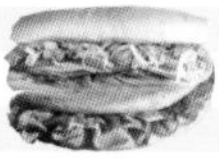
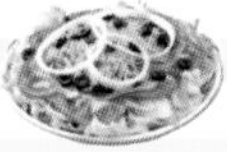

In-N-Out Burger® (Nov '20)

Burgers:	C	F	Cb
Hamburger: with Onion	390	19	39
w/ Mstrd & Ketchup, w/out Spread	310	10	41
Protein Style with Lettuce Wrap, without Bun, with Lettuce	240	17	11
Cheeseburger: with Onion	480	27	39
w/ Mstrd & Ketchup, w/out Spread	400	18	41
Protein Style with Lettuce Wrap, without Bun, with Lettuce	330	25	11
Double Double: with Onion	670	41	39
w/ Mstrd & Ketchup, w/oit Spread	590	32	41
Protein Style with Lettuce Wrap, without Bun, with Lettuce	520	39	11
French Fries, 4.5 oz	370	15	52
Hot Cocoa: 8 fl.oz	130	3	26
with Marshmallows, 8 fl.oz	150	3	32
Shakes: *Per 15 fl.oz*			
Chocolate	580	28	84
Strawberry	590	24	114
Vanilla	580	30	65

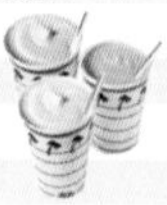

IHOP® (Nov '20)

Pancakes:	C	F	Cb
Cannoli (3)	970	44	125
Double Blueberry (4)	610	16	101
NY Cheesecake (4)	910	35	125
Orig. Buttermilk (3)	430	17	56
Strawberry Banana (4)	650	15	115
Griddle Faves: *With Menu Set Toppings*			
French Toast: Original	740	36	84
Strawberry Banana	840	31	121
Stuffed, Plain	920	40	125
Waffles, Belgian	590	29	69
Crepes: *With Set Toppings*			
Chicken Florentine, w/ Swiss Cheese	790	45	44
German Crepes	610	32	65
Strawb. & Cream	710	29	96
Swedish	600	28	72
Omelettes: *Without Side Choices or Additions*			
Big Steak	830	55	20
Chicken Fajita	910	57	25
Garden	800	61	17
Spicy Poblano	1020	76	30
Spinach & Mushroom	910	71	22
Combos: *With Two B'Milk Pancakes*			
Chicken & Pancakes & IHOP Sauce	1100	59	96
Sirloin Tips & Fried Egg, w H. Browns	1070	56	82
Smokehouse, with Poached Egg	940	68	42
T-Bone Steak (12 oz), w/ Fried Egg	990	45	63
Ultimate Steakburgers: *With Standard Ingredients, without Sides or Dressings*			
Big Brunch	1000	64	58
Cowboy BBQ	950	54	75
The Classic	670	42	41
Sandwiches: *With Standard Ingredients, without Sides or Dressing*			
BLTA on Sourdough	1160	85	73
Philly Cheese Steak Stacker on Hoagie	820	40	63
Spicy Buffalo Chicken on Brioche	630	31	58
Turkey Cheddar Club on Sourdough	1180	78	66
Entrees: *As Served, without Sides, Dressing or Bread*			
Fried Chicken	980	54	30
Grilled Tilapia	240	10	2
Pot Roast	370	20	15
Smoked Sausage	660	60	9
55+ Lunch: *Without Soup, Salad or Dressing*			
BLT Sandwich, on White Bread	410	28	27
Grilled Cheese S'wich, on Sourdough	6830	31	61
Sides: Crispy Breakfast Potatoes	290	13	37
Crispy Potato Pancakes	370	24	35
French Fries	320	15	41
Hash Browns	210	14	19
Onion Rings	530	30	60

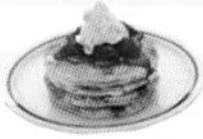
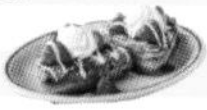
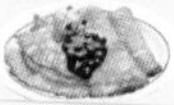
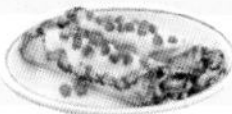
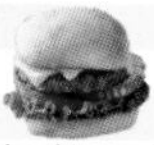
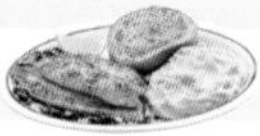
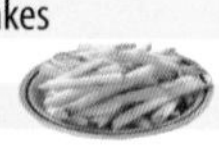

For Complete Menu & Data ~ see CalorieKing.com

Updated Nutrition Data ~ www.CalorieKing.com
Persons with Diabetes ~ See Disclaimer (Page 22)

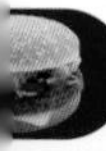

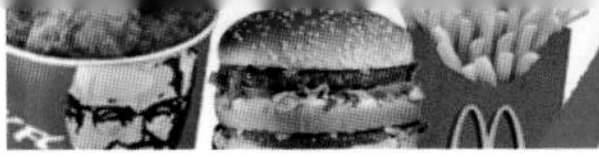

Jack in the Box® (Nov '20)

Sandwiches & Burgers:	C	F	Cb
Bacon Swiss Buttery Jack	**890**	59	48
Bacon Ultimate Cheeseburger	**930**	65	32
BBQ Bacon Double Cheeseburger	**710**	42	53
BBQ Bacon Triple Cheeseburger	**850**	53	54
Classic Buttery Jack	**860**	58	51
Double Jack	**830**	58	34
Jumbo Jack	**520**	33	32
Jumbo Jack Cheeseburger	**600**	40	33
Junior Bacon Cheeseburger	**480**	31	32
Sourdough Jack	**700**	45	39
Spicy Sriracha Burger	**620**	45	38
Ultimate Cheeseburger	**840**	59	31
Chicken & Fish Sandwiches:			
Chicken Fajita Pita	**330**	9	35
Chicken Sandwich	**510**	31	42
Homestyle Ranch Chicken Club	**630**	28	61
Jack's Spicy Chkn S'wich	**550**	29	48
with Cheese	**630**	35	49
Sourdough Grilled Chicken Club	**580**	30	38
Chicken: Crispy Strips (4), 6.9 oz	**565**	24	53
Nuggets, 5 pieces	**240**	17	13
Popcorn: Classic, 4.6 oz	**260**	9	25
Spicy, 4.6 oz	**260**	9	24
Jack's Chicken Teriyaki Bowl:			
with White Rice	**630**	6	109
with Brown Rice	**680**	15	104
Breakfast:			
Biscuit: Bacon, Egg & Cheese	**410**	25	26
Sausage, Egg & Cheese	**535**	38	27
Breakfast Jack: Bacon	**380**	21	30
Ham	**350**	18	30
Sausage	**485**	33	29
Burrito: Meat Lovers	**810**	51	50
Grand Sausage	**1070**	72	70
Croissants: Sausage	**555**	39	32
Supreme	**450**	27	32
Hash Browns, 2.2 oz	**185**	13	17
Mini Pancakes (8)	**145**	2	28
Sandwiches: Extreme Sausage	**650**	49	29
Grilled Sourdough Swiss	**580**	34	36
Loaded	**705**	47	36
Ultimate	**520**	31	30
Late Night: *Includes Fries, Tacos & Beverage*			
Chick-N-Tater Melt	**2030**	110	220
Spicy Nacho Chicken Sandwich	**1530**	80	155
Srircha Curly Fry Burger	**1715**	87	196
Stacked Grilled Chees Burger	**1890**	94	213

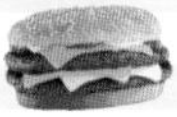
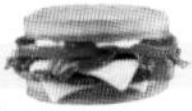
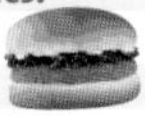
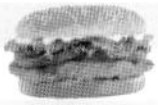
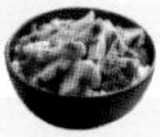
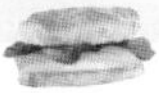
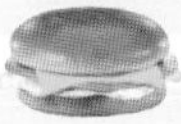
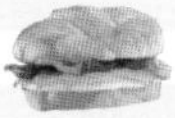
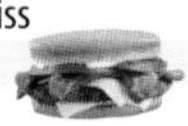

Jack in the Box® cont... (Nov '20)

Snacks & Sides:	C	F	Cb
Bacon Cheddar Potato Wedges	**650**	40	57
Egg Roll (1)	**145**	7	15
Onion Rings (8), 4.2 oz	**445**	24	52
Stuffed Jalapenos: 3 Pieces	**220**	12	21
7 Pieces	**510**	29	49
Two Tacos	**345**	18	32
Fries:			
French Fries: Small	**300**	14	40
Medium	**430**	20	58
Large	**550**	25	75
Seasoned Curly Fries: Small	**280**	16	30
Medium	**430**	25	46
Large	**480**	28	52
Salads: *Without Dressing, Croutons or Corn Sticks*			
Chicken Club: Crispy Chicken	**320**	28	34
Grilled Chicken	**230**	8	12
Side Salad	**20**	0	4
Southwest Chicken: Crispy Chicken	**500**	23	50
Grilled Chicken	**340**	13	25
Croutons, 0.5 oz	**70**	3	9
Dressing: Creamy S'thwest, 1.75 oz	**190**	19	3
Ranch, 1.75 oz	**250**	25	5
Low Fat Balsamic Vinaigrette, 1.5 oz	**25**	1.5	3
Desserts: Mini Churros (5)	**345**	18	42
Choc. Overload Cake	**300**	7	57
New York Style Cheesecake	**310**	17	32
Ice Cream Shakes: *16 fl.oz, with Whipped Topping*			
Chocolate	**780**	28	103
Oreo Cookie	**795**	42	92
Strawberry	**760**	38	97
Vanilla	**685**	38	78

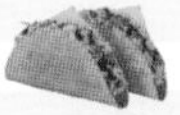
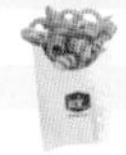
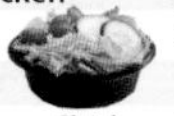
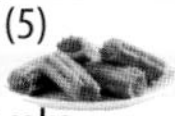
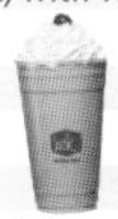

For Complete Nutritional Data ~ see CalorieKing.com

Jack's® (Nov '20)

Burgers & Sandwiches:	C	F	Cb
Big Bacon	**800**	57	36
Big Jack Burger	**720**	47	43
Cheeseburger	**440**	23	38
Double Cheeseburger	**680**	43	38
Grilled Chicken S'wich	**410**	17	35
Hamburger	**400**	19	38
Chicken: Chicken Breast	**480**	29	20
Fingers Dinner, 3 piece with Fries	**610**	27	56
Fries, large	**380**	23	39
Sides: Coleslaw, 4 oz	**210**	18	13
Mashed Potatoes, 4 oz	**140**	3.5	26
Breakfast: Hash Browns	**360**	25	31
Bacon Egg & Cheese Biscuit	**520**	36	32
Big Breakfast Sandwich	**800**	57	36

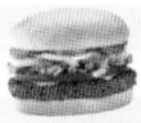
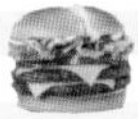
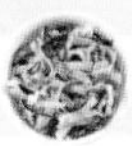

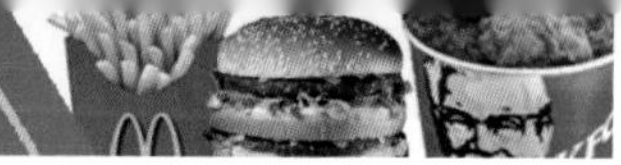

Jamba Juice® (Nov '20)

Freshly Squeezed Juice: 16 fl.oz	C	F	Cb
Orange Carrot Twist	210	1	48
Purely Carrot	190	1	45
Purely Orange	220	1	52

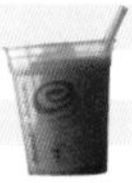

Smoothies: Per 16 fl.oz	C	F	Cb
Classic: Caribbean Passion	260	1	63
Mango-A-Go-Go	300	1	73
Orange Dream Machine	310	1.5	68
Razzamatazz	270	1	65
Strawberry Surf Rider	250	1.5	60
Strawberries Wild	240	0	57
Watermelon Breeze	300	1	72
Plant-Based: Amazing Greens	360	13	57
Apple 'n Greens	250	1	58
Greens 'n ginger	230	1	56
Mega Mango	210	0.5	50
Peach Perfection	210	0	51
Strawberry Whirl	210	0.5	51
Power: Acai Super-Antioxidant	340	4	69
Lotta Horchata	190	2.5	38
La Vida Mocha	270	2	58
PB & Banana Protein	540	22	51
PB Chocolate Love	400	14	64
Soy Protein Berry Workout	300	1	58

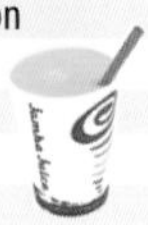
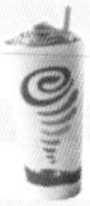
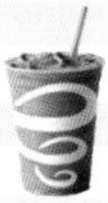

Tasty Bites:	C	F	Cb
Artisan Flat Bread: *Per Flatbread*			
Four Cheese	350	11	44
Spicy 'n Sweet Chicken	330	11	38
Baked Goods: *Per Item*			
Apple Cinnamon Pretzel	390	4.5	78
Cheddar Tomato Twist	250	5	41
Sourdough Parmesan Pretzel	420	11	69
Sweet Belgian Waffle	310	15	39
Breakfast Sandwiches:			
Bacon, Rstd Tom., Spinach & Feta	250	9	30
Roasted Tomato, Spinach & Feta	240	8	30
Breakfast Wraps: Spinach 'n Chse	240	7	30
Turkey Sausage 'n Cheese	320	15	30
PB Banana Toast	360	12	56
Steel-Cut Oatmeal: *Without Add-Ons*			
Plain	170	2.5	31

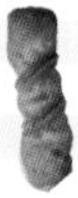

Energy Bowls: Per 16 fl.oz without Add-Ons	C	F	Cb
Acai Primo	510	10	101
Chunky Strawberry	580	16	94
Island Pitaya	480	8	102
Nutty Almond Butter	430	16	68
PB Wow Cacao	690	27	101
Peachy Green Godess	510	18	82
Vanilla Blue Sky	330	9	62

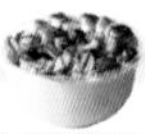
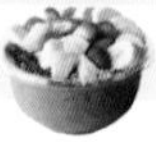

Jersey Mike's Subs® (Nov '20)

Cold Subs: Per Regular, on White, without Vinegar, Oil or Mayo Unless Indicated	C	F	Cb
#1 BLT, with Mayo	700	40	65
#2 Jersey Shore Favorite	570	16	68
#3 Ham & Provolone	570	15	67
#5 Super Sub	580	15	69
#6 Roast Beef & Provolone	630	16	67
#7 Turkey & Provolone	530	12	65
#8 Club Sub with Mayonnaise	850	44	67
#9 Club Supreme w/ Mayonnaise	880	44	66
#10 Albacore Tuna	780	42	67
#13 Original Italian	700	26	70
#14 Veggie	690	30	68
***Hot Subs:** Per Reg., on White Roll, w/ Standard Menu Components*			
#15 Meatball & Cheese	810	38	79
#17: Mike's Philly	720	29	68
#19 BBQ Beef	670	10	87
#20 Grilled Pastrami Reuben	730	30	72
#42 Chipotle Chicken Cheese Steak	940	53	70
#43 Chipotle Cheese Steak	1000	59	68
#55 Big Kahuna Chkn Cheese Steak	720	27	72
#56 Big Kahuna Cheese Steak	770	33	70
French Fries: 5 oz	310	19	34
6 oz	370	23	41
***Salad:** Without Dressing*			
Grilled Chicken	810	25	52
Tossed	190	2	41
***Breakfast Subs:** On White Bread, w/ Standard Menu Components, without Ketchup*			
#2: Mini Bacon, Egg & Cheese	490	25	41
#3: Mini Sausage, Egg & Cheese	890	63	41
#4: Ham, Egg & Cheese	510	22	43
#5: Steak, Egg & Cheese	540	22	41
***Kid's:** On White Bun, with Standard Menu Components, without Condiments*			
Ham Sub	230	5	33
Salami Sub	260	9	33
Turkey Sub	230	4.5	32
Desserts:			
Brownie, regular	500	28	63
Choc. Chip Cookie, mini	180	9	26
Tastykake: Butterscotch Krimpet	320	9	58
Chocolate Cupcake, regular	340	10	59
Cream Filled, regular	390	14	62

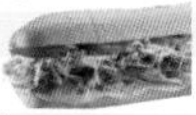
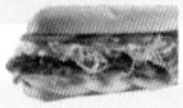
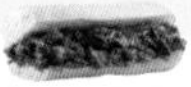
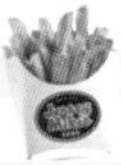
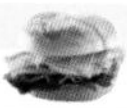
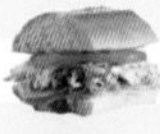
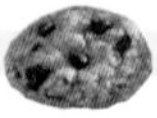

Updated Nutrition Data ~ www.CalorieKing.com
Persons with Diabetes ~ See Disclaimer (Page 22)

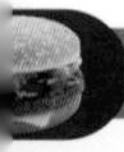

Jimmy John's® (Nov '20)

Item	C	F	Cb
***Original Subs:** (8") Figures Based on French Bread w/ Standard Menu Board Toppings*			
#1 Pepe	**650**	30	60
#2 Big John	**550**	22	57
#3 Totally Tuna	**550**	22	61
#4 Turkey Tom	**530**	19	58
#5 Vito	**630**	27	61
#6 Vegetarian	**730**	39	60
JJBLT	**590**	28	57
***Favorite Subs :** (8") Figures Based on 9 Grain Baguette w/ Standard Menu Set Toppings*			
#7 Smoked Ham Club	**1200**	75	75
#8 Billy Club	**960**	51	71
#9 Italian Night	**1080**	64	75
#10 Hunter's Club	**970**	52	68
#11 Country Club	**930**	48	72
#12 Beach Club	**1000**	58	72
#13 Gourmet Veggie Club	**990**	57	68
#14 Bootlegger	**830**	40	69
#15 Club Tuna	**910**	51	73
#16 Club Lulu	**830**	44	69
#17 Ultimate Porker	**840**	45	70
***Plain Slims:** Figures Based on French Bread without Toppings, Dressing or Mayo*			
Slim 1 Ham & Provolone Cheese	**580**	14	77
Slim 2 Roast Beef	**480**	6	74
Slim 3 Tuna Salad	**640**	23	78
Slim 4 Turkey Breast	**460**	3	75
Slim 5 Salami Capicola & Cheese	**670**	23	76
Slim 6 Double Provolone	**630**	21	75
Sides:			
Jimmy Chips: Average	**290**	17	33
Thinny	**260**	11	39
Cookies: Raisin Oatmeal, 3 oz	**370**	13	57
Triple Chocolate Chunk, 3 oz	**410**	19	56
Jumbo Kosher Dill Pickle, 6.9 oz	**20**	0	3

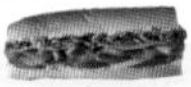
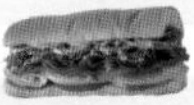
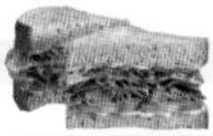
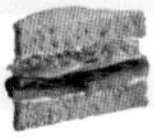
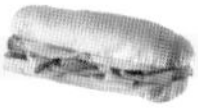
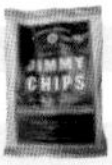

Johnny Rockets® (Nov '20)

Item	C	F	Cb
Starters:			
Chili Bowl	**620**	50	20
Fries: Plain	**330**	10	50
Bacon Cheese	**630**	30	60
Cheese	**540**	30	60
Chili Cheese	**820**	50	70
Onion Rings	**630**	30	80
Tots: Plain	**740**	50	70
Bacon Cheese	**1050**	70	80
Cheese	**960**	70	80
Chili Cheese	**1230**	90	90

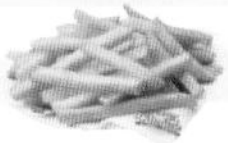
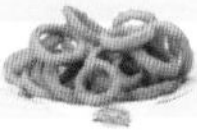

Johnny Rockets® cont... (Nov '20)

Item	C	F	Cb
***Burgers:** Per Regular Size Bun*			
Bacon Cheddar/Route 66:			
Beef Burger	**780**	50	40
Boca Veggie Burger	**680**	40	50
Grilled Chicken	**720**	40	40
Original: Beef Burger	**680**	40	40
Gardein	**640**	40	70
Rocket: Beef Burger	**690**	40	40
Boca Veggie Burger	**590**	30	50
Turkey	**810**	60	40
Smokehouse: Beef Burger	**800**	40	70
Boca Veggie Burger	**710**	30	80
Gardein Burger	**760**	40	90
Spicy Houston:			
Beef Burger	**640**	40	40
Grilled Chicken	**540**	20	40
Turkey	**730**	50	40
Chicken, Tenders, BBQ Sauce	**670**	20	90
Hot Dogs:			
Rocket Dog	**480**	30	40
Rocket Chili Dog	**670**	50	40
Philly Cheese Steak, Beef	**780**	40	60
Melts:			
BBQ Chicken	**940**	30	100
Tuna on Sourdough	**650**	40	50
***Sandwiches:** On sourdough, without Substitutions*			
BLT	**690**	50	50
Fried Chicken Club	**910**	50	70
Grilled Chicken Club	**800**	40	50
Grilled Cheddar Cheese	**600**	40	50
Sourdough Burger Melt	**680**	40	50
***Salads:** Without Dressing*			
Crispy Chicken Club	**420**	20	20
Grilled Chicken Club	**400**	20	10
Garden Salad	**150**	10	10
***Breakfast:** Standard, without Subsititutions*			
French Toast: 2 slices	**620**	10	100
3 slices	**800**	20	130
Pancakes: B'milk (2) w/ Sausage	**1020**	50	110
Buttermilk (2), with Bacon	**700**	20	110
Scramblers: Bacon Denver	**1130**	60	80
Biscuits, Sausage & Gravy	**2010**	130	120
Cheesy Bacon Lovers	**1170**	70	80
Philly Cheesesteak	**1270**	70	80
***Shakes:** Without Malt*			
Banana	**830**	40	90
Chocolate	**910**	40	110
Hershey's Chocolate	**920**	40	110
Oreo Cookies & Cream	**1020**	50	120
Peanut Butter Banana	**1050**	60	100

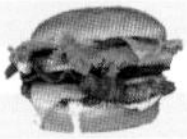
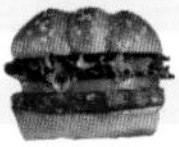
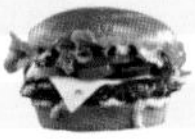
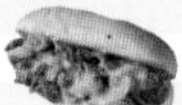
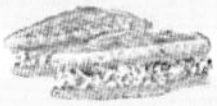
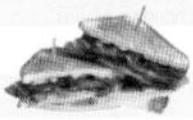
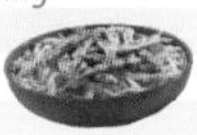
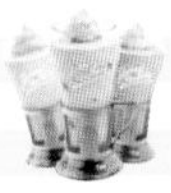

For Complete Menu & Data ~ see CalorieKing.com

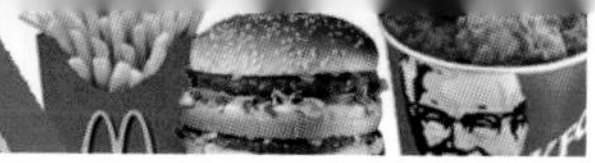

KFC® (Nov '20)

Chicken On The Bone: Per Piece	C	F	Cb
Original Recipe: Breast, 6 oz	390	21	11
Drumstick, 1.87 oz	130	8	4
Thigh, 3.7 oz	280	19	8
Whole Wing, 1.5 oz	130	8	3
Extra Crispy: Breast, 6.3 oz	530	35	18
Drumstick, 1.9 oz	170	12	5
Thigh, 3.5 oz	330	23	9
Whole Wing, 1.7 oz	170	13	5
Kentucky Grilled: Breast, 4.6 oz	210	7	0
Drumstick, 1.4 oz	80	4	0
Thigh, 2.5 oz	150	9	0
Whole Wing, 1 oz	70	3	0
Spicy Crispy: Breast, 5.2 oz	350	20	11
Drumstick, 1.6 oz	130	8	5
Thigh, 2.8 oz	270	20	10
Whole Wing, 1.2 oz	120	8	5
Chicken:			
Fried Wings: Buffalo, 1.2 oz	100	7	3
Honey BBQ, 1.35 oz	100	6	8
Nashville Hot, 1.2 oz	130	11	4
Unsauced, 1 oz	80	6	3
Nashville Hot:			
Extra Crispy: Breast, 7.4 oz	770	60	21
Drumstick, 2.3 oz	250	21	6
Thigh, 4.72 oz	500	40	11
Grilled:			
Breast, 4.86 oz	260	12	1
Thigh, 2.6 oz	180	12	0
Spicy Crispy:			
Breast, 6 oz	540	40	14
Thigh, 3.3 oz	390	32	12
Popcorn Nuggets: Kids	290	19	19
Large	620	39	39
Famous Bowls & Pot Pie:			
Chicken Pot Pie, 14 oz	720	41	60
Famous Bowl:			
Snack Size	270	14	27
Large	740	35	81
Salads: W/out Dressing or Croutons			
Caesar, Side	40	2	2
House Side Salad	15	0	3
Dressings & Add-Ins:			
Creamy Parmesan Caesar, 2 oz	260	26	4
Light Italian, 1 oz	15	0.5	2
Original Ranch Fat Free, 1.5 oz	35	0	8
Croutons, Parmesan Garlic, 1 pouch	60	3	8

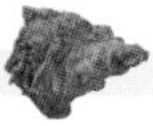
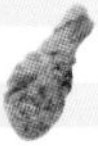
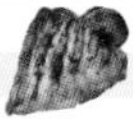
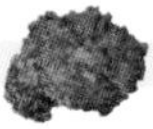
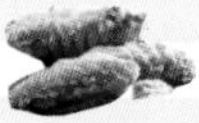
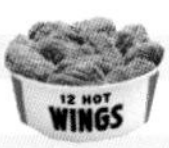

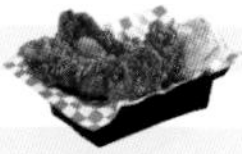
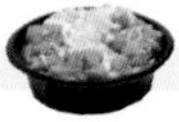
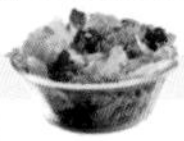

KFC® cont... (Nov '20)

Dipping Sauces & Condiments: Per 0.9 oz Container	C	F	Cb
Buttermilk Ranch Sauce	100	10	2
Colonel's Buttery Spread	35	4	0
Creamy Buffalo Sauce	70	7	2
Finger Linkin' Good; Honey Mstrd, av.	125	11	5
Honey Sauce; Ketchup	30	0	8
Lemon Juice, 0.14 oz	5	0	1
Strawberry Jam	35	0	9
Summertime BBQ Sce	40	0	9
Sweet & Tangy Sauce	45	0	12
Sandwiches:			
Chicken Littles: Regular	300	15	27
Buffalo; Honey BBQ, average	315	16	29
Nashville Hot	340	19	27
Colonel's Crispy Sandwich:			
Regular	470	24	39
Buffalo	500	27	39
Honey BBQ	510	25	48
Nashville Hot	540	32	40
Crispy Twister	630	34	53
Honey BBQ	350	3.5	55
Homestyle Sides: Per Single Portion			
BBQ Baked Beans, 4.25 oz	190	1	34
Coleslaw, 4.2 oz	170	12	14
Corn on the Cob, 2.5 oz	70	0.5	17
Mac. & Cheese, 4.8 oz	140	6	17
Mashed Potatoes, 4.2 oz	110	3.5	17
Mashed Potatoes with Gravy, 5 oz	130	4.5	20
Potato Wedges, 3.8 oz	270	13	34
Sweet Kernel Corn, 2.75 oz	70	0.5	16
Kids: Chicken Little, w/ Mac & Cheese, & 1% Choc Milk	700	30	85
Extra Crispy Tenders, with Potato Wedges & 1% Choc Milk	600	22	80
Desserts:			
Apple Turnover, 2.9 oz	230	10	32
Cafe Valley: Choc. Chip Cake, 1 slice	300	15	39
Mini Choc. Chip Cake (1)	300	12	49
Lemon Cake, 1 slice	220	10	30
Chocolate Chip Cookie (1)	120	6	18
Oreo Cookies & Creme Pie	270	13	35
Reese's Peanut Butter Pie, 2.6 oz	300	17	33

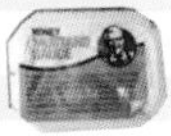
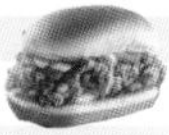
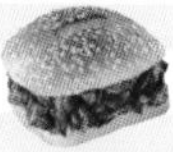
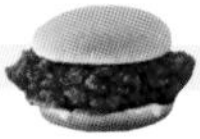
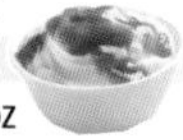
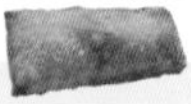
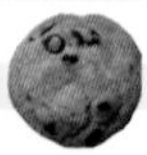

Updated Nutrition Data ~ www.CalorieKing.com
Persons with Diabetes ~ See Disclaimer (Page 22)

Krispy Kreme® (Nov '20)

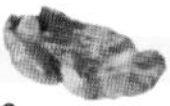
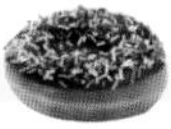
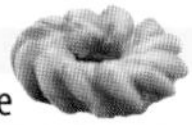
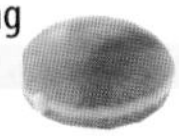
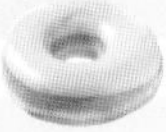
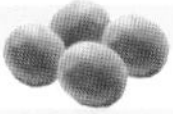
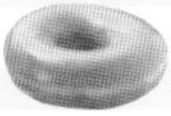
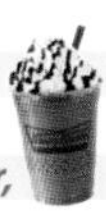
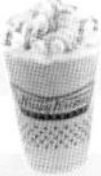
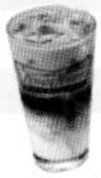

Doughnuts:	C	F	Cb
Apple Fritter	350	19	42
Chocolate Iced: Cake	340	19	40
Custard Filled	300	15	37
Glazed	240	11	33
with Sprinkles	250	11	36
Kreme Filling	350	19	41
Cinnamon Apple Filled	270	15	31
Cinnamon Bun	270	16	29
Cinnamon Sugar	190	11	21
Cruller: Glazed Cake	240	15	25
Chocolate Iced Glazed Cake	240	15	25
Double Dark Chocolate	370	20	46
Dulche De Leche	300	16	35
Glazed: Kreme Filling	340	19	40
Lemon Filled	290	15	37
Maple Iced	240	11	34
Sour Cream Cake	300	15	40
Strawberry Iced	190	11	22
Powdered Cake	310	19	32
Powdered Strawberry Filled	270	15	30
Powdered Lemon Kreme	290	17	32
Glazed Doughnut Holes:			
Blueberry Cake (4)	180	7	28
Original (5)	210	12	25
Original Glazed:			
Regular	190	11	22
Mini size (3)	250	13	30
Hot:			
Chocolate, w/ 2% Milk, 12 fl.oz	390	14	57
Mocha Latte, w/ Skim Milk, 12 fl.oz	260	4.5	42
Frozen Coffees: With Whipped Cream			
Caramel Latte, 12 fl.oz	350	11	58
Mocha, 12 fl.oz	330	11	52
Vanilla Latte, 12 fl.oz	330	10	54
Frozen Lemonade Chiller, 12 fl.oz	200	0	52
Iced: Per 12 fl.oz with Skim Milk & Whipped Cream,			
Caramel Latte	310	8	52
Caramel Mocha	250	10	33
Mocha	250	7	38
Skinny Iced Lattes:			
With Skimmed Milk:			
Caramel, 12 fl.oz	160	1.5	29
Vanilla, 12 fl.oz	70	0	12

For Complete Menu & Data ~ See CalorieKing.com

Krystal® (Nov '20)

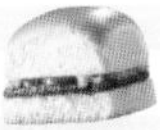
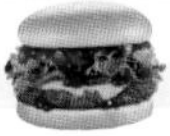
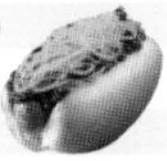
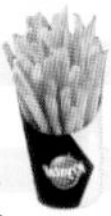
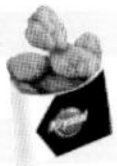
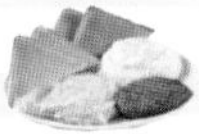
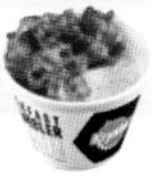
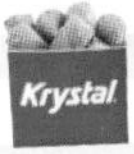
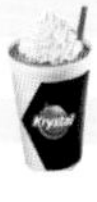

Krystals:	C	F	Cb
Original	130	6	15
with Cheese	150	8	15
Double	190	11	16
with Cheese	150	8	16
Bacon Cheese	190	10	16
Chik, regular	280	16	23
Pups: Chili Cheese Pup	300	20	16
Classic	170	10	14
Corn	290	21	18
Fries:			
French Fries: Small	140	9	14
Medium	240	15	24
Large	300	19	30
Loaded: Chili Cheese Fries	670	47	40
Junk Yard	800	59	42
Nuggets: 4 pieces	240	19	8
10 pieces	600	47	20
Sauce:			
Honey Mustard; Ranch, average	130	12	2
Swt & Sour/Baby Rays BBQ, av.	60	0	15
Wings, Spicy (12)	1170	90	36
Breakfast:			
3 Egg Plates:			
Eggs, Bacon & Biscuit	480	30	29
Eggs, Sausage & Biscuit	520	36	28
Biscuits: Bacon, Egg & Cheese	380	23	28
Chik	380	21	36
Sausage, Egg & Cheese	410	29	28
Scramblers:			
Original: with Bacon	300	19	17
with Sausage	340	24	16
Low-Carb Scramblers:			
with Bacon	300	23	3
with Sausage	360	34	2
Sides: Grits, bowl	210	5	36
Tots, regular	330	23	28
Dessert, Apple Turnover	290	18	31
Hand-Spun Shakes: Regular			
Chocolate	650	18	114
Oreo	650	22	101
Strawberry	560	17	92
Vanilla	510	17	80

For Complete Menu & Data ~ see CalorieKing.com

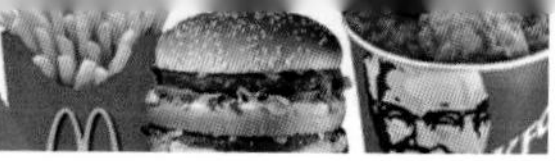

LaRosa's Pizzeria® (Nov '20)

Classic Pizzas:	C	F	Cb
Hand Tossed: *Per Slice, ⅛ of 12" Medium Pizza*			
Chicken Bacon Ranch	340	18	29
Double Pepperoni	290	13	30
Garlic Chicken	280	12	30
Hawaiian	290	11	33
Zesty BBQ Chicken	290	10	34
Traditional: *Per Slice, 1/12 of 14" Large Pizza*			
Chicken Bacon Ranch	290	18	18
Double Pepperoni	230	13	19
Hawaiian	240	12	21
Zesty BBQ Chicken	240	11	23
Deluxe Pizzas:			
Hand Tossed: *Per Slice, ⅛ of 14" Large Pizza*			
Buddy	500	25	47
Meat	570	30	46
Original	490	23	47
Veggie	360	11	49
Pan: *Per Slice, ⅛ of 14" Large Pizza*			
Buddy	510	26	47
Meat	580	32	46
Original	500	25	47
Veggie	370	12	49
Hoagies: With White Bun & Provolone Cheese			
Baked Meatball & Pasta Sauce	810	36	89
Fried Cod with Tartar Sauce	820	37	79
Steak w/ Tomato, Onion & Mayo	880	48	71
Pasta Entrees: Without Bread, Soup or Salad			
Lasagna, with Meat Sauce	1050	62	76
Ravioli: Cheese, with Pasta Sauce	750	29	89
Meat, with Pasta Sauce	730	26	89
Ziti: Chicken Alfredo	890	27	112
Sausage Pelucci w/ Spag. Sce	1040	42	136
Salad : Entree, w/out Dressing or Breadstick			
Antipasto,	400	28	13
Crispy Chicken	500	27	36
Grilled Chicken	280	11	11
JoJo BLT	160	11	9
Tossed Garden	160	9	11
Salad Dressings: Per 2 oz Cup			
Blue Cheese	280	30	2
Honey French	250	19	18
Italian	320	34	4
Soup: With 2 Packets Saltine Crackers			
Baked Onion	220	9	29
Minestrone	120	1.5	24

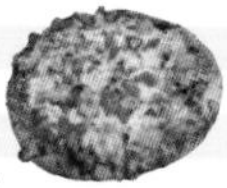
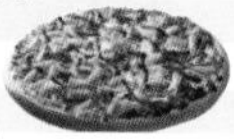
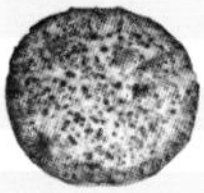
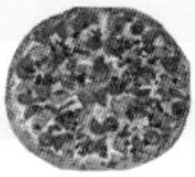
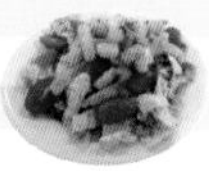

LaRosa's Pizzeria® cont... (Nov '20)

Appetizers:	C	F	Cb
Cheesy Flatbread, w/ Pizza Sauce	1480	88	117
Fried Mozz. Chse Stick w/ Pizza Sce	640	35	46
Garlic Fries, w/ Ranch Dressing	900	62	77
Onion Twists, w/ Diablo Sauce	1110	72	107
Rondo:			
Pepperoni, with Pizza Sauce	1380	79	116
Spinach, with Pizza Sauce	1260	66	115
Wings, with Sauce: BBQ (5)	400	23	19
Diablo (5)	470	31	17
Garlic-Romano (5)	580	47	10

La Salsa Fresh Mexican® (Nov '20)

Breakfast:			
Burritos: Chicken	660	30	56
Steak	700	36	55
Huevos Ranchero Platter:			
Chicken	500	14	59
Chorizo	610	27	61
Steak	550	20	58
Taco	200	10	14
Burritos: Without Chips			
Black Beans & Cheese:	720	37	62
with Carnitas	820	41	62
with Grilled Chicken	810	40	63
California Steak, w/ Black Beans	830	39	81
Grande, Black Beans,			
with Carnitas/Chicken/Steak, av.	760	31	79
Pinto Beans & Cheese: Plain	810	37	79
with Chicken	910	40	80
with Steak	970	49	80
Overstuffed Burrito:			
with Carnitas	860	35	56
with Grilled Chicken	860	32	59
with Steak	980	49	58
Platters:			
Enchiladas:			
Pinto Beans: Carnitas; Chicken, av.	985	53	59
Cheese	850	49	58
Steak	1070	63	59
Taquitos & Quesadillas:			
Pinto Beans: Carnitas; Chicken, av.	1600	76	134
Cheese	1470	72	129
Steak	1660	84	134
Three Pepper Fajita Flour Tortilla:			
Black Beans: Carnitas	700	29	55
Chicken	690	27	58
Steak	820	44	57
Tacos: Without Chips			
Baja Grilled Fish	260	12	23
Baja Shrimp	250	9	23
Guadalajara Carnitas	300	17	22

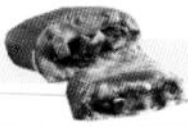
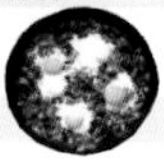
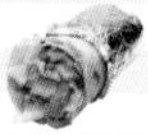
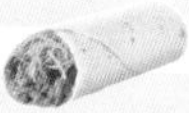
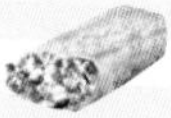
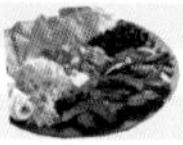
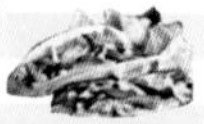

Updated Nutrition Data ~ www.CalorieKing.com
Persons with Diabetes ~ See Disclaimer (Page 22)

La Salsa Fresh Mex® cont... (Nov '20)

Favorites: Without Chips	C	F	Cb
Classic Quesadillas: Carnitas	980	58	59
Cheese	880	54	59
Chicken	980	57	60
Steak	1040	65	60
Fire Roasted Bowls:			
Black Beans: Carnitas	510	18	54
Chicken	500	16	55
Steak	570	25	55
Nachos:			
Black Beans: with Carnitas	1150	56	93
with Chicken	1150	54	95
with Steak	1210	63	94
Pinto Beans:			
with Carnitas	1190	56	101
with Chicken	1170	54	98
with Steak	1230	63	98
Stuffed Fajitas: Carnitas	930	49	59
Cheese	830	45	59
Chicken	930	48	60
Steak	990	57	60

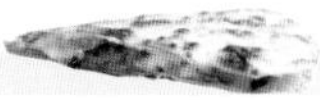
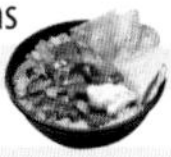
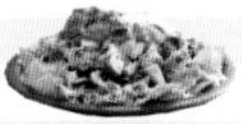
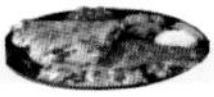

Little Caesars® (Nov '20)

14" Pizza: Per Slice, ⅛ Pizza	C	F	Cb
Classic: Beef	270	10	31
Cheese	245	10	31
Pepperoni	275	11	31
Sausage	270	11	31
Specialty Deep!Deep! Dish:			
3 Meat Treat	433	22	40
Hula Hawaiian, Ham/Bacon, av.	345	12	43
Ultimate Supreme	380	16	42
Veggie	340	12	41
Caesar Wings: Per 8 Wing			
BBQ	620	35	32
Buffalo	510	35	3
Garlic Parmesan	670	51	5
Oven Roasted	510	35	3
Caesar Dips: Per 1.5 oz Container			
Buffalo Ranch	230	23	4
Butter Garlic	370	42	0
Cheezy Jalapeno	210	21	3
Ranch	230	23	4
Bread: Crazy Bread, 1 stick	100	3	16
Italian Cheese Bread	135	5.5	15
Crazy Sauce, 1 cup	30	0	7

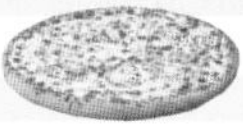
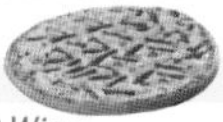
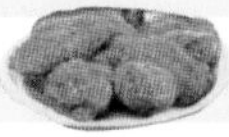
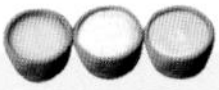
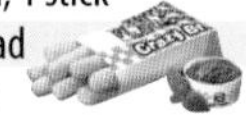

Long John Silver's® (Nov '20)

Chicken Tenders,	C	F	Cb
1 piece 2.1 oz	150	7	11
Sandwiches & Tacos:			
Baja: Fish Taco	410	21	40
Grilled: Salmon	210	9	23
Grilled Shrimp	210	10	21
Seasoned Grilled Salmon	180	4	21
Sweet Chili Salmon	190	5	22
Seafood: Without Sides			
Baked Cod, 1 piece, 6 oz	160	1	1
Battered: Alaskan Pollock, 1 piece, 3.2 oz	200	10	16
Cod, 1 piece, 3 oz	190	11	9
Shrimp, 3 pieces	100	7	5
Breaded Clam Strips	340	20	35
Lobster Stuffed Crab Cake (1), 2.2 oz	280	15	26
Popcorn Shrimp, 3 oz	210	9	24
Sauces & Condiments:			
Dipping Sauces: BBQ, 1 oz	40	0	10
Cocktail, 0.9 oz	20	0	4
Marinara, 1 oz	15	0	4
Sweet & Sour 1 oz	45	0	12
Other Sauces & Condiments:			
Honey Mustard, 0.4 oz packet	60	6	2
Ketchup, 1oz pouch	30	0	8
Louisiana Hot Sauce, 1 tsp	0	0	0
Malt Vinegar, 0.5 oz	0	0	0
Tartar Sauce, 0.5 oz packet	40	4	3
Sides: Baked Potato, 12 oz	295	0	67
Battered Onion Rings, 4 oz	480	35	39
Breaded Mozzarella Sticks (3)	370	23	24
Broccoli Cheese Bites, 5 pieces	310	24	18
Brocc. Chse Soup, 1 bowl, 7.4 oz	220	18	8
Clam Chowder, 1 bowl, 8 oz	230	16	16
Cole Slaw, 4 oz	170	11	18
Corn Kernels, 4 oz	160	8	9
Crumblies, 1 oz	170	12	13
Green Beans, 4 oz	25	0	4
Hushpuppies, 2 pcs	150	7	19
Jalapeno Peppers (1)	15	0	2
Macaroni & Cheese, 4 oz	150	6	19
Rice, 5 oz	180	1	37
Fries, 3.7 oz	350	17	44
Dessert: Choc. Chip Cookie (1)	190	11	22
Chocolate Cream Pie, 1 slice	280	17	28
Strawberry Swirl Cheesecake, 1 sl.	320	17	35

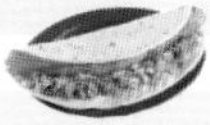
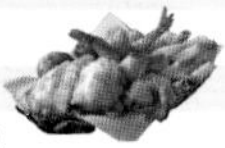
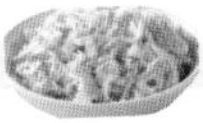
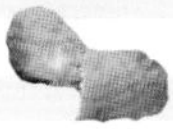

For Complete Menu & Data ~ see CalorieKing.com

Macaroni Grill® (Nov '20)

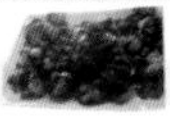
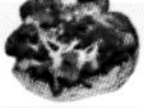
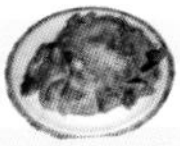
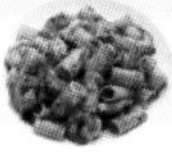
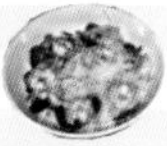
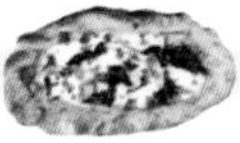

Antipasti: As Served	C	F	Cb
Baked Prosciutto & Mozzarella	**610**	36	35
Calamari Fritti	**760**	55	33
Crispy Brussels Sprouts	**370**	25	37
Crispy Fresh Mozzarella	**820**	79	17
Goat Cheese Peppadew Peppers	**350**	11	56
Mushroom Arancini	**610**	40	40
Spinach Artichoke Dip	**1100**	61	109
Stuffed Mushrooms	**510**	38	20
Meals: With Menu Set Sides			
Carne: Braised Lamb Shank	**1390**	101	29
Gr. Steak & Potatoes: Rosemary Butt.	**1250**	94	34
with Oreganata Sauce	**1220**	85	42
Grilled Pork Chop,			
with Wild Mushroom Risotto	**1420**	93	48
Porterhouse Steak	**1480**	115	16
Chicken: Caprese	**560**	22	40
Lunch Portion	**1050**	76	59
Marsala	**790**	32	61
Lunch Portion	**670**	26	74
Parmesan	**1610**	92	120
Lunch Portion	**960**	96	97
Scaloppine	**1240**	76	83
Pasta: Butternut Tortellaci	**980**	66	63
Eggplant Parmesan	**1340**	90	103
Fettuccine Alfredo	**1140**	56	114
Lasagna Bolognese	**1110**	67	69
Mushroom Ravioli	**930**	66	53
Penne Rustica	**1060**	52	82
Truffle Mac & Cheese	**1060**	89	24
Seafood: Grilled Salmon	**930**	45	82
Lobster Ravioli	**920**	74	36
Parmesan-Crusted Sole	**1180**	66	115
Pasta Di Mare	**1030**	43	101
Shrimp Portofino	**1200**	78	93
Shrimp Scampi	**1180**	88	56
Brick Oven Pizza: Per Whole Meal, as Served			
Cheese	**1170**	41	146
Farmhouse	**1350**	60	136
Margherita	**1140**	41	146
Pepperoni	**1280**	76	143
Kids: Chicken Strips with Fries	**1250**	73	108
Macaroni & Cheese	**540**	31	44
Pepperoni Pizza	**570**	19	70
Spaghetti, with Pomodoro Sauce	**290**	8	43

Macaroni Grill® cont... (Nov '20)

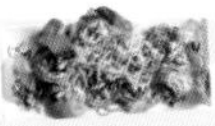
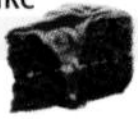

Salads: Includes Menu Set Dressing	C	F	Cb
Parmesan Crusted Chicken	**1080**	48	100
Entree: Bibb & Bleu with Shrimp	**590**	43	18
with Salmon	**830**	57	14
Side Salads:			
Bibb & Bleu	**270**	22	9
Florentine	**500**	29	44
Fresh Green	**190**	16	11
Dessert: Decadent Choc. Cake	**1090**	88	79
Lemon Passion	**740**	45	77
New York Style Cheesecake	**690**	41	70
Romano's Cannoli	**640**	32	69
Tiramisu	**600**	39	54

Manhattan Bagel® (Nov '20)

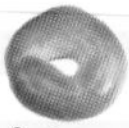

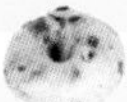
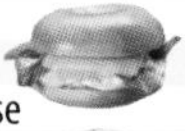
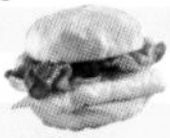
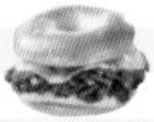
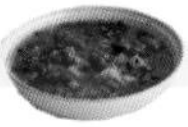

Bagels: Per Bagel	C	F	Cb
Plain; Salt	**310**	1	64
Honey Whole Wheat	**260**	3	49
Californian: Blueberry, 3.8 oz	**300**	1	65
Chocolate Chip, 3.8 oz	**290**	2.5	58
Cinnamon Raisin, 4 oz	**290**	1	63
Egg, 3.6 oz	**300**	5	54
Everything; Poppy, av., 3.7 oz	**275**	2.5	56
Pumpernickel, 3.6 oz	**240**	1.5	53
Gourmet: Asiago, 4.4 oz	**340**	4	64
Blueberry Glaze, 4.6 oz	**370**	1	79
Super Cinnamon, 4.6 oz	**360**	1	77
Cream Cheese: Plain; Lox, av.	**115**	12	3
Scallion, 1.3 oz	**140**	12	5
Breakfast:			
Bagel Sandwich: *On Plain Bagel*			
Egg & Cheese	**530**	19	64
Egg Bacon & Cheese	**580**	23	64
Egg, Pork Roll & Cheese	**770**	37	66
Wrap, Ranchero	**800**	45	61
Pizza Bagel, 9.1 oz	**520**	13	78
Sandwiches:			
Deli: Chicken Salad Croissant	**680**	44	60
Ham & Swiss on Sesame Bagel	**600**	21	69
Roast Beef on Cheddar Roll	**510**	12	68
Signature Lunch Sandwiches:			
Chelsea Chicken, on Asiago Roll	**750**	37	59
East Side Reuben, on Marble Rye	**580**	27	54
Steak: Bronx Bomber	**580**	27	54
Manhattan Chsesteak	**660**	30	59
SoHo Chkn Caesar Wrap	**580**	21	59
Thintastic: Avocado BLT	**440**	23	48
Turkey	**330**	7	42
Soup: Boston Clam Chowder	**360**	17	40
Chicken Noodle	**250**	7	30
Cream of Broccoli	**320**	18	27
Timberline Chili	**240**	8	27

Updated Nutrition Data ~ www.CalorieKing.com
Persons with Diabetes ~ See Disclaimer (Page 22)

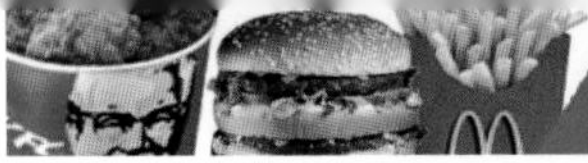

Marie Callender's® (Nov '20)

Appetizers: As Served	C	F	Cb
Crispy Chicken Tenders, 12.9 oz	870	47	72
Crispy Green Beans, 10.5 oz	810	52	75
Mozzarella Sticks, 8.6 oz	690	42	46
Onion Rings	1150	63	129
***Burgers and Sandwiches:** With Fries*			
Original Burger	1290	87	84
Albacore Tuna Melt	1430	92	99
Callender's Cheeseburger	1450	99	85
Frisco Chkn Breast On Parm Sourd.	1290	81	95
Meatloaf on Parm. Sourdough	1250	78	96
Roasted Turkey Croissant Club	1450	97	95
***Main Meals:** With Menu Set Sides*			
Comfort Classics:			
Braised & Slow Rstd Pot Roast	740	39	39
Chicken & Broccoli Fettuccine	1090	49	98
Crispy Fish & Shrimp Platter	1700	97	143
Home-Style Beef Stroganoff	850	30	99
Home-Style Meatloaf Dinner	610	35	34
Honey Ginger Glazed Salmon	570	30	29
Roasted Turkey Dinner	730	36	65
Shrimp & Chicken Carbonara	1140	50	93
Pies, Chicken Pot Pie, w/out sides	1140	79	70
Savory Skillets:			
Kickin' Chicken Bacon Broccoli	720	37	40
Spicy Beef & Chicken	790	54	27
Thai Shrimp	730	43	52
Salads:			
Cobb without Dressing	570	31	15
Combo Caesar with Caesar Dressing	240	18	9
Honey Mstd Chkn Crunch w/ dressing	950	61	54
Trad. Caesar w/ Caesar Dressing	490	35	28
Sides: Cornbread, w/ Honey Spread	340	21	33
French Fries, 4 oz	380	20	45
Loaded Mashed Potatoes, 6.2 oz	340	23	23
Macaroni & Cheese, 6.4 oz	230	9	26
Tater Tots, 5 oz	330	20	33
***Soups:** Per Bowl*			
Chicken Tortilla	230	10	26
Clam Chowder	270	13	22
Hearty Vegetable	90	3	13
Potato Cheese	590	40	49
***Breakfast:** With Menu Set Items*			
Classics: Croissant Sandwich	1100	70	76
Eggs Bened., Calif.	830	53	66
Triple Egg Dare Ya	1380	71	132

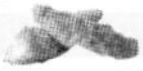

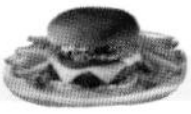

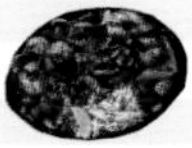

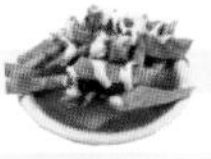

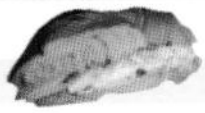

Marie Callender's® cont... (Nov '20)

***Breakfast (Cont.):** W/ Set Menu Sides*	C	F	Cb
Griddle Greats: Belgian Waffles	600	19	99
Banana Cream Pie Pancakes	800	28	118
Buttermilk Pancakes (3)	670	28	92
Old Fashioned French Toast	830	31	123
Omelets, w/out Tater Tots: BTA	1210	66	103
Oh My	1340	74	98
Veggie	570	37	23
Quiche: Bacon, 1 sl.	990	79	45
Ham, 1 slice	1030	83	40
Vegetable, 1 slice	990	80	42
***Desserts:** Per Slice Unless Indicated*			
Pies: Cream Cheese	620	38	63
Banana Cream, with Meringue	510	24	66
Chocolate Cream, with Meringue	570	25	77
Kahlula Cream Cheese	670	36	76
Tradtnl NY Style Cheesecake, slice	740	52	58

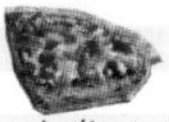

Max & Erma's® (Nov '20)

Shareables: As Served	C	F	Cb
Baja Fish Taco: Crispy	1070	35	138
Grilled	680	20	84
Chicken Fajita Quesadilla	1250	78	80
Potato Skins	1970	95	231
Spinach Dip	710	46	57
Wings with Blue Cheese Dressing:			
Cherry Cola BBQ	1990	120	95
Sweet Chili	1830	120	53
***Burgers & Sanwiches:** Without Fries*			
BBQ Pulled Pork Sandwich	760	33	71
Big Ol' Buffalo Chicken Sandwich	1370	71	144
Bodalicious Bacon Burger	1230	83	59
Cola BBQ Bacon Burger	1510	99	94
Garbage Burger, 6 oz	1680	126	61
Reuben Grill Sandwich	1060	58	84
Sauteed Mushrm & Swiss Burger	1200	85	53
Smokehouse Chicken Sandwich	1010	56	76
Tortilla Burger	1270	92	52
Turkey Avocado Swiss Burger	830	55	35
***Salads:** Entrée Size, w/ Dressing, without Breadstick*			
3rd Street	1160	100	41
Grilled Chicken Santa Fe	1090	83	46
Village	410	39	13
Sides: Baked Potato	220	0	51
Creamy Coleslaw	160	12	14
Fresh Fruit Salad	100	0	25
Mashed Potatoes	260	11	36
Seasoned Fries	360	17	49
Steamed Broccoli	30	0	6
Tater Tot	320	19	33
Dessert: Banana Cream Pie	790	37	107
Chocolate Cake a la Mode	1600	82	206

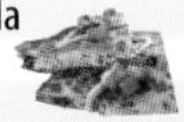

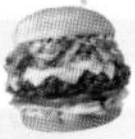

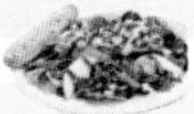

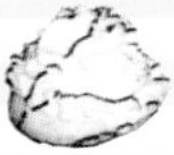

For Complete Menu & Data ~ See CalorieKing.com

McAlister's Deli® (Nov '20)

Sandwiches: Standard Components	C	F	Cb
Black Angus Club	**850**	42	74
Four Cheese Melt	**670**	31	62
French Dip	**530**	15	43
Grilled Chicken Club	**830**	35	78
Harvest Chicken Salad	**680**	44	53
McAlister's Club	**820**	37	78
New Yorker	**750**	25	64
Reuben	**900**	41	76
The Rachel	**800**	31	77
Giant Spuds: Bl. Angus Roast Beef	**1020**	31	134
Chipotle Chicken & Bacon	**1200**	46	139
Spud Max	**1070**	40	135
Sides: Mac & Cheese	**220**	12	20
Mashed Potatoes	**150**	6	22
Potato Salad	**250**	17	22
Steamed Broccoli	**80**	6	6
Tomato & Cucumber Salad	**70**	4	6

Mellow Mushroom® (Nov '20)

Burger,	C	F	Cb
Ritz Burger	**1140**	75	60
Calzones: Chicken & Cheese	**1350**	43	158
Steak & Cheese	**1410**	50	158
Hoagies, Whole: Chicken & Chse	**1090**	49	95
Italian	**1240**	73	88
Meatball	**820**	29	93
Mushroom Club	**1450**	77	101
Steak & Cheese	**1170**	61	96
Tofu	**970**	49	97
Munchies:			
Garlic Cheese Bread	**830**	42	83
Magic Mushroom Soup	**350**	24	15
Meatball Trio	**360**	24	11
Rstd Red Potatoes	**150**	3	27
Spinach & Artichoke Dip	**760**	44	67
Tomato Bisque	**290**	22	18
Wings: BBQ (10)	**700**	35	41
Sweet Thai Chili (10)	**780**	33	60
Pizzas: With Baked Crust, Per Medium Slice			
Buffalo Chicken	**520**	31	46
Funky Q Chicken	**450**	20	51
Kosmic Karma	**420**	22	47
Salads: Per Regular Size			
Caesar, with Caesar Dressing	**810**	71	30
Greek, without Dressing	**300**	17	20
Dressing, Balsamic Vinaigrette, 1 oz	**90**	8	5
Desserts: Choc Chunk Cookie Sundae, with Triple Choc. Chunk Cookie	**990**	53	120
Half Baked Brownie Supreme	**800**	48	83
Oatmeal Raisin Cookie Sundae	**870**	41	112
PB Cookie Sundae	**970**	56	102

McDonald's® (Nov '20)

Beef Burgers:	C	F	Cb
Big Mac	**550**	30	45
Cheeseburger: Regular	**300**	13	32
Double	**440**	23	34
Hamburger	**250**	9	31
McDouble	**390**	18	33
Quarter Pounder: with Cheese	**510**	25	42
with Cheese Deluxe	**620**	36	44
with Cheese & Bacon	**620**	33	44
Double, with Cheese	**720**	40	43
Burger Meal Combos: Includes Medium Fries + Coke			
Big Mac Meal	**1090**	45	147
Cheeseburger Meal	**840**	28	134
Quarter Pounder w/ Cheese	**1050**	40	144
Chicken Sandwiches:			
Aritsan Grilled Chicken	**430**	15	40
Buttermilk Crispy Chicken	**600**	29	58
McChicken	**400**	21	39
Filet-O-Fish, regular bun	**380**	18	38
Chicken:			
McNuggets: 4 pieces	**170**	10	10
6 pieces	**250**	15	15
10 pieces	**420**	25	25
Sauces: Per Packet			
Creamy Ranch	**110**	12	1
Honey Mustard	**50**	3	6
Spicy Buffalo	**30**	3	1
Sweet 'N Sour; Tangy BBQ	**50**	0	12
Tangy BBQ	**40**	0	11
French Fries: Kids, 1.3 oz	**110**	5	15
Small, 2.6 oz	**220**	10	29
Medium, 3.9 oz	**320**	15	43
Large, 5.9 oz	**490**	23	66
Ketchup, packet	**10**	0	2
Breakfast:			
Bacon, Egg & Cheese Bagel	**550**	25	54
Big Breakfast:			
with Reg. Biscuit	**750**	49	53
with Hotcakes	**1340**	64	155
Biscuits: *Regular*			
Bacon, Egg & Cheese	**460**	5	39
Sausage	**460**	30	36
Sausage with Egg	**530**	34	38
Burrito, Sausage	**300**	16	26
Fruit 'N Yogurt Parfait	**210**	3	40

Updated Nutrition Data ~ www.CalorieKing.com
Persons with Diabetes ~ See Disclaimer (Page 22)

McDonald's® cont... (Nov '20)

Breakfast (Cont):	C	F	Cb
Fruit & Maple Oatmeal:			
with brown sugar	**310**	4	62
Hash Browns, (1), 2 oz	**150**	9	16
Hotcakes: Plain (3)	**330**	8	56
with Syrup and Whipped Butter	**590**	15	102
McGriddle:			
Bacon, Egg & Cheese	**420**	18	45
Sausage	**430**	24	42
Sausage, Egg & Cheese	**550**	32	45
McMuffin: Egg	**300**	12	30
Sausage	**400**	25	29
Sausage with Egg	**480**	30	30
Happy Meals: *With Kid's fries, 1% Fat Milk Jug & Apple Slices*			
w/ Chicken McNuggets:			
4 pieces	**395**	18	41
6 pieces	**475**	23	46
w/ Hamburger	**475**	17	62
Salads: *Without Dressing*			
Bacon Ranch: Grilled Chicken	**300**	13	8
Buttermilk Crispy Chicken	**470**	27	26
Southwest: Grilled Chicken	**330**	11	26
Buttermilk Crispy Chicken	**500**	25	44
Side Salad	**15**	0	3
Snacks: Apple Slices	**15**	0	4
Donut Sticks, 12 pieces	**730**	31	101
Yoplait Go-Gurt, Strawberry, tube	**45**	0.5	7
Desserts: Baked Apple Pie	**240**	11	35
Chocolate Chip Cookie	**170**	8	22
Kiddie Cone	**45**	1	8
Vanilla Cone	**200**	5	32
McFlurry: with M&M's	**640**	22	96
with Oreo Cookies	**510**	17	80
Sundaes:			
Hot Caramel, 6.4 oz	**340**	8	60
Hot Fudge, 6.3 oz	**330**	10	52
Strawberry, 6.3 oz	**270**	6	49
Iced Tea, all sizes	**0**	0	0
Sweet Tea, Small	**90**	0	21
Medium	**110**	0	28
Large	**160**	0	38
Juices:			
Minute Maid Orange:			
Small	**150**	0	36
Medium	**200**	0	45
Honest Kids Appley	**35**	0	8
Milk Jug: 1% Low-Fat, 8 fl.oz	**100**	2.5	12
Low Fat, red. sug. Choc. Mlk, 8 fl.oz	**130**	2.5	18

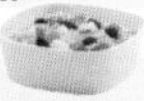
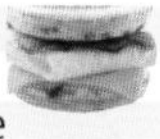
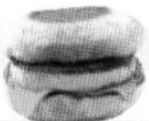
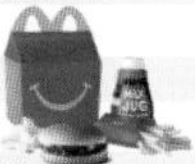
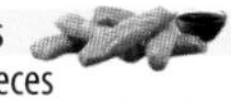
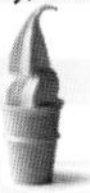
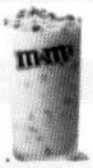
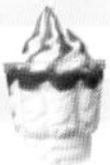
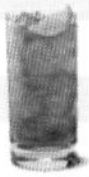
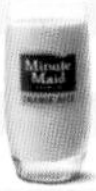

McDonald's® cont... (Nov '20)

Shakes:	C	F	Cb
Chocolate:			
Small, 12 fl.oz	**530**	15	87
Medium, 16 fl.oz	**630**	17	104
Large, 22 fl.oz cup	**840**	22	142
Strawb./Vanilla, avg:			
Small, 12 fl.oz	**500**	15	80
Medium 16 fl.oz	**590**	18	95
Large, 22 fl.oz	**800**	23	130
Slushies: *All Flavors*			
Small	**190**	0	51
Medium	**250**	0	68
Large	**350**	0	93
Soda: *With Ice, approximately 30%*			
Coca-Cola:			
Extra Small, 12 fl.oz cup	**110**	0	28
Small, 16 fl.oz cup	**150**	0	39
Medium, 21 fl.oz cup	**220**	0	59
Large, 30 fl.oz cup	**290**	0	80
Dr Pepper:			
Extra Small, 12 fl.oz cup	**100**	0	27
Small, 16 fl.oz cup	**140**	0	38
Medium, 21 fl.oz cup	**200**	0	54
Large, 30 fl.oz cup	**280**	0	75
Sprite: Extra Small, 12 fl.oz cup	**90**	0	27
Small, 16 fl.oz cup	**120**	0	36
Medium, 21 fl.oz	**170**	0	51
Large, 30 fl.oz	**230**	0	69
Sprite, Tropic Berry, 21 fl.oz	**190**	0	51
McCafe:			
Frappes: *With Whipped Cream & Toppings*			
Caramel; Mocha, average:			
Small	**420**	17	60
Medium	**510**	21	72
Hot Chocolate: *With Whipped Cream & Toppings*			
Whole Milk: Small	**370**	14	52
Medium	**450**	17	63
Hot Mocha: *With Whipped Cream & Toppings*			
Whole Milk: Small	**300**	10	46
Medium	**380**	12	57
Iced Coffee:			
Regular: Small, 16 fl.oz	**140**	5	24
Medium, 22 fl.oz	**180**	7	30
Large, 30 fl.oz	**260**	9	45
Caramel: Small, 16 fl.oz	**140**	5	23
Medium, 22 fl.oz	**190**	7	31
Iced Mocha: *With Whipped Cream & Toppings*			
Small	**280**	11	39
Medium	**330**	12	48
Smoothies: *Av. All Flavors*			
Small, 16 fl oz cup	**190**	1	44
Medium, 16 fl oz cup	**240**	1	55

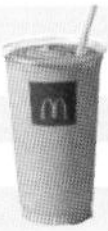
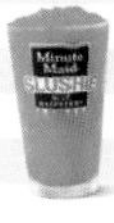
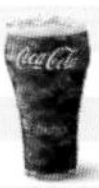
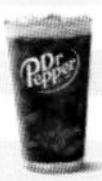
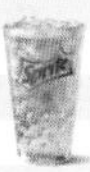
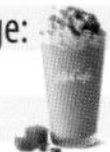
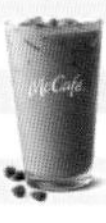
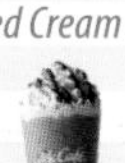
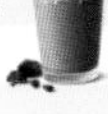

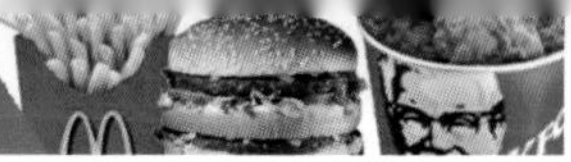

Mimi's Cafe® (Nov '20)

Bakery:	C	F	Cb
Croissants: Just Baked All Butter	360	20	38
Almond	370	20	40
Muffins: Blueberry Crumble	590	30	74
Buttermilk Spice	575	21	85
Carrot Raisin Nut	520	27	64
Chocolate Chip	865	44	105
Breakfast: Without Potatoes			
Eggs Benedicts: Original	645	39	34
Corned Beef Hash	730	44	46
Smoked Salmon	605	39	33
French Toast Items: *Without Side Options*			
Brioche	595	23	74
Cinnamon Roll	715	29	95
Griddlecakes: *With Eggs, Any Style*			
Berry	1030	38	135
Buttermilk	1025	44	120
3 Egg Omelets: *With Roasted Potatoes*			
Bacon Avocado	920	65	30
Hickory-Smoked Ham & Cheese	675	45	27
Mushroom Bacon & Brie	775	56	28
Smoked Salmon	555	35	24
Waffle: *With Pork Sausage*			
Malted	785	55	46
Malted Berry	790	49	61
Lunch & Dinner: Without Side Choices			
Burgers: Brioche Cheeseburger	775	41	56
Hickory Bacon Cheddar	945	50	68
Mushroom & Brie	890	51	51
The French Quarter	1285	90	48
Sandwiches:			
French Dip	585	14	70
Grilled Chicken Pesto Baguette	920	47	56
Parisian Ham Baguette	520	8	73
Turkey Hummus	560	25	54
West Coast Reuben	1335	72	99
Entrees:			
Beer Battered Fish & Fries	1185	78	79
Coastal Shrimp Pasta	1035	53	99
French Pot Roast	515	32	22
Mimi's Meatloaf	445	25	15
Slow Roasted Turkey	700	29	69
Sides: Broccoli	115	9	5
Coleslaw	250	23	7
French Fries	125	3	22
Garlic Spinach	70	4	4
Mashed Potatoes	130	4	21
Potatoes au Gratin	490	32	32
Roasted Potatoes	150	5	23

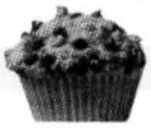
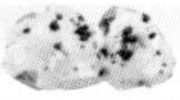
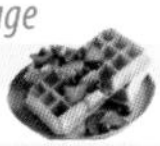
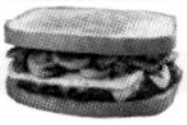
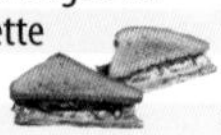
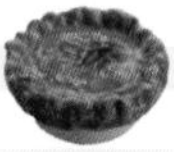
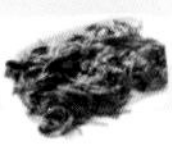

Mr. Goodcents® (Nov '20)

Cold Subs:	C	F	Cb
Per 8" Wheat Bread Sub with Standard Toppings			
Bologna	670	41	60
Centsable	600	31	62
Garden Veggie	510	24	66
Goodcents Original	670	38	61
Oven Roasted Chicken Breast	490	18	60
Penny Club	510	19	61
Pepperoni	840	56	58
Tuna Salad	620	32	64
Toasted Sub: Per 8" Wheat Bread Sub with Standard Toppings			
Chicken Bacon Ranch	730	33	55
Meatball	720	29	69
Pasta: Without Garlic Bread			
with Meatballs	910	33	119
Chicken Alfredo	990	44	103
Chicken Parmesan	840	25	108
Garlic Bread, 1 piece, 2 4 oz	290	12	44
Soup: Per 16 oz Bowl			
Broccoli Cheese	360	28	16
Chicken Homestyle Noodle	140	4	20
Saltine Crackers for soup bowls	110	2	17

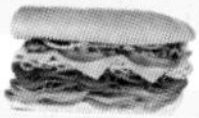
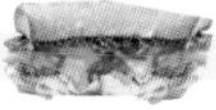
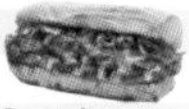
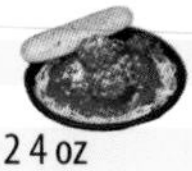

Mr. Hero® (Nov '20)

7" Subs & Burgers:	C	F	Cb
Burgers: Cheeseburger	720	49	44
Romanburger	805	56	46
Romanburger BTE	1000	73	48
Chicken Subs:			
Chicken Bacon Ranch	590	29	43
Chicken Philly	510	22	45
Deli Subs: *Per 7" Sub with Menu Board Toppings*			
Italiano	550	26	54
Original Italian	520	27	50
Tuna 'N Cheese	670	53	45
Turkey	330	2.5	49
Steak Subs: Hatta Potatta	720	45	53
Sicilian Parm	710	46	40
Sir Racha Bourbon	635	35	48
Zesty Bacon & Swiss	670	41	39
Sides: Per Regular Size			
Chicken Nuggets, 5 pce	275	19	12
Coleslaw, 3 oz	130	9	11
Mozzarella Sticks	565	35	43
Onion Petals	545	36	52
Potato Waffers	360	27	29
Kids: Cheeseburger Meal	510	32	43
Nugget Meal	470	33	32
Desserts: Brownie	500	28	63
Funnel Cake Fries, Regular, with sauce	285	5.5	57

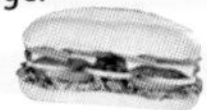
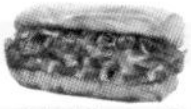
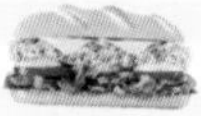
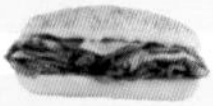
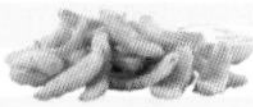
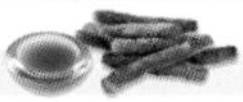

Mrs Fields Cookies® (Nov '20)

Brownies: Per 2.15 oz Brownie	C	F	Cb
Butterscotch Blondie	**260**	10	38
Double Fudge; Pecan Fudge, av.	**265**	14	33
Special Walnut Fudge & Blondie	**260**	13	35
Toffee/Walnut Fudge, average	**265**	14	33
Brownie Bites:			
Butterscotch Blondie (3)	**200**	8	29
Double/Toffee Fudge (3)	**200**	10	27
Coffee Cake,			
Chocolate Chip, small, 2.35 oz	**240**	11	30
Bite Size Nibblers Cookies:			
Cinnamon Sugar (3)	**180**	8	25
Peanut Butter (3)	**170**	9	19
Semi-Sweet Chocolate (3)	**170**	8	23
Triple Chocolate (3)	**160**	8	22
White Chunk Macadamia (3)	**180**	9	22
Cookies: Butter	**200**	8	28
Cut Out	**280**	11	44
Debra's Special	**200**	9	27
Oatmeal, Raisins & Walnuts	**200**	9	27
Peanut Butter	**200**	12	24
Semi-Sweet: Chocolate	**210**	10	29
with Walnuts	**220**	11	28
Triple Chocolate	**210**	10	28
White Chunk Macadamia	**230**	12	28
Muffins: Blueberry	**190**	9	24
Chocolate Chip	**200**	10	26

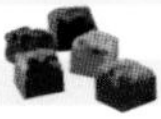
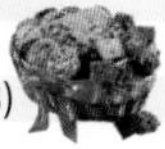
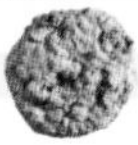
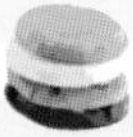

For Complete Nutritional Data ~ see CalorieKing.com

My Favorite Muffin® (Nov '20)

Muffins: Per Large Muffin	C	F	Cb
Large: Blueberry	**590**	28	78
Boston Cream Pie	**740**	33	105
Chocolate Chip	**790**	39	100
Carrot Cake	**850**	42	112
Deep Dish Apple Pie	**560**	22	85
Lemon Poppy Seed	**670**	32	90
Pumpkin Spice	**600**	26	86
Strawberry Cheesecake	**580**	31	67

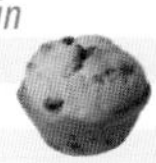
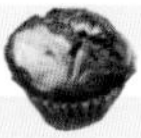

Nathan's Famous® (Nov '20)

Burgers:	C	F	Cb
Super Cheeseburger, 5 oz	**850**	49	49
Cheesesteak, Original Philly, 10.5 oz	**600**	27	49
Chicken:			
Sandwiches: Grilled Chicken, 8.2 oz	**430**	17	42
Krispy Chicken, 8.5 oz	**600**	29	60
Tenders, Krispy,3 pieces, 6.3 oz	**520**	31	32
Wings, Original Buffalo, 5 pcs	**700**	62	3

Nathan's Famous® cont... (Nov '20)

Hot Dogs: With Natural Casings	C	F	Cb
Original, 3.5 oz	**290**	18	24
Chili, 5.5 oz	**410**	27	30
Chili Cheese, 6.5 oz	**450**	29	33
Hot Dog Nuggets, 6 pieces, 3.5 oz	**350**	27	20
Corn Dog, on a stick, 3.2 oz	**360**	19	39
Fries: Per Regular Size			
Bacon Cheese	**720**	51	49
Cheese	**600**	42	48
Chili	**660**	48	49
Chili Cheese	**720**	52	53
French Fries	**540**	39	43
Onion Rings, regular	**460**	31	39
Salads: Grilled Chicken, 19 oz	**300**	7	35
Krispy Chicken, 19 oz	**500**	27	33

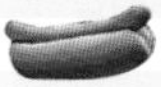

New York Fries® ~ *See CalorieKing.com*

Ninety Nine® (Nov '20)

Standout Starters: As Served	C	F	Cb
Boneless Wings & Skins Sampler	**1850**	123	87
Mozzarella Moons	**870**	52	63
Outrageous Pot. Skins	**1470**	101	84
Burgers: Without Sides			
Bacon & Cheese	**870**	43	58
Cheeseburger	**750**	34	58
Plain Burger	**690**	28	59
Vermont Cheddar	**970**	54	61
Sandwiches:: Without Sides			
Apple BBQ Chicken Sandwich	**690**	28	58
Open Face Pub Steak Sandwich	**700**	39	36
Entrees:			
Braised Short Rib Taco with Rice	**1100**	55	113
Cntry Fried Chkn, Mashed Pot & Bisc.	**1240**	55	150
Garlic Parm. Chicken Mac & Cheese	**1200**	67	185
Grilled Angus Sirloin w/ Mashed Pot.	**1330**	87	92
New Eng. Fried Shrimp w/ Fries & Slaw	**1110**	67	94
Ranch Crusted Chicken w/out sides	**610**	42	27
S'west Fajita Bowl with Shrimp	**750**	35	85
Sundried Tomato Chkn Kabobs w/ Rice	**820**	32	66
Sides: Baked Potato, plain	**250**	3	51
with butter	**350**	15	52
Broccoli Florets	**50**	0.5	9
Coleslaw	**150**	12	10
Corn	**140**	5	26
French Fries	**1040**	64	107
Honey Butter Biscuit	**250**	12	33
House Salad without dressing	**110**	3	18
Russet Mashed Potatoes	**260**	11	36
Dessert, Midnight Fudge Cake	**780**	40	96

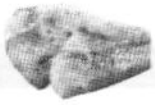
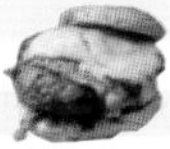
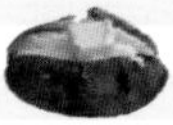

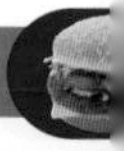

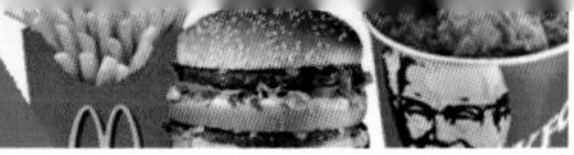

Noodles & Company® (Nov '20)

Asian Noodles: Per Reguar Size	C	F	Cb
Grilled Orange Chicken Lo Mein	840	28	106
Pad Thai	1040	42	143
Spicy Korean Beef Noodles	880	34	112
Classic Noodles: *Regular Size*			
Alfredo MontAmore Parm Chkn	1410	84	110
Buttered Noodles	760	35	98
Penne Rosa, w/ Parmesan/Feta	720	24	103
Pesto Cavatappi, w/ Feta	730	31	93
Spaghetti & Meatballs	980	48	102
Steak Stroganoff	1200	67	116
Macs: *Per Regular Size*			
BBQ Pork Mac	1210	47	129
Buffalo Chicken Mac	1100	39	128
Wisconsin Mac & Cheese	980	38	119
Zucchini Truffle Mac	510	33	31
Zoodles & Caulifloodles: *Per Regular*			
Cauliflower Rigatoni Fresca w/ Shrimp	880	39	102
Zucchini Pesto with Grilled Chicken	480	29	18
Zucchini Shrimp Scampi	430	25	26
Salads: *Per Regular Size*			
Grilled Chicken Caesar	420	27	18
Chicken Veracru	650	47	30
The Med, with Chicken	390	16	33
Soups: *Per Regular Size*			
Thai Chicken	370	22	31
Tomato Basil Bisque	430	28	37
Dessert: Chocolate Chunk Cookie	450	21	64
Rice Crispy	540	19	87
Snoodledoodle Cookie	450	20	64

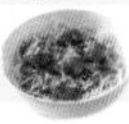
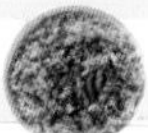
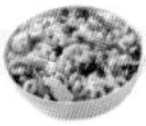
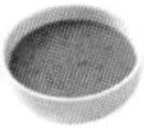
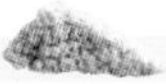

O'Charley's® (Nov '20)

Appetizers: As Served	C	F	Cb
Chicken Tenders, Chipotle	1160	40	107
Nashville Deviled Eggs	720	61	24
Spicy Jack Cheese Wedges (7)	720	48	44
Top Shelf Combo Platter	1880	132	74
Burgers: *Without Sides*			
Better Cheddar Bacon	1000	68	49
Classic Cheeseburger	930	61	47
Chicken & Pasta: *Without Sides*			
Chicken Tenders & Fries	1410	85	74
Chicken Tender Dinner: Buffalo	1070	64	31
Chipotle	1040	40	77
Nashville Hot	1260	87	44
Garlic Shrimp Pasta	950	43	104
New Orleans Cajun Chicken Pasta	1170	61	99
Peach Chutney Chicken	470	8	69

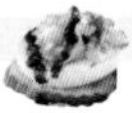
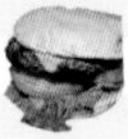
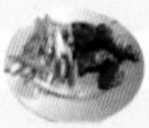

O'Charley's® cont... (Nov '20)

Classic Combos: Without Sides	C	F	Cb
BBQ Ribs & Tenders	950	37	84
Steak & Chicken Tenders, 6 oz	1030	67	26
Steak & Gr. Atlantic Salmon, 6 oz	750	33	5
Steak & Half Rack Baby Back Ribs	890	49	48
Ribs & Steak: *Without Sides*			
Baby Back Ribs: Regular	1220	62	95
Carolina Gold	1220	62	96
Nashville Hot	1540	110	63
BBQ Ribs Platter	4960	249	381
Slow Roasted Prime Rib:			
8oz	830	70	3
12 oz	1140	95	3
16 oz	1460	120	4
Steak: Bacon & Bourbon Glazed Filet	640	42	28
Filet Mignon, w/ Garlic Butter	580	47	1
Grilled Top Sirloin, 6 oz	270	18	0
Louisiana Sirloin	600	43	3
Ribeye Steak, 10 oz	720	56	1
Sandwiches: *Without Sides Unless Indicated*			
Carolina BBQ Chicken	650	22	74
Classic French Dip	1020	44	79
Club Sandwich	950	85	91
Nashville Hot Chicken, with Fries	2000	101	119
Seafoodl Favorites: *Without Sides Unless Indicated*			
Grilled Blackened Atl. Salmon, 9 oz	500	31	3
Grilled Salmon Bowl	990	70	44
Hand Battered Fish & Chips	1420	92	85
Hand Breaded Catfish, w/ Fries & Slaw	1720	124	103
Sides: Baked Potato (1)	200	1	50
Bacon Smashed Potatoe	350	16	44
Broccoli, 5 oz	110	8	6
Coleslaw	200	15	12
French Fries, 6 oz	400	24	40
Loaded Baked Potato, 1 portion	490	27	53
Mac & Cheese	450	22	47
Seasoned Rice Pilaf	160	4	27
Sweet Potato Fries, 1 portion	280	19	27
Salads: *Per Full Salad, with Dressing*			
California Chicken	1020	67	71
Classic Cobb	1140	92	36
Southern Fried Chicken	1550	110	48
Southern Pecan Chicken Tender	1550	106	95
Signature Soup: *Per Bowl*			
Chicken Harvest	210	13	20
Chicken Tortilla	190	7	20
Desserts: *Per slice*			
Country Apple Pie	630	35	77
Double-Crust Cherry Pie	600	35	69
French Silk Pie	580	43	49
Goo Goo Crunch Pie	1450	93	155
Ooey Gooey Caramel Pie	640	39	76
Southern Pecan Pie	730	45	78

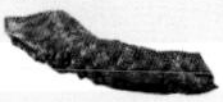
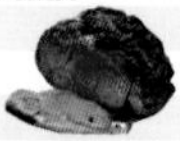
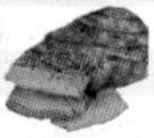
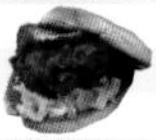
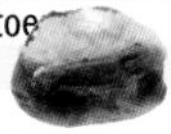
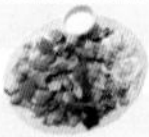
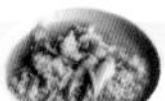

Updated Nutrition Data ~ www.CalorieKing.com
Persons with Diabetes ~ See Disclaimer (Page 22)

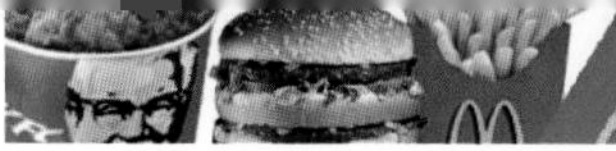

Old Spaghetti Factory® (Nov '20)

Appetizers: As Served	C	F	Cb
Spinach & Artichoke Dip	640	46	44
Sicilian Garlic Cheese Bread	1220	78	97
with Bacon	1450	95	97
Entrées, Lunch/Dinner:			
Founder's Favorites:			
Baked Lasagna, 17.6 oz	820	45	61
Garlic Mizithra, 17 oz	1360	85	102
Tenderloin w/ Mizithra & Brocc.	1260	87	59
Manager Favorites:			
Marinara: Clam, 15 oz	690	18	107
Meat, 15 oz	600	8	108
Mushroom, 16.5 oz	610	10	109
Signature Pasta:			
Angel Hair Pomodoro, 16.6 oz	570	8	98
Fettuccine Alfredo, 13.3 oz	1090	72	91
Spinach & Cheese Ravioli, 11 oz	470	16	63
Spaghetti: w/ Clam Sauce, 15 oz	790	29	107
with Marina Sauce, 15 oz	570	7	106
with Meat Sauce, 15 oz	650	11	108
with Sicilian Meatballs, 21 oz	1040	36	115
Soup: Clam Chowder, 9 oz	320	25	10
Cream of Broccoli, 9 oz	210	12	20
Dessert, Tiramisu, 4.5 oz	295	14	43

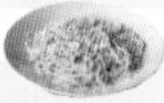
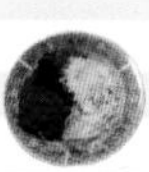
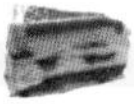

Olive Garden® (Nov '20)

Appetizers:	C	F	Cb
Calamari	670	42	48
Sauce: Marinara	45	2.5	6
Ranch	250	27	2
Fried Mozzarella	860	59	48
Lasagna Fritta	1070	71	73
Lunch: Fettuccine Alfredo	650	45	47
Chicken Parmigiana	660	29	65
Eggplant Parmigiana	660	32	74
Lasagna Classico	640	36	39
Shrimp Scampi	480	19	53
Dinner Entrees: Chicken Alfredo	1620	100	96
Five Cheese Ziti al Forno	1220	71	103
Tour of Italy	1520	96	92
Sides: French Fries	260	13	32
Steamed Broccoli	35	0	7
Desserts: Choc. Brownie Lasagna	910	52	44
Black Tie Mousse Cake	750	50	76
Lemon Cream Cake	550	31	60
Tiramisu	470	27	54
Zeppoli, without sauce	810	28	119

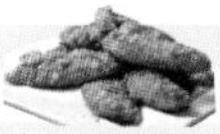
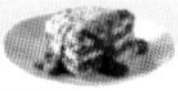

On the Border® (Nov '20)

Appetizers: As Served	C	F	Cb
Border Sampler	2000	134	109
Fajita Quesadillas:			
Chicken	1190	82	58
Steak	1280	96	55
Stacked Nachos	2030	129	145
Burritos: Without Bean, Rice or Sauce			
Classic Chicken Tinga	690	31	58
Classic Ground Beef	840	47	55
Chimichangas: Without Beans, Rice or Sauce			
Chicken Tinga	810	43	57
Ground Beef	960	55	66
Enchiladas: Without Bean or Rice			
Border Queso: Seasoned Beef	510	29	35
Shredded Beef	440	22	34
Salads: W/out Dressing			
Fajita: Chicken	430	20	27
Steak	500	28	30
Grande Taco Salad: Chkn Tinga	630	39	42
Ground Beef	710	49	40
Tacos: Without Beans or Rice			
Brisket Tacos (2)	850	42	79
Dos XX Fish Tacos (3)	1510	102	105
Southwest Chicken Tacos (3)	1510	105	82
Sides: Black Beans	200	1	36
Cilantro Lime Rice	180	2	37
Corn Tortillas (3)	170	2	35
Mexican Rice	220	6	37
Refried Beans	220	7	30
Dressings: Ranch	230	24	2
Smoked Jalapeno Vinaigrette	120	10	9

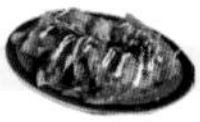
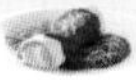
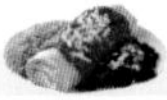
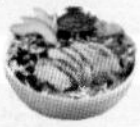
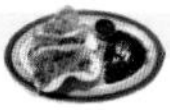
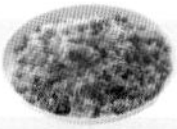

For Complete Nutritional Data ~ see CalorieKing.com

Orange Julius® (Nov '20)

Julius Originals: Per Medium Size	C	F	Cb
Mango Pineapple	320	0	78
Orange Julius	260	0	63
Pina Colada	540	7	117
Strawberry Banana	460	7	98
Premium Fruit Smoothies: Per Medium Size			
Mango Pineapple	350	0.5	82
Pomegranate Berry Blast	390	.5	91
Strawberry	370	0.5	86
Sunshine Orange	390	0.5	91
Light Smoothies: Per Medium Size			
3 Berry Daylight	210	0	51
Berry Pomegranate Twilight	210	0	51
Boost, Banana, Small drink	30	0	7

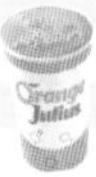

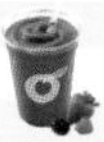

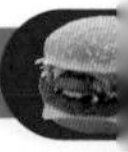

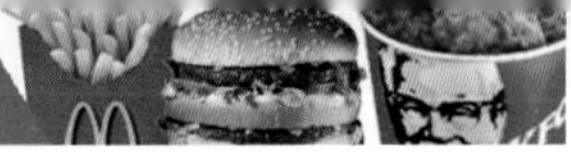

Outback Steakhouse® (Nov '20)

Aussie-Tizers: Per Regular Size, with Selected Dressing/Sauce	C	F	Cb
Alice Springs Chicken Quesadillas	**1630**	98	91
Aussie Cheese Fries: Small	**1170**	83	70
Large	**1770**	117	124
Bloomin' Onion	**1950**	155	123
Crab Cakes	**740**	60	19
Kookaburra Wings (medium), reg.	**1420**	123	13
Seared Peppered Ahi, large	**430**	26	17
Steakhouse Quesadilla, regular	**1590**	107	78
Volcano Shrimp	**960**	73	55
***Forkless Features:** Without Sides*			
Classic Cheeseburger	**710**	43	42
Cripsy Chicken Sandwich	**880**	52	69
Steakhouse Philly S'wich	**1040**	61	54
The Bloomin' Burger	**1160**	83	58
Chicken & Ribs:			
Alice Springs Chicken & Fries, 5 oz	**930**	52	69
Baby Back Ribs & Fries, full order	**1820**	115	78
Grilled Chkn On The Barbie, 8 oz,	**360**	7	16
with Fresh Mixed Veggies	**520**	16	34
Parmesan-Herb Crusted Chicken,	**510**	23	13
with Mixed Veggies	**670**	33	30
Queensland Chicken & Shrimp Pasta	**1210**	55	99
***Signature Steaks:** Without Sides*			
Melbourne Porterhouse, 20 oz	**1010**	71	4
Outback Centre Cut Sirloin: 6 oz	**210**	7	0
9 oz Sirloin	**320**	10	0.5
Ribeye, 10 oz	**540**	35	0
Victoria's Filet Mignon, 6 oz	**240**	9	0
***Straight From The Sea:** Without Sides*			
Bacon Bourbon Salmon, 10 oz	**650**	42	6
Halibut Fish & Chips	**1040**	43	104
Lobster Tails (2), grilled	**650**	45	2
Entree Salads:			
Aussie Cobb Salad, without dressing:			
with Crispy Chicken	**750**	43	45
with Grilled Chicken	**510**	27	14
Brisbane Caesar, with dressing:			
with Grilled Chicken	**560**	40	14
with Grilled Shrimp	**560**	40	16
Steakhouse, with dressing	**1000**	67	47
***Side Salads:** With Dressing*			
Caesar	**270**	25	8
House: Base Salad	**100**	6	9
add Blue Cheese Vinaigrette	**230**	21	12
add Caesar Dressing	**200**	21	2
add Creamy Blue Cheese	**240**	25	0.5
add Honey Mustard	**230**	21	12
add Thousand Island	**250**	25	6

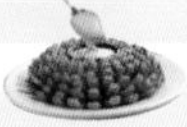

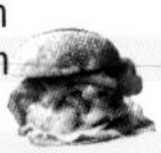

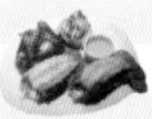

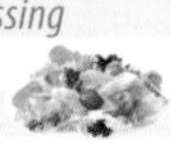

Outback Steakhouse® cont...(Nov '20)

Soups:	C	F	Cb
Baked Potato: Cup	**280**	17	23
Bowl	**520**	32	47
Chicken Tortilla Soup: Cup	**170**	9	13
Bowl	**260**	14	21
Clam Chowder: Cup	**350**	22	22
Bowl	**710**	44	44
French Onion	**420**	29	21
Sides:			
Aussie Fries	**410**	17	57
Baked Potato, with all toppings	**390**	12	58
Fresh Seasonal Mixed Veggies	**160**	10	17
Grilled Asparagus	**60**	4	4
Homestyle Mashed Pot.	**240**	15	20
Steamed Broccoli	**150**	10	14
Steamed Rice	**270**	0	59
Sweet Potato, with all toppings	**410**	11	72
***Kid's Menu:** Without Sides or Drink*			
Entrees: Boomerang Cheeseburger	**600**	36	40
Chicken Fingers	**400**	20	31
Grilled Cheese-A-Roo	**580**	21	77
Grilled Chicken on the Barbie	**160**	3.5	0
Junior Ribs	**500**	21	2
Mac-A-Roo 'N Cheese	**510**	19	65
***Desserts:** Per Whole Dish*			
Chocolate Thunder	**1500**	101	138
Double Chocolate Mini Parfait	**590**	39	54
NY Style Cheesecake, w/ Choc. Sce	**1080**	73	92
Triple Layer Carrot Cake	**1290**	68	174

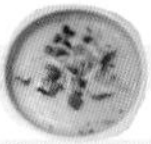

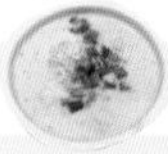

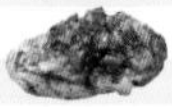

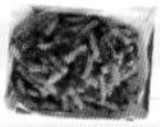

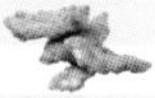

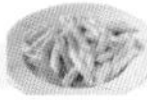

For Complete Menu & Data ~ see CalorieKing.com

Panda Express® (Nov '20)

Appetizers:	C	F	Cb
Chicken Egg Roll (1), 2.75 oz	**200**	10	20
Chicken Potsticker (3), 3.3 oz	**160**	6	20
Cream Cheese Rangoon (3), 2.4 oz	**190**	8	24
Veggie Spring Rolls (2), 3.4 oz	**190**	8	27
Entrées:			
Beef: Beijing Beef, 5.6 oz	**470**	26	46
Black Pepper Angus Steak, 5.3 oz	**180**	7	10
Broccoli Beef, 5.4 oz	**150**	7	13
Shanghai Angus Steak	**310**	19	17
Chicken:			
Black Pepper, 6.3 oz	**280**	19	15
Breast: String Bean, 5.6 oz	**190**	9	13
SweetFire, 5.8 oz	**380**	15	47
Mushroom, 5.7 oz	**220**	4	10
Orange, 5.7 oz	**490**	23	51
Potato, 5.2 oz	**190**	1	18

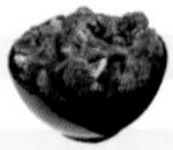

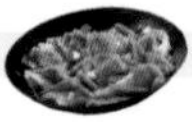

Updated Nutrition Data ~ www.CalorieKing.com
Persons with Diabetes ~ See Disclaimer (Page 22)

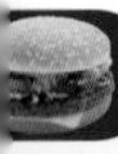

Panda Express® cont... (Nov '20)

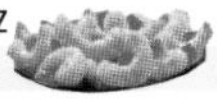
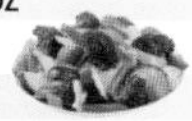

Entrees (Cont):	C	F	Cb
Shrimp: Firecracker Shrimp, 4.5 oz	110	3.5	7
Golden Treasure, 5 oz	360	18	35
Honey Walnut, 3.7 oz	360	23	35
Steamed Ginger Fish, 6 oz	200	12	8
Vegetables: Eggplant Tofu, 6.1 oz	340	24	23
Super Greens, 3.5 oz	45	2	5
Sides: Chow Fun, 8.5 oz	410	9	73
Chow Mein, 9.4 oz	510	20	80
Fried Rice, 9.3 oz	520	16	85
Steamed Brown Rice, 10.4 oz	420	4	86
Steamed White Rice, 8.1 oz	380	0	87
Hot & Sour Soup: Cup, 12.2 oz	120	5	14
Bowl, 17.4 oz	170	6	20
Dessert, Choc Chip Chunk Cookie	160	7	25

Panera Bread® (Nov '20)

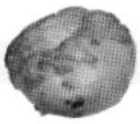
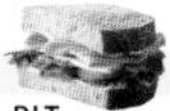
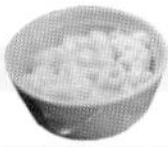
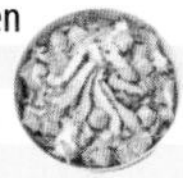

Bagels:	C	F	Cb
Asiago Cheese	320	5	55
Cinnamon Crunch	420	6	82
Breakfast Sandwiches:			
Avocado, Egg White & Spinach, on Flat Sprouted Grain Bagel	350	14	40
Bacon, Egg & Cheese on Brioche	450	25	33
Bacon, Scr. Egg & Chees on Brioche	470	26	33
Steak & Egg on Everthing Bagel	530	18	59
Sandwiches: Per Full Sandwich			
Bacon Turkey Bravo on Tomato Basil	620	23	58
Heritage Ham & Swiss, on Cntry Rustic	610	26	53
Mediterranean Veggie on Tomato Basil	470	13	68
Roasted Turkey & Avocado BLT, on Country Rustic	690	35	54
The Cuban on Artisan Ciabatta	880	34	87
Tstd Frontega Chicken on Gr. Focaccia	790	30	86
Entree:			
Baja Grain Bowl with Chicken	740	35	82
BBQ Chicken Mac & Cheese Bread Bowl	1270	41	173
Chicken Tortellini Alfredo Bowl	750	39	68
Mac & Cheese:			
Small, 1 cup	590	41	38
Large, 2 cups	1180	81	76
Salads: Full Size, with Dressing, without Bread			
Asian Sesame w/ Chicken	430	22	28
Chicken Caesar	460	28	20
Fuji Apple with Chicken	580	34	38
Greek	410	36	15
Strawberry Poppyseed with Chkn	360	14	34

Panera Bread® cont... (Nov '20)

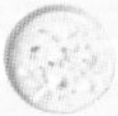
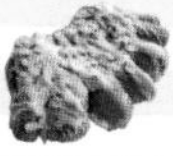

Soups: Per Cup, without Bread	C	F	Cb
Baked Potato	260	14	29
Black Bean	90	1	27
Broccoli Cheddar	230	13	19
Cream of Chicken & Wild Rice	210	11	21
Ten Vegetables	60	1	10
Vegetarian Creamy Tomato	230	15	24
Pastries & Sweets:			
Bear Claw	500	23	66
Cheese Brittany	310	16	37
Cherry Cheese Brittany	290	13	41
Chocolate Croissant	380	22	39
Brownie, (1)	400	13	68
Cake, Cinnamon Crumb Coffee, slice	520	28	61
Cookie, Chocolate Chunk (1)	630	33	85
Oatmeal Raisin with Berries (1)	350	13	54
Muffin: Choc. Chip	640	28	91
Blueberry with Fresh Blueberries	460	18	69

Papa Gino's® (Nov '20)

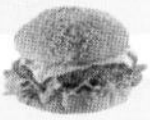
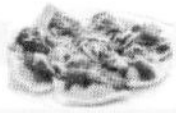
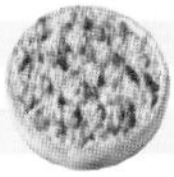
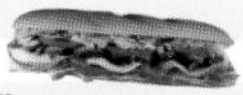
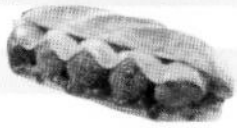
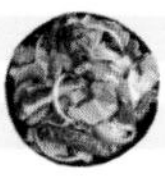

Burgers:	C	F	Cb
Cheeseburger	550	31	37
Classic Double	1000	65	43
Hamburger	520	28	36
French Fries, side, 1 serving	280	12	40
Pasta: Fettuccine Alfredo	760	23	108
Mac & Cheese	780	38	68
Penne & Meatballs	840	27	126
Ravioli	530	13	76
Pizzas:			
Thin Crust: *Per Slice, ⅛ Large Pizza*			
Boss BBQ Chicken	310	11	39
Cheese	230	7	32
Crispy Buffalo, w/ Blue Cheese	370	18	36
Meat Combo	390	16	44
Pepperoni	280	11	32
Super Veggie	250	8	35
Works	310	13	33
Subs: Per Small Sub			
BLT	720	45	60
Chicken Breast Filet	1050	51	101
Chicken Parm	1050	41	109
Italian	790	43	59
Meatball Parmesan	1140	69	85
Tuna	800	55	54
Turkey	430	5	7
Turkey Club	740	37	62
Salads: Without Dressing or Breadstick			
BBQ Chicken Tender	530	24	50
Buffalo Chicken Tenders	390	17	36
Chicken Cobb BLT	450	23	24
Dressings: Blue Cheese	270	28	3
Caesar	200	22	1
Greek	210	24	1

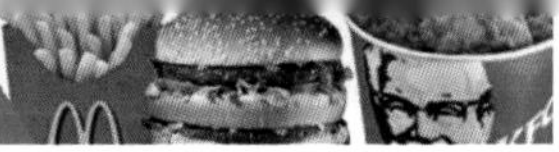

Papa John's® (Nov '20)

Pizzas:	C	F	Cb
Original Crust (14"): *Per ⅛ of Large 14" Pizza*			
BBQ Chicken & Bacon	340	11	45
Cheese	290	10	38
Chicken & Veggie	260	7	38
Chicken BBQ	350	11	45
Double Bacon Six Cheese	350	14	38
Garden Fresh	280	9	39
Gr. Chicken & Bacon	270	7	37
Hawaiian BBQ Chicken	360	11	47
Pepperoni	320	13	38
Pepperoni Sausage & Six Cheese	390	20	36
Spicy Italian	380	18	38
The Works	340	14	39
Papadias: Italian	940	53	76
Meatball Pepperoni	940	49	79
Philly Cheesesteak	810	35	80
Wings: *Per 8 Wings, with Dipping Sauce*			
BBQ	880	57	20
Honey Chipotle	900	57	27
Spicy Buffalo	840	58	8
Chicken Poppers: 5 Poppers	270	10	21
10 Poppers	530	21	42
15 Poppers	800	31	64
Sides:			
Breadsticks, 1 X 12"	130	2	24
Garlic Parmesan, 1 X 12"	160	5	24
Cheesesticks, 1 X 10"	90	4	10
Desserts: Chocolate Chip Cookie	200	10	27
Double Chocolate Chip Brownie	240	12	34

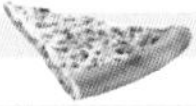

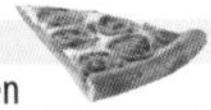

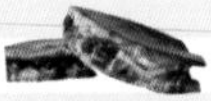

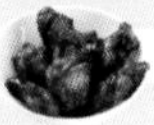

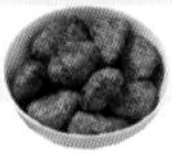

Papa Murphy's® (Nov '20)

Pizzas:	C	F	Cb
Original Crust: *Per 1/12 of Family Size Pizza*			
BBQ Chicken	340	13	35
Chicken Garlic	320	15	29
Cowboy	360	19	31
Garden Veggie	270	11	31
Gourmet Vegetarian	320	16	30
Hawaiian	270	10	32
Murphy's Combo	340	18	31
Papa's Favorite	350	17	33
Pepperoni	290	14	29
Rancher	310	14	30
Thai Chicken	330	12	39
Stuffed Pizzas: *Per 1/16 of Family Size Pizza*			
5 Meat	450	18	49
Big Murphy	440	18	50
Chicago Style	450	18	49
Chicken and Bacon	440	17	48

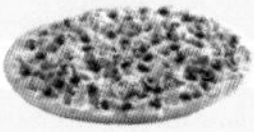

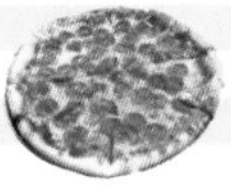

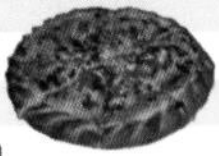

Papa Murphy's® cont... (Nov '20)

Pizzas (Cont):	C	F	Cb
Salads: *Per Whole Salad, w/out Dressing or Croutons*			
Caesar	100	5	7
Club	270	16	12
Garden	190	11	13
Italian	270	19	11
Mediterranean	320	17	23
Desserts:			
Choc. Chip Cookie, ⅛ slice	170	11	34
Cinnamon Wheel, ⅛ slice	250	7	42
S'mores Dessert Bar	130	7	25

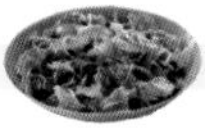

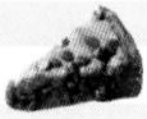

Pei Wei Asian Diner® (Nov '20)

Shareables: *Without Sauce*			
Crab Wonton (1)	85	5	7
Trad'nl Edamame, lge	320	13	19
Vegetable Spring Rolls (4)	480	24	60
Vietnamese Chkn Salad Lettuce Wraps	310	12	31
Sauce: Lettuce Wrap, 2 oz	60	3	3
Sweet Chile, 2 oz	80	0	20
Thai Peanut Dipping Sce, 2 oz	230	15	20
House-Rolled Sushi Rolls: *Per 4 Roll*			
Mango California	190	4	28
Spicy Tuna Roll	180	8	24
Noodle Bowls:			
Dan Dan	990	40	110
Chicken Lo Mein	1170	42	123
Chicken Pad Thai	1490	42	167
Lo Mein without Chicken	940	24	114
Pad Thai without Chicken	1120	37	164
Salad Bowls: *With Dressing*			
Asian Chopped Chicken	660	35	44
Spicy Polynesian Poke Bowl	760	33	90
Soup: Hot & Sour, bowl	180	6	15
Thai Wonton, bowl	140	4	43
Kid's Wei:			
Honey Seared:			
Crispy Tempura Chkn	980	30	63
Five-Spice Tofu & Steamed Veggies	710	8	59
Teriyaki: Grass-Fed Steak	790	21	58
Steamed Chicken	750	17	57
Wei Better Orange: Shrimp	620	33	67
Five-Spice Tofu & Fresh Vegegables	600	29	65
Fresh Vegetables Only	380	15	55
Dessert: Fudge Brownie	430	22	57
Fortune Cookie	25	0	5
Thai Donuts	500	19	75
Sauce for Donuts, 2 oz	260	6	44

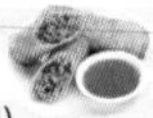

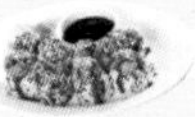

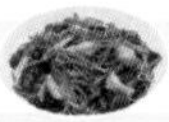

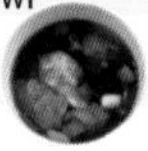

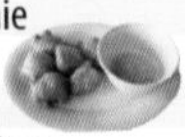

Pepe's Mexican® ~ see CalorieKing.com

Updated Nutrition Data ~ www.CalorieKing.com
Persons with Diabetes ~ See Disclaimer (Page 22)

Perkins® (Nov '20)

Breakfast: Without Side Choices	C	F	Cb
Classic: Country Fried Steak & Eggs	740	45	47
Hearty Man's Combo	800	69	11
Magnificent Seven	770	45	68
Eggs Benedict	660	34	59
Omelets:			
Everything	550	40	14
Farmer's	660	54	8
Granny's Country	640	41	34
Griddle Greats: Belgian Waffle	460	26	49
Blueberry Pancakes (3)	570	26	73
Buttermilk Pancakes (3)	540	26	66
Platters: Belgian Waffle	620	38	51
Brioche French Toast	730	33	68
Cinnamon Roll French Toast	810	45	73
French Toast	620	32	53

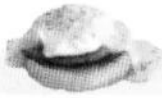
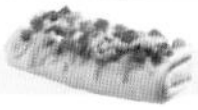
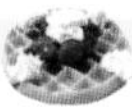

Syrups & Toppings:			
Apricot Syrup, 2 oz	120	0	30
Glazed Blueberries, 6 oz	200	0	51
Glazed Strawberries, 6 oz	140	0	36
Pancake/Twinberry Syrup, 2 oz, av.	130	0	33
Sugar Free Pancake Syrup, 2 oz	20	0	6
Side Choices: Bacon, 4 slices	140	12	0
Blueberry Muffin, with butter	650	33	81
Breakfast Potatoes, 5 oz	280	17	30
English Muffin, with butter	230	11	28
Fresh Cut Fruit, 4 oz	70	0	19
Ham, grilled, 5.6 oz	160	4.5	6
Hash Browns, 4.3 oz	210	13	22
Homestyle Potatoes, 6.8 oz	210	3	40
Jumbo Biscuits (2), with butter	650	36	68
Oatmeal, with butter blend, 2% Milk & Brown Sugar	390	15	57
Sausage Patties (2)	380	38	1
Smoked Sausage, 4.1 oz	380	34	8
Sticky Bun, with butter	790	41	98
White Toast (2), with butter	310	16	34
Whole Wheat Toast (2), with butter	310	13	38
Burgers: Without Sides			
BBQ Tangler	1140	70	75
Classic Burger	760	45	48
Classic Cheeseburger	910	59	48
Sandwiches: Without Sides			
Chicken Strips Melt, on Sourdough	1290	80	88
Country Club Melt, on Sourdough	990	57	64
Pot Roast Melt, on Sourdough	1040	62	65
Reuben Melt, on Rye	1090	61	79

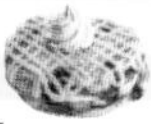
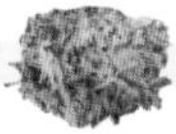
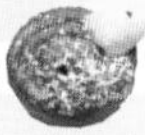
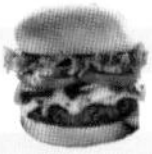

Perkins® cont... (Nov '20)

Lunch & Dinners:	C	F	Cb
Comfort Classics: *Without Sides*			
Chicken Strips	800	43	59
Country Fried Steak	570	32	45
Fish 'n Chips, with Tartar Sauce	1290	85	97
Grilled Garlic Tilapia & Shrimp	550	20	57
Grilled Salmon	430	29	2
Turkey & Dressing, w/- Cranb. Sce	430	20	21
Supper Skillets: *With Menu Set Sides*			
Hibachi Fried Chicken	780	29	103
Hibachi Gr. Shrimp	610	20	85
Steak & Pepper	800	43	58
Sides: Applesauce, 3 oz	40	0	9
Baked Potato,with Sour Cream	300	12	42
Buttered Corn	150	8	17
French Fries, 7 oz	570	36	56
Green Beans & Bacon, 4 oz	45	2.5	4
Herb Rice Pilaf, 6.5 oz	270	6	50
H'style Seasoned Potato, 6.8 oz	210	3	40
Macaroni & Five Cheese, 5.2 oz	300	16	26
Mashed Potatoes & Gravy, 8.6 oz	240	9	34
Sauteed Spinach, 4 oz	70	3.5	4
Tater Tots	470	28	47
Soups: Per Bowl, Includes Crackers			
Chicken Noodle	260	6	37
Loaded Potato; Tomato Basil	460	26	46
Salads: With Set Dressing Unless Indicated			
Honey Mstrd Chicken Crunch	980	63	63
Southwest Avocado	820	50	61
Turkey BLT w/out dressing	380	19	11
55 Plus Lunch/Dinner: Without Sides			
Cheeseburger	690	39	41
Pork Chop Dinner	560	32	8
Pot Roast Dinner	560	31	16
Dessert: As Served			
Muffins: *Includes Whipped Butter Blend*			
Apple Cinnamon	630	33	76
Banana Nut	790	46	85
Blueberry	650	33	81
Pies: *Per Slice*			
Banana Cream Pie	700	46	67
Caramel Apple, 7.2 oz	500	22	68
Cherry	580	27	75
Chocolate French Silk	760	54	66
Southern Pecan, 5.5 oz	670	33	86
Wildberry, no sugar added, 7 oz	470	27	50

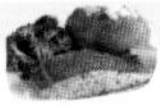
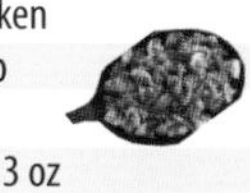
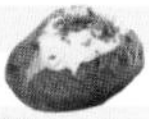
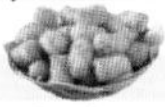
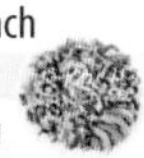
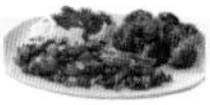
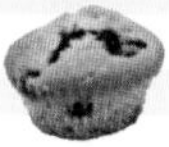
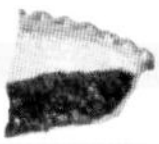

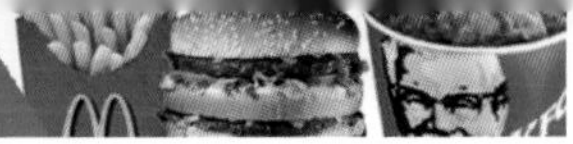

Peter Piper Pizza® (Nov '20)

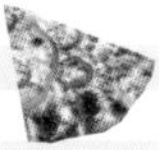
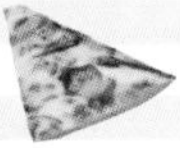
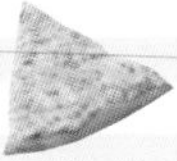
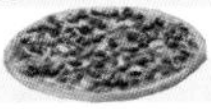
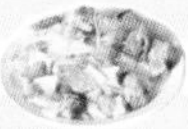
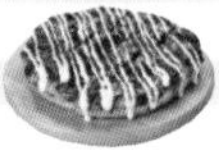

Signature Pizzas:	C	F	Cb
Original Crust: *Per 1/8 of Large 14" Pizza*			
5 Meat Supreme	**360**	15	39
California Veggie	**290**	9	41
Cheese	**320**	11	39
Chicago Classic	**330**	13	40
Hearty Hawaiian	**310**	9	41
New York 3 Cheese w/ Pepperoni	**390**	18	39
Pizza Mexicana	**390**	18	39
Spinach Chkn Alfredo	**350**	15	37
The Werx	**310**	11	40
Veggie Harvest	**300**	9	42
Original Crust: *Per 1/12 of Extra Large 16" Pizza*			
5 Meat Supreme	**350**	16	34
California Veggie	**250**	8	35
Cheese	**280**	10	34
Chicago Classic	**300**	12	35
Hearty Hawaiian	**270**	8	36
New York 3 Cheese w/ Pepperoni	**350**	16	34
Pizza Mexicana	**340**	15	34
Spinach Chkn Alfredo	**310**	14	32
The Werx	**290**	11	34
Veggie Harvest	**260**	8	36
Pasta: *With Breadstick*			
Mac & Pepperoni	**1670**	91	168
Meaty Ziti	**1240**	78	79
Spinach Alfredo	**1640**	89	153
Salads: *Small Size, without Dressing*			
Caesar, with Croutons	**320**	14	35
Chopped Italian	**260**	19	10
Wings & More:			
Bone In Wings (10), without sauce	**1160**	97	0
Boneless Wings, 10 oz, w/out sauce	**880**	58	47
Cheddar Bacon Roll (1)	**350**	18	34
Garlic Cheese Bread, 3.25 oz	**390**	17	45
Handmade Breadsticks, with Marinara Sauce (6)	**1190**	31	199
Loaded Tots	**1280**	102	70
Dipping Sauces:			
BBQ	**240**	0	60
Buffalo	**120**	9	6
Ranch	**320**	36	2
Sweet Chili	**200**	0	46
Xtra Hot Buffalo	**90**	6	5
Dessert:			
Cinnamon Crunch, small slice	**380**	9	69
Vanilla Soft Serve: Cone	**200**	6	35
Cup	**180**	6	31

P.F. Chang's® (Nov '20)

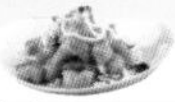
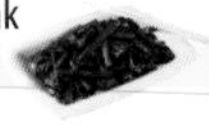
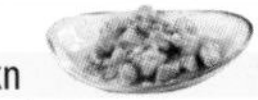
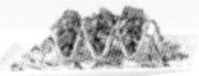
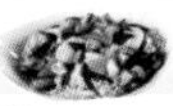
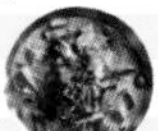
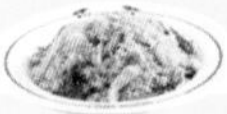
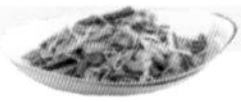
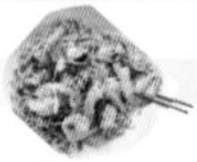

Shareables/Sides:	C	F	Cb
Calamari & Vegetables Tempura	**960**	73	61
Chang's BBQ Spare Ribs	**870**	28	35
Chang's Chicken Lettuce Wraps	**660**	27	66
Chang's Vegetarian Lettuce Wraps	**570**	29	51
Crispy Green Beans	**990**	78	70
Dynamite Shrimp	**640**	48	36
Edamame with Kosher Salt	**400**	17	25
Kung Pao Brussels Sprouts	**720**	42	84
Entrées:			
Beef: *Per Whole Meal*			
Beef with Broccoli	**670**	33	46
Korean Bulgogi Steak	**1370**	58	121
Mongolian	**770**	42	39
Pepper Steak	**640**	36	29
Chicken: *Per Whole Dish, without Rice*			
Chang's Spicy	**840**	33	77
Crispy Honey Chkn	**1120**	60	87
Ginger Chicken with Broccoli	**480**	12	41
Kung Pao	**960**	58	46
Sesame Chicken	**870**	36	75
Sweet & Sour Chicken	**860**	41	86
Seafood: *Per Whole Meal, without Rice*			
Crispy Honey Shrimp	**1020**	55	79
Kung Pao Shrimp	**760**	52	40
Miso Glazed Salmon	**660**	37	30
Oolong Chilean Sea Bass	**560**	35	30
Salt & Pepper Prawns	**500**	22	37
Shrimp with Lobster Sce	**500**	27	22
Vegetarian: *Without Rice*			
Buddha's Feast: Steamed	**260**	4	32
Stir-Fried	**380**	8	53
Thai Harvest Curry	**1070**	74	74
Noodles & Rice:			
Fried Rice: Combo	**1200**	35	160
with Beef	**1140**	33	155
with Chicken	**1100**	26	159
with Pork	**1190**	37	161
with Shrimp	**1000**	20	154
Lo Mein: Beef	**980**	31	127
Chicken	**950**	24	130
Combo	**1050**	33	132
Pork	**1030**	35	133
Shrimp	**850**	18	126
Vegetables	**760**	13	135
Singapore Street Noodles	**1260**	17	224

Updated Nutrition Data ~ www.CalorieKing.com
Persons with Diabetes ~ See Disclaimer (Page 22)

P.F. Chang's® cont... (Nov '20)

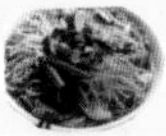

Noodles & Rice (Cont):	C	F	Cb
Pad Thai: Chicken	1230	33	181
Combo	1210	32	181
Shrimp	1180	31	181

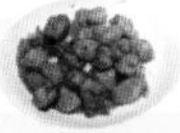

Lunch Bowls: *Without Rice*	C	F	Cb
Beef & Brocoli	370	19	29
Honey Chicken	1120	41	136
Mongolian Beef	490	28	89
Spicy Chicken	680	27	127
Rice: Brown, 6 oz	190	0	40
Fried	300	6	53
White, 6 oz	220	0	49

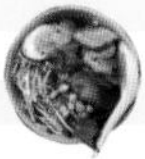

	C	F	Cb
Ramen: Poached Pork	310	24	3
Spicy Miso	660	15	109
Tonkotsu	700	22	106

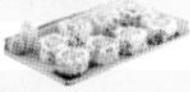

	C	F	Cb
Sushi: California Roll	360	16	47
Kung Pao Dragon Roll	490	24	55
Shrimp Tempura Roll	560	25	65
Spicy Tuna Roll	280	6	39

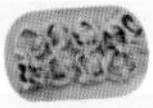

	C	F	Cb
Salad: Asian Caesar	410	30	20
Mandarin Crunch	750	46	75
Add: Chicken	160	5	4
Salmon	240	16	0

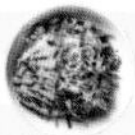

	C	F	Cb
Soup: Egg Drop, bowl	270	7	42
Hot & Sour	470	12	63
Wonton	570	17	53
Dessert: Banana Spring Rolls	940	35	149
New York Style Cheese Cake	940	61	80
The Great Wall of Chocolate	1700	71	259
Vietnamese Chocolate Lava Cake	820	48	97

Pita Pit® ~ *See CalorieKing.com*

Pizza Hut® (Nov '20)

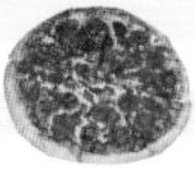

Hand-Tossed Style: *Per ⅛ of Medium 12" Pizza*	C	F	Cb
Cheese	210	8	26
Chicken-Bacon Parmesan	230	9	25
Meat Lover's	280	15	26
Pepperoni	220	10	25
Pepperoni Lover's	270	13	26
Supreme	240	10	26
Ultimate Cheese Lover's	230	10	25
Veggie Lover's	200	6	26

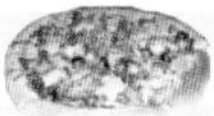

Original Pan: Per ⅛ of Medium 12" Pizza	C	F	Cb
Cheese	260	12	28
Meat Lover's	320	18	28
Pepperoni	260	13	27
Pepperoni Lover's	320	17	28
Supreme	280	14	28
Ultimate Cheese Lover's	280	14	27
Veggie Lover's	240	10	29

Pizza Hut® cont... (Nov '20)

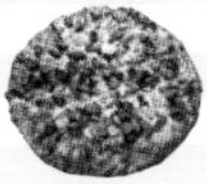

Personal Pan: *Per ¼ of 6" Pizza*	C	F	Cb
Backyard BBQ Chicken	180	6	25
Meat Lover's	210	12	17
Pepperoni	150	7	17
Pepperoni Lover's	180	9	17
Supreme	170	9	17
Ultimate Cheese Lover's	170	8	17
Veggie Lover's	140	5	18

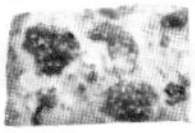

Rectangle Slices: *Per Slice, ⅛ of Pizza*	C	F	Cb
Backyard BBQ Chicken	260	9	34
Buffalo Chicken	240	8	32
Cheese	240	10	29
Pepperoni	250	11	28
Veggie Lovers	220	8	29

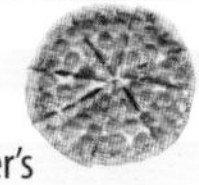

Thin 'n Crispy: *Per ⅛ of Medium 12" Pizza*	C	F	Cb
Backyard BBQ Chicken	210	7	27
Cheese	180	7	22
Chicken-Bacon Parmesan	220	10	21
Meat Lover's	260	14	22
Pepperoni Lover's	250	13	22
Supreme	210	9	23
Ultimate Cheese Lover's	210	10	21
Veggie Lover's	170	6	24
Pastas, Tuscani:			
Creamy Chicken Alfredo, 9.9 oz	990	57	77
Meaty Marinara, 9.6 oz	880	40	88

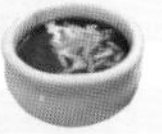

Soup: *Per Bowl with Crackers*	C	F	Cb
Broccoli & Cheese	530	37	35
Creamy Tomato Basil	390	23	37
Loaded Baked Potato	600	40	41

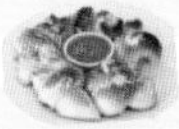

	C	F	Cb
Sides: Baked Bone Out Wing (1)	60	2	4
Breadstick (1), without sauce	140	4.5	19
Buffalo Chicken Nachos	1110	50	132
Cheesy Dip 'N Cheese	660	36	78
Fried Onion Rings, with Ketchup	860	50	93
Garlic Bread, 1 piece	140	8	15
Stuffed Garlic Knot	80	2.5	10
Stuffed Pizza Roller	230	10	27

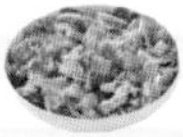

Salad: *Entree Size, without Dressing*	C	F	Cb
Asian	330	15	24
BLT	400	26	26
Chicken Caesar	470	25	27
Harvest	470	19	48
Zesty Italian	370	22	30
Dressing: Blue Cheese, entree size	450	48	3
Buttermilk Ranch, 1.5 oz	200	22	2
Honey French,1.5 oz	190	15	13
Desserts: Fried Apple Pie	170	9	22
Hershey's: Chocolate Chip Cookie	300	14	45
Triple Choc. Brownie, ⅙ square	380	16	56
New York Style Cheesecake, slice	840	57	69

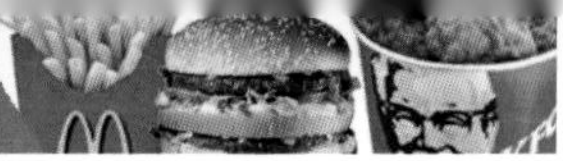

Pizza Ranch® (Nov '20)

Pizza:	C	F	Cb
Original Crust: *Per Slice, 1/10 of Medium Pizza*			
Bacon Cheeseburger	180	7	20
BBQ Chicken	170	6	20
Bronco	200	8	19
Buffalo Chicken	1890	9	18
Chicken Bacon Ranch	230	12	18
Macaroni 'N' Cheese	210	9	22
Prairie (Veggie)	170	6	20
Stampede	200	9	20
Sweet Swine	170	6	21
Taco Texan	220	9	27
Thin Crust: *Per 1/10 Slice of Medium Pizza*			
BBQ Chicken	150	7	12
Bronco	180	10	12
Mac 'N' Cheese	190	11	15
Ranch Wraps:			
BBQ Chicken	1560	75	130
Caesar Chicken	1680	106	96
Chicken Bacon	2090	146	98
Sides: Biscuit	200	10	23
Coleslaw	180	16	11
Corn	150	1	35
Mashed Potatoes & Gravy, 8 oz	120	5	16
Ranch Potato Wedges (8)	680	40	71
Salads: Chef	460	20	12
Chicken Fiesta	200	8	11
Garden	110	6	10
Taco	600	36	50

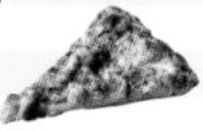
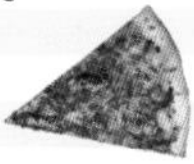
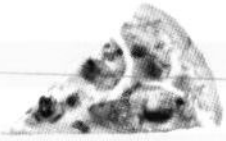
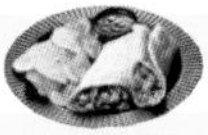
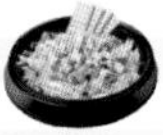

For Complete Menu & Data ~ see CalorieKing.com

Pollo Tropical® ~ *See CalorieKing.com*

Popeye's® (Nov '20)

Chicken Pieces: *Mild & Spicy with Skin*	C	F	Cb
Breast	380	20	16
Leg	160	9	5
Thigh	280	21	7
Wing	210	14	8
Nuggets: 6 pieces	225	14	15
9 Pieces	340	20	23
Tenders: Mild/Spicy, 3 pieces	445	21	29
5 pieces	740	34	48
Sandwiches & Wraps: Each			
Classic Chicken	700	42	50
Loaded Chicken Wrap	310	12	35
Spicy Chicken	700	42	50
Seafood: Catfish Fillets, 2 pieces	460	29	27
Butterfly Shrimp (8)	420	25	34
Popcorn Shrimp, 4 oz	390	25	28

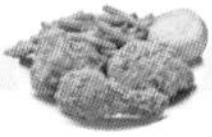
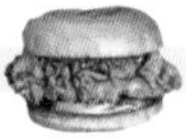

Popeye's® cont... (Nov '20)

Sides:	C	F	Cb
Biscuit	205	13	20
Cajun Fries, regular	270	14	33
Cajun Rice, regular	185	6	24
Cole Slaw, regular	140	10	12
Corn on the Cob (1)	210	6	34
Mashed Potatoes, with Cajun Gravy	110	4	18
Onion Rings, regular	280	19	25
Red Beans & Rice, regular	245	16	22
Breakfast:			
Biscuits: Bacon	400	25	37
Chicken	490	26	47
Egg	510	29	41
Egg & Sausage	690	45	43
Sausage	540	36	41
Sausage & Gravy	510	33	42
Grits	370	5	80
Hash Rounds	360	20	41
Desserts:			
Edward's Sliced Pecan Pie, 3.4 oz	410	21	52
Mardi Gras Cheesecake, 3 oz	320	21	29
Mississippi Mud Cake, 3 oz	260	7	50
Sweet Potato Pie 3.4 oz	350	19	41

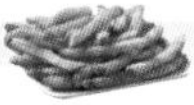
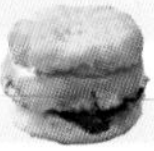
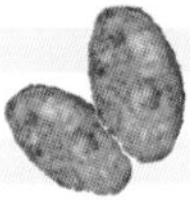

Port of Subs® (Nov '20)

Figures Based on West Coast Outlets	C	F	Cb
Classic Subs: *Per 8" White Sub with Standard Menu Components*			
#1 Ham, Salami, Capicolla, Pepperoni, Provolone	630	26	64
#2 Ham & Turkey, Provolone	540	15	65
#3 Salami & Turkey, Provolone	580	20	65
#4 Ham, Salami, Provolone	550	20	63
#5 Smoked Ham, Turkey, Cheddar	580	17	65
#6 Vegetarian, 3 Chse	670	34	68
#7 Roast Beef, Prov.	540	14	61
#8 Turkey, Provolone	560	15	66
#10 Rstd Chicken Breast, Provolone	530	14	64
#11 Ham, American Cheese	530	16	64
#12 Salami, Provolone	590	25	63
#13 Pepprd Pastrami Turkey, Swiss	560	15	65
#15 Salami, Pepperoni, Provolone	600	27	63
#16 Chkn, Pepperoni, Pepper Jack	570	22	62
#17 Tuna, Provolone	700	29	65
#18 Roast Beef,Turkey, Provolone	550	14	64

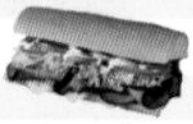

Updated Nutrition Data ~ www.CalorieKing.com
Persons with Diabetes ~ See Disclaimer (Page 22)

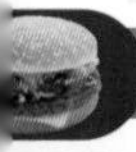

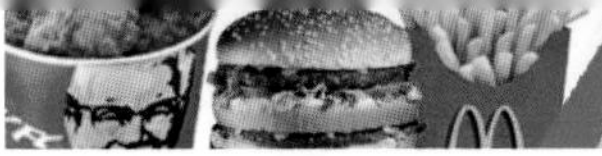

Port of Subs® cont... (Nov '20)

Figures Based on West Coast Outlets

	C	F	Cb
***Hot Subs:** Per 8" White Sub with Provolone , without Additional Toppings*			
Melts: Buffalo Chicken	590	13	60
Chicken	590	13	60
Teriyaki Chicken	670	13	77
Pastrami	780	39	64
NY Steak	650	28	59
Ultimate BLT	740	38	67
***Flatbreads:** With Provolone without Sauce*			
All American Club	430	18	37
Melts: Pastrami	550	30	37
NY Steak	450	22	33
Pulled Pork	390	13	33
Ultimate BLT	470	26	38
***Wraps:** On Wheat Wrap with Povolone & Standard Menu Components*			
Grilled Chicken Caesar	670	25	60
Pastrami Melt	850	47	62
Ultimate BLT	800	46	65
***Fresh Salads:** Standard Components, w/out Dressing*			
Caesar	70	2.5	10
Chef	260	15	13
Garden	70	2.5	9
Grilled Chicken	280	7	11
Gr. Chicken Caesar	280	7	11
Spinach	60	2.5	8
Tuna	360	20	13
***Salad Dressings:** Per 2 fl.oz*			
Caesar; Ranch, average	220	23	3
Honey Mustard	260	26	10
***Sides:** Per Regular, 8 oz*			
Macaroni Salad	520	36	44
Potato Salad	380	21	47
Soup: Boston Clam Chowder, small	200	9	22
Chicken & Wild Rice, small	190	8	21
Chicken Noodle, small	90	2.5	12
Cream of Broccoli, small	200	12	17
New England Clam Chowder, small	180	7	22
***Breakfast Sub:** With American Cheese & Egg*			
5" Wheat Bread:			
Peppered Bacon	470	23	40
Smoked Ham	390	15	39
Turkey Sausage	480	22	38
Flatbread: Peppered Bacon	480	25	37
Smoked Ham	400	17	35
Turkey Sausage	490	24	35
Desserts:			
Chocolate Chunk Cookie, 4 oz	500	23	71
Jumbo Brownie	760	36	109
Oatmeal Raisin Cookie, 4 oz	480	20	69
White Choc.Macadamia Nut Cookie	530	26	67

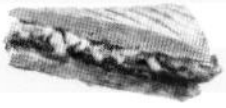
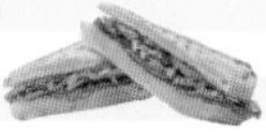
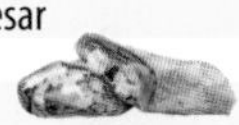
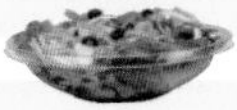
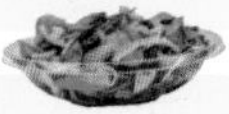
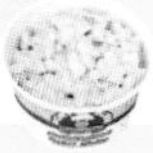
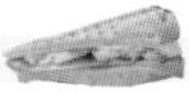
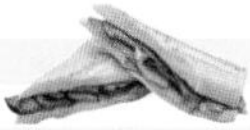

Pret A Manger® (Nov '20)

East Coast Outlets.

	C	F	Cb
Baguettes:			
Balsamic Chicken & Mozzarella	590	21	62
Chicken Caesar & Bacon	730	35	62
Ham & Cheese	600	24	62
Italian	610	28	63
***Hot Food:** Per Pack*			
Chipotle Chicken Grain Bowl	400	6	67
Spinach & Tomato Mac & Cheese	580	21	78
Pots: Banana & Honey	360	11	54
Blueberry & Granola	360	13	39
Little Cup of Goodness	300	10	38
Sunshine Bowl	390	12	63
***Sandwiches:** OnMultigrain Bread*			
Balsamic Chicken & Avocado	470	20	47
California Club	490	20	53
Carrot & Hummus	480	18	69
Cheddar & Tomato	460	23	46
Chicken & Bacon	630	34	39
Egg Salad & Arugula	490	27	42
Super Veggie	400	18	51
Tuna Salad	670	34	54
***Soups:** Per Small*			
Chicken Noodle	110	2.5	12
Moroccan Lentil	220	10	25
Tomato Feta	130	7	13
Turkey Chili	210	4.5	28
***Salads:** With Set Dressing*			
Chicken Avocado	670	51	30
Mediterranean Mezze	570	34	55
Salmon & Mango Grain	570	30	56
Steak & Gorgonzola	590	47	19
Veggie Fiesta	530	31	54
Breakfast:			
Coconut Oatmeal, w/out Toppings	250	11	32
Add Almond & Dried Cranberries	60	3	8
Egg Salad & Avocado Baguette	420	22	42
Egg White & Veggie Brioche	330	13	35
Egg & Cheddar Brioche	370	17	33
Ham & Spinach Frittata	400	24	5
Southern Breakfast Wrap	380	14	45
***Bakery:** Per Pack*			
Croissants: Almond	370	21	39
Pain au Chocolate	310	17	33
Pain au Raisin	390	20	46
Cookies: Carrot Cake, 2.5 oz	270	14	35
Chocolate Chunk, 2.5 oz	310	16	41
Harvest, 2.5 oz	280	12	40
Muffin, Blueberry, 4.5 oz	420	16	63

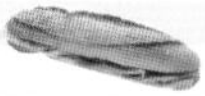
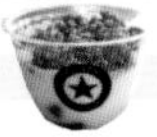
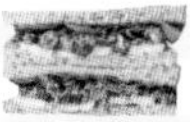
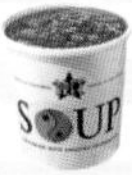

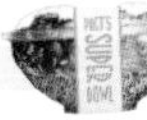
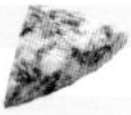
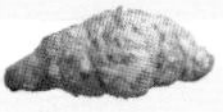
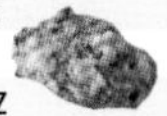

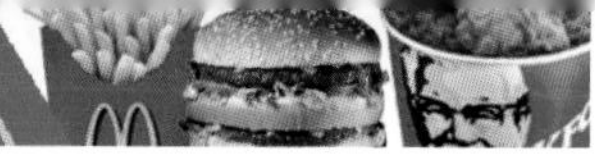

Pretzelmaker® (Nov '20)

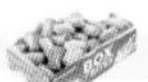
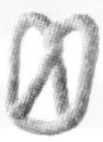
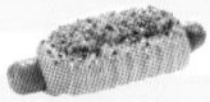
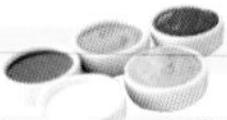
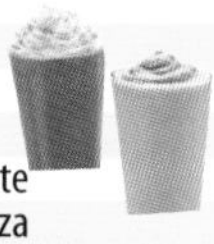

Pretzels: Per Small Serving	C	F	Cb
Bites: Salted, 6 oz	500	14	85
Cinn. Sugar, 6 oz	530	14	90
Whole: Plain, 4 oz	310	3	66
Cinnamon Sugar, 5 oz	450	12	79
Garlic, 5 oz	430	12	74
Parmesan, 5 oz	450	15	66
Ranch, 5 oz	440	12	72
Pretzel Dogs: Regular	420	23	31
Mini (8)	430	29	33
Jalapeno (1), 6 oz	450	24	34
Sauces: Per 2 oz			
Caramel	100	1	22
Cheddar/Nacho Cheese, average	80	6	5
Cream Cheese	200	20	2
Pizza Sauce	30	1	6
Vanilla Glaze	170	0	42
Beverages: Per 20 oz Unless Indicated			
Blended Drinks:			
Cool Cappuccino	430	22	58
Mango Madness	500	16	90
Mocha Mania	580	22	94
Power Pomegranate	490	16	86
Strawberry Bananza	500	16	85
Fresh Lemonade: Original, 20 oz	140	0	38
Strawberry; Raspberry, 20 oz, av.	210	0	52

Qdoba® (Nov '20)

Make Your Own Burrito:	C	F	Cb
Meat: Chorizo; Ground Beef, av. 3.5 oz	200	12	5
Grilled: Adobo Chicken, 3.5 oz	150	9	2
Smoked Brisket; Steak, av., 3.5 oz	250	17	4
Pulled Pork, 3.5 oz	140	4	9
Other Burrito Fillings: 3 Chse, 2 oz	90	8	3
Black Beans, 4 oz	140	1	24
Brown Rice, 4 oz	170	1	35
Cilantro Lime Rice, 4 oz	190	3	38
Corn Tortilla Strips, 4 oz	560	26	75
Fajita Veggies, 2 oz	35	2	4
Pico De Gallo, 2 oz	10	0	3
Pinto Beans, 4 oz	130	1	23
Romaine Lettucce, 3.5 oz	15	0	3
Salsas, average	20	0	4
Seasoned Potatoes, 2 oz	140	4	9
Shredded Cheese, 1 oz	110	9	1
Shredded Lettuce, 0.25 oz	7	0	1
Smashed Guacamole, 2 oz	90	7	5
Sour Cream, 1 oz	50	5	3
Tortillas: Corn, 5.5"	60	1	11
Crispy Taco Shell	60	3	8
Crunchy Flour Tortilla Bowl	390	22	41
Flour Tortilla: 5.5"	70	2	12
10"	210	5	36
12.5"	300	7	52

Qdoba® cont...® (Nov '20)

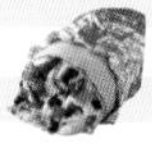
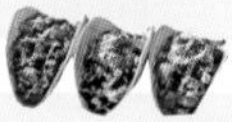
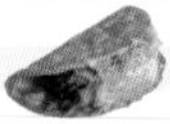

Signature Eats:	C	F	Cb
Bowls: Chicken Protein	10	29	48
Chicken Queso	780	34	75
Impossible Fajita	580	15	85
Burrito, Chicken Cheese	1080	41	127
Quesadills, Steak Fajita	1130	68	72
Street Style Tacos:			
Chicken:			
Corn Tacos (3)	470	22	50
Flour Tacos (3)	520	25	52
Soup, Tortilla, 8 oz	100	5	11
Kid's Meals: Burrito	80	5	67
Quesadilla	60	12	25
Taco: with Beef	220	12	11
with Chicken	200	11	11
Beans with Cheese, side	160	3	24
Desserts:			
Chocolate Chunk Cookie, 1.9 oz	260	14	34
Double Chocolate Brownie, 3.1 oz	360	16	52

Quiznos Subs® (Nov '20)

Subs: Per 8" Regular Japaleno Cheddar Sub, with Standard Menu Toppings Unless Indicated

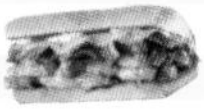
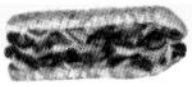
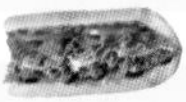
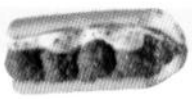
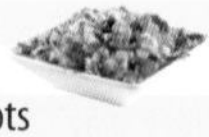

Chicken:	C	F	Cb
Apple Harvest	790	32	97
Baja	800	32	76
Carbonara	890	42	73
Honey Mustard	850	36	80
Mesquite	800	33	73
Southwest Chicken	860	45	73
Steak:			
Black Angus Steak,			
On Rosemary Parmesan	780	27	88
Chipotle Steak & Cheddar	840	44	73
French Dip	760	30	79
Peppercorn Steak	840	42	76
Deli Classic:			
Classic Italian	890	48	79
Spicy Monterey	600	15	81
Tuna Melt	660	22	76
Turkey Ranch & Swiss	670	25	73
Veggie Guacamole	810	44	81
Salads: Per Full Size With Set Dressing			
Apple Harvest Chkn	520	29	48
Chef	590	46	13
Italian	700	57	18
Sides: Classic Tater Tots	210	11	25
Loaded	320	19	25
Side Salad with Red Wine Vinaigrette	270	26	9

continued next page...

Quiznos Subs® cont... (Nov '20)

Savory Soups: Per Regular	C	F	Cb
Broccoli Cheese	**220**	14	18
Chicken Noodle	**120**	4	14
Chili	**290**	10	34
Tomato Bisque	**290**	21	21
Breakfast:			
Biscuit: Egg & Cheddar	**460**	31	31
Sausage, Egg & Cheddar	**630**	48	31
Subs:			
Bacon, Egg & Cheddar	**370**	17	34
Ham, Egg & Cheddar	**340**	14	36
Sausage, Egg & Cheddar	**550**	37	35
Desserts: Chocolate Brownie	**440**	23	56
Chocolate Chunk Cookie, 3 oz	**400**	18	57
Cinnamon Sugar Cookie	**400**	17	58
Oatmeal Raisin Cookie	**360**	12	58

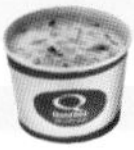
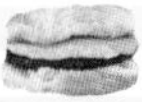
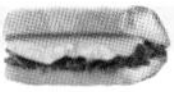

Rally's/Checkers® (Nov '20)

Burgers/Sandwiches:	C	F	Cb
Bacon Roadhouse	**680**	47	37
Baconzilla	**910**	62	43
Big Buford	**660**	39	39
Cheese Champ	**430**	21	39
Crispy Chicken Filet	**350**	11	42
Double Crispy Fish	**570**	33	52
Classic Wings: Buffalo, 5 pieces	**360**	23	3
Honey BBQ, 5 pieces	**430**	23	19
Garlic Parmesan, 5 pcs	**510**	40	3
Fries: Regular, medium	**500**	24	63
Chili Cheese Fries	**590**	30	72
Fully Loaded Fries	**870**	56	72

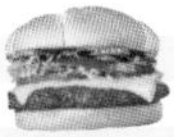
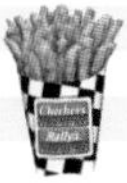

Ranch One® (Nov '20)

Sandwiches:	C	F	Cb
Chicken & Cheese	**390**	12	40
Chicken Philly, 9.3 oz	**410**	13	40
Grilled Classic Chicken, 9.4 oz	**680**	47	37
Original Crispy Chicken, 11.5 oz	**640**	31	60
Other Favorites:			
Chicken Fajitas, 10 oz	**540**	24	53
Chicken Platter, with Rice, 11.9 oz	**270**	6	28
Popcorn Chicken:			
Small, 5.5 oz	**310**	10	30
Large, 7.5 oz	**420**	14	40
Salads: Completed			
Grilled Chicken Caesar, 13.3 oz	**430**	30	14
Southwest Chicken, 17.5 oz	**680**	43	44
Fries:			
Medium, 5.8 oz	**380**	19	43
Large, 10.9 oz	**530**	27	58
Cheese Fries: Medium, 7.3 oz	**490**	27	46
Large, 11 oz	**760**	44	66

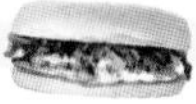
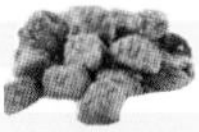
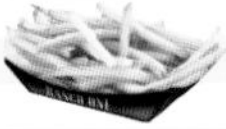

Red Hot & Blue® (Nov '20)

Starters:	C	F	Cb
Catfish Fingers	**590**	19	75
Nachos, with Chili	**1005**	51	103
Smokin Buffalo Wings	**1045**	85	28
Burgers:			
ALL IN	**915**	52	46
Classic Blues	**665**	32	44
Ribs, Full Slab:			
Dry	**1870**	144	28
Sweet	**1895**	142	44
Favorite Entrees: Delta Catfish	**835**	42	57
Delta Surf & Turf	**1025**	68	38
Southern Fried Chicken Crispers	**760**	35	50
Rib & Crispers Platter	**1060**	68	39
BBQ Platters: Five Meat	**935**	63	15
Delta Double with Memphis Chkn	**900**	54	12
Pulled Pork	**325**	21	7
Smoked Sausage	**965**	68	36
Sandwiches:			
Fried Delta Catfish	**655**	25	71
Grilled Chicken	**360**	6	40
Pulled Pork	**370**	15	37
Ribwich Combo	**685**	39	42
Sides: BBQ Beans	**255**	2	48
Collard Greens	**50**	2	7
Fried Ocra	**190**	8	29
Mashed Potatoes, with gravy	**310**	14	44
Memphis Fries, 6 oz	**345**	19	38
Potato Salad	**405**	28	33
Sweet Potato	**495**	0	114
Sweet Potato Fries	**375**	19	49
Salads: Grilled Chicken Caesar	**770**	46	47
Southern Fried Chicken	**710**	31	60

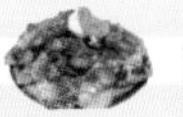
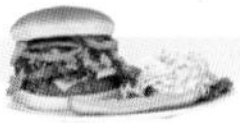
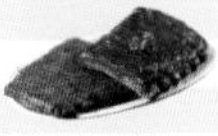
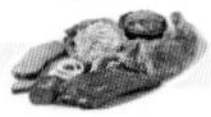
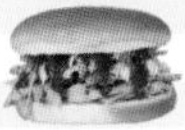
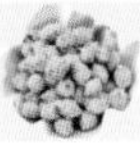
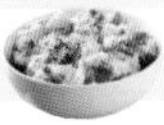

Red Lobster® (Sept '19)

Appetizers: As Served	C	F	Cb
Lobster & Langostino Pizza	**700**	35	59
Mozzarella Cheesesticks	**700**	40	56
Oysters Half Shell (12), raw	**530**	11	85
Parrot Isle Jumbo Cocktail Shrimp	**610**	39	52
Seafood Stuffed Mushrooms	**390**	22	18
Signature Jumbo Shrimp Cocktail	**130**	0	11
Sweet Chili Shrimp	**960**	66	68
Land & Sea: With Menu Set Sides & Sauce			
Cajun Chicken Linguini, full	**1340**	60	116
Maple Glazed Chicken Dinner	**490**	7	51
Rock Lobster & NY Strip (12 oz)	**1250**	83	27
Steak: Grilled Filet Mignon (6 oz)	**460**	23	26
Grilled Sirloin (7 oz)	**480**	22	26
Wood-Grilled Shrimp & Sirloin	**560**	25	27

continued next page...

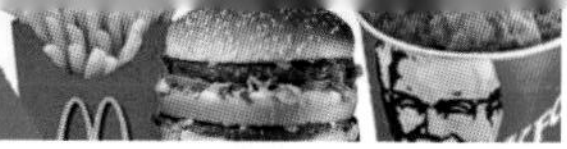

Red Lobster® cont... (Sept '19)

Lunch Classics:
With Menu Fixed Sides & Dipping Sauce

	C	F	Cb
Cajun Chicken Linguini, half order	**690**	30	62
Crab Linguini Alfredo, half order	**610**	28	57
Crunchy Popcorn Shrimp	**430**	19	49
Farm-Raised Catfish, Blackened	**210**	10	2
Garlic Shrimp Scampi	**220**	18	3
Hand Breaded Shrimp	**240**	11	23
Maple Glazed Chicken	**360**	5	50
Sailor's Platter	**450**	18	18
Wild Caught Flounder:			
Golden Fried	**710**	50	38
Oven Broiled	**210**	5	1
Savor The Sea:			
Bar Harbour Lobster Bake	**1250**	56	106
Seafarer's Feast	**1140**	73	69
Seaside Shrimp Trio	**1100**	58	94
Ultimate Feast	**1120**	69	68
Sides:			
Baked Potato, Plain	**210**	2	45
Broccoli	**40**	0	8
Cheddar Bay Biscuit	**160**	10	16
Coleslaw	**150**	10	13
Creamy Lobster Mashed Potatoes	**330**	18	31
French Fries	**290**	12	42
Garden Salad, without dressing	**100**	5	10
Mashed Potatoes	**190**	9	24
Rice Pilaf	**160**	3	30
Tomato Mozzarella Caprese	**160**	11	9
Salads:			
Caesar Salad: *With Caesar Dressing*			
with Gr. Chicken	**640**	48	19
with Gr. Shrimp	**610**	50	18
With Salmon	**830**	65	18
Sauces: 100% Pure Melted Butter	**300**	33	0
Blue Cheese Dressing	**230**	24	2
Caesar Dressing	**300**	32	0
Cocktail Sauce	**45**	0	11
Honey Mustard Dressing	**200**	18	9
Marinara Sauce	**35**	2	4
Desserts:			
Brownie Overload	**1020**	57	121
Chocolate Wave	**1110**	62	134
Key Lime Pie	**400**	14	59
Warm Apple Crostada	**590**	30	74

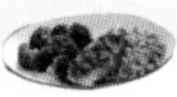
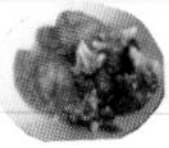
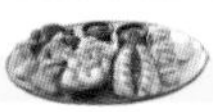
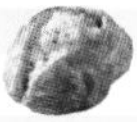
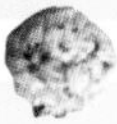
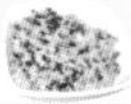
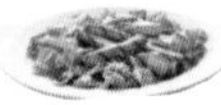
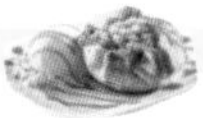

For Complete Nutritional Data ~ see CalorieKing.com

Red Robin® (Nov '20)

Nutritional Information varies between restaurants. Please refer to Red Robin's website for further information.

	C	F	Cb
Appetizers:			
Fried Pickle Nickels	**740**	50	62
Pretzel Bites	**810**	40	95
The O-Ring Shorty	**910**	56	94
Towering Onion Rings	**1290**	57	179
Jump Starters: *Without Dressing*			
Cheese Sticks	**550**	30	43
Fresh Fried Zucchini Sticks	**520**	43	28
Fried Jalapeono Coins	**560**	41	38
Sweet Potato Fries	**410**	14	68
Wings:			
Bone In Bar: with Buzz Sauce	**1260**	88	26
with Banzai Sauce	**1200**	70	49
with Whisky River Sauce	**1280**	76	58
Boneless: with Buzz Sauce	**990**	55	71
with Whisky River Sauce	**1010**	42	103
Burgers: *Without Fries or other Options*			
Finest: Black & Bleu	**850**	53	52
Smoke & Pepper	**790**	41	58
The MadLove	**1050**	58	71
The Master Cheese	**790**	45	48
The Southern Charm	**1130**	67	82
Gourmet:			
Burnin' Love	**910**	61	56
Guacamole Bacon	**930**	58	51
Keep It Simple, Beef	**530**	24	44
Red Robin Gourmet Cheeseburger	**800**	47	56
Royal Red Robin	**1110**	78	49
Sauteed 'Shroom	**770**	40	53
Veggie Burger	**750**	44	69
Veggie Vegan Burger	**320**	17	35
Whiskey River BBQ	**1140**	75	73
Tavern Menu Burgers:			
Haystack Double	**680**	43	39
Red's Double	**590**	36	32
The Big: Cowboy Ranch	**810**	46	60
Haystack	**930**	58	62
Pig Out	**1080**	70	63
Veggie Vegan Burger,			
with Steamed Broccoli	**260**	11	34
Entrées: *With Menu Set Sides*			
Arctic Cod Fish & Steak Fries	**1520**	89	135
Clucks & Fries	**1330**	82	104
Buffalo Style	**1630**	113	106
Ensenada Chicken Platter	**470**	18	20
Pub Mac 'N' Cheese w/ Caesar Salad	**1040**	68	75

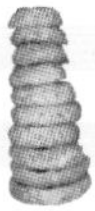
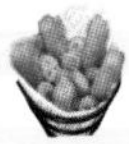
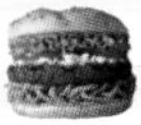
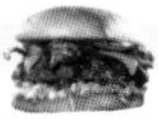
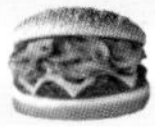
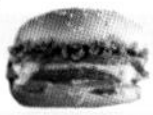
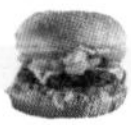

Updated Nutrition Data ~ www.CalorieKing.com
Persons with Diabetes ~ See Disclaimer (Page 22)

Red Robin® cont... (Nov '20)

S'wiches & Wraps: Without Sides	C	F	Cb
BLTA Croissant	680	41	50
Caesars Chicken Wrap	820	50	59
Whiskey River BBQ Chicken Wrap	1030	58	81
Soups:			
Chicken Tortilla: Cup	200	9	19
Bowl	390	19	37
Clam Chowder:			
Cup	210	15	12
Bowl	420	31	25
Red's Chili:			
Cup	210	9	18
Bowl	430	18	36
***Salads:** Without Dressing Unless Indicated*			
Avo-Cobb-O	510	26	25
Crispy Chicken Tender	880	50	60
Mighty Caesar, with Caesar Dressing	750	61	20
Simply Grilled Chicken	280	8	20
Southwest	900	63	41
Sides: Bottomless Steak Fries	360	16	49
Caesar Side, with dressing	230	21	8
Mac 'n' Cheese	290	16	26
Onion: Rings	280	1	61
Straws	200	14	16
Sauteed Mushrooms	140	7	13
Steamed Broccoli	30	0.5	6
Yukon Chips	500	35	41
Zucchini Fries	260	17	23
Desserts:			
Gooey Chocolate Brownie Cake	950	37	150
Mountain High Mudd Pie	1360	59	193

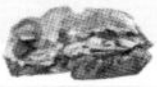
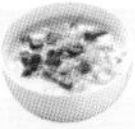
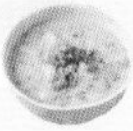
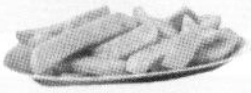
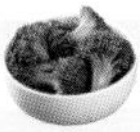

Roly Poly® (Nov '20)

Wraps: *Per 6" White Tortilla Unless Indicated*	C	F	Cb
Chicken: Basil Cashew Chicken	300	10	30
Chicken Caesar	310	11	30
Chicken Fajita	315	9	28
Santa Fe Chicken	305	11	28
Beef/Ham: Philly Melt	280	11	25
Ranch Roast	320	15	28
Tuna: Classic Tuna Melt	340	17	26
Popeyes Tuna on Wheat	305	10	31
Texas/Thai Hot Tuna, average	300	11	30
Turkey: Applejack	320	12	30
California	330	12	30
Veggie & Cheese:			
California Humer	305	13	32
Nutty Avocado on Wheat Tortilla	265	12	35
***Salads:** Without Dressing*			
Alpine Chef	315	16	13
Chipotle Caesar	520	25	21
Just Veggies	95	0	19
Walnut Spinach	420	33	14

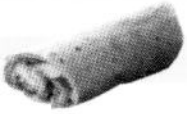
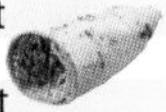
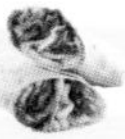
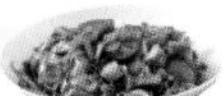

Round Table Pizza® (Nov '20)

Appetizers:	C	F	Cb
Boneless Wings, Oven Roasted:			
with BBQ Sauce (1)	100	2	13
with Buffalo Sauce (1)	90	3.5	8
Garlic Bread: 1 piece	70	3.5	9
with Cheese, 1 piece	110	6	9
Garlic Parmesan Twists, 1 twist	170	5	25
***Pizzas:** Per 1/12 of Large 14" Pizza*			
Original Crust: Cheese	230	10	24
Gourmet Veggie	230	10	25
Guinevere's Garden Delight	220	8	26
Hawaiian	220	8	27
Italian Garlic Supreme	270	14	24
King Arthur Supreme	270	13	26
Maui Zaui Chicken	260	11	28
Montague's All Meat Marvel	290	15	24
Smokehouse Combo, Pepperoni	290	14	27
Triple Play Pepperoni	250	12	24
Pan Crust: BBQ Dragon	330	16	37
Gourmet: Chkn & Garlic	290	10	35
Veggie	280	10	35
Guinevere's Garden Delight	270	9	36
Hawaiian	280	8	37
Hearty Bacon Supreme	330	14	34
King Arthur Supreme	320	13	35
MacDougal	190	1.5	38
Montague's All Meat Marvel	340	16	35
Pepperoni	300	12	34
Triple Play Pepperoni	310	13	34
Skinny Crust: BBQ Chicken	260	12	24
Chicken Garlic Gourmet	220	11	19
Garden Pesto	230	12	20
Gourmet Veggie	210	10	20
Hawaiian	210	8	22
King Arthur Supreme	260	14	21
MacDougal	100	1	20
Smokehouse Combo, Chicken	260	12	22
West Coast Combo	250	14	19
Sandwiches: Chicken Club	670	27	58
Ham Club	670	30	59
Hero	800	41	59
Meatball	750	37	70
RT Pizza Veggie	550	21	62
Salami	970	59	59
Turkey Club	650	27	59
Tukey Pesto	710	37	56

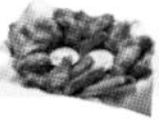
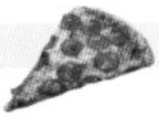
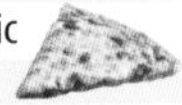
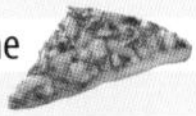
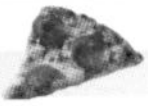
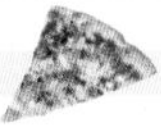
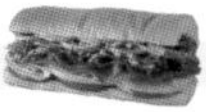
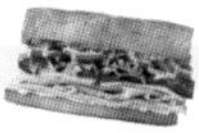

For Complete Nutritional Data ~ see CalorieKing.com

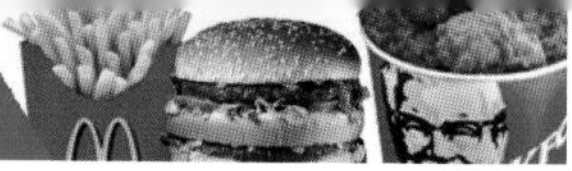

Rubio's Coastal Grill® (Nov '20)

Burritos: Flour Tortilla, w/o Chips	C	F	Cb
Beef: California, with Steak	1120	63	88
Especial, with Steak	930	39	103
Chicken, Especial, with Chicken	880	34	105
Seafood: Ancho Shrimp	830	34	103
Beer Battered Fish	940	55	83
Classic Grilled Shrimp	880	35	101
Grilled Wild Alaska Salmon	830	36	95
Grilled Wild Mahi Mahi	830	36	93
Shrimp & Bacon	1010	52	93
Tacos: With Corn Tortilla Unless Indicated			
Chicken: *Per One Taco*			
Classic All Natural	250	12	21
Grilled Gourmet	350	19	22
Seafood: *Per One Taco*			
Grilled: Wild Mahi Mahi, Flour Tortilla	270	13	23
Wild Alask. Salmon	230	10	23
Wild Mahi Mahi	230	9	22
House Blackened: Mahi Mahi	240	10	24
Mango Wild Gropher	270	14	23
Salsa Verde Shrimp, Flour Tortilla	290	17	23
Steak, Grilled: *Per One Taco*			
Classic	270	14	20
Gourmet	370	21	22
Street	120	5	9
Sides:			
Black Beans: Reg., 4 oz	100	2	15
Large, 9.4 oz	280	2.5	46
Citrus Rice: Reg., 2.3 oz	100	1.5	21
Large, 6 oz	270	3.5	55
Mexican Rice: Regular, 2.3 oz	100	1.5	20
Large, 6 oz	270	4	53
No Fried Pinto Beans: Reg., 4 oz	110	1	17
Large, 10.9 oz	300	2	51
Tortilla Chips: Regular, 1.8 oz	210	2.5	43
Large, 4 oz	460	5	96
Salsas, average all varieties	15	0	3
Salad & Bowls: Entrée Size, Includes Dressing			
Keto Style:			
Balsamic & Grilled Veggie	380	32	24
Keto, with Salmon	620	44	21
Keto, with Steak	620	44	21
Chopped:	380	30	19
Keto, with Salmon	500	36	14
Keto, with Steak	500	36	14
Mango Avocado	460	33	39

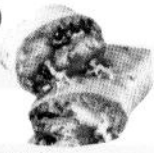
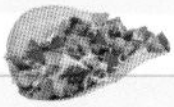
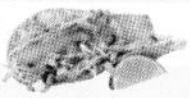
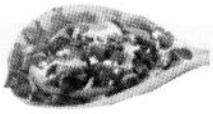
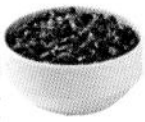
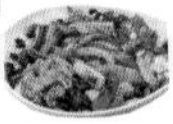
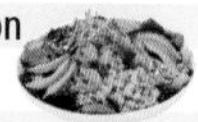

Ruby Tuesday® (Nov '20)

Shareables: As Served	C	F	Cb
Bang' Shrimp: Classic	570	38	34
Spicy	920	74	39
Classic Sampler	1500	72	152
Spinach Artichoke Dip	900	57	72
Burgers: Without Fries			
Bacon Cheeseburger	815	47	36
Classic	665	35	36
Classic Cheeseburger	720	39	36
Hickory Bourbon Bacon	950	53	46
Mushroom & Swiss	870	50	40
Smokehouse	975	52	61
Lunch/Dinner Entrees: Single, Without Sides			
Chicken: Asiago Bacon	480	27	9
Parmesan	1525	69	135
Fresco	370	22	2
Hickory Bourbon	250	5	18
Pasta: Cajun Chicken & Shrimp	600	21	41
Chicken & Broccoli	1395	81	101
Parmesan Shrimp	505	20	48
Ribs & Chops:			
Hickory Boubon Pork Chop	570	22	23
Classic BBQ Ribs: Half Rack	470	22	21
Full Rack	940	47	42
Texas Dusted Ribs: Half Rack	590	33	24
Full Rack	1100	68	30
Seafood: Blackened Tilapia	195	3	1
Grilled Salmon	325	17	0
Hickory Bourbon Salmon	410	17	18
New Orleans Seafood	335	11	3
Steak:			
Asiago Peppercorn Sirloin, 8 oz	355	16	7
Hickory B'rbon Bacon Sirloin, 6 oz	280	7	10
Ribeye, 12 oz	725	56	0
Top Sirloin, 8 oz	355	19	2
Lunch Combos:			
Chicken Quesadilla	850	41	46
Sandwiches: Crispy Chicken	715	31	67
with Pimento	1095	64	75
Sliders:			
Classic Cheeseburger:			
with Fries	790	41	70
with Tater Tots	745	38	65
Crispy Chicken Club:			
with Fries	845	42	78
with Tater Tots	800	39	73
Salads: Crispy Ranch with Dressing	710	45	41
Grilled Chicken Caesar w/ Dressing	515	35	16

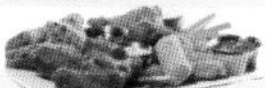
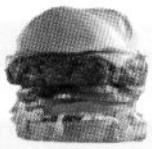
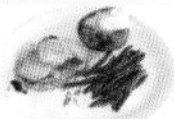
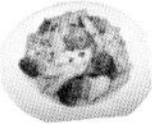
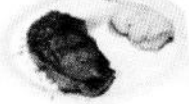
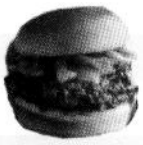
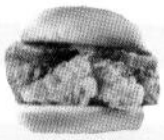

Updated Nutrition Data ~ www.CalorieKing.com
Persons with Diabetes ~ See Disclaimer (Page 22)

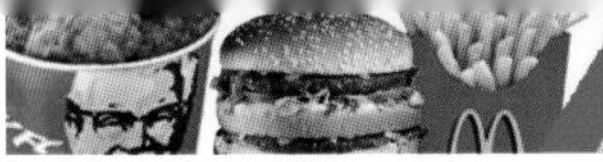

Ruby Tuesday® cont... (Nov '20)

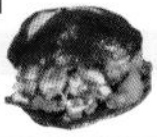
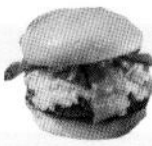
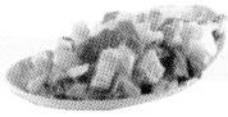
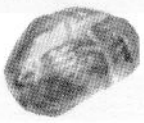
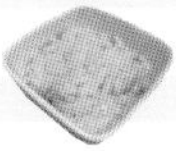
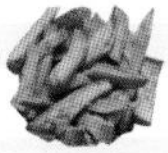
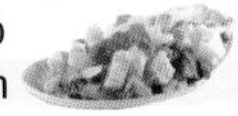
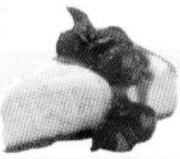

Lunch Combos Cont:	C	F	Cb
Soup: Broccoli Cheese	260	18	17
Garden Vegetable	85	1	16
Roasted Tomato	270	14	24
Turkey Burger	650	35	36
Sandwiches: *Without French Fries*			
Avocado Grilled Chicken	710	35	38
Avocado Turkey Burger	825	49	38
Cajun Grilled Chicken	800	50	37
Crispy Chicken: Classic	715	31	67
with Pimentos	1095	64	75
Spicy	1060	67	72
with Pimentos	1445	100	80
Sides:			
Braised Green Beans	50	2	6
Caesar Salad, with Caesar Dressing	590	52	17
Coleslaw	215	17	16
Dirty Rice	240	7	28
French Fries	505	24	63
Fresh: Baked Potato	250	3	51
Grilled Zucchini	20	0	2
Steamed Broccoli	45	1	4
Garden Salad, without Dressing	265	18	13
Loaded Baked Potato	560	27	51
Mac 'N Cheese	560	29	46
Mashed Potatoes	295	16	32
Onion Rings	340	19	37
Sweet Potato	240	12	29
Sweet Potato Fries	445	23	55
Tater Tots	365	16	45
White Rice	190	1	40
Salads: *With Dressing*			
BBQ Chicken Cobb	625	31	25
Crispy Chkn Ranch	1030	67	56
Grilled Chicken Caesar	855	53	33
Desserts: *As Served*			
Apple Crumble Skillet	875	46	103
Cake: Chocolate Fall	1310	65	164
Chocolate Lava	620	31	76
Pineapple Upside Down	495	19	73
Chocolate Chip Cookie Skillet	1350	69	172
New York Cheesecake	975	61	90

For Complete Menu ~ see CalorieKing.com

Runza® (Nov '20)

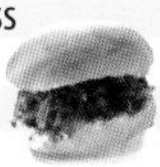
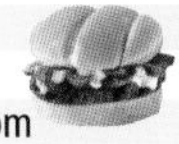
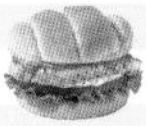
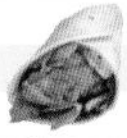
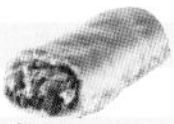
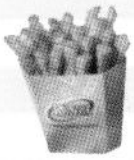
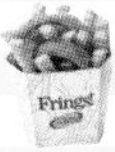
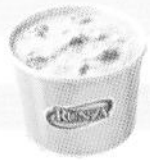
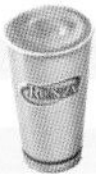

Burgers:	C	F	Cb
¼ LB: BBQ Bacon & Swiss	530	32	26
Bacon Cheeseburger	490	28	23
Cheeseburger	410	22	23
French Onion	490	29	26
Hamburger	350	18	21
Spicy Jack	570	38	23
Swiss Cheese Mushroom	480	29	24
Chicken Sandwiches:			
BBQ Grilled	400	11	40
Buffalo Grilled	360	11	37
Spicy Jack Grilled	530	28	26
Wraps: Buffalo Jr.	330	17	32
Ranch Jr.	330	17	31
Chicken Strips, 2 pieces	220	12	14
Runza Sandwiches: Original	530	20	67
Cheese Runza	590	25	69
Original Vegetarian	530	9	94
Spicy Jack Runza	750	41	69
SW Black Bean Vegetarian	470	12	76
Swiss Cheese Mushroom Runza	620	28	68
Sides: Chili	290	11	26
French Fries: Small	210	9	28
Medium	300	13	40
Large	440	19	59
French Onion Dip	70	5	3
Frings, Medium	320	17	39
Onion Rings: Medium	320	19	35
Large	550	31	58
Side Salad	20	0	4
Salads: *Without Dressing*			
Southwest Chicken Salad, w/ Salsa	360	18	32
Sweet Berry Chicken	400	20	20
Dressings: Honey Mustard	200	18	9
SW Ranch	220	24	4
Soups: *Per Bowl*			
Boston Clam Chowder	280	15	29
Broccoli Cheese	240	16	20
Chicken Tortilla	150	6	16
Potato Bacon	260	14	30
Kids: Chicken Strip Meal, w/o drink	430	21	42
Junior: Cheeseburger, plain	260	13	18
Hamburger, plain	200	9	16
Swiss Cheese Mushroom Burger	300	17	17
Desserts:			
Chocolate Chip Cookie	370	18	53
Ice Cream Cones, all flavors	210	6	32
Shake, Cappuccino, regular	490	12	82
Sundaes: Caramel; Chocolate	300	7	51
Turtle	360	13	53

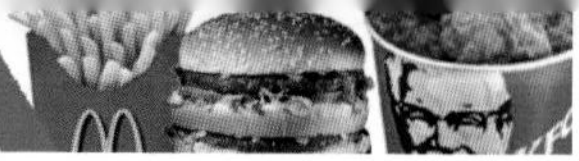

7-Eleven® (Sept '18)

Breakfast Sandwiches:	C	F	Cb
Biscuits:			
Sausage, 3.3 oz	330	22	28
Spicy Chicken, 4.5 oz	270	14	30
Croissants:			
Sausage, Egg & Cheese, 4.7 oz	450	32	23
English Muffin:			
Egg, Bacon & Chse, 4.5 oz	300	14	28
Egg, Cheese & Sausage, 5 oz	390	25	24
Salads: Per Container			
Balsamic Garden Salad, with Chicken, 6.5 oz	170	9	18
BLT, 8 oz	270	18	12
Caprese Salad, 4.5 oz	150	11	7
Chicken Caesar, 7.5 oz	390	28	17
Chicken Caesar Pasta Salad, 9 oz	540	24	61
Kale & Quinoa Salad, 6 oz	300	18	30
Mediterranean Pasta Salad, 8.5 oz	490	29	49
Side, 5 oz	30	0	7
Sandwiches/Melts:			
Chicken, Bacon Ranch Melt, 7.4 oz	560	22	56
Chicken Salad Sandwich, 6.6 oz	470	21	49
Double Cheeseburger, with American Cheese, 9.6 oz	800	54	35
Egg Salad Sandwich, 6.8 oz	480	24	50
Go!Smart Turkey Sandwich	300	2.5	48
Grilled Chicken Sandwich, w/ Honey Mustard BBQ Sauce, 6 oz	340	10	39
Italian Melt, 7.8 oz	610	39	38
Southwest Turkey Sandwich, 8 oz	560	28	48
Steak & Cheese Melt, 7.8 oz	680	35	57
Sides:			
Hash Brown (1), 2 oz	100	5	12
Potato Wedges (6), 0.7 oz	240	4.5	27
Taquitos,			
Chicken & Monterey Jack, (2), 5.3 oz	330	12	44
Drinks: Cappuccino, 8 fl.oz	180	4	36
Caramel Macchiato, 8 fl.oz	190	5	34
Cuban Coffee, with milk, 8 fl.oz	200	7	34
French Vanilla Cappuccino, 8 fl.oz	190	6	34
Skinny, 8 fl.oz	140	4.5	30
Hot Chocolate, 8 fl.oz	170	2.5	37
Peppermint Mocha, 8 fl.oz	180	4	36
Pumpkin Spice Late, 8 fl.oz	190	6	35
Slurpees, average all flavors:			
12 oz cup	95	0	26
22 oz cup	175	0	44
28 oz cup	220	0	56
Sugar Free, 12 oz cup	30	0	9

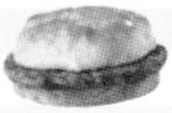

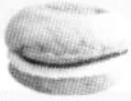

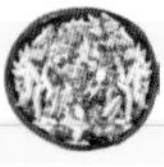

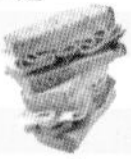

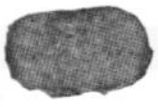

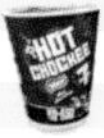

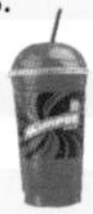

Saladworks® (Nov '20)

Salads: W/out Dressing or Bread	C	F	Cb
Bently	290	15	11
Buffalo Bleu	350	12	29
Chicken Caesar	370	15	29
Cobb	370	23	19
Farmhouse	270	12	28
Fire Roasted Cabo	350	17	25
Mandarin Chicken	230	4	25
Mediterranean	330	23	16
Sophie's	310	13	35
Thai Chicken	200	6	20
Tivoli	470	21	41
Turkey Club	290	2	38
Paninis: Buffalo Chicken	870	36	85
Caprese	940	47	94
Chicken Parmesan	870	32	93
Turkey Melt	1020	49	90
Sandwiches: Avocado BLT	830	55	60
Chicken Salad	370	9	28
Tuna Salad	410	8	54
West Coast Turkey	580	30	51
Wraps: Bentley	550	21	63
Buffalo Bleu	660	20	82
Chicken Caesar	610	20	81
Cobb	690	33	71
Farmhouse	590	20	82
Fire Roasted Cabo	670	25	78
Mandarin Chicken	530	12	83
Mediterranean	650	34	92
Sophie's Salad	550	17	81
Thai Chicken	410	9	70
Tivoli	610	28	63
Turkey Club	460	14	61
Soups: Per Medium Serve, without Bread Roll			
Baked Potato	340	23	28
Broccoli Cheddar	280	19	18
Chicken Dumpling	180	6	21
Chicken Noodle	180	5	18
Chicken Tortilla	260	14	19
Homestyle Tomato	300	21	25
Lasagna, with Turkey Sausage	230	11	21
Maine Lobster Bisque	470	39	21
New England Clam Chowder	370	26	22

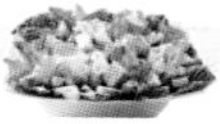

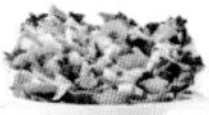

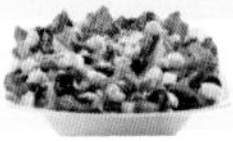

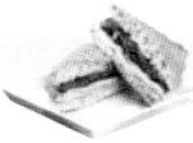

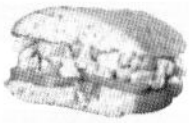

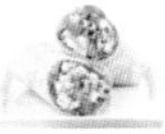

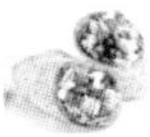

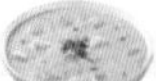

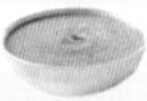

Updated Nutrition Data ~ www.CalorieKing.com
Persons with Diabetes ~ See Disclaimer (Page 22)

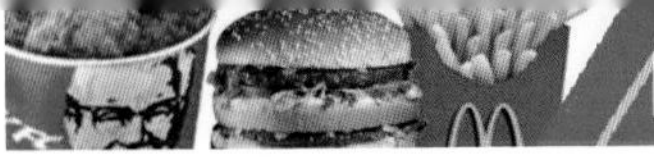

Sandella's® (Nov '20)

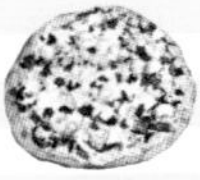
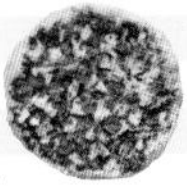

Grilled Flatbread:	C	F	Cb
BBQ Cheese	430	9	67
Bacon & Cheddar	630	34	54
Chicken Fajita	500	18	52
Chicken Parmesan	560	20	55
El Paso	710	19	97
Ham & Cheddar	570	25	51
Meatball	630	29	56
Olympian	480	26	53
Pesto & Peppers	530	27	52
Spinach & Artichoke	610	33	54
Thai Chicken	630	24	66
Tomato Bacon	580	26	58
***Paninis:** With Standard Toppings*			
Americana	580	25	54
Arizona Chicken	660	23	78
BBQ Chicken	490	2	92
Beef Fajita	630	27	58
Bistro Ham & Brie	560	19	70
Brazilian Beef, without cheese	500	6	86
Holiday Ham	770	21	110
Napoli Chicken	440	17	49
Pastrami Melt	670	33	55
Philly Cheese	590	25	55
Spinach & Bacon	610	29	65
Toasted Caprese	380	14	50
***Quesadillas:** With Standard Toppings*			
Barbecue	570	18	66
Beef Fajita	570	22	55
Buffalo Chicken	510	20	49
Thai Veggie	570	27	60
***Salads:** With ½ Flatbread, without Dressing*			
Apple Walnut	370	13	60
Napa Valley	770	60	54
Panzanella	190	3	36
Siesta	310	15	44
Thai Chicken	330	13	35
***Rice Bowls:** Includes Flatbread & Standard Toppings*			
Asian Chicken & Broccoli	680	3	138
Mesquite BBQ	930	21	140
Southwest Veggie	810	20	126
Thai Peanut Saute	680	16	116
***Wraps:** With Standard Toppings*			
California Turkey	410	10	55
Greek Salad	370	13	55
Nut & Honey	800	32	116
Seven Layer	570	23	66
Swiss Salad	500	20	62
Texas Beef	420	10	58
The Russian	400	7	60
Veggie & Cheese	450	19	52

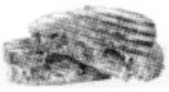
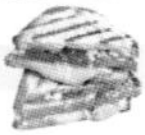
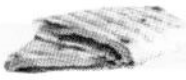
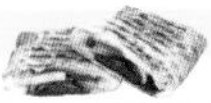
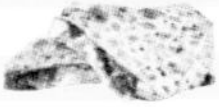
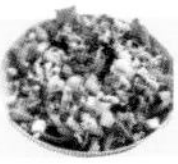
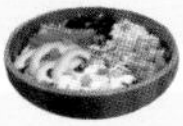
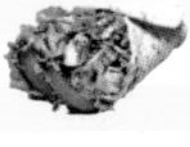

Sarku Japan® (Nov '20)

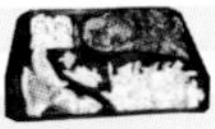
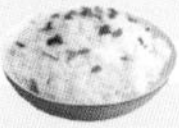
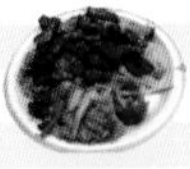

Bento Box:	C	F	Cb
Fried Rice: Beef	830	32	98
Chicken	820	35	95
Shrimp	750	27	96
D'Lite Meals, Vegetarian:			
Fried Rice	430	10	79
Noodles	640	14	109
Steamed Rice	410	6	83
***Teriyaki Meals:** With Steamed Rice*			
Beef	580	16	80
Beef & Shrimp	690	21	85
Chicken	640	24	79
Chicken & Shrimp	750	29	85
Shrimp	530	12	80
Sushi Rolls: California	330	8	57
Chicken Teriyaki	360	11	53
Dancing Eel	430	13	61
Green Dragon	650	35	71
Philadelphia	430	18	49
Rainbow	360	7	51
Rock & Roll	550	21	66
Salmon	220	5	33
Tuna	190	0	33
Sauce, Teriyaki, 1.5 oz	45	0	9
Sides: Chicken Egg Roll	160	6	21
Dumplings (6)	260	12	29
Edamame	170	7	11
Miso Soup	50	2	6
Seaweed Salad	70	2	13
Shrimp Tempura (3)	390	30	23
Vegetable Spring Roll	190	9	15

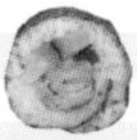
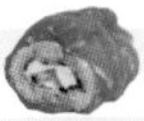
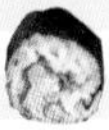
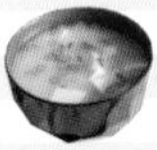

Schlotzsky's® (Nov '20)

***Sandwiches:** Per Medium*	C	F	Cb
Angus Beef & Cheese	780	30	81
Beef Bacon Smokecheesy	810	43	77
Chicken Bacon Smokecheesy	860	31	80
Chipotle Chicken	530	9	78
Cuban Brisket	770	30	75
Deluxe Original	980	47	81
Fiesta Chicken	810	31	78
Fresh Veggie	500	14	74
Ham & Cheese, Original	730	25	81
Smoked Turkey Breast	500	6	80
The Original	780	34	78
The Sicilian	730	43	42
The Tuscan	700	35	49
Turkey Bacon Club	770	30	81
Turkey Original	820	33	81
Turkey & Guacamole	520	11	78

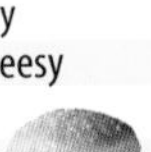
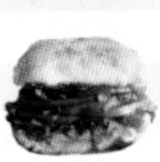
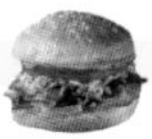

continued next page...

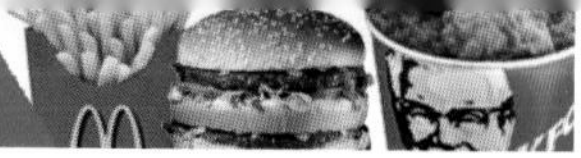

Schlotzsky's® cont... (Nov '20)

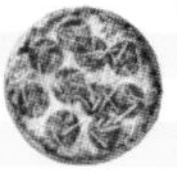

Pizzas: Per 10" Pizza	C	F	Cb
BBQ Chkn & Jalapeno	**920**	21	148
Combination Special	**960**	38	119
Grilled Chicken & Pesto	**910**	29	114
Pepperoni & Double Cheese	**980**	42	115
Macs: Brisketeer	**1090**	49	69
Double Cheese	**830**	43	69
Poultry In Motion	**1130**	47	70
Shrimpy The Best	**1070**	45	71
Smokey Brisketeer	**1120**	50	74
Salads: *Without Dressing or Breadsticks*			
Chicken Caesar	**680**	17	29
Cranberry, Apple, Pecan & Chicken	**640**	27	68
Southwest Chicken	**600**	29	44
Turkey Avocado Cobb	**610**	33	42
Dressing: Blue Cheese, 3 oz	**460**	49	3
Caesar, 3 oz	**430**	45	2
Italian, 3 oz	**280**	28	3
Thousand Island, 3 oz	**360**	12	5
Soup: *Per 10 oz Bowl*			
Broccoli Cheese	**185**	12	14
Chicken & Wild Rice	**280**	14	25
Chicken Tortilla	**315**	16	27
Loaded Potato	**385**	31	29
Timberline Chili	**380**	21	27
Tomato Basil	**320**	26	21
Chips:			
Baked: Regular; BBQ	**140**	4	26
Other varieties, average	**230**	14	24
Kidz Meals: *Without Cookie or Drink*			
Cheese Pizza	**540**	17	78
Ham Sandwich	**220**	2	40
Pepperoni Pizza	**590**	22	78
Turkey Sandwich	**220**	1.5	40
Desserts:			
Brownie (1)	**420**	23	46
Cookies: Chocolate Chip (1)	**160**	7	24
Oatmeal Raisin; Sugar, (1), av.	**155**	5	24
Breakfast: *Per Whole Burrito/Sandwich*			
Burritos: Bacon	**460**	22	41
Ham	**490**	21	44
Sausage	**570**	31	41
Veggie	**430**	19	44
Sandwiches: Bacon; Veggie	**500**	21	51
Ham	**530**	22	50
Sausage	**650**	32	49
Tacos: Bacon; Sausage, average	**250**	14	19
Ham	**290**	17	18
Veggie	**220**	10	21
Sides:			
Hash Brown, 1 piece	**60**	5	8
Mixed Fruit, 1 scoop	**20**	0	5

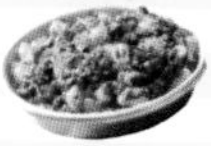

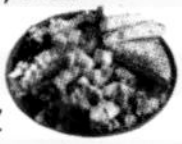

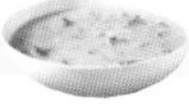

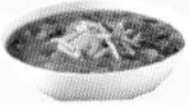

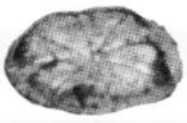

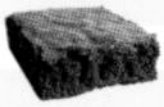

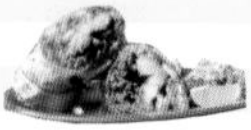

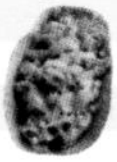

Second Cup® ~ *see CalorieKing.com*

Shake Shack® (Nov '20)

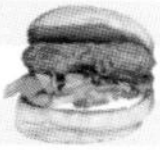

Burgers: Per Single Burger	C	F	Cb
Bacon Cheeseburger	**540**	33	25
Cheeseburger	**470**	28	25
Crackle Shack	**580**	37	25
Green Chile CheddarShack	**510**	30	28
Hamburger, without toppings	**400**	22	24
Lockhart Link	**810**	60	27
Shack Stack	**800**	49	50
Shroom Burger	**550**	31	49
SmokeShack	**610**	39	28
Veggie Shack	**530**	27	56
Vegan Style	**390**	22	50
Chicken: Bites (6)	**300**	15	18
Hot Chick'N Sandwich	**560**	31	38
Flat-Top Dogs: Chicken Dog	**310**	13	27
Garden Dog	**220**	10	28
Hot Dog	**390**	26	25
Shack-Cago Dog	**410**	26	29
Fries: Bacon Cheese	**840**	52	65
Cheese	**710**	44	64
Regular	**470**	22	63
Floats, Creamsicle; Purple Cow, av.	**450**	15	77
Shakes:			
Chocolate	**750**	45	76
Salted Caramel	**840**	42	99
Vanilla	**680**	36	72
Breakfast: Bacon Sandwich	**440**	27	25
Egg & Cheese Sandwich	**370**	23	25
Sausage Sandwich	**560**	37	28

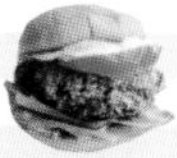

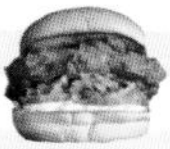

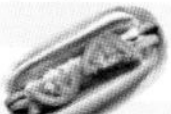

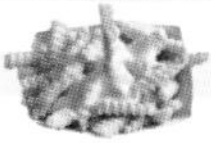

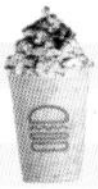

Shakey's® (Nov '20)

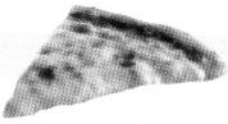

Pizzas: Per Slice, 1/10 Medium Size 12" Pizza	C	F	Cb
Big Island: Pan Crust	**210**	6	30
Thin Crust	**160**	6	19
California Pizzarito: Pan Crust	**265**	12	30
Thin Crust	**215**	11	19
Cheese: Pan Crust	**190**	5	30
Thin Crust	**135**	5	17
Firehouse: Pan Crust	**280**	13	30
Thin Crust	**230**	12	20
Garden Veggie: Pan Crust	**205**	6	30
Thin Crust	**150**	6	19
Rustic Garlic Chicken: Pan Crust	**215**	6	30
Thin Crust	**160**	6	18
Shakey's Special: Pan Crust	**255**	11	30
Thin Crust	**200**	10	18
Texas BBQ Chicken: Pan Crust	**220**	6	32
Thin Crust	**165**	5	20
Ultimate Meat: Pan Crust	**310**	15	30
Thin Crust	**260**	14	20

Shakey's® cont... (Nov '20)

Golden Fried Chicken: Per Piece	C	F	Cb
Breast	360	11	16
Leg	175	10	6
Thigh	350	24	9
Wing	130	9	4
***Rice:** Per ½ Cup*			
Mexican Fiesta	100	0	22
Pilaf	120	3	22
Sides & Extras: Enchilada (1)	80	2	37
Boneless Chicken Strip (1)	125	7	10
Garlic Bread, 1 piece	180	4	30
Macaroni & Cheese, 1 cup	350	17	33
Macaroni Salad, ½ cup	220	14	19
Mashed Potatoes, ½ cup	65	1	13
Mojo Potatoes, 5 pieces	215	11	5

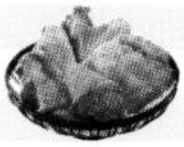
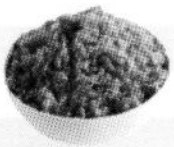
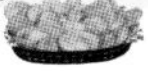

Shari's® (Nov '20)

***Breakfast:** As Served*	C	F	Cb
Bacon & Eggs without extras	290	22	1
Buttermilk Pancakes	800	27	123
Cheese & Ham Omelette	670	52	7
Country Sausage Benedict	1470	102	90
Double Smoked Sausage & Egg	450	32	6
French Toast, Traditional	960	62	82
Meat Lover's Skillet	1100	86	38
Oatmeal	570	21	88
Sausage & Eggs Only	630	57	1
Shari's Sampler	1610	105	116
Ultimate Country Fried Steak	1060	72	67
Waffle	340	14	48
***Lunch:** Without Side Choices*			
Chicken Strips	340	18	23
Salads: *Entrée Size, with Dressing*			
Caesar	460	40	15
Northwest Steak	890	50	65
Rustic Tuscan Chicken	510	32	21
Sandwiches: *Per Whole Sandwich*			
BLT on Texas Toast	540	26	51
Cajun Chicken Avocado Club	1360	74	115
Cuban on Ciabatta Roll	680	30	60
Grilled Ham & Four Cheese Melt, on Sourdough	1140	68	78
Hot Turkey on Whole Wheat	1040	31	129
Prime Rib Dip on French Roll	680	33	63
Traditional Club	1310	72	114
***Dinner:** With Menu Set Sides*			
Beer Battered Fish & Chips	1600	119	104
Chopped Steak	930	50	50
Country Fried Steak	1010	63	83
Grilled Lemon Chicken	450	17	17
Slow Roasted Turkey	980	50	109
Wild Alaskan Salmon, grilled	470	28	19

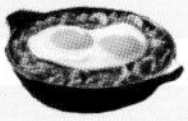
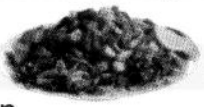
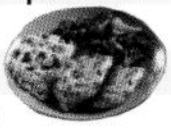

Shari's® cont... (Nov '20)

Sides, Add-Ons:	C	F	Cb
Baked Potato: Plain	210	5	37
with Sour Cream & Butter	330	18	38
Broccoli	130	11	7
Coleslaw	140	10	11
French Fries	490	32	48
Loaded Baked Potato	330	15	38
Loaded Mashed Potatoes	410	21	42
Rice Pilaf	90	5	10
Shrimp Skewer	90	1	1
Stuffed Hash Browns	420	28	32
Tater Tots	370	26	33
Desserts:			
Pies:			
Banana Cream Dream	450	26	48
Chocolate Cream Supreme	510	30	54
Creamy Caramel Pecan Crunch	730	49	67
Peanut Butter Chocolate Silk	620	45	51
Tropical Coconut Cream	580	37	63

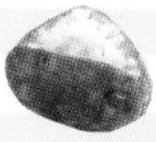
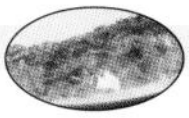
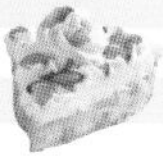

Sheetz® (Nov '20)

Breakfast Sandwiches:	C	F	Cb
Dreamy Bacon Croissant	400	25	28
Twisted BLT	710	42	53
Walker Breakfast Ranger	550	23	58
Burgerz: Big Mozz	670	33	57
Boss Bacon	790	56	35
Cowboy	730	39	56
Twisted Swiss	760	45	50
***Hot Dogs:** With Standard Hot Dog*			
BLT	450	28	33
Junkyard	340	16	38
Philly	360	19	39
Shmokehouse	390	20	40
Mac & Cheese Platter: Boom Chicka	510	27	40
Meatball	610	37	35
Morning	500	30	38
Sandwichez:			
Deli: Boom Boom BLT	820	46	52
Ciabatta Bing	620	34	54
Garden of Eatin	470	18	59
Grilled Chicken Breast: Big Mozz	600	19	60
Carolina Slaw	490	17	46
Twisted Brunch	800	42	54
Shwingz: with BBq Sauce (6)	540	28	39
with Boom Boom Sauce	700	55	20
with Garlic Parmesan Sauce	660	50	18
with Spicy Asian Sauce	540	30	37

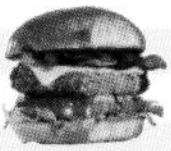
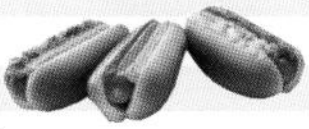
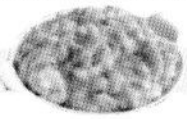
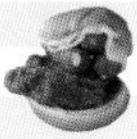

continued next page...

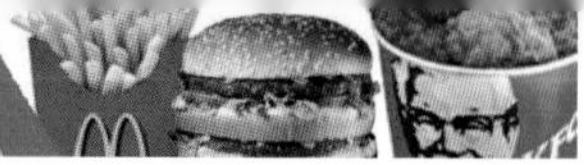

Sheetz® cont... (Nov '20)

Subz: Per Half	C	F	Cb
Big Philly Sub, on Pretzel Sub	**590**	19	71
Cali Turkey Flatbread Sub	**820**	43	65
Southwest Veggie, on White Sub	**470**	20	61
Sidez:			
Coleslaw	**250**	11	35
Crispy Chicken Stripz, w/out sauce:			
3 pieces	**330**	11	39
5 pieces	**550**	18	65
Fryz, without sauce, 1 cup	**390**	13	64
Hard Cooked Egg (1)	**70**	4.5	0
Jalapeno Poppers, without Sauce	**330**	18	35
Loaded Fryz, without toppings	**600**	20	97
Mac & Cheese, without toppings	**190**	7	25
Onion Rings, without sauce, 1 cup	**470**	27	52
Popcorn Chicken, without Sauce:			
Regular	**300**	14	28
Large	**610**	28	55
***Beverages:** With 2% Milk & Chocoalte Sauce*			
Caramel Hot Chocolate	**700**	23	109
Hot Chocolate	**730**	22	118

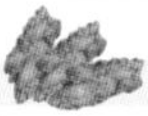
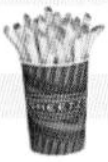
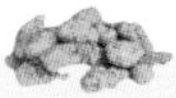

Sizzler® (Nov '20)

Menus May Vary. Please Check Your Local Outlet For Menu Choices And Further Nutritional Information.

Burgers & Sandwiches:	C	F	Cb
Classic ⅓ lb Burger	**830**	57	44
Mega Bacon Burger	**940**	61	49
Smokey Bacon Burger	**950**	5	47
***Entrees:** Without Sides, Condiments, Dipping Sauce or Optional Accompaniments*			
Chicken: *Small Plate*			
Italian Herb Chicken	**230**	6	1
Malibu Chicken	**680**	60	14
Combo Nation:			
Classic Steak Trio	**1270**	89	48
Steak & Jumbo Crispy Shrimp (8)	**720**	32	47
Steak & Lobster	**720**	51	2
Steak & Malibu Chicken	**920**	73	14
Ribs:			
BBQ: 6 bones	**1870**	145	32
3 Bones & BBQ Chicken, 7 oz	**1170**	70	34

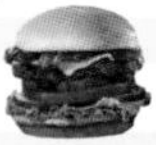
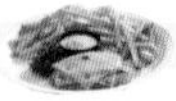
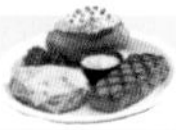
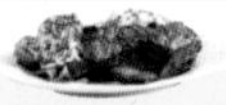

Sizzler® cont... (Nov '20)

Entrees (Cont):	C	F	Cb
Seafood: Grilled Salmon, 6 oz	**370**	23	3
Cilantro Lime Barramundi	**470**	17	37
Jumbo Shrimp Skewers (2)	**440**	15	29
Steaks:			
New York Strip, 12 oz	**830**	61	2
Ribeye, 14 oz	**1100**	88	3
Tri-Tip Sirloin, 8 oz	**340**	16	0.5
Steak Toppings: Grilled Onions	**80**	6	7
Sauteed Button Mushrooms	**180**	17	5
Sides: Cheese Toast	**290**	19	22
Cilantro Lime Rice	**150**	0	31
Garlic Mashed Potatoes	**200**	3.5	39
Rice Pilaf	**170**	3.5	31
Salted Baked Potato	**510**	30	55
Loaded	**760**	57	55
Street Fries	**500**	31	52
Vegetable Medley	**80**	4.5	8
Yeast Roll	**190**	7	29

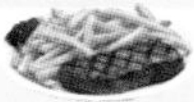
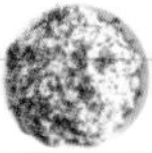
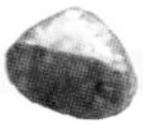

Skyline Chili® (Nov '20)

Burritos:	C	F	Cb
Chili Deluxe	**610**	33	38
Original	**610**	31	54
Coneys/Sandwiches:			
Coneys: Cheese, w/ onions & mstrd	**350**	23	25
Coney, plain	**220**	13	22
Sandwiches: Chili Cheese, with onions & mustard	**290**	17	24
Chili, with onions & mustard	**180**	8	23
***Ways:** Per Regular Serving*			
Chili Spaghetti with Bean & Onion:			
Small	**250**	10	34
Regular	**490**	19	68
Large	**670**	26	94
Bowls: Chili	**200**	12	0
Loaded Chili	**480**	28	20
Vegetarian Black Beans & Rice	**400**	14	48
Steamed Potatoes:			
3-Way Potato	**620**	26	65
Cheddar Potato	**630**	33	65
Sour Cream Potato	**460**	19	65
***Salads:** Without Dressing*			
Buffalo Chicken	**220**	11	12
Greek	**210**	12	17
Fries: Chili Cheese	**840**	53	61
Regular Fries	**430**	24	51

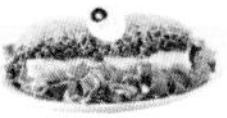
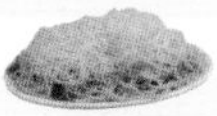
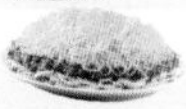
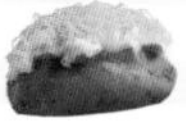
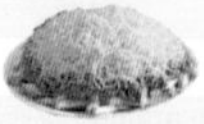

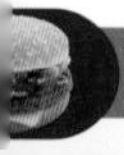

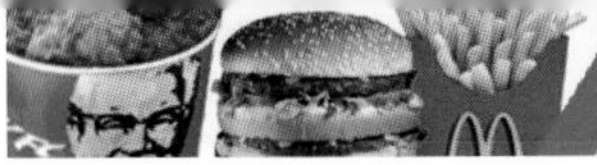

Smoothie King® (Nov '20)

Fruit Smoothies: Per 20 oz Cup

	C	F	Cb
Break Time Blends: *With Turbinado*			
Angel Food	350	0	84
Banana Boat	480	6	99
Caribbean Way	390	0	98
Coffe D-Lite: Mocha	350	5	61
Vanilla	270	5	44
Passion Passport	410	0	102
Pineapple Surf	420	1.5	99
Fitness Blends: *Without Turbinado*			
HIIT Fit:			
Chocolate Cinnamon	420	15	44
Veggie Mango	400	15	41
Keto Champ: Berry	430	31	19
Chocolate	430	31	18
Coffee	420	31	14
Original High Protein:			
Banana	340	12	35
Chocolate	400	12	44
Pineapple	320	12	29
Peanut Power Plus: Chocolate:	600	24	77
Strawberry	680	23	110
The Activator: Chocolate	210	2.5	21
Blueberry Strawberry	260	1.5	39
Strawberry Banana	200	2	24
The Hulk: With Turbinado			
Chocolate; Vanilla	710	32	101
Strawberry	850	32	136
Slim Blends: *With Stevia*			
Metabolism Boost: Mango Ginger	280	3.5	49
Strawberry Pineapple	280	3	51
Slim-N-Trim: Chocolate	220	2.5	36
Strawberry	150	2.5	26
Vanilla	180	2.5	34
The Shredder: Strawberry	310	2.5	46
Vanilla	230	4	17
Wellness Blends: *Without Turbinado*			
Blueberry Heaven	260	1.5	57
Vegan: Mango Kale	330	6	66
Dark Chocolate Banana	350	1.5	81
Pineapple Spinach	360	6	75

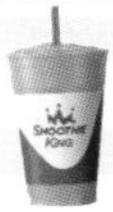
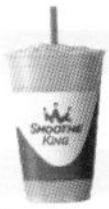
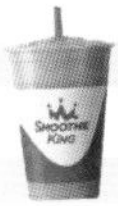
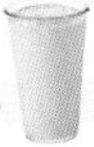
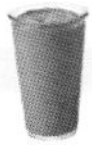
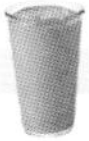
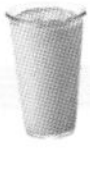
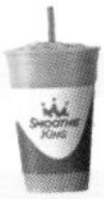

Snappy Tomato® (Nov '20)

Snappetizers:	C	F	Cb
Bone In Wings (6)	460	34	4
Flatbread, medium, ⅙ flatbread	270	12	33
Wedge Fries, plain	220	10	28
Hoagies:			
Italian Combo	650	23	69
Steak & Cheese	760	35	73
Veggie Melt	490	11	74
Pasta: Plain Spaghetti/Rigatoni, av.	350	1.5	70
Toppings: Bacon	120	8	1
Black or Green Olives	50	4.5	2
Cheese	90	7	1
Chicken	120	2.5	1
Pepperoni	140	10	0
Tomatoes	5	0	1
Sauce: Ranch	570	60	8
Snappy	80	2	8
Salads: Crispy Chkn, w/o dressing	280	9	24
Garden, without dressing	90	4.5	11
Grilled Chicken, w/out dressing	160	2.5	10
Dessert: Cinnabread, med., ⅙ slice	340	13	55
Raspberry Cinnabread, ⅙ slice	360	13	60

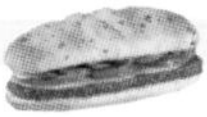
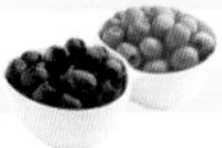

Sonic Drive-In® (Nov '20)

Burgers:	C	F	Cb
Bacon Cheeseburger, with Mayo	770	46	53
Bacon Dble Cheeseburger, w/ Mayo	1030	65	54
Cheeseburger: w/ Mayo	680	39	54
with Ketchup	600	28	58
¼ lb Double Chseburger w/ Mayo	960	59	55
Jalap. Dble Chseburger, w/ Mstrd	850	48	54
Jr. Burger	330	16	32
Veggie Burger: w/ Mayo	530	22	69
with Musard	430	11	69
Chicken:			
Sandwiches: Classic Crispy Chicken	550	30	48
Classic Grilled Chkn	470	22	39
Crispy Tender Chicken	440	22	41
Boneless Wings: *6 Pieces*			
Asian Sweet Chili	470	24	32
Honey BBQ	470	24	33
Buffalo	440	28	17
Tenders: Crispy, 3 pieces	260	12	16
5 pieces	430	20	27

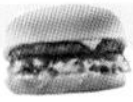
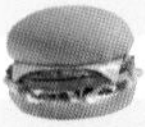
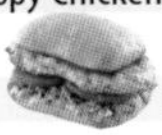
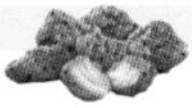

continued next page....

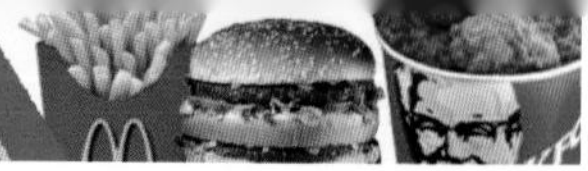

Sonic Drive-In® cont... (Nov '20)

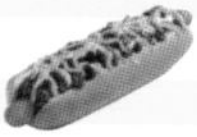

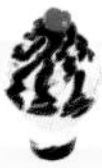

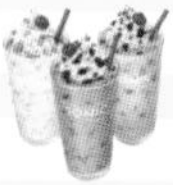

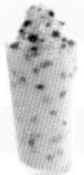

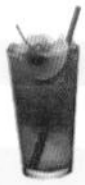

Coneys & 6" Hot Dogs:	C	F	Cb
All American Dog	410	21	41
Chicago Dog	400	20	41
Chili Cheese Coney	470	29	34
New York Dog	400	23	35
Ice Cream Cone,			
Vanilla	250	12	30
Ice Cream Sundaes:			
Caramel	490	22	61
Chocolate	430	22	51
Hot Fudge	520	26	65
Strawberry	440	21	55
Add Ons: Peanuts	40	3.5	2
Whipped Topping	70	5	5
Classic Shakes: *Per Medium*			
Caramel	830	41	97
Chocolate	810	43	95
Fresh Banana	850	41	108
Hot Fudge	940	48	113
Peanut Butter	940	58	89
Strawberry	790	41	92
Vanilla	820	45	89
Master Shakes: *Per Medium*			
Cheesecake	840	43	101
Oreo Cheesecake	1030	51	131
Oreo Chocolate	1000	51	125
Oreo Peanut Butter	1130	66	118
Strawberry Cheesecake	890	43	112
Sonic Blast: *Per Medium*			
Butterfingers Pieces	980	48	118
Choc. Chip Cookie Dough	920	45	118
M&M's Minis Choc. Candy	1060	54	127
Oreo Pieces	860	44	103
Reese's Peanut Butter Cups	990	55	110
Snickers Bars	890	46	103
All Natural Lemonade: Small	160	0	42
Medium	270	0	69
Large	400	0	105
Limeade Slush: Small	190	0	52
Medium	280	0	74
Large	430	0	116
Cold Brew Coffee: *Per Medium*			
Original: No add ins	260	13	32
French Vanilla	300	13	42

For Complete Nutritional Data ~ see CalorieKing.com

Southern Tsunami® (Nov '20)

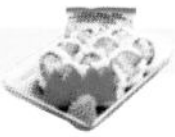

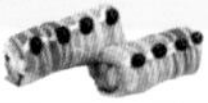

Appetizers:	C	F	Cb
Calamari Salad, 4 oz	140	1	15
Edamame, 3 oz	120	4.5	10
Grilled Dumplings: Chicken, 5.2 oz	270	7	38
Shrimp, 5.9 oz	320	12	42
Veetables, 5.9 oz	320	10	47
Seabreeze Salad, 4 oz	90	2.5	17
Bowls:			
Cold: Orange chicken	900	18	155
Sesame Chicken	920	20	156
Spicy Teriyaki Chicken	880	16	141
Teriyaki Chicken	860	16	136
Hot: *With White Rice*			
Premium Chirashi: Chicken	810	26	118
Kani Kama	780	25	125
Salmon & Tuna	820	29	116
Premium Hawaiian Poke: Tuna	600	8	97
Tuna & Salmon	660	16	97
Tuna, Salmon & Albacore	640	13	97
Ramen Grab-N-Go: *Per Bowl*			
Spicy Tonkotsu Noodle	500	15	72
Tonkotsu Noodle	450	13	66
Rolls: *With White Rice*			
Classic Rolls: California, 10.5oz	440	8	80
Cream Cheese:			
Imitation Crab, 15 pieces	500	14	80
Salmon, 15 pieces	560	20	74
Crunchy Shrimp, 6 pieces	250	9	36
Hawaiian, 5 pieces	240	9	34
Inari, 10 oz	530	16	101
Ocean Crab, 7 pieces	220	4.5	37
Hybrid:			
Berry Roll, 9 oz	400	13	66
Blueberry Roll, 5 pieces	250	9	30
Classic Yummy Roll, 5 pieces	280	12	39
Crunchy Tempura Roll, 10 oz	480	17	70
Done Deal Roll, 10.8 oz	520	22	65
Dynamite Roll, 5 pieces	240	1	28
Spicy Jumbo Roll, 9 oz	460	16	64

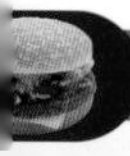

Updated Nutrition Data ~ www.CalorieKing.com
Persons with Diabetes ~ See Disclaimer (Page 22)

Southern Tsunami® cont... (Nov '20)

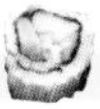

One Roll:	C	F	Cb
California, 10 pieces	320	6	59
California Salad Roll, 10 pieces	350	9	59
Cream Cheese Roll:			
Imitation Crab, 10 pieces	370	10	59
Salmon, 10 pieces	410	15	54
Crunchy CA Roll, 10 pieces	520	24	67
Crunchy, 10 pieces	620	28	80
Crunchy Dragon: Orange, 10 pieces	570	27	64
Red, 10 pieces	570	27	64
White, 10 pieces	550	25	71
Crunchy Shrimp Tempura, 10 pcs	620	30	77
Dragon, 10 pieces	490	22	66
Eel, 10 pieces	360	8	59
Rainbow Roll:			
Albacore, Salmon, Tuna, 10 pcs	450	13	59
Salmon, Shrimp, Tuna, 10 pcs	430	13	59
Wraps: Berry , 4 pieces	80	3	12
Califormia, 4 pieces	110	6	13
Smoked Salmon Roll, 3.5 oz	160	10	11
Spicy California Wrap, 3 pieces	110	7	10
Spicy Chicken Roll, 3.5 oz	120	6	11
Spicy Salmon, 4 pieces	140	9	11
Summer Roll 2, 1 piece, 3.5 oz	90	2.5	14
Teriyaki Chicken Roll, 1 piece, 3.5 oz	110	3	14
Vegetable Wrap, 4 pieces	80	3.5	11

Starbucks® (Nov '19)

Brewed Coffee: *Per16 fl.oz Grande,without Whipped Cream*

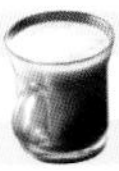

Caffe Misto:	C	F	Cb
with Almond Milk	50	3.5	4
with Coconut Milk	70	4.5	7
with Nonfat Milk	70	0	10
with Soy Milk	100	3	13
with Whole Milk	130	7	10

Chocolate: *Per 16 fl.oz Grande without Whipped Cream*

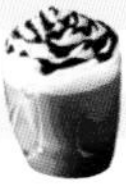

Hot Chocolate:	C	F	Cb
with 2% Milk	320	9	47
with Almond Milk	240	8	38
with Coconut Milk	270	10	42
with Soy Milk	320	8	51
with Whole Milk	360	13	47

Starbucks® cont... (Nov '19)

Vanilla Creme (Hot):

Per 16 fl.oz Grande w/out Whipped Cream

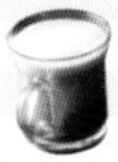

	C	F	Cb
with 2% Milk	270	7	37
with Coconut Milk	210	9	33
with Nonfat Milk, 16 fl.oz	210	0	38
with Soy Milk	260	6	42
with Whole Milk	310	12	37

Hot Espresso Beverages:

Per 16 fl.oz Grande without Whipped Cream

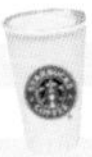
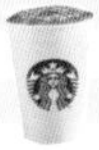
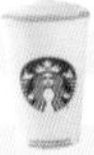

	C	F	Cb
Caffe Latte: with Almond Milk	100	6	9
with Coconut Milk	140	8	14
with Nonfat Milk	130	0	20
with Soy Milk	190	6	24
with Whole Milk	230	12	19
Caffe Mocha: with Almond Milk	220	7	34
with Coconut Milk	250	9	39
with Nonfat Milk	250	2.5	42
with Soy Milk	290	7	46
with Whole Milk	330	12	42
Cappuccino: with Almond Milk	100	6	9
with Coconut Milk	140	8	14
with Nonfat Milk	80	0	12
with Soy Milk	120	3.5	16
with Whole Milk	140	7	12
Caramel Macchiato: w/ Alm. Milk	170	6	27
with Coconut Milk	200	8	32
with Nonfat Milk	200	1.5	36
with Soy Milk	250	6	39
with Whole Milk	280	11	35
Cinn. Dolce Latte: w/ Alm. Milk	190	6	32
with Coconut Milk	220	7	37
with Nonfat Milk	220	0	42
with Whole Milk	310	11	41
Espresso: 1 Doppio, 2 fl.oz	10	0	2
1 Solo, 1 fl.oz	5	0	1
Espresso Con Panna, 1 Solo, 1 fl.oz	30	2.5	2
Latte Macchiato: with 2% Milk	190	7	19
with Soy Milk	180	5	23
with Whole Milk	220	11	19

Iced Espresso: *Per 16 fl.oz Grande w/out Whipped Cream*

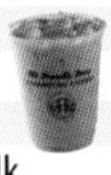
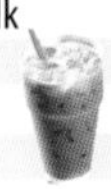

	C	F	Cb
Caffe Latte: with Coconut Milk	90	5	10
with Nonfat Milk	90	0	13
with Soy Milk	130	3.5	17
with Whole Milk	150	7	13
Vanilla Latte: with 2% Milk	190	4	30
with Coconut Milk	160	4.5	28
with Nonfat Milk	160	0	31
with Whole Milk	210	6	30

continued next page...

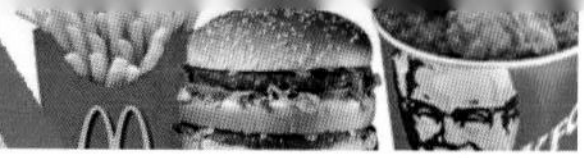

Starbucks® cont... (Nov '19)

Frappuccino Blended Coffee: Per 16 fl.oz Grande w/ Whole Milk, w/out Whipped Cream	C	F	Cb
Caffe Vanilla	**320**	3	69
Caramel	**280**	3.5	60
Coffee	**240**	3	50
Java Chip	**350**	7	68
Mocha	**300**	4	51
White Chocolate Mocha	**300**	5	61
***Frappuccino Blended Creme:** Per 16 fl.oz Grande, with Whole Milk and Whipped Cream*			
Chai Creme	**360**	15	52
Double Chocolaty Chip Creme	**420**	20	57
Vanilla Bean Creme	**400**	16	60
***Refreshers:** Per 16 oz Grande*			
Mango Dragonfruit Lemonade	**140**	0	33
Pink Drink	**140**	2.5	27
Strawberry Acai	**90**	0	23
Violet Drink	**110**	3	22
***Teas:** Per 16 fl.oz Grande, with Whole Milk*			
Hot Tea Latte: Chai Latte	**270**	7	45
Matcha Green Tea, sweetened	**280**	11	34
Iced Tea Latte: Chai	**260**	7	44
Matcha Green Tea, sweetened	**230**	8	29
Drink Extras:			
Caramel Drizzle, 1 teaspoon	**15**	0.5	2
Flavored Syrup: 1 pump	**20**	0	5
Sugar-Free, 1 pump	**0**	0	0
Mocha Syrup, 1 pump	**25**	0.5	6
Sweetened Whipped Cream:			
Grande/Venti, cold drinks, av.	**115**	11	3
Grande/Venti, hot drinks	**70**	7	2
Breakfast:			
Bacon & Gyuyere Sous Vide Egg Bites	**300**	20	9
Chicken Sausage & Bacon Biscuit	**450**	22	35
Classic Oatmeal	**160**	2.5	28
Cold Sandwich,			
Chipotle Chkn Wrap	**470**	19	55
Warm Sandwiches:			
Chicken Caprese	**500**	18	58
Chicken & Double Smoked Bacon			
Crispy Grilled Cheese on Sourdough	**540**	29	47
Ham & Swiss Panini	**490**	24	42
Tomato & Mozzarella	**350**	13	43
Turkey & Basil Pesto	**540**	21	55
Greek Yogurt Parfait,			
Berry Trio, 5.8 oz	**240**	2.5	39

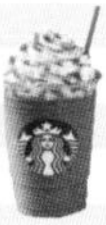
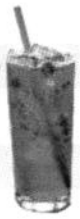
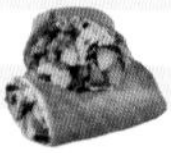
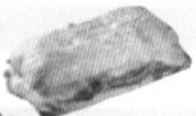

Starbucks® cont... (Nov '19)

***Bakery:** Each*	C	F	Cb
Bagels: Blueberry, 3.8 oz	**270**	1	57
Cinnamon Raisin, 3.5 oz	**270**	1	58
Vegan, Sprouted Grain, 4 oz	**330**	6	57
Brownie, Double Choc. Chunk, 3.6 oz	**480**	28	55
Cakes: Blueberry Oat, 4.5 oz	**390**	12	71
Classic Coffee, 3.8 oz	**330**	15	43
Confetti Sugar Cookie, 3.25 oz	**410**	21	54
Croissants: Almond 3.5 oz	**420**	22	45
Chocolate, 2.8 oz	**340**	20	38
Dessert Bars:			
Cocoa M'mallow Dream	**250**	4.5	50
Marshmallow, 2 oz	**230**	5	44
Doughnut, Old Fash. Glazed. 4 oz	**480**	27	56
Muffin, Blueberry, 3.9 oz	**360**	15	52

Bottled Drinks ~ See Page 37

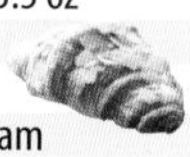

Steak Escape® (Nov '20)

***Cheesesteaks:** Per Medium*	C	F	Cb
Bourbon & Bacon	**1100**	64	89
Grand Escape	**690**	28	66
Original Philly	**710**	30	68
Sriracha	**790**	34	73
***Sandwiches:** Per Medium*			
Chicken Bacon Club	**980**	58	62
Crispy Buffalo Chicken	**1020**	48	90
Grandest Chicken	**680**	22	65
Simply Chicken	**550**	13	60
***Subs:** Per Medium*			
Cubano	**910**	47	66
Hangover	**890**	39	76
Italian Hottie	**920**	48	66
Wraps: Crispy Buffalo Chicken	**930**	47	81
Cubano	**820**	46	57
Grandest Chicken	**590**	21	56
Italian Hottie	**770**	43	57
Ragin' Cajun Chicken	**610**	26	54
Fries: Buffalo Chicken; Cajun Bleu	**950**	60	83
Loaded Cheese & Bacon, small	**920**	63	79
Naked, regular	**650**	34	78
Sriracha Steak	**900**	53	87
Salads:			
Bourbon & Bacon	**720**	54	33
Cubano	**530**	38	10
Hangover	**630**	29	50
Potatoes: Bourbon & Bacon	**1020**	54	101
Delerious Dagwood	**1100**	66	74
Simply Chicken	**460**	4	72
Triple Cheesesteak	**910**	45	78

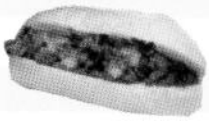
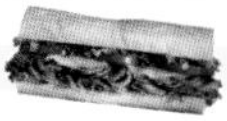
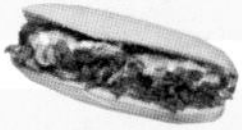
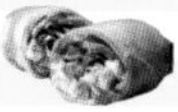
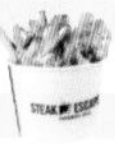
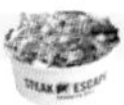
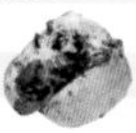

For Complete Nutritional Data ~ see CalorieKing.com

Updated Nutrition Data ~ www.CalorieKing.com
Persons with Diabetes ~ See Disclaimer (Page 22)

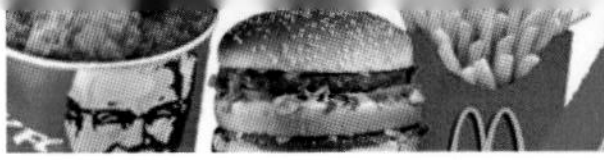

Steak 'n Shake® (Nov '20)

Steakburgers: Without Fries	C	F	Cb
Bacon Lovers	870	55	34
Bacon 'n Cheese: Single	460	26	29
Double	600	38	29
Triple	1030	74	32
Garlic Double	730	50	33
Jalapeno Crunch	690	43	39
Portobello & Swiss	740	50	36
Royale	750	49	33
Single Burger with Cheese	390	20	32
The Original: Double	460	26	33
with Cheese	530	32	32
Western BBQ 'N Bacon	790	43	54
Chili: 3-way	710	21	98
5-way	1160	57	103
Chili Deluxe: Bowl	1000	56	71
Cup	500	28	36
Chili Mac: Regular	1200	61	112
Supreme	1410	78	114
Melts: Frisco	960	66	51
Veggie, with Portobellos	620	45	44
Sandwiches: Fish	470	19	18
Grilled Cheese	620	43	41
Grilled Chicken	360	7	37
Spicy Chicken	480	16	48
Steak Franks:			
Chili Cheese Frank	710	44	46
Steak Frank, footlong, with mustard	390	23	32
Salad, Garden, without dressing	310	19	18
Fries: Per Regular			
Reg.; Cajun; Parm. & Garlic Herb, av.	450	24	54
Cheese Fries	590	35	63
Chili Cheese Fries	760	39	83
Sides: Baked Beans	310	0	64
Coleslaw	160	11	13
Onion Rings, regular	330	17	39
Breakfast:			
Breakfast Bowl with Hash Browns	460	42	11
Bagel Sandwich: with Bacon	450	16	53
with Sausage	690	37	53
Banana Pancakes	970	16	189
Biscuits: Bacon	380	25	33
Bacon, Egg & Cheese	520	35	34
Sausage, Egg & Cheese	760	56	34
Hash Browns, Shredded	300	28	15
Milk Shakes: Per Regular			
Banana	700	17	126
Birthday Cake	840	26	136
Reese's Choc. Peanut Butter	980	47	118
White Chocolate	630	18	105

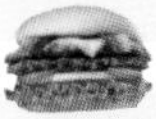
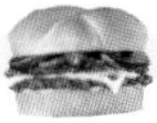
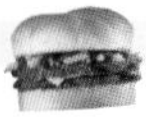
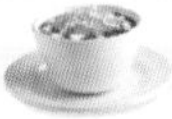
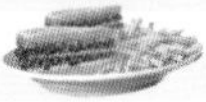
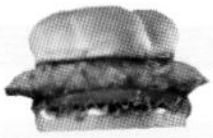
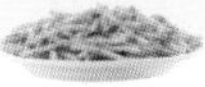
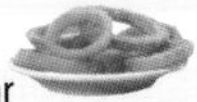
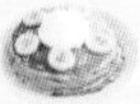
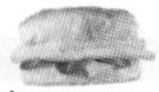
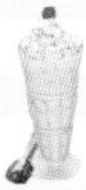

Subway® (Nov '20)

Sandwiches On 6" 9-Grain Sub:	C	F	Cb
Includes cucumbers, green peppers, lettuce, red onions, spinach & tomatoes. Without any condiments			
Black Forest Ham	260	4	42
Chicken & Bacon Ranch Melt	550	26	45
Cold Cut Combo	340	12	44
Oven Rstd Chicken	310	6	40
Roast Beef	280	4.5	40
Rotisserie Style Chkn	310	6	40
Steak & Cheese	250	3	41
Subway Club	280	4	41
Sweet Onion Chicken Teriyaki	320	4	52
Turkey Breast	250	3	41
Veggie Delite	190	2	39
Sandwiches On Ciabatta: *Includes cucumbers, green peppers, lettuce, red onions & tomatoes. Without any condiments*			
Black Forest Ham	390	6	63
Chicken & Bacon Ranch Melt	660	28	63
Classic Tuna	580	27	60
Meatball Marinara	560	20	70
Oven Rstd Chicken	400	6	61
Steak & Cheese	460	13	61
Turkey Breast	390	5	62
Sandwiches On Italian Sub: *Includes cucumbers, green peppers, lettuce, red onions & tomatoes. Without any condiments*			
Classic Tuna	450	25	38
Italian B.M.T.	380	17	40
Meatball Marinara	430	18	48
Spicy Italian	450	24	40
Sandwiches On Tomato Basil Wraps: *Includes cucumbers, green peppers, lettuce, red onions, spinach & tomatoes. Without any condiments*			
Black Forest Ham	380	10	55
Cold Cut Combo	380	10	53
Italian BMT	490	22	55
Oven Roasted Chicken	380	10	53
Roast Beef	400	10	53
Rotisserie Style Chicken	430	12	53
Spicy Italian	560	30	55
Subway Sub	400	10	55
Sweet Onion Chicken Teriyaki	320	4	52
Turkey Breast	370	9	55
Veggie Delite	310	8	53

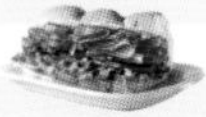
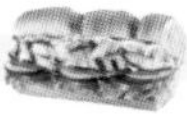
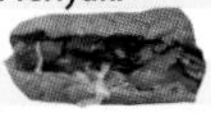
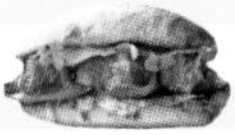
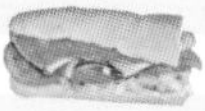
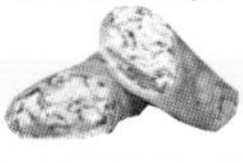
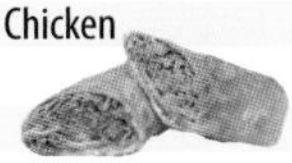

continued next page....

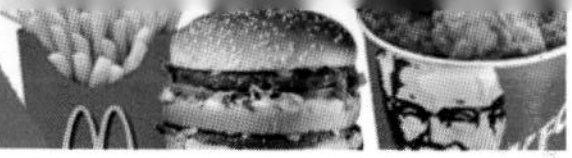

Subway® cont... (Nov '20)

Sliders: W/- Menu Set Components	C	F	Cb
Ham & Jack	**150**	4.5	18
Italian Spice	**230**	14	18
Little Cheesesteak	**170**	7	19
Turkey	**200**	10	18
Sandwich Condiments & Extras: *For 6" Sandwiches*			
Bacon Strips, 0.5 oz	**70**	6	1
Cheese: American, 0.4 oz	**40**	4	1
Cheddar; Swiss, 0.5 oz, av.	**55**	4.5	0
Chipotle Southwest Sauce, 0.5 oz	**80**	7	1
Honey Mustard Sce, Fat-Free, 0.5 oz	**20**	0	4
Mayonnaise: 1 Tbsp, 0.5 oz	**100**	11	0
Light, 1 Tbsp, 0.5 oz	**50**	5	1
Olive Oil Blend, 0.2 oz	**45**	5	0
Ranch Dressing, 0.5 oz	**70**	8	1
Sweet Onion, Fat-Free, 0.63 oz	**30**	0	8
Yellow Mustard, 0.5 oz	**10**	0	1
Signature Wraps: *On Tomato Basil Wrap With Set Menu Board Components*			
Chipotle Southwest Steak & Cheese	**740**	35	63
Cold Cut Combo	**560**	27	57
Italian BMT	**680**	37	58
M'ball Marinara	**790**	39	77
Spicy Italian	**820**	52	57
Chopped Salads (6g Fat or Less): *Figures based on lettuce, tomatoes, spinach, onions, green peppers olives & cucumbers. Dressing or croutons not included.*			
Black Forest Ham	**120**	3	13
Oven Rstd Chicken	**130**	2.5	12
Roast Beef; Subway Club	**140**	3.5	12
Rotisserie Style Chicken	**170**	5	11
Turkey Breast	**120**	2	13
Veggie Delite	**60**	1	11
Breakfast:			
Omelet Sandwiches on Artisan Flatbread: *With Regular Egg & American Cheese*			
Bacon, Egg & Cheese	**450**	20	45
Black Forest Ham, Egg & Chse	**410**	16	45
Egg & Cheese	**380**	15	44
Steak, Egg & Chse	**440**	18	46

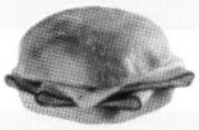

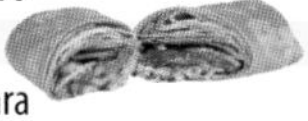
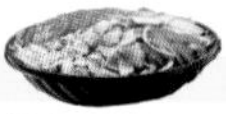
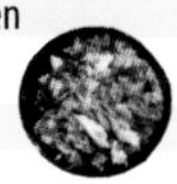
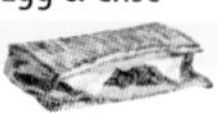

Swiss Chalet® (Nov '20)

Canadian Outlets	C	F	Cb
Starters: Chkn Spring Rolls, 8 oz	**460**	10	63
Chalet Wings (10), without Sce	**560**	34	13
Cheese Perogies, 9.45 oz	**510**	15	80
Cheesy Spinach Dip, 13.2 oz	**920**	90	108
Garlic Cheese Loaf, 13 oz	**1270**	79	100
Kale Caesar Salad, no protein, 5 oz	**380**	9	14
Burgers: *With Mayo, Without Sides*			
Classic Hamburger	**580**	28	47
Lightlife Burger	**450**	17	52
Veggie Burger	**390**	11	51
Ribs: *With Dinner Roll & Coleslaw*			
BBQ Side Ribs: ⅓ Rack	**700**	33	63
½ Rack	**820**	40	59
Full Rack	**1360**	71	87
BBQ Back Ribs: ½ Rack	**820**	40	59
Full Rack	**1270**	62	87
Main Menu:			
Chicken Strips: 3 pieces	**620**	26	65
5 pieces	**930**	43	88
Crispy Chicken: 2 pieces	**890**	35	69
3 pieces	**1110**	46	69
Double Leg Rotiss. Chkn Dinner	**950**	53	31
Rotisserie Chicken Pot Pie	**840**	38	78
Rotisserie Beef/Chkn: *W/Dinner Roll & Chalet Sauce*			
¼ Dark Meat Chicken, 11.4 oz	**480**	18	31
¼ White Meat Chicken, 12.9 oz	**520**	16	31
½ Chicken, 22 oz	**1060**	45	31
Sandwiches/Wraps:			
Crispy Chicken Caesar Wrap	**1180**	33	61
Hot Rotisserie Beef Sandwich	**550**	20	56
Hot Rotisserie Chicken Sandwich			
Rotisserie Chicken Club Wrap	**720**	34	55
The Southern Canuck	**690**	22	69
Teriyaki Stir Fry: Rotisserie Chicken	**840**	35	72
Shrimp	**760**	36	72
Vegetarian	**640**	30	72
Entree Salads: *As Served*			
Beet with Crispy Chicken	**920**	58	71
Asian Sesame w/ Rotiserie. Chicken	**580**	23	35
Kale Caesar: w/ Rotisserie Chicken	**860**	24	14
with Chicken & Bacon	**980**	34	14

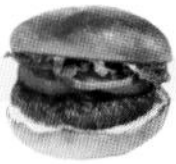
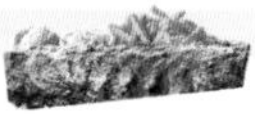
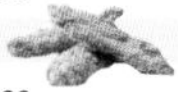
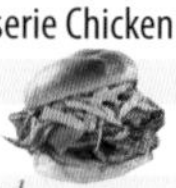

Updated Nutrition Data ~ www.CalorieKing.com
Persons with Diabetes ~ See Disclaimer (Page 22)

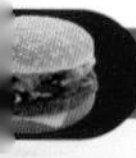

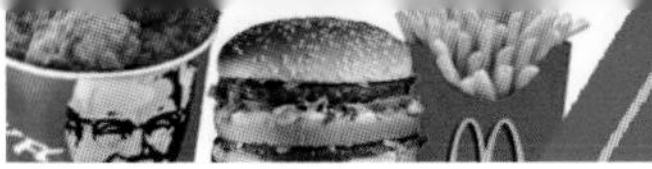

Swiss Chalet® cont... (Nov '20)

Sides: Per Serving	C	F	Cb
Baked Potato w/ Sour Crm & Onions	410	11	73
Creamy Mashed Potatoes w/ Gravy	200	4	42
Garden Salad without dressing	30	0.2	6
Garlic Green Beans	230	19	13
Jasmine Rice	500	0	110
Kale Caesar Salad with Bacon	480	15	16
Multigrain Dinner Roll	130	1	26
Poutine	800	47	76
with Rotisserie Chicken	940	51	76
Seasoned Rice Pilaf	630	13	119
Sweet Potato Fries	710	37	93
White Dinner Roll	130	1	26
Fries: Fresh Cut, 8 oz	550	30	68
Harvey's, 8 oz	630	26	96
Parm Glazed, 9 oz	790	56	69
Dressings: Blue Cheese, 2 oz	200	20	4
Caesar, 2 oz	320	3	0
Ranch, 2 oz	250	25	4
Sweet Onion, 2.25 oz	170	12	17
Sauce: Chalet Dipping, 4 oz	25	0.5	5
Plum, 2 oz	120	0.1	27
Smoky BBQ, 2 oz	110	0.2	24
Desserts/Pies: Slice			
Apple Pie, 6 oz	440	20	62
Cheesecake w/ Strawb Sce, 6.8 oz	550	22	77
Coconut Cream Pie, 6.7 oz	490	28	54
Lemon Meringue Pie, 6.7 oz	410	15	64
Pecan Pie, 4.4 oz	540	29	65

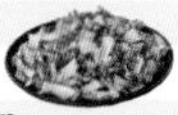
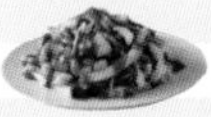
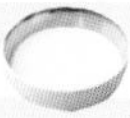
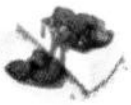

Taco Bell® (Nov '20)

Burritos: W/ Standard Components	C	F	Cb
7-Layer, no meat	420	15	58
Bean	350	9	54
Beefy 5-Layer	490	18	63
Beefy Fritos	440	18	57
Beefy Nacho Loaded Griller	370	15	48
Black Bean	370	11	56
Burrito Supreme Beef	390	14	51
Cheesy Bean & Rice	410	16	56
Cheesy Potato Griller	340	13	50
Chili Cheese, no meat	370	17	40
Quesarito	650	33	68
Shredded Chicken	420	20	47
Nachos, Triple Layer	320	15	40
Power Menu: With Standard Menu Component			
Power Bowls: Fire Grilled Chicken	480	20	50
Steak	490	20	51
Veggie	430	18	57

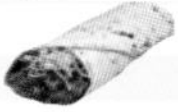
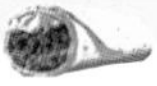
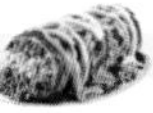
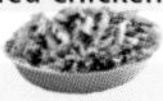

Taco Bell® cont... (Nov '20)

Specialties: W/Standard Components	C	F	Cb
Chalupa Supreme:			
Grilled Steak	330	16	32
Fire Grilled Chicken	330	16	31
Seasoned Beef	350	18	33
Cheesy Gordita Crunch,			
Shredded Chicken	480	27	39
Gordita Crunch Supreme:			
Fire Grilled Chicken	500	27	41
Grilled Steak	500	27	42
Seasoned Beef	520	29	43
Shredded Chicken	510	29	41
MexiMelt, Seasoned Beef	250	13	19
Nachos BellGrande, Seas'nd Beef	740	38	82
Quesadillas: 3 Cheese	450	25	37
Seasoned Beef	520	30	40
Shredded Chicken	510	29	38
Taco Salads: Fiesta, Seasoned Beef	740	38	75
Expr. Fiesta, Shredded Chicken	530	23	58
Tacos: With Standard Menu Components			
Crunchy: Seasoned Beef	170	9	13
Supreme, S'nd Beef	190	11	15
Soft: Grilled Steak	200	10	17
Shredded Chicken: Regular	170	8	16
Supreme	200	9	18
Spicy Potato, no meat	230	12	27
Sides: Regular Size			
Black Beans & Rice	170	3.5	31
Cheesy Fiesta Potatoes	230	12	28
Chips & Guacamole	230	15	23
Chips & Nacho Cheese Sauce	220	13	24
Chips & Pico de Gallo	180	9	22
Pintos 'n Cheese	170	6	20
Seasoned Rice	120	2	23
Breakfast: With Standard Menu Components			
Crunchwrap: Bacon & Egg	650	41	51
Sausage Patty & Egg	690	45	51
Grilled Fiesta Potato Burrito:			
Bacon & Egg	400	19	44
Grilled Steak & Egg	390	16	44
Quesadillas: Bacon & Egg	510	28	37
Sausage Crumbles & Egg	500	29	37
Steak & Egg	500	26	38
Sweets: Cinnabon Delights:			
4 Pack	310	18	35
12 Pack (serves 4)	930	53	104
Cinnamon Twist	170	6	27

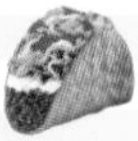
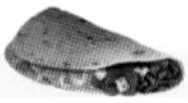
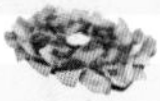
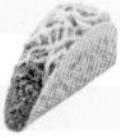
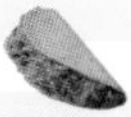
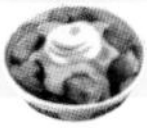
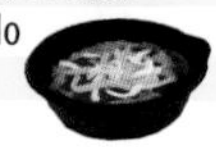
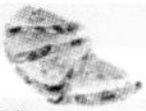
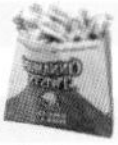

Note: Nutritional data in New York outlets may vary slightly. Please check Taco Bell website

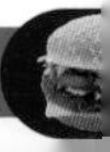

Taco Cabana® (Nov '20)

Burritos: *Includes Flour Tortilla, Rice, Refried Beans, Romaine, Meat, Shredded Cheese, Pico de Gallo & Sour Cream*

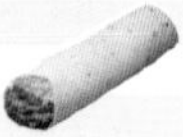

	C	F	Cb
Beef Cabana	720	29	79
Brisket Canana	790	40	76
Chicken Cabana	770	30	81
Flame Grilled Chicken Fajita	730	26	79
Steak	750	31	79
Cabana Bowls: *Includes Shell, Rice, Lettuce, Meat, Shredded Cheese, Pico de Gallo & Sour Cream*			
Beef	710	36	64
Brisket	780	48	60
Chkn/Chkn Breast, av.	740	35	65
Steak	740	39	63
Enchiladas: Beef (1)	200	11	14
Cheese (1)	320	23	13
Chicken (1)	280	13	21
Quesadillas: *Small, with Lettuce, Guac. & Sour Cream*			
Brisket	920	63	51
Cheese	770	50	51
Flame-Gr. Chkn Fajita	840	52	52
Steak	850	55	52
Tacos:			
Crispy: Beef	180	8	15
Shredded Chicken	200	9	16
Soft: Bean & Cheese	300	14	31
Beef, ground	210	9	21
Black Bean	220	5	38
Brisket	280	13	31
Carne Guisada	210	8	20
Chkn Breast Fajita, flame grilled	210	6	21
Shredded Chicken	240	9	23
Steak	220	9	21
Street, Beef (3)	460	25	40
Salads: *Includes Shell, Lettuce Meat, Shredded Cheese, Pico de Gallo & Sour Cream*			
Beef, ground	570	34	37
Chicken, shredded	610	35	39
Chicken Fajita, flame grilled	570	31	36
Steak	600	36	36
Sides & Add-Ons:			
Borracho Beans, reg.	290	6	40
Combo Chips & Queso/Guacamole	490	29	50
Guacamole, 3 oz	110	9	7
Queso, 3 oz	110	8	5
Refried Beans with Cheese, reg	530	29	49
Rice, regular	310	6	58
Salsa, all flavors, 1 oz	5	0	1
Sour Cream, 3 oz	160	15	3
Tortillas, Corn, 0.9 oz	60	1	13

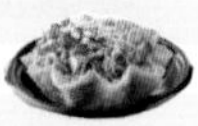
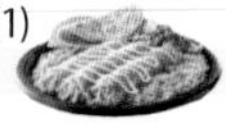
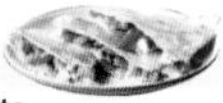
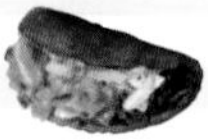
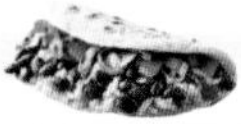
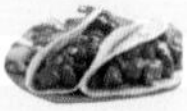
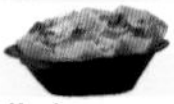
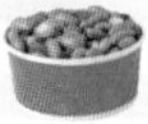
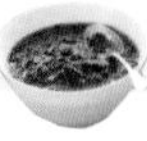

Taco Del Mar® (Nov '20)

Burritos: *Includes Flour Tortilla, Rice, Refr. Beans, Protein, Cheese, Pico de Gallo & Sour Crm*

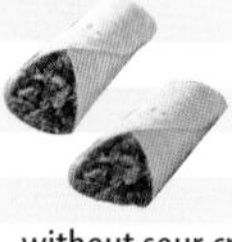

	C	F	Cb
Regular: Chicken	910	31	115
Ground Beef	950	37	116
Pork	900	31	115
Shredded Beef	910	31	116
Steak	870	27	117
Vegan with guac., without sour cream, cheese or meat	680	15	115
Veggie with guac., without meat	840	29	119
Burrito Bowls: *Per Regular Bowl, with Rice, Refried Beans, Protein, Cheese, Pico de Gallo & Sour Cream*			
Beef, shredded	640	30	64
Chicken	600	24	63
Pork	590	24	63
Steak	560	20	65
Vegan, with guacamole, without meat, cheeese or sour cream	370	8	63
Veggie with guacole, without meat	530	22	67
Nachos: *Includes Chips , Refried Beans, Protein, Cheese, Pico de Gallo, Guacamole & Sour Cream*			
Beef: Ground	1210	78	90
Shredded	1160	71	90
Cheese	1040	66	88
Chicken; Pork, av.	1160	72	89
Fish	1200	74	100
Steak	1130	68	91
Enchilada Platters: *Includes 2 Soft Corn Tortillas, Protein, Cheese, Rice, Ench. Sce. Refr. Beans, Lettuce, Pico de Gallo, Guacamole &, Sour Cream*			
Beef, ground (2)	890	37	106
Cheese (2)	810	32	105
Chicken (2)	850	31	105
Fish (2)	880	33	116
Pork (2)	830	30	104
Steak (2)	810	27	107
Quesadillas: *Includes Flour Tortilla, Meat, Cheese & Pico*			
Beef, shredded	710	34	59
Cheese	590	29	57
Chicken	720	35	58
Fish	750	37	69
Pork	700	34	58
Steak	680	31	60
Taco Salads: *Includes Shell, Cheese, Refried Beans, Lettuce, Meat , Sour Cream & Pico de Gallo*			
Beef, ground	750	45	60
Chicken	710	38	59
Fish	730	41	70
Pork	690	38	58
Steak	670	35	61

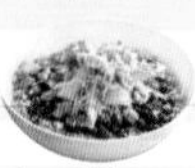
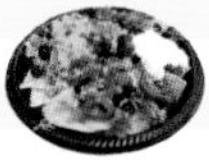
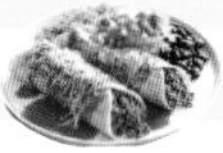
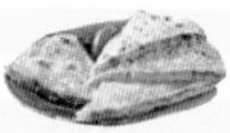
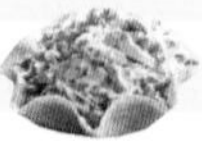

Note: Nutritional Information varies from state to state. Please refer to Taco Del Mar Website

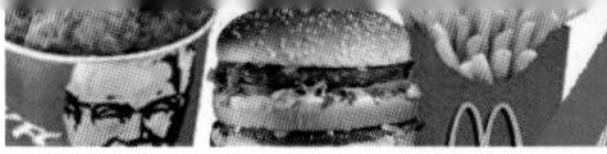

Taco John's® (Nov '20)

	C	F	Cb
Burritos:			
Bean, 6.6 oz	360	10	54
Combination, 6.6 oz	400	15	48
Grilled Beef, 8.7 oz	590	31	54
Grilled Chicken, 8.7 oz	580	28	53
Meat & Potato: Beef, 8.35 oz	510	24	59
Chicken, 8.35 oz	480	19	58
Crunchy Chicken, 8.85 oz	580	25	68
Super, Beef, 8.85 oz	440	18	51
Super Nachos:			
Beef, 12.62 oz	800	43	82
Sirloin Steak, 13.1 oz	810	42	81
Quesadillas:			
Cheese, 5.5 oz	450	24	40
Chicken, 8.6 oz	530	25	48
Super Potato Oles, reg., 16.86 oz	1090	67	98
Tacos: Crispy Beef, 3.25 oz	170	10	11
Combination, 6.6 oz	400	15	48
Softshell Taco: Beef, 4 oz	210	10	21
Chicken, 4 oz	180	5	20
Single Street: Chkn, 3.25	170	6	17
Sirloin Steak, 3.25	180	8	17
Stuffed Grilled Beef, 7.4 oz	540	25	60
Taco Bravo Beef, 6.5 oz	320	13	36
Salads: *Without Dressing*			
Beef Taco Salad	540	33	45
Chicken Taco Salad	500	27	44
Crunch Chicken	630	36	58
Sides:			
Black Beans & Rice, 6 oz	200	3	36
Chips & Nachos, 5 oz	380	20	45
Potato Oles: Small	480	27	52
Medium	670	38	73
Large	860	49	94
Refried Beans, 9.5 oz	320	7	45
Side Salad, without dressing 3.2 oz	40	2.5	3
Condiments: *Guacamole, 2.5 oz*			
Bacon Ranch Dressing, 1.5 oz	120	9	10
House Dressing, 1.5 oz	70	7	2
Nacho Cheese Sauce, 3 oz	110	9	5
Pico de Gallo, 1 oz	10	0	2
Salsa, average 1 oz	7	0	1
Sour Cream, 2.5 oz	140	13	4
Breakfast:			
Burritos: Bacon & Potato, 7.7 oz	540	25	57
Bacon Scrambler, 8.7 oz	550	25	59
Sausage Scrambler, 8.7 oz	650	33	60
Potato Ole Scrambler, Ssg, 116.8 oz	1190	79	88
Desserts: Churro Bites, 2.7 oz	280	13	37
Mexican Donut Bites, 3.2 oz	290	12	47

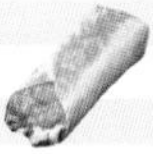
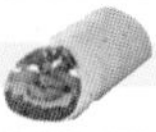
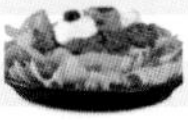
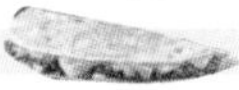
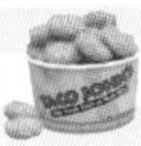
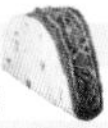
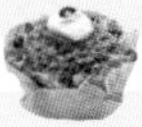
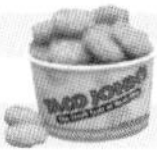
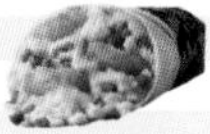

Taco Mayo® (Nov '20)

	C	F	Cb
Burritos:			
Bean	450	14	63
Chicken Burrito Supreme	420	19	40
Double Smothered Dble Queso:			
Beef	930	43	88
Chicken	850	39	83
Mexicali Gr. Chicken	635	38	48
Super: Regular	525	21	56
Beef	525	21	56
Mexicali Bowls: Chipotle Chicken	1225	71	91
Insalata Little Big	275	16	14
Little Big	450	18	41
Queso Chicken	1035	48	92
Nachos:			
Classic: Beef Supreme	790	38	81
Cheese	370	20	44
Chicken Supreme	710	34	77
Ultimate Grande	990	51	93
Quesadillas: Beef Melt	655	35	45
Chicken Melt	575	30	41
Chicken Platter	690	40	45
Tacos: Crispy Beef	160	9	10
Fish	280	13	27
Soft Taco: Beef	230	10	19
Chicken	185	8	16
Taco Burger	360	15	32
Tamale Ole	715	38	64
Salads: *As Per Menu Description*			
Beef	665	33	55
Chicken	445	26	31
Sides: Cheddar & Chips	555	31	62
Guacamole	185	16	11
Guacamole & Chips	575	35	63
Mexicali Rice	180	10	17
Mixed Fruit Cup	60	0	16
Queso & Chips	575	30	62
Potato Locos, small	400	25	37
Refried Beans	225	4	34
Kids Meals:			
Burritos: with Fruit Cup	505	14	78
with Potato Loco	845	39	99
Quesadillas: with Fruit Cup	270	12	31
with Potato Loco	605	37	52
Tacos:			
Crispy: Beef with Fruit Cup	220	7.5	29
with Potato Loco	560	33	50
Soft: Beef w/ Fruit Cup	290	10	35
with Potato Loco	630	36	56

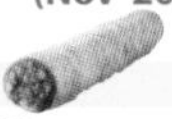
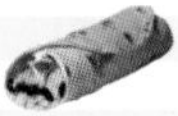
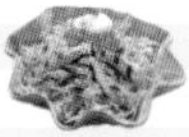
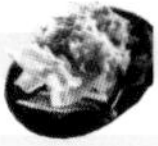
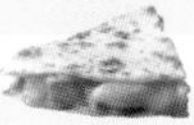
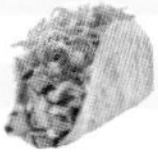
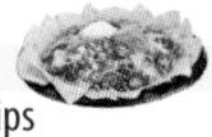
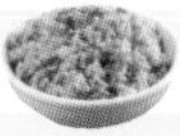
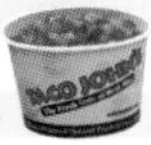
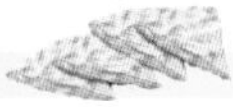
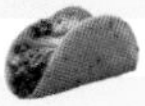

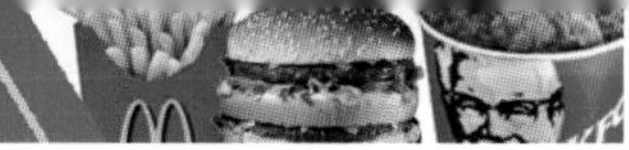

Taco Time® (Nov '20)

Burritos:	C	F	Cb
5 Alarm	420	15	58
Chicken B.L.T.	600	31	46
Sweet Pork	550	18	72
Big Juan: Chicken	590	16	79
Seasoned Beef	650	22	83
Casita: Chicken	450	16	44
Seasoned Beef	510	22	48
Crisp Burrito:			
Chicken	380	17	39
Meat	390	17	43
Pinto Bean	380	13	53
Soft Burrito: Pinto Bean	380	10	56
Seasoned Beef	420	16	46
Veggie	440	17	60
Nachos: Original	900	39	91
Chicken	970	39	92
Seasoned Beef	1020	45	96
Optionals:			
Green Chili Pork Carnita: Burrito	460	18	43
Chimichanga	590	21	65
Enchiladas	340	12	26
Soup, Enchilada, 8 oz	130	0.5	20
Quesadillas: Cheese	450	23	39
Chicken	520	24	42
Tacos:			
Soft Tacos: Chicken	360	10	42
Junior	300	13	29
Pork	440	16	43
Super Soft Tacos: Chicken	500	16	61
Pork	590	21	62
Seasoned Beef	560	21	65
Fries:			
Mexi: Small, 3.2 oz	190	12	19
Regular, 4.7 oz	300	19	29
Stuffed: Small, 4.5 oz	320	20	29
Regular, 6.6 oz	460	28	42
Salads:			
Fiesta, Chicken, 12.3 oz	340	11	37
Taco: Chicken, 8 oz	310	14	26
Seasoned Beef, 7.5 oz	360	19	28
Breakfast:			
Burritos: *Regular Size*			
Bacon & Egg	450	20	48
Egg & Cheese	370	16	40
Enchilada	450	20	46
Sausage & Egg	560	30	48
Ultimate	760	48	50
Quesadilla	300	17	18
Taters & Gravy, regular	410	27	36
Churros: Plain	210	16	15
Bavarian Cream	320	8	54
Cinnamon Crustos	320	5	64

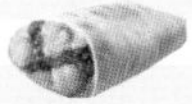
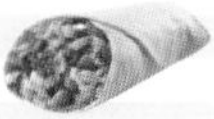
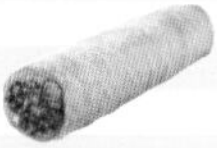
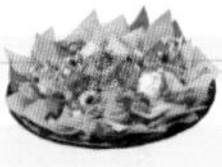
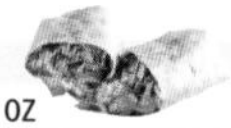
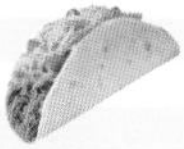
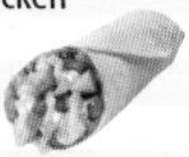
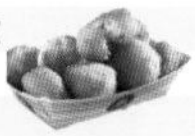
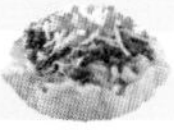
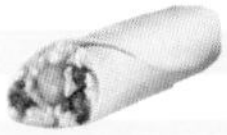
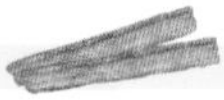

TCBY® (Nov '20)

Soft Serve Frozen Yogurt:	C	F	Cb
Per ½ Cup, 4 fl.oz			
Dairy Free/Sorbet:			
Chocolate Almond	100	1	28
Coconut	125	5	18
Kiwi Strawberry Sorbet	90	0	22
Mango Sorbet	95	0	24
Orange Sorbet	90	0	23
Watermelon Sorbet	100	0	25
No Sugar Added, av. all flavors	63	0	18
Super Fro Yo: Bananas Foster	90	0	23
Cake Batter; Golden Vanilla	105	2	22
Chocolate	100	1.5	22
Dutch Chocolate	95	0	23
Graham Cracker	105	2	25
Greek Honey Vanilla	100	0	20
New York Cheesecake	115	2	23
Old Fashioned Vanilla	90	0	23
Peppermint	140	2	22
White Chocolate Mousse	120	1.5	24
Hand-Scooped Frozen Yogurt:			
Dairy Free, Psychedelic Sorbet	130	0	33
Gluten Free:			
Butter Pecan: Kid's, 4 fl.oz	220	10	27
Small, 6.4 fl.oz	350	16	43
Regular, 12.8 fl.oz	705	32	86
Chocolate Chocolate:			
Kid's, 4 fl.oz	120	2.5	20
Small, 6.4 fl.oz	190	4	38
Regular, 12.8 fl.oz	385	8	76
Peanut Butter Delight:			
Kid's, 4 fl.oz	250	13	30
Small, 6.4 fl.oz	400	21	48
Regular, 12.8 fl.oz	800	42	96
Pralines & Cream: Kid's 4 fl.oz	210	6	27
Small, 6.4 fl.oz	335	10	43
Regular, 12.8 fl oz	670	19	86
Vanilla Bean:			
Kid's, 4 fl.oz	170	4.5	27
Small, 6.4 fl.oz	270	7	43
Regular, 12.8 fl.oz	545	14	86
Other Flavors:			
Cookies & Cream:			
Kid's, 4 fl.oz	200	6	32
Small, 6.4 fl.oz	320	10	51
Regular, 12.8 fl.oz	640	19	102

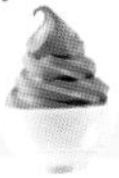
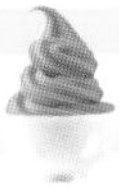
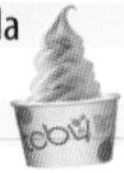

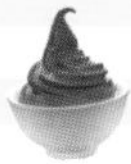
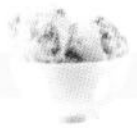
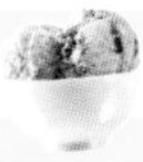
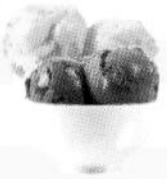
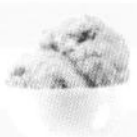
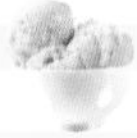

Updated Nutrition Data ~ www.CalorieKing.com
Persons with Diabetes ~ See Disclaimer (Page 22)

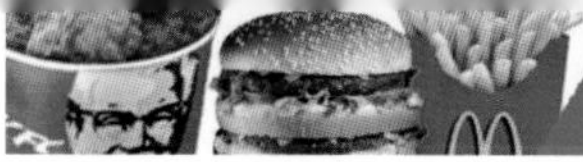

TGI Friday's® (Nov '20)

Appetizers/Snacks:	C	F	Cb
Bucket of Bones	**1570**	82	120
Chips & Salsa	**280**	13	49
Chicken Quesadilla	**1620**	110	83
Giant Onion Rings	**1190**	55	155
Loaded Potato Skins,			
with Ranch Sour Cream	**1510**	73	179
Mozzarella Sticks, with Marinara	**840**	52	54
Pan Seared Potstickers,			
with Szechuan Sauce	**590**	25	72
Spinach Artichoke Dip	**720**	50	63
Burgers: *Without Sides*			
Bacon Cheeseburger	**840**	54	47
Beyond Meat Cheeseburger	**890**	57	55
Cheeseburger	**780**	0	44
Signat. Whiskey-Glazed	**1110**	55	110
Green Style:			
Bacon Cheeseburger	**580**	43	12
Beyond Meat	**630**	46	19
Chicken & Seafood:			
Crispy Checken Tenders, with Slaw,			
Fries & Honey Mustard	**1040**	70	73
Fried Shrimp, with Fries,			
Coleslaw & Cocktail Sauce	**1020**	51	111
Parmesan Crusted Chicken, with			
Mashed Pot. & Lemon Butter Sce	**1010**	49	54
Sizzling Street Noodles	**1520**	39	230
Pasta: Cajun Shrimp & Chicken,			
with Breadstick	**1600**	83	132
Chicken Parmesan, full order	**1890**	107	154
Shrimp & Lobster	**1680**	89	140
Ribs: *With Coleslaw & Seasoned Fries*			
Apple Butter: Half Rack	**830**	54	65
Full Rack	**1220**	81	81
Whiskey Glazed: Half Rack	**1100**	51	129
Full Rack	**1630**	75	178
Sandwiches: *Without Sides*			
Bacon Ranch Chicken	**690**	31	42
Southern Fried Chicken	**970**	62	62
Whiskey Glazed Chicken	**1110**	57	100
Steaks: *With Mashed Potatoes & Lemon Butter Broccoli*			
Centre Cut Sirloin:			
w/ Parm. Butter	**640**	41	34
w/ Whiskey Glaze	**710**	31	76
Filet Mignon: with Parm Butter	**750**	39	33
with Whiskey Glaze	**880**	35	75

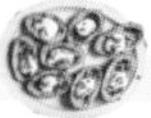

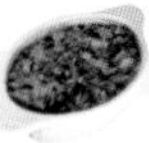

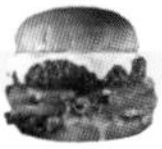

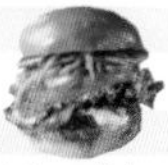

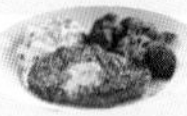

TGI Friday's® cont... (Nov '20)

Salads:	C	F	Cb
BBQ Chicken w/ BBQ Ranch Dressing	**990**	56	73
Caesar: 6 oz Sirloin & Caesar Drssng	**770**	62	20
w/ Beyond Meat Patty & Caesar Drsng	**1060**	89	28
Chinese Chkn: Beyond Meat Patty	**1300**	97	76
with Grilled Salmon & Caesar Drsng	**870**	69	24
Million $ Cobb: Gr Chkn & Ranch	**1020**	74	26
with Gr. Salmon & Ranch Dressing	**1110**	85	30
Soups: French Onion	**590**	18	84
New England Clam Chowder	**500**	30	45
Tomato Basil	**300**	24	20
White Cheddar Broccoli Cheese	**280**	20	18
Add Ons: Cheddar Mac & Cheese	**630**	35	52
Coleslaw	**100**	8	5
Giant Onion Rings	**510**	26	61
House Salad with Breadstick	**270**	12	34
Jasmine Rice	**420**	11	72
Lemon Butter Broccoli	**150**	11	11
Mashed Potatoes	**220**	11	21
Seasoned Fries	**320**	16	40
Sweet Potato Fries	**390**	20	50
Desserts: *Per Whole Dish*			
Brownie Obsession	**1180**	58	154
Oreo Madness	**670**	29	98
Red Velvet Cake	**1690**	92	199
Signature Slushes:			
Blue Raspberry	**170**	0	42
Mango Peach Lemonade	**170**	0	44
Red Bull Passion, regular	**210**	0	54
Strawberry Lemonade	**150**	0	38

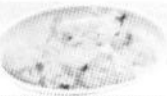

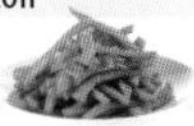

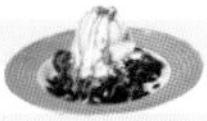

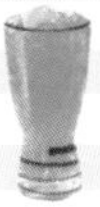

Thundercloud Subs® (Nov '20)

Subs: *Small, w/ Standard Toppings*	C	F	Cb
Classic: BLT	**365**	17	35
Genoa Salami	**265**	6	35
Roast Beef	**290**	4	35
Smoked Chicken	**270**	4	35
Turkey	**255**	4	36
Signature Subs:			
Club	**445**	19	38
California Club	**475**	23	40
NY Italian	**540**	30	37
Office Favorite	**790**	39	71
Texas Tuna	**675**	44	39
Veggie Delite, with Hummus	**385**	19	52

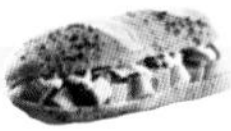

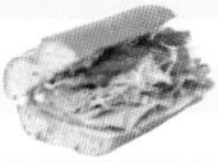

T.J. Cinnamons® (Nov '20)

Bakery:	C	F	Cb
Orig. Gourmet Cinn. Roll, 7.8 oz	**840**	42	106
Pecan Stick Bun, 8.3 oz	**940**	49	111

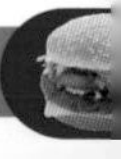

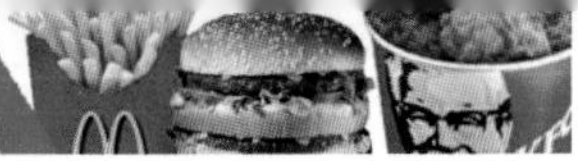

Tim Hortons® (Nov '20)

Breakfast:	C	F	Cb
Bagel BELT	560	24	62
Biscuit Sandwich:			
Angus Steak & Egg	400	20	34
Bacon, Egg & Cheese	420	23	33
Sausage, Egg & Cheese	530	34	33
Turkey, Egg & Cheese	350	16	31
Grilled Breakfast Wrap: Farmer's	680	42	54
Steak & Cheddar	440	21	40
Oatmeal, with Mixed Berries, reg.	210	3	44
Hash Brown, 1.9 oz	130	7	16
Lunch:			
Chili, regular	480	27	26
Pasta, Mac & Cheese	490	27	48
Soup: *Per Regular Size*			
Broccoli Cheddar	270	15	23
Chicken Noodle Soup	160	2	30
Clam Chowder	270	10	32
Hearty Vegetable Soup	110	0.5	20
Potato Bacon Cheddar Soup	380	23	31
Roasted Red Pepper & Gouda	310	20	24
Turkey & Wild Rice	180	2	35
Wraps:			
Grilled Chicken Fajita	430	19	39
Steak Fajita	430	20	40
Sides,			
Kettle Cooked Potato Chips, 1.4 oz	220	14	22
Cinnamon Roll, glazed	350	13	51
Cookies: Chocolate Chunk	210	9	32
Oatmeal Raisin Spice	210	8	32
Peanut Butter	250	15	24
Donuts: Apple Fritter	290	8	48
Blueberry Bloom	240	9	37
Caramel Apple Fritter	300	8	52
Chocolate Dip	190	7	29
Double Chocolate	270	15	32
Double Strawbery	230	5	40
Honey Cruller	310	18	37
Strawberry Cream	290	10	45
Muffins: Chocolate Caramel	410	15	64
Wild Blueberry	340	11	57
Whole Grain Pecan Banana Bread	350	11	60
Timbits: Apple Fritter (1)	50	1.5	9
Chocolate Glazed (1)	70	3	10
Honey Dip (1)	45	1	8
Old Fashioned Glazed (1)	70	2.5	10
Sour Cream Glazed (1)	90	4.5	12
Strawberry Filled (1)	50	1	8

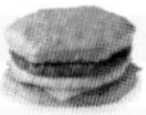
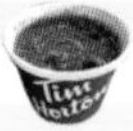
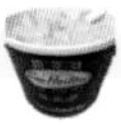
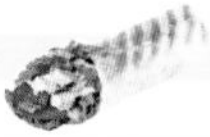
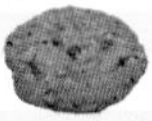
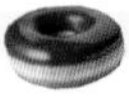
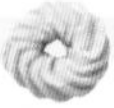
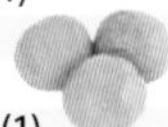

Tim Hortons® cont... (Nov '20)

Beverages:	C	F	Cb
Frozen, all flavors, 16 fl.oz	530	27	70
Hot: Cappuccino, 15 fl.oz	100	0	15
Mocha Latte, 15 fl.oz	230	7	32
Iced: Coffee, 20 fl.oz	110	7	11
Latte, 20 fl.oz	240	7	35
Mocha Latte, 20 fl.oz	390	9	68

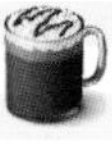
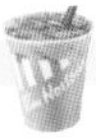

Togo's® (Nov '20)

California Outlet ~ Please check local outlet for menu items and nutritional information

	C	F	Cb
***Cold Sandwiches:** Per Regular 6", with Menu Set Components on White Bread*			
#2: Ham & Swiss	690	28	70
#3:Turkey & Cheddar	800	39	68
#4: Turkey, Salami & Cheddar	980	56	68
#5: Turkey & Cranbery	650	18	86
#7: Roast Beef	700	21	67
#8: Roast Beef & Turkey	880	40	69
#16: The Italian	880	47	70
#20: Albacore Tuna	670	27	72
#23: Salami & Provolone	1020	61	68
***Hot Sandwiches:** Per Regular 6", with Menu Set Components on White Bread*			
#1: Chicken & Cheddar			
#6: Meatball	890	40	81
#9: Pastrami	740	34	73
#32: Pepperjack Melt	1010	59	73
***Wraps:** Per Whole 12" Spinach Tortilla Wrap, with Menu Set Components*			
Asian Chicken	650	28	70
Bacon Ranch Chicken	680	33	55
Cali Veggie	810	49	63
Chicken Caesar	570	21	62
Greek Veggie	760	45	78
Santa Fe Chicken	710	34	69
***Salads:** Per Full Salad, with Dressing*			
Asian Chicken	670	43	44
Chicken Caesar	450	26	22
Farmer's Market	480	39	26
Santa Fe Chicken	780	55	37
***Soups:** Per Regular, 10 fl.oz*			
Broccoli Cheddar	220	14	16
Chicken Noodle	120	3.5	15
Chicken Tortilla	160	5	20
Chili	240	8	23
Garden Vegetable	120	4.5	18
Brownie, Choc. Chunk, 3 oz	440	23	56
Cookies: Choc. Chunk, 3 oz	410	21	54
Oatmeal Raisin, 3 oz	370	13	58

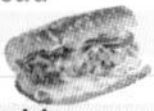
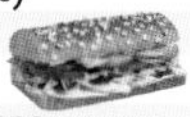
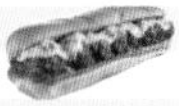
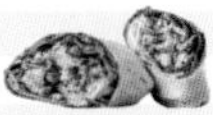
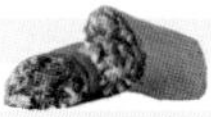
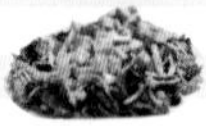
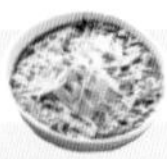

Updated Nutrition Data ~ www.CalorieKing.com
Persons with Diabetes ~ See Disclaimer (Page 22)

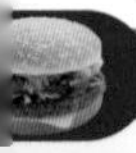

Tropical Smoothie Cafe® (Nov '20)

Menu & Nutrition Differ from Outlets to Outlet. Please Check Instore. Figures below Based On Irvine, CA

	C	F	Cb
Breakfast:			
All American Omelet Wrap	430	20	37
Peanut Butter Crunch Flatbread	590	24	77
Southwest Omelet Wrap	580	36	38
Bowls: Baja Chicken	470	21	37
Buffalo Chicken	420	25	16
Caribbean Jerk Chicken	440	12	52
Hummus Veggie	620	42	48
Pressed Sandwiches: Cuban	790	42	64
Chicken Caprese	730	30	64
with Bacon	790	35	64
Quesadillas: Island Chicken	570	27	51
Santa Fe Chicken	600	28	50
Three Cheese Chicken	550	27	41
Toasted Sandwiches: *Per Whole Ciabatta Sandwich*			
Turkey Apple Dijon	640	31	52
Turkey Bacon Ranch	560	20	59
Tropical Chicken Salad	610	33	52
Toasted Wraps: *In Flour Tortilla*			
Baja Chicken	640	24	67
Buffalo Chicken	510	21	44
Caribbean Jerk Chkn	590	17	74
Hummus Veggie	740	38	83
Supergreen Caesar Chicken	610	31	42
Thai Chicken	500	15	62
Classic Smoothies: *Per 24 oz with Turbinado*			
Bahama Mama	500	4.5	117
Beach Bum	550	5	129
Blimey Limey	440	0	111
Blueberry Bliss	340	5	86
Health Nut, with Soy	530	4.5	101
Lean Machine	490	0	124
Mocha Madness	660	5	152
Muscle Blaster, with Pea	520	2	98
Peanut Paradise, with Pea	740	17	107
Peanut Butter Cup	710	20	127
Sunrise	390	0	98
Sunrise Sunset	360	0	89

Tubby's® (Nov '20)

Subs: *Per Regular 8" Sub, with Standard Ingredients, without Added Sauce or Dressing*

	C	F	Cb
Deli-Subs:			
Ham & Cheese	540	11	78
Turkey Breast & Cheese	550	11	77
Turkey Club	630	17	77
Grilled Burger Subs:			
Cheeseburger Italiano	790	35	78
Pizza Burger	810	36	81
Taco	960	44	89

Tubby's® cont... (Nov '20)

Subs (Cont): *Per Reg. 8" Sub, with Standard Ingredients, without Added Sauce or Dressing*

	C	F	Cb
Grilled Chicken Subs: Gr. Chicken	450	4.5	75
Chicken & Broccoli	550	11	78
Chicken & Cheddar	540	11	75
Crispy Chicken	860	37	97
Grilled Steak Subs:			
Loaded Steak	650	18	81
Pepper Steak & Cheese	630	17	77
Mushroom, Steak & Cheese	620	17	77
Steak & Cheese	620	17	76
Specialty Subs: BLT	570	21	72
Cold Veggie	490	10	86
Tuna	570	11	76
Sides: Breaded Mushrooms	410	22	47
French Fries	390	24	39
Mac & Cheese Bites	510	37	34
Mozzarella Sticks	490	26	42

Uno Pizzeria & Grill® (Nov '20)

	C	F	Cb
Appetizers: *Per Whole Dish*			
Mozzarella Sticks	1090	57	107
Muchos Nachos	1700	71	199
Shrimp & Crab Dip	1160	84	66
Burgers: *Without Friess*			
Bacon Cheddar	1350	99	35
Cheddar Burger	1110	81	35
Uno	1000	72	35
Entrees:			
Chicken: *Without Sides or Breadstick*			
Baked Stuffed Spinoccoli	330	15	6
Herb Rubbed Chicken	310	20	1
Romano Crusted Chicken Parm.	1120	42	128
Pasta: *With Housemade Bread*			
Chicken Spinoccoli	1260	62	105
Deep Dish Mac & Cheese	1740	103	140
Shrimp Scampi	1190	54	128
Steak & Seafood: *Without Sides or Breadstick*			
Grilled Shrimp & Sirloin	690	45	1
Shrimp Skewer	130	8	1
Sirloin, 10 oz	560	37	0
Sirloin Steak Tips	470	20	4
Deep Dish Individual Pizza: *Per Slice, ⅙ Pizza*			
Chicago Classic	360	26	19
Numero Uno	300	19	20
Prima Pepperoni	280	15	8
Sides: French Fries, 7.5 oz	450	33	35
House Made Bread	120	1	18
Jumbo Onion Rings, 7.5 oz	370	7	68
Loaded Mashed Potatoes	420	26	37
Red Bliss Mashed Potatoes	280	14	36
Roasted Seasonal Veggies, 7.2 oz	70	4	8
Dessert: All American	640	28	90
Uno Deep Dish Sundae	1520	74	206

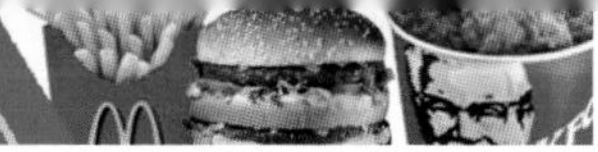

Villa Italian Kitchen® (Nov '20)

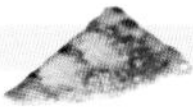
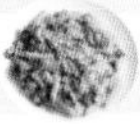
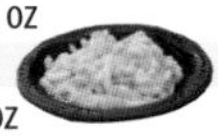
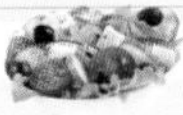

Pizzas: Per Slice	C	F	Cb
Neapolitan: Buffalo	770	46	52
Deluxe	530	22	55
Sausage & Pepperoni	550	25	53
Stuffed: Baked Ziti	845	33	97
Spinach & Mushroom	735	33	79
Entrees:			
Chicken Pasta Primavera, 16 oz	505	20	58
Fettuccini Alfredo, 14 oz	765	38	85
Mac & Cheese, 14 oz	725	54	39
Pasta Primavera, 16 oz	495	21	66
Spaghetti & Meatballs, 18 oz	840	28	112
Sides: Caesar Salad, 4 oz	90	5	9
Garlic Roll	260	10	34
Garden Salad, 3 oz	15	1	3
Greek Salad, 6 oz	125	10	7
Roasted Potatoes, 6 oz	210	12	24
Sauteed Vegetables, 6oz	85	6	6

Vocelli Pizza® (Nov '20)

Pizzas:

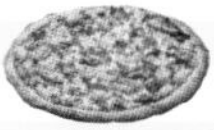
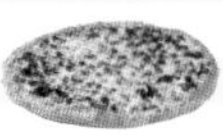
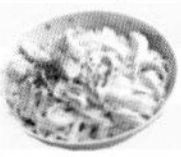
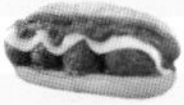
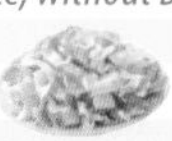
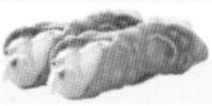

Artisan: *Per ⅛ of Medium Pizza, with Menu Set Components*	C	F	Cb
BBQ Chicken	290	10	35
Chicken Carbonara	270	11	27
Chicken Pesto	260	10	27
Deluxe	260	11	29
Hawaiian	280	11	29
Meat Magnifico	290	13	28
Philly Steak	270	12	28
Quattro Cheese	260	10	27
Spring Veggie	220	7	29
Linguini Pasta: *Single Serving*			
Chicken Alfredo	1200	54	129
Chicken Parmesan	960	26	144
Chicken Pesto	1230	57	128
House Baked Subs: On Italian Bread			
Buffalo Chicken	950	39	86
Chkn Parmesan	990	39	105
Meatball	1170	55	103
Salads: Per Regular Size, without Dressing			
Chicken Caesar	180	4	14
Mediterranean	230	11	22
Tuscan Grilled Chicken	320	13	22
Desserts: Cannoli	150	7	17
Chocolate Cake	320	14	46
Double Fudge Chunk Brownie	500	28	62

Wahoo's Fish Taco® (Nov '20)

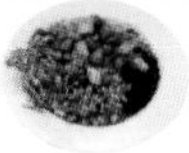
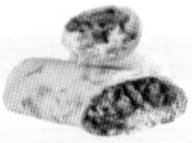
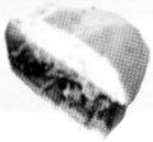
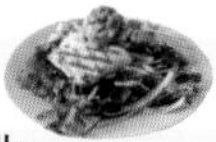

Banzai Bowls: With White Rice & Black Beans	C	F	Cb
Blackened: Chicken	720	14	104
Fish	675	9	104
Carne Asada	795	24	102
Carnitas	890	26	105
Salmon	705	14	102
Burritos: With Brown Rice & White Beans			
Outer Reef: Blackened Chicken	765	32	79
Blackened Fish	725	28	79
Mushroom	700	32	81
Shrimp	705	28	79
Tofu	715	30	81
Side Kicks, Soft Corn Tortillas, each	145	2	29
Shredder Sandwiches: With White Rice & White Beans			
Blackened or Charbroiled:			
Chicken, average	1045	36	140
Fish	1000	32	140
Carne Asada	1110	44	140
Wahoo Salads:			
Banzai Veggie	415	24	35
Carne Asada	690	48	22
Chicken, Blackened/Charbroiled, av.	540	32	22
Carnitas	750	46	25
Salmon	550	32	22
Tofu	40	31	30
Soup, Chicken Tortilla	130	6	11

For Complete Nutritional Data ~ see CalorieKing.com

WAWA® (Nov '20)

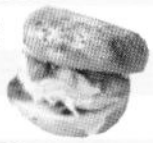
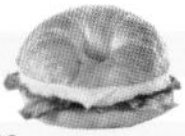
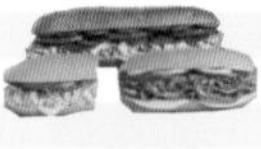

Breakfast Sizzlis:	C	F	Cb
Bagels: Bacon, Egg & Cheese	410	18	42
Dble Bacon Dble Cheese	540	28	44
Pork Roll, Egg & Cheese	420	19	42
Sausage, Egg & Cheese	510	29	42
Biscuit, Sausage, Egg & Cheese	670	45	48
Croissants:			
Bacon, Egg & Cheese	420	28	27
Chorizo	500	36	28
Sausage, Egg & Cheese	520	39	27
Muffin, Sausage, Egg & Cheese	450	30	28
Sourdough Melts: With Egg Omelet & Cheddar Cheese			
Fully Loaded; Bacon, Turkey & Egg, av.	870	38	78
Spicy Sausage & Egg	980	54	77
Western	670	22	78
Cold Hoagies: On Shorti Roll w/out Any Toppings/Spread			
Egg Salad	560	32	51
Italian	420	14	47
Roast Beef	400	4	45
Roasted Veggie	300	5	51
Tuna Salad	560	28	55

Updated Nutrition Data ~ www.CalorieKing.com
Persons with Diabetes ~ See Disclaimer (Page 22)

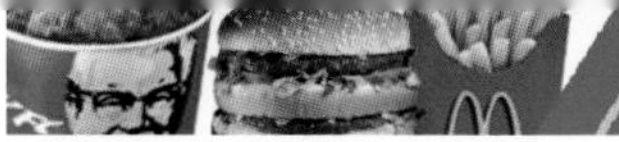

WAWA® cont... (Nov '20)

	C	F	Cb
***Hot Hoagies:** On Classic Roll, without Toppings or Spread*			
Beef Steak	600	21	64
Chicken Steak	510	11	64
Meatball	1050	60	91
***Quesadillas:** Without Toppings*			
Beef & Cheddar Cheese	560	28	44
Chicken & Cheddar Cheese	500	21	44
***Soups:** Per Medium Serving without Toppings*			
Baked Potato w/ith Cheddar & Bacon	400	27	26
Broccoli Cheddar Soup	300	22	15
Chicken Noodle	190	6	20
New Eng. Clam Chowder	310	20	23
Tomato Soup	330	22	28
***Sides:** Per Medium*			
Beyond Meatball	280	14	12
Buffalo Mac & Cheese	510	26	49
Mashed Potatoes	470	27	47
Meatballs in a Cup	480	38	20
Rice & Beans	270	3.5	49
Rice	240	0	52
Bakery: Apple Fritter	510	19	79
Coffee Roll	430	14	68
Muffins: Banana Walnut	610	33	74
Blueberry	570	28	72
Chocolate Chip	680	34	86
***Hot Beverages:** Per 16 oz, without Extras*			
Hot Cappuccino, with 2% milk	130	5	13
Mocha Latte, with 2% milk	330	7	63
Milkshake, Chocolate, w/ Crm, 16 oz	970	50	119

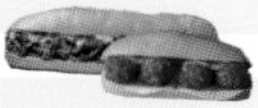
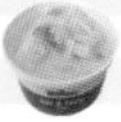
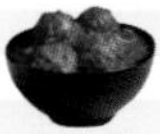
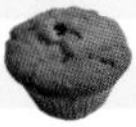

Wendy's® (Nov '20)

	C	F	Cb
Breakfast:			
Biscuits:			
Bacon, Egg & Cheese	420	27	27
Honey Butter Chicken	500	29	44
Sausage, Egg & Cheese	610	45	28
Croissants: Bacon, Egg & Swiss	410	23	34
Maple Bacon Chicken	560	30	51
Sausage, Egg & Swiss	600	41	34
Hamburgers:			
Bacon Jalapeno Cheeseburger:			
Single	740	47	44
Double	980	65	45
Baconator	920	60	38
Big Bacon Classic: Single	630	38	39
Double	870	56	40
Daves: Single	570	34	38
Double	810	51	39
Jr.: Bacon Cheeseburger	380	23	26
Cheeseburger	280	13	26
Cheeseburger Deluxe	340	19	27
Son of Baconator	630	40	35

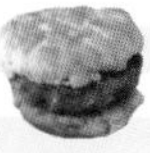
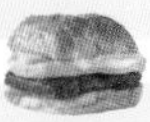
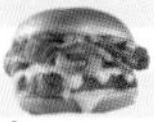
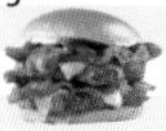
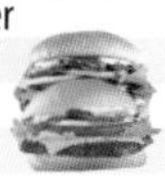

Wendy's® cont... (Nov '20)

	C	F	Cb
Sandwiches:			
Crispy: Chicken	330	16	33
Chicken BLT	420	24	34
Grilled: Avocado BLT Chicken	590	30	37
Bacon Jalapeno Chicken	590	28	42
Barbecue Chicken	520	18	49
Chicken	370	10	36
Homestyle: Asiago Ranch Chkn Club	640	32	51
Avocado BLT Chicken	720	40	53
Bacon Jalapeno Chicken	720	39	59
Barbecue Chicken	650	28	66
Chicken	510	22	51
Spicy: Avocado BLT Chicken	730	39	55
Barbecue Chicken	650	26	67
Chicken	500	22	49
Chicken Nuggets:			
Crispy Nuggets: 4 pieces	170	11	10
6 pieces	250	16	14
Spicy Nuggets: 4 pcs	190	12	9
6 pieces	280	18	13
***Dipping Sauces:** Per 1 oz*			
Barbecue	45	0	11
Buttermilk Ranch	120	12	2
Creamy Sriracha	120	12	3
Honey Mustard	90	7	7
Sweet & Sour	45	0	12
***Fresh-Made Salads:** Full Size with Menu Set Dressing*			
Apple Pecan Grilled Chicken	520	23	41
Parmesan Caesar Chicken	480	29	9
Southwest Avocado Chicken	520	34	15
Taco	610	27	67
Sides:			
Baconator Fries	490	27	46
Bacon Jalapeno Fries	560	35	47
Baked Potatoes:			
Bacon Cheese	440	13	64
Cheese	450	14	65
Chili & Cheese	460	11	73
Sour Cream & Chives	320	2.5	63
Chili Cheese Fries	510	25	55
French Fries: Jr.	230	10	30
Small, 4 oz	320	15	43
Medium, 5 oz	420	19	56
Large, 6.5 oz	530	24	70
Rich Meaty Chili: Small	160	4	19
Large	250	6	29
Frosty:			
Chocolate; Vanilla, average:			
Small	345	9	57
Medium	460	12	77
Large	580	15	96

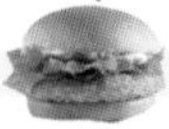
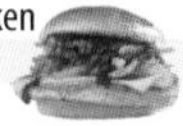
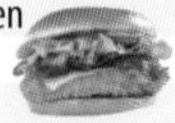
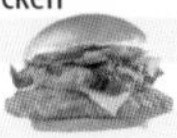
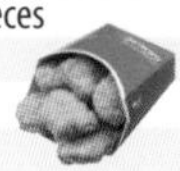

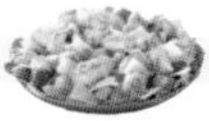
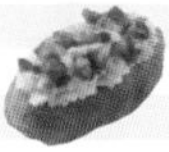
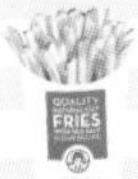

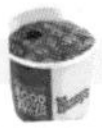
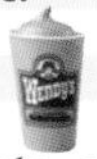

For Complete Nutritional Data ~ see CalorieKing.com

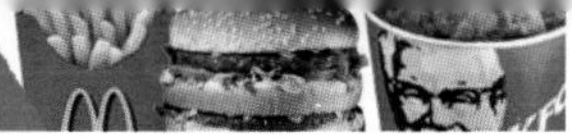

Whataburger® (Nov '20)

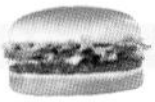
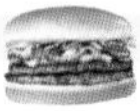
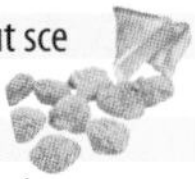
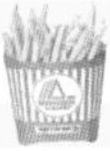
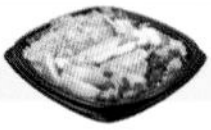
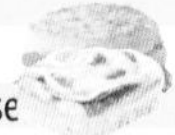
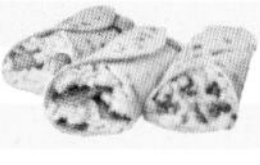
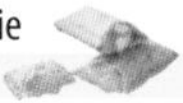
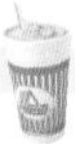

Burgers & Sandwiches:	C	F	Cb
Whataburger:			
#1 Original	**590**	25	62
#2 Double Meat	**835**	44	62
#3 Triple Meat	**1075**	63	62
#4 Jalapeno & Cheese	**680**	32	63
#5 Bacon & Cheese	**750**	37	62
#6 Double Meat Jr.	**420**	20	36
#7 Whataburger Jr.	**310**	11	36
All Time Favorites:			
Avocado Bacon Burger	**815**	49	51
Green Chili Double Burger	**990**	58	59
Honey BBQ Chicken Strip Sandwich	**910**	42	87
Mushroom Swiss Burger	**1110**	69	59
Patty Melt	**950**	61	45
Whatachick'n:			
Bites: 6 pieces, w/out sce	**450**	22	33
9 pieces w/o sce	**640**	31	45
Sandwich	**520**	19	56
Strips, 3 pieces, w/out sce	**490**	29	32
French Fries: Small, 3 oz	**280**	14	35
Medium, 4.5 oz	**420**	21	52
Large, 6 oz	**560**	28	70
Onion Rings: Medium, 3.2 oz	**300**	17	32
Large, 4.8 oz	**450**	25	49
Salad: Without Dressing			
Apple & Cranberry Grilled Chicken	**385**	12	38
Garden	**160**	9	10
with Whatachick'n	**400**	20	22
Breakfast:			
Buttermilk Biscuit:			
Bacon, Egg & Cheese	**500**	32	32
Sausage, Egg & Cheese	**665**	48	32
Honey Butter Chicken	**560**	33	51
Cinnamon Roll	**580**	17	94
Taquitos: *Without Cheese*			
with Bacon	**395**	23	28
with Chorizo	**405**	25	28
with Potato	**405**	21	38
with Sausage	**395**	23	28
Desserts:			
Chocolate Chunk Cookie	**230**	11	31
Hot Apple Pie, 3 oz	**270**	14	34
Malts: Chocolate, 20 oz	**570**	11	107
Vanilla, 20 oz	**520**	12	93
Shake, Chocolate, 20 oz	**550**	12	101

White Castle® (Nov '20)

Note: Nutritional Information varies from state to state. Please check instore

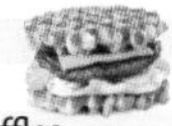
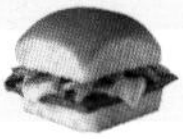
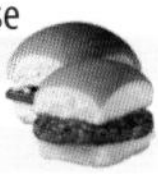
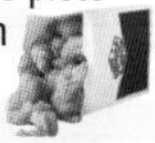
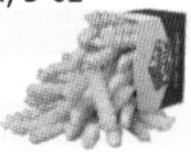
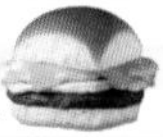
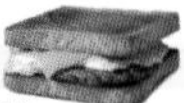
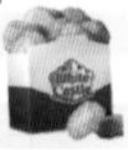

Sliders:	C	F	Cb
Bacon Cheese	**220**	14	15
Cheese	**170**	9	16
Crispy Chicken & Waffles	**350**	18	36
Crispy Chicken Breast with Cheese	**230**	10	22
Chicken Ring with Cheese	**230**	10	22
Double Original	**250**	13	24
Double Smoked Cheddar Cheese	**320**	19	26
Impossible with Smoked Cheddar	**240**	14	18
without Cheese	**210**	11	17
Fish with Cheese	**320**	22	22
Impossible	**210**	11	17
Jalapeno Cheese	**170**	9	16
Panko Surf & Turf with Cheese	**550**	36	34
Surf & Turf with Cheese	**520**	36	31
The Original	**140**	7	16
Veggie: with Ranch	**320**	23	23
with Honey Mustard	**210**	10	27
Sides: Chicken Rings, 3 piece	**160**	10	6
Clam Strips, medium	**410**	34	9
Fish Nibblers: Small	**320**	16	28
Medium	**590**	29	51
Mozzarella Cheese Sticks (3)	**460**	33	26
Onion Chips, medium	**930**	65	73
Onion Rings, small, 5 oz	**480**	33	40
Fries:			
Cheese, 7 oz	**400**	27	35
French: Kids, 4 oz	**250**	16	24
Small, 5.2 oz	**350**	21	34
Medium, 9.4 oz	**630**	39	60
Loaded Fries, 5.7 oz	**460**	38	20
Breakfast: With Cheddar Cheese			
Sliders: Bacon, Egg & Cheese	**260**	17	15
Bologna, Egg & Cheese	**350**	24	17
Egg & Cheese	**200**	12	15
Orig., w/ Egg & Chse	**270**	18	16
Sausage, Egg & Chse	**350**	26	15
Toasted Sandwiches:			
Bacon, Egg & Chse	**380**	23	29
Egg & Cheese	**270**	13	29
Sausage, Egg & Chse	**420**	27	29
Waffle Sliders:			
with Bacon, Egg & Cheese	**390**	26	27
with Sausage, Egg & Cheese	**490**	36	28
Hash Round Nibblers:			
Small	**360**	28	25
Medium	**600**	46	42
Dessert:			
On A Stick: Fudge Dipped Brownie	**250**	12	33
Fudge Dipped Cheesecake	**180**	10	21

Updated Nutrition Data ~ www.CalorieKing.com
Persons with Diabetes ~ See Disclaimer (Page 22)

Wienerschnitzel® (Nov '20)

Hot Dogs: On Hot Dog Bun	C	F	Cb
Original: Chicago Dog	330	15	37
Chili Dog	300	15	30
Chili Cheese Dog	350	20	30
Deluxe Dog	290	14	30
Junkyard Dog	430	24	42
Kraut Dog	280	14	29
Mustard Dog	280	14	28
Street Dog	350	20	30
Hot Dog Substitute, add to Original:			
All Beef Dog	100	10	1
Polish Sausage	140	12	2
Pretzel Bun Substitute, add to Orig.	80	1	15
Burgers:			
BBQ Bacon Chseburger	610	34	33
Chili Cheeseburger	450	24	27
Classic with Thousand Island Drssng	460	25	30
Specialties:			
Corn Dog	230	13	21
Fritos Pie	490	31	40
Polish Sausage Sandwich	500	34	36
Sides: Per Regular			
Chili Cheese Fries	530	29	53
Bacon Ranch	630	39	54
Thousand Island	710	45	60
French Fries: Small	310	16	38
Medium	440	23	54
Large	750	39	92
Breakfast:			
Biscuits: Egg, Bacon, Cheese	490	30	36
Egg, Sausage, Cheese	580	39	40
Burritos:			
Egg, Bacon, Cheese	420	20	38
Egg, Sausage, Cheese	510	29	42
Desserts:			
Classic Banana Split	760	24	131
Cones: With Sprinkles	240	9	40
Chocolate Dipped	350	21	40
Freezee,			
Oreo; M&M, Reese's, av.	630	25	98
Shakes, Chocolate with Oreo	950	35	155
Sundaes:			
Caramel; Choc; Hot Fudge, av.	395	15	64
Strawberry	370	14	59

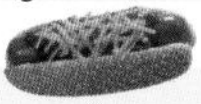
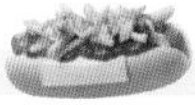
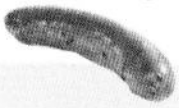
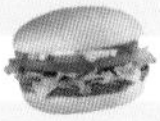
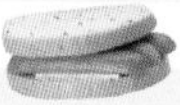
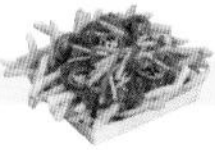
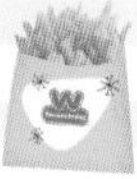

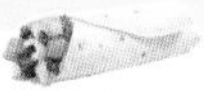
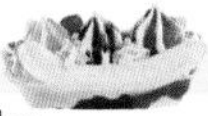
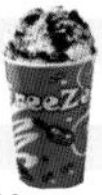

Winchell's® (Nov '20)

Donuts: Per Donut	C	F	Cb
Buttermilk Bars, Choc Iced/Glazed	420	19	61
Jelly Filled:			
Apple with Cinnamon Crumb	370	15	53
Raspberry with Glaze	390	13	61
Strawberry with Sugar	380	13	60
Old Fashioned, Glazed; Maple Iced	410	17	60
Raised Ring: Chocolate Iced	270	10	41
Coconut	240	12	30

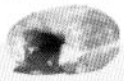

WingStreet (Nov '20)

Chicken: Without Dipping Sauce

Bone Out Wings: *Per Wing*	C	F	Cb
Buffalo, Mild	90	4	10
Garlic Parmesan	130	9	6
Honey BBQ	100	4	11
Ranch Rub	80	4	6
Traditional Bone In Wings: *Per Wing*			
Buffalo, Medium/Hot	100	4.5	5
Garlic Parmesan	140	11	0.5
Spicy Garlic	120	8	3
Sandwiches: Honey BBQ with Fries	1720	78	210
Honey BBQ with Bacon & Fries	1890	94	210
Fries:			
Regular, with Ketchup	500	24	67
Straight Cut, all var., with Ketchup	510	24	69

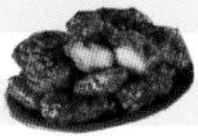
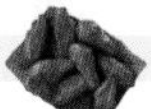

Woody's Bar-B-Q® (Sept '19)

Starters:	C	F	Cb
Breaded Wings (10)	700	47	13
Beef Chili Cheese Fries	805	38	63
Dinner Entrees: Without Sides			
½ Chicken	840	56	0
Baby Back Combo	680	48	1
Baby Back Ribs	520	40	2
Beef Prime Rib	760	62	1
New York Strip	490	36	2
Pork Sampler	1010	62	4
Ribeye Steak	735	54	2
Sandwiches: Per Regular, without Sides			
Beef	390	14	28
Pork	490	26	29
Wraps: Without Sides			
Beef BBQ	380	13	31
Pork BBQ	440	21	31
Extras: BBQ Beans	170	8	20
Cobettes	80	1	18
French Fries	185	7	28
Garlic Toast	120	6	14
Green Beans	50	2.5	6
Okra	95	1	21
Squash	140	1	28

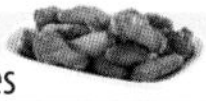
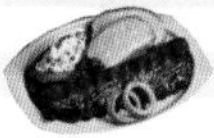
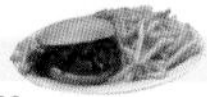
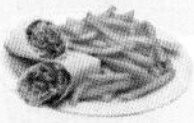
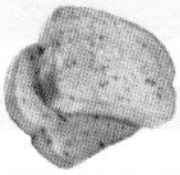

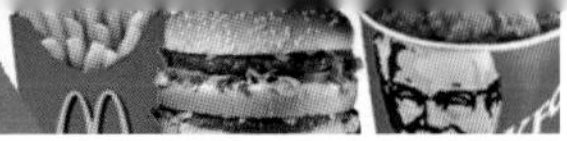

Yard House® (Nov '20)

	C	F	Cb
***Appetizers:** With Sides & Sauce*			
California Roll	1000	56	97
Chicken Nachos	2470	158	155
Chicken Lettuce Wraps	760	31	88
Poke Nachos	870	59	51
Spinach Cheese Dip	1280	98	73
Snacks: Devilled Eggs	400	31	18
Guacamole & Chips	760	49	75
Hot Spicy Edamame	500	41	19
Sweet Potato Fries	660	35	78
Truffle Fries	500	24	63
***Grilled Burgers:** Without Fries*			
BBQ Bacon Cheddar Burger	1220	82	54
Black Truffle Cheeseburger	980	61	48
Kurobuta Pork Burger	1000	60	62
Fries, 1 Serving	360	14	52
***House Favorites:** With Sides & Sauce*			
Fish & Chips	1360	95	85
Mac & Cheese, with Chicken, full	1980	137	115
Parmesan Crusted Pork Loin	1130	45	81
Spicy Jambalaya Pasta, full	1370	73	104
Pizza: Margherita	1080	44	125
The Carnivore	1520	81	111
***Seafood:** With Sides & Sauce*			
Ginger Crusted Salmon	990	57	66
Lobster Garlic Noodles	1030	57	77
***Soups:** Per Bowl*			
Chicken Tortilla	1060	83	46
Clam Chowder	480	35	29
***Salads:** Full Entree Size, with Dressing*			
Cobb Chicken	1020	71	29
Kale, Grilled Shrimp Caesar	730	48	34
Dessert: Mini Trio Sampler	1230	66	153
Brownies: Caramel	960	40	139
S'mores	1360	52	213

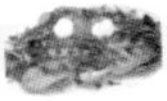
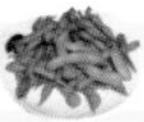
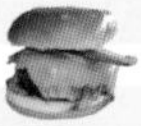
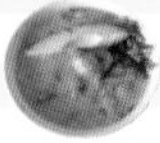
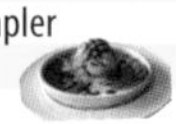

For Complete Nutritional Data ~ see CalorieKing.com

Yoshinoya® (Nov '20)

	C	F	Cb
***Entrees:** As Served*			
Angus Steak Bowl: Regular	570	11	97
Large	850	17	144
Beef Bowl: Regular	730	27	91
Large	1040	38	131
With Vegetables: Regular	650	20	95
Large	960	29	141
Teriyaki Chicken Bowl:			
Regular, without Skin	740	15	110
Large, without Skin	1090	21	166
Grilled Tilapia:			
with Rice & Coleslaw	570	13	91
with Rice, Veggies & Teriyaki Sce	590	12	100
Sides, Clam Chowder Soup	210	7	34
Kid's Meals: Beef	350	11	48
Teriyaki Chicken without skin	340	6	53

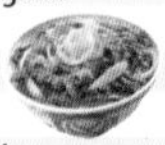
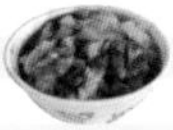

Zaxby's® (Nov '20)

	C	F	Cb
***Zappertizers:** With Menu Set Sauce*			
Cheddar Bites with Marinara Sauce	790	50	55
Spicy Fried Mushrooms w/ Ranch Sce	520	41	31
Tater Chips with Ranch Sauce	880	62	66
***Zalads:** With Texas Toast, Without Dressing*			
Blackened Blue	530	24	34
Buffalo Blue	680	35	48
Fried Cobb Zalad	820	47	47
Fried House Zalad	700	38	46
Grilled: Caesar Zalad	550	23	31
Grilled Cobb Zalad	700	36	35
Grilled House Zalad	580	27	35
***Dressings:** Per 1.25 oz Serving*			
Blue Cheese	180	19	2
Caesar	90	9	2
Honey Mustard	150	14	6
Mediterranean	140	13	4
Ranch	160	16	1
Thousand Island	230	23	3
Most Popular:			
Boneless Wings & Things	1480	88	109
Buffalo Boneless Wings & Things	1490	90	107
Buffalo Chicken Finger Plate (4)	1220	68	100
Chicken Finger Plate (4)	1190	66	101
Traditional Wings & Things	1530	96	90
***Sandwich Meals:** With Menu Set Components*			
Cajun Club	920	44	82
Chicken Finger	1000	50	97
Grilled Chicken	820	32	85
Kickin' Chicken	1070	55	102
Nibblerz	1280	63	132
Zaxby's Club	1150	62	101
Wings & Fingers:			
Boneless Wings (5): Insane	340	17	25
Sweet & Sour	390	17	36
Teriyaki	370	16	32
Traditional Wings (5): BBQ	440	24	17
HHM	480	33	8
Torch	400	25	6
Chicken Fingers 5:: Original	530	26	23
Wimpy	520	22	29
Sides:			
Crinkle Fries: Basket	850	46	99
Regular	330	14	47
Tater Chips	350	22	33
Texas Toast:			
1 Slice, 1.5 oz	150	7	19
Basket, 4.5 oz	450	21	57
Kidz Meals: Kiddie Cheese	820	44	87
Kiddie Finger	700	39	61
Kidz Nibbler	630	29	76

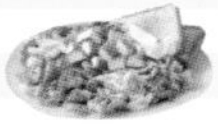
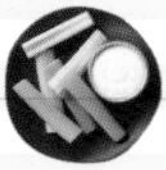
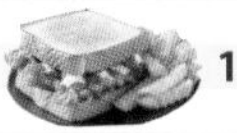
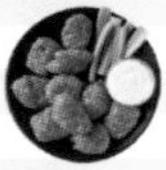
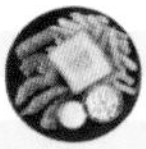
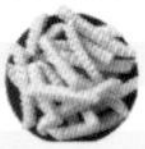
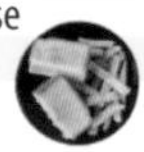

Zero Sub's® ~ *see CalorieKing.com*

Updated Nutrition Data ~ www.CalorieKing.com
Persons with Diabetes ~ See Disclaimer (Page 22)

Notes on Cholesterol

- **Cholesterol** is a white waxy substance produced mainly by our liver. It is also found in animal food products. Plant foods have no cholesterol.
- **Cholesterol is essential to life.** It is a structural part of every body cell wall and is the building block for vitamin D, sex hormones, and bile acids which help in the digestion of dietary fats. **Cholesterol is also vital for a healthy brain** (which contains some 20% of total body cholesterol).
- **The body makes sufficient cholesterol** for its needs and does not rely on cholesterol in the diet. Dietary fats have a major influence on blood cholesterol levels. (See next page)
- **A high blood cholesterol level increases** the risk of atherosclerosis - the thickening of arteries that can reduce or block blood flow to the heart, brain, eyes, kidneys, sex organs and other body parts.

  This in turn increases the risk of heart attack, stroke, blindness, kidney failure, impotence and other blood circulatory problems.

  Other risk factors which increase the risk of atherosclerosis include high blood pressure, smoking, obesity and uncontrolled diabetes.

Heart Attack Warning Signals

Many victims die before reaching the hospital by ignoring warning signals and delaying medical help.

Symptoms vary and commonly include:

- **Chest pain,** vice-like squeezing or burning sensation in center of the chest or between the shoulder blades, or in the mid-back. Pain may even feel like severe indigestion.
- **Pain** may be felt in the arms, shoulders, neck or jaw.
- **Shortness of breath** often occurs with or before chest discomfort.
- **Other signs,** with or without pain, include a cold sweat, nausea or light-headedness.

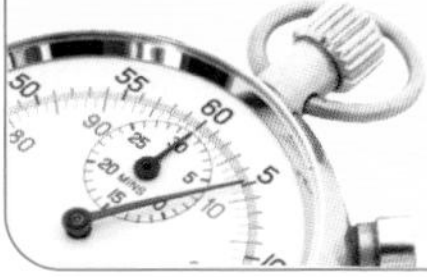

If you experience any of the above symptoms call IMMEDIATELY for medical help. Every minute counts.

***Call 9-1-1** or your emergency number*

Blood Cholesterol

CHECK YOUR RISK!

Total Cholesterol Level (mg/dl)		Risk of Heart Attack
240 and above	~	**High Risk**
200 - 239	~	**Borderline/High**
Below 200	~	**Desirable**

- **Know your cholesterol level, particularly if there is a family history of heart disease or stroke. If your level is high, see your doctor.**
- **All adults should have their cholesterol, HDL and triglycerides tested at least every 5 years.**

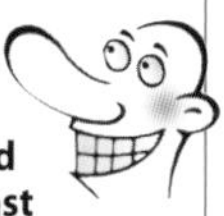

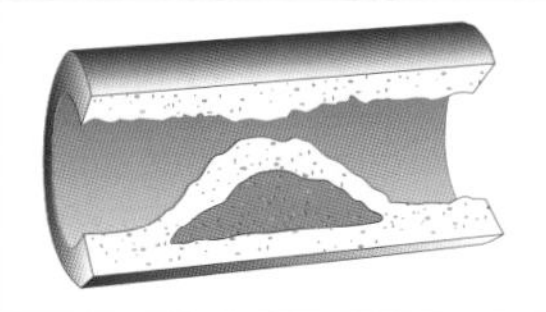

▲ **Atherosclerosis can clog arteries and impede blood flow to the heart or other body organs.**

▼ **A thrombus (blood clot) can form on unstable, festering athero-sclerotic plaque and rapidly block blood flow. A heart attack or stroke can result.**

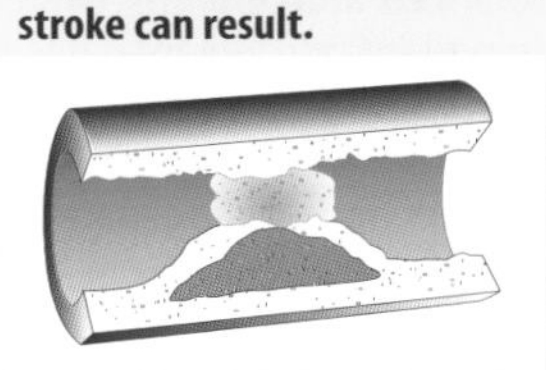

Fats & Cholesterol Guide

The amount and type of dietary fat has the greatest influence on blood cholesterol levels.

Fats in food are a mixture of 3 basic types: saturated, monounsaturated, and polyunsaturated. Animal fats are mainly saturated while plant oils and fish oils are mainly mono- and polyunsaturated.

Saturated fats have subgroups known as long-chain, medium-chain, and short-chain fats. Most of the long chain fats raise blood cholesterol, and increase the risk of blood clots and thrombosis leading to artery blockage.

Long-chain saturated fats are found mainly in full-cream milk, cheese, butter, cream, fatty meats and sausages, and processed foods.

Medium-chain fats (MCT) have little effect on LDL-cholesterol but may raise "good" HDL.

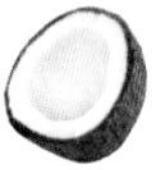

***Note: Coconut oil** has some MCT but is mainly saturated fat – so limit use.*

Monounsaturated fats tend to more selectively lower 'bad' LDL cholesterol and maintain the protective 'good' HDL cholesterol in the bloodstream – but only if they replace saturated fats in the diet. Foods rich in monounsaturates include canola and olive oils, canola margarine, peanuts, and avocados.

Polyunsaturated fats consist of two main classes. **Omega-6** polyunsaturates tend to lower blood cholesterol. Rich sources include safflower, sunflower and corn oils.

Omega-3 polyunsaturated fats can lower blood cholesterol; significantly lower blood triglycerides; and reduce the rise of thrombosis, heart arrythmmia, and artery spasm.

Best practical omega-3 sources include canola oil and margarine, soybean oil and fish.

A balanced intake of the two omega classes is important for optimal health. For most Americans, slightly increasing omega-3 intake would help attain a more ideal balance.

Trans fats from hydrogenated vegetable oils and shortenings should also be avoided. They are common in commercial baked and fried food products such as cakes, muffins, pastries, doughnuts, fried snacks and french fries.

DIETARY FATS COMPARISON

■ Saturated Fat ■ Monounsaturated Fat

Polyunsaturated Fats:

■ Linoleic (Omega-6) ■ Alpha-Linolenic (Omega-3)

OILS — **PERCENTAGE CONTENT**

OILS	Saturated	Monounsaturated	Linoleic (Omega-6)	Alpha-Linolenic (Omega-3)
CANOLA OIL	7	63	20	10
LINSEED/FLAX OIL	9	19	17	55
SAFFLOWER OIL	9	14	77	
GRAPESEED OIL	10	22	68	
SUNFLOWER OIL	11	23	66	
CORN OIL	14	32	52	2
OLIVE OIL	14	76	10	
SOYBEAN OIL	15	23	54	8
PEANUT OIL	19	45	34	2
COTTONSEED OIL	26	16	58	
PALM OIL	51	39	10	

SPREADS & FATS

Saturated Fat includes 'Trans Fats' ❑ WATER CONTENT

SPREADS & FATS	Saturated	Monounsaturated	Linoleic (Omega-6)	Alpha-Linolenic (Omega-3)	Water Content
LIGHT MARGARINE	14	14	21		51
CANOLA MARGARINE	18	45	12	6	19
POLYUNSATURATED MARG	24	20	36		20
BUTTER	57	18	2		24
LARD	41	47	12		
BEEF FAT	44	37	4		15

GOOD SOURCES OF OMEGA-3 FATS

Plant Sources	Omega-3 Fats (Grams)
Canola Oil, 1 Tbsp, ½ fl.oz	1.5g
Flaxseed Oil, 1 Tbsp	8g
Soybean Oil, 1 Tbsp	1.2g
Canola Margarine, 1 Tbsp, ½ oz	1g
Soybeans, cooked, ½ cup, 4 oz	0.5g
Walnuts, ½ oz	0.5g

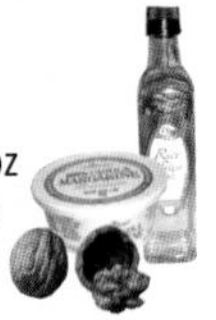

FISH - *Per 4 oz Serving*

High Content: Salmon (Chinook), Tuna, 3g
Trout (Lake), Sardines, Herring, Mackerel 3g

Medium Content:
Salmon, (Pink/Red/Coho), 4 oz 2g

Fair Content: *Per 4 oz Serving*

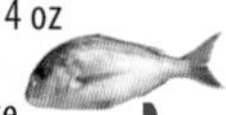

Bass, Catfish, Cod, Grouper, Hake, Halibut, Kingfish, Perch, Pollock, Shark, Trout (Rainbow), Tuna, Crab, Oysters, Blue Mussels, Shrimp, Squid } 0.5-1g

How Much Is Needed?

As little as 1-2 grams daily of omega-3 fats may benefit general health. High doses of fish-oil supplements should only be taken as directed by your Healthcare provider.

Dietary Cholesterol

Cholesterol in food varies in its effect on blood cholesterol level (BCL) from person to person. Much depends on the amount and type of fat and fiber eaten at the same meal.

Any elevating effect of dietary cholesterol on BCL is more likely to occur when the diet is high in saturated fat. Little elevation, if any, generally occurs when dietary fats are balanced in favor of mono- and poly-unsaturated fats (including omega-3 fats).

Example: While fish does contain cholesterol, the omega-3 fats can prevent any increase in BCL. Conversely, a meal containing no cholesterol but rich in saturated fat may result in a significant increase in BCL - as well as impairing artery wall functions.

Consequently, the need to be overly concerned about dietary cholesterol is being de-emphasized in favor of simply limiting total fat, saturated fat, and trans fat in particular – and substituting unsaturated fats (including omega-3 fats).

Note: Persons with familial (genetic) hyper-cholesterolemia should limit cholesterol; and ideally follow a plant-based diet.

The liver usually cuts back its own cholesterol production in response to cholesterol in the diet. Many people can consume high-cholesterol foods without concern.

However, it is difficult to identify just who is at risk - the so-called 'hyper-responders'. Because over 50% of Americans have a BCL above ideal levels, it may be prudent to limit cholesterol intake to less than 300mg daily, as well as to adopt a heart-healthy diet.

This limitation still allows the inclusion of most foods that are regularly eaten – even the overly maligned egg.

Avocados (like all plant foods) contain no cholesterol. Their fats are mainly monounsaturated and can lower blood cholesterol.

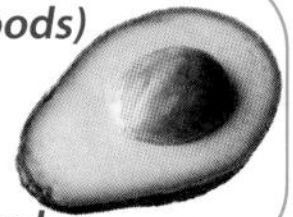

CHOLESTEROL COUNTER

Cholesterol is found only in foods of animal origin. Plant foods contain no cholesterol.

	Cholesterol mg
Meat - Average all types:	
Lean Meat, cooked, 120g	100
Fatty Meat, cooked, 120g	100
Fat, thick strip, 60g	40

Note: While lean meat and fat have similar amounts of cholesterol, choose lean meat to limit fat intake.

	Cholesterol mg
Chicken/Turkey, average, 120g	100
Organ Meats: Liver, fried, 4 oz	500
Brains, beef, pan fried, 3 oz	1700
Sausages: Frankfurter, 40g	25
Salami, 2 slices, 55g	40
Bacon: 3 slices, cooked, 30g	20
Fish: Fish fillets, average, ckd, 120g	70
Tuna/Salmon, canned, 100g	50
Scallops, 9 medium, 3 oz	30
Prawns, raw, 100g	110
Oysters, raw, 6 medium, 85g	45
Crayfish, Crab, cooked, 100g	70
Eggs (Chicken), 1 large	210
1 medium	180
Egg White, *Scramblers*	0
Milk/Yoghurt: Whole, 1 cup, 250ml	30
Light/low-fat Milk (1%), 1 cup	10
Skim/Non-fat, 1 cup	10
Soy Milk, Tofu, Tempeh	0
Cheese: Natural/Hard/Cream, 30g	30
Cottage, low-fat, 2 Tbsp, 40g	5
Cream Cheese, 30g	25
Fats: Butter, 1 Tbsp, 20g	45
Margarine, Oils (vegetable)	0
Mayonnaise, 1 Tbsp	10
Cream: Heavy, whipping, 2 Tbsp, 40g	40
Light/Sour, 2 Tbsp	10
Ice Cream: Full-fat (10-11%), 100ml/50g	20
Low-fat (less than 4%), 50g	5
Fruit, Vegetables, Avocados	0
Nuts, Seeds, Grains	0
Coffee, Tea, Beer, Wine	0

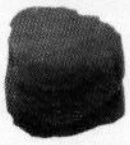
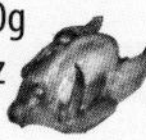
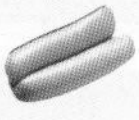
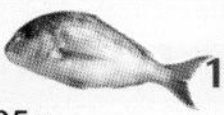
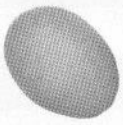
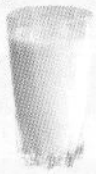
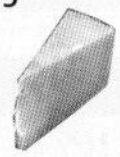
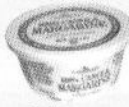
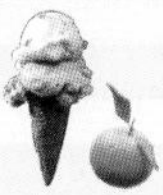

For Comprehensive Food Listings ~ see www.CalorieKing.com

Blood Cholesterol ~ Diet Tips

DIETARY TIPS TO LOWER BLOOD CHOLESTEROL

1. **Maintain a healthy weight.**
   If overweight, lose weight with a sensible, low-fat meal plan and daily exercise.

2. **Reduce saturated fat intake by:**

   (a) eating less dairy fat. Choose low-fat or fat-reduced milk, yogurt, soy drinks, and cheese.

   (b) replacing saturated fats with whole foods rich in monounsaturated and polyunsaturated fats – such as fish, nuts, seeds, avocado and olives.

   Limit vegetable oils but choose mainly extra virgin olive oil and black seed oil. Avoid frying which can oxidize fats and harm health.

   (c) eating less fat from meat and poultry. Choose lean cuts of meat and skinless chicken. Go easy on lunch meats, salami and fatty sausages.

   Eat more fish, particularly higher fat fish such as salmon, herring, albacore tuna and sardines. They contain omega-3 fats that benefit the heart and all body cells.

   (d) eating less saturated and trans fats from baked and fried fast-foods. Avoid deep-fried foods. Avoid donuts, cakes, pastries and cookies unless made with healthier fats and oils.

3. **Increase your soluble fiber intake.**
   Foods rich in soluble fiber include beans, lentils, chickpeas, hummus, nuts, seeds, psyllium-seed husks and psyllium-fiber supplements. Oat bran, rice bran and barley are also good sources; as are fruit, vegetables, nopales (cactus leaves) and avocados. *(See Fiber Guide - Page 264-269)*

4. **Eat more soy bean foods such as:**
   soy drinks, tofu, tempeh (cultured soy beans), soy flour, soy vegetarian foods and edamame (fresh green soybeans).

   Soy protein in place of animal protein can significantly decrease high blood cholesterol levels, LDL cholesterol and blood triglycerides while maintaining 'good' HDL cholesterol.

5. **Eat more fruit, vegetables, and whole grains** in place of high-fat foods.
   Aim for 2 fruits and 5 servings of vegetables per day. They also contain valuable antioxidants. The fat of avocados (and most nuts) is mainly unsaturated and can lower blood cholesterol levels.

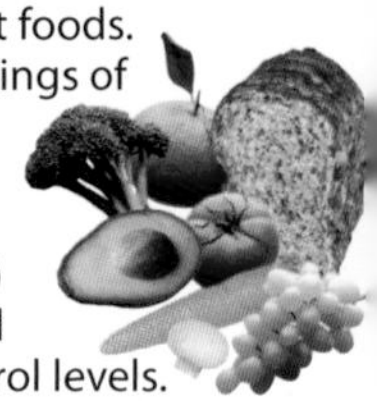

6. **Limit cholesterol to 300mg per day.**
   (Extra Notes ~ See Previous Page)

7. **Avoid brewed unfiltered coffee**
   (espresso; plunger-style). Several cups per day may raise blood cholesterol. Filtered coffee is fine.

8. **Spread your food intake over the day.**
   Have 3-4 smaller meals per day rather than just 1-2 very large meals. Nibbling, versus gorging, favors lower blood cholesterol.

   Eat most food during the day and less at night.

ALCOHOL – WINE

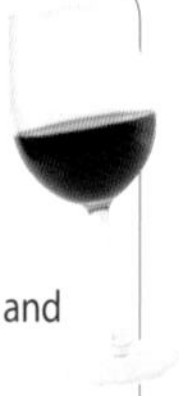

Alcohol is a mixed bag. Moderate amounts of 1-2 drinks daily appear to reduce the risk of heart attack and ischemic stroke in older persons.

However, larger amounts increase the risk of high blood pressure, obesity, heart failure and hemorrhagic stroke, and can aggravate hypertriglyceridemia: as well as many other health hazards. *(See Alcohol Guide – Page 23)*

The speculative benefits of moderate alcohol intake have been overstated in the media. The overriding harmful effects of excess alcohol do not allow its recommendation for any aspects of health promotion.

Fruit, Vegetables & Tea Also Protect:

Red wine and red grapes (more so than white) contain antioxidants which may help protect cholesterol in the blood from becoming oxidized.

Most fruits, vegetables, whole-grains, nuts and tea also contain protective antioxidants.

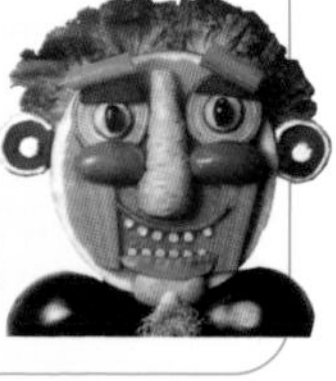

How Fats Affect Blood Flow

Fats in the diet affect more than blood cholesterol levels. They can also strongly influence blood clot formation and thrombosis, as well as blood flow and ultimate oxygen delivery to body parts and organs. While advanced atherosclerosis can impede blood flow to the heart and other organs, it is thrombosis (complete blockage by blood clots) or arterial spasm which commonly results in a heart attack or stroke. **Plant and fish oils rich in omega-3 fats** lessen the risk of blood clots, thrombus formation, and artery spasm by reducing platelet stickiness and adhesion to artery walls. This also reduces inflammation of the artery wall lining. This in turn reduces the risk of atherosclerotic plaque becoming unstable and reactive.

Omega-3 fats also improve blood flow by reducing blood viscosity and increasing the flexibility of red blood cells that need to flex and twist on themselves in order to squeeze through tiny narrow capillaries often half their diameter.

A diet high in saturated fats (longer chain) has the opposite effect by stiffening red blood cell membranes and increasing blood viscosity, thereby hindering blood flow.

Stiff red blood cells may also form aggregates that resemble coin stacks. In narrow blood vessels, this further impedes blood flow and impairs oxygen release through the much-lessened surface area of red blood cell membranes exposed to blood.

Note: Smoking, lack of exercise, and stress can have similar adverse effects on thrombosis, red blood cell flexibility, and blood flow.

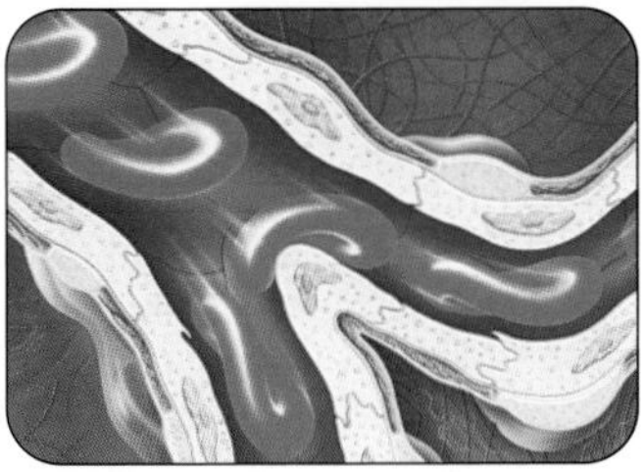

▲ *Picture of Healthy Blood Flow*

Flexible red blood cells twist and slide through tiny capillaries - often half the diameter of red blood cells.

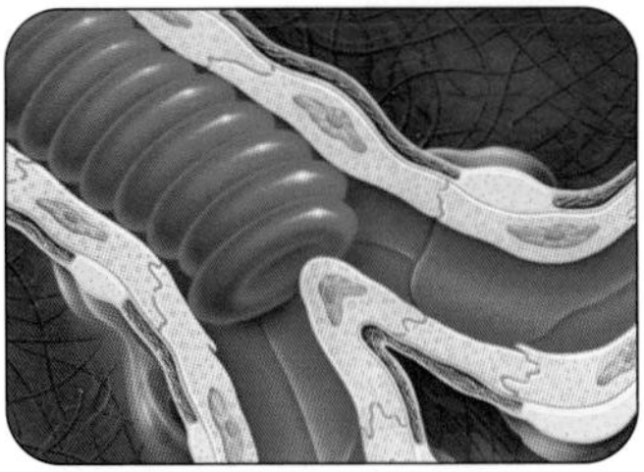

▲ *A Not-So-Healthy Picture!*

Red blood cells have lost their flexibility and ability to twist and slip through capillaries. They are stacked up, thereby impeding blood flow.

A diet high in saturated fats can contribute to this picture - as can smoking, lack of exercise, and stress.

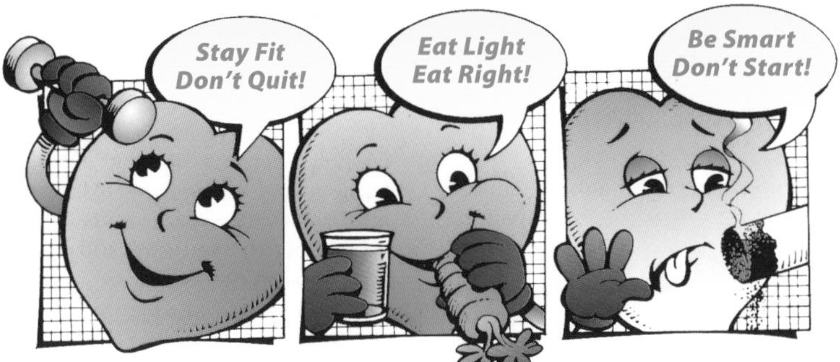

Fiber Guide

Introduction

Fiber

Fiber is the general term for those parts of plant food that we cannot digest (although bacteria in the large bowel partly digests fiber through fermentation). It is not found in foods of animal origin (meats, dairy products).

Fiber promotes intestinal health, bowel regularity, can benefit diabetes and blood cholesterol levels, and may help prevent colon cancer. High-fiber foods also assist weight control.

Most Americans don't eat enough fiber – less than 20 grams/day – instead of a healthier 25 to 35 grams/day.

A fiber-rich diet assists the growth of friendly gut microbes that can benefit our metabolism, weight and blood glucose levels – as well as hunger, mood and our immune system.

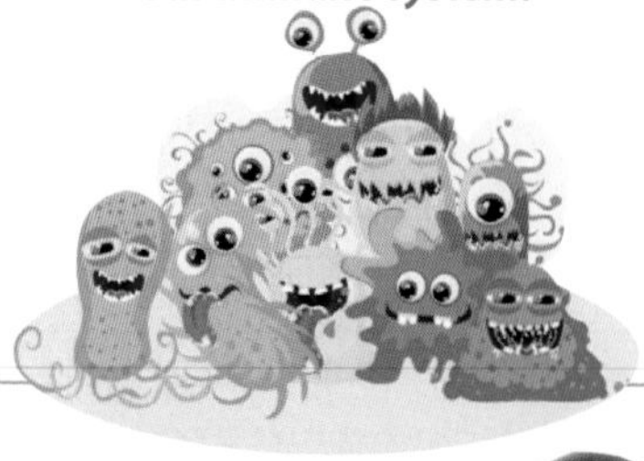

Types of Fiber

Plant foods contain a mixture of different fibers in varying proportions. Insoluble and soluble fiber categories are based on their solubility in water. All types of fiber are beneficial to the body.

- **Insoluble fibers** (cellulose, hemi-celluloses, lignin) make up the structural parts of plant cell walls.

  Best food sources are wheat bran, corn bran, rice bran, wholegrain cereals and breads, beans and peas, nuts, seeds, and the skins of fruits and vegetables.

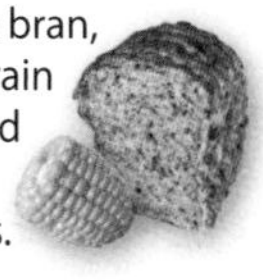

These fibers absorb many times their own weight in water. They create a soft bulk and hasten the passage of waste products through the intestines.

They promote bowel regularity, and aid in the prevention and treatment of uncomplicated forms of **constipation, diverticulosis and hemorrhoids.**

The risk of colon cancer may also be reduced by fiber's diluting effect on potentially harmful substances.

- **Soluble fibers (pectin, gums, mucilages)** are found mainly within plant cells, soy milk (whole bean) and products.

Best Sources of Soluble Fiber:

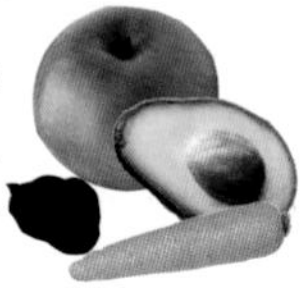

Fruits and vegetables, oat bran, barley, beans and peas, prunes, psyllium and flax seed.

These fibers form a gel which slows both stomach emptying and the absorption of sugars from the intestines. **This helps to control blood sugar levels.**

Weight control is also aided by the slower emptying of the stomach and the feeling of **fullness provided by soluble fiber.**

Soluble fiber can also lower blood cholesterol by binding bile acids and excreting them. More body cholesterol must then be broken down to supply bile acids for emulsification of dietary fats. **Rice bran, while not high in soluble fiber, can also lower blood cholesterol.**

- **Resistant starch** is that part of starchy foods (approx. 10%) which is tightly bound by fiber and resists normal digestion. Friendly bacteria in the large bowel ferment and change the resistant starch into short-chain fatty acids, which are important to bowel health and may protect against colon cancer.

Starchy foods include bread, cereals, rice, pasta, potatoes and legumes.

Fiber & Weight Control

Fiber can assist weight control in several ways. Fiber-rich foods such as fresh fruit and vegetables, potatoes and wholegrain bread contain few calories for their large volume (due to their low-fat, high-water content).

Their bulk fills the stomach and satisfies the appetite much sooner than fiber-depleted foods. The extra chewing time also contributes to satiety, and gives the stomach time to register a feeling of fullness. Excessive calories are less likely to be consumed.

Fiber-depleted foods and drinks are more concentrated in calories; e.g. fats, sugar, candy, soft drinks, fruit juices, alcohol. They require little or no chewing. Large amounts with excessive calories can be consumed before the appetite is satisfied.

Example: Whereas one fresh apple might satisfy the appetite, an apple juice drink with the equivalent sugars and calories of 2-3 apples only minimally satisfies the appetite. (See illustration below.)

High-fiber foods fill the stomach. Fewer calories are consumed.

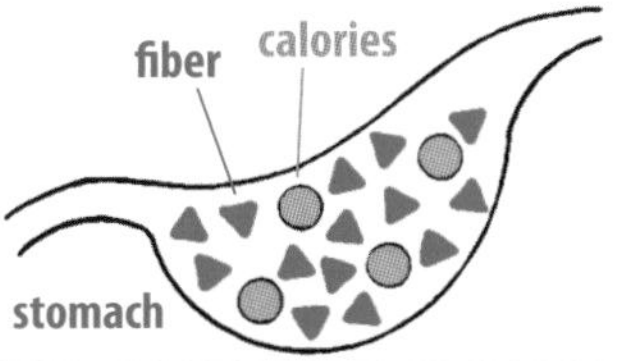

Low-fiber foods are more concentrated in calories. More food must be eaten to fill the stomach.

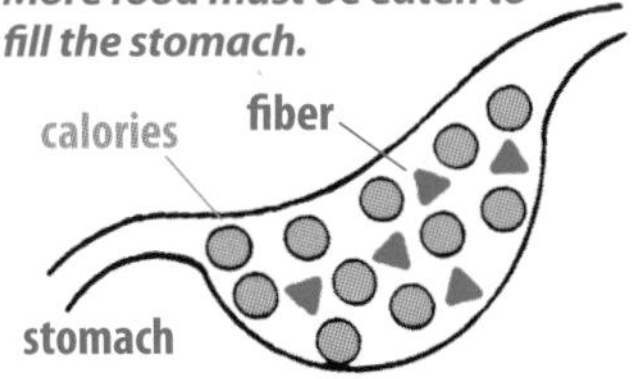

EFFECTS OF REMOVING FIBER FROM FOOD

2-3 pieces of fresh fruit produces 1 glass of fruit juice. The removal of fiber concentrates the sugars and calories.

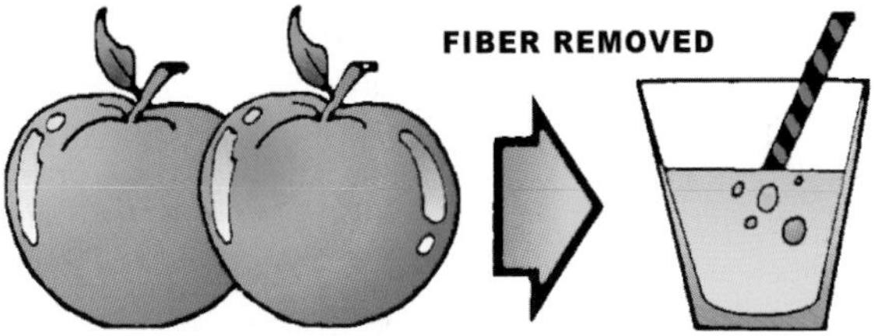

FRESH FRUIT	(Comparison)	FRUIT JUICE
Higher Fiber	✦	Negligible Fiber
Low Calorie Density	✦	High Calorie Density
Long Eating Time	✦	No Eating Time (Drink)
Satisfies Hunger	✦	Does Not Satisfy Hunger
Sugars Slowly Absorbed	✦	Sugars More Quickly Absorbed
Less Insulin Required	✦	More Insulin Required
Supports Gut Microbes	✦	Fewer Benefits to Microbes

Constipation

Constipation can reasonably be defined as a failure to have a bowel movement at least every second day – and just as importantly, without straining or pain.

Typically, constipated stools are too hard, too narrow and too small.

The **main cause** is simply a lack of dietary fiber. Other contributing factors include insufficient fluids, too little exercise, emotional stress, gastrointestinal disease, lack of proper dentition to chew high-fiber foods, and some medications (e.g. some antacids, antidepressants, pain medications).

Note: Check with your doctor to rule out any underlying medical problem – especially if you have a change in bowel habits in middle-age or later years.

DESIRABLE FIBER INTAKE

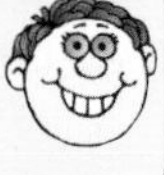

Adults: 25-35gm per day
Children (under 18): Age + 5gm
Example: 6-year old (6 + 5)= 11gm

SAMPLE FOOD QUANTITIES

For 35 Grams of Fiber/Day

		Fiber
	Breakfast Cereal (higher-fiber)	5g
plus	4 slices wholegrain Bread	6g
plus	3 servings fresh Fruit	9g
plus	1 medium Potato (w. skin)	4g
or	1 cup Brown Rice	
or	½ cup wholegrain Pasta	
plus	3-4 servings Veggies/Salad	6g
plus	1 cup Bean Soup	5g
or	¼ cup Baked/Soy Beans	
or	½ cup Corn/Peas/Lentils	
or	1¼ oz Almonds (natural)	
or	3 medium Figs	

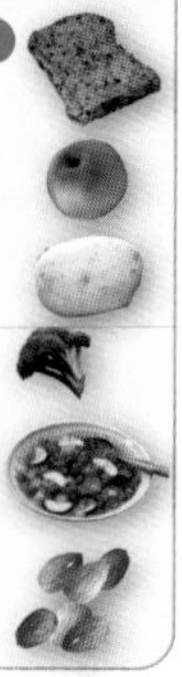

HINTS TO INCREASE FIBER AND AVOID CONSTIPATION

1. **Breakfast is an important** contributor to daily fiber intake. Eat high-fiber breakfast cereals (bran-based cereals, oatmeal etc.). Add 1-2 tablespoons of unprocessed bran.

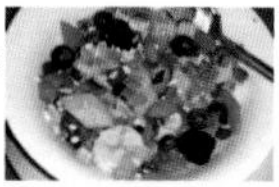

   Dried fruits, chopped nuts, soy grits, and seeds are also excellent additions to cereals.

   Note: A gradual increase in fiber will prevent bloating, gas or pain. People intolerant to bran may benefit from psyllium-based fiber supplements and cereals.

2. **Drink adequate water daily.** Fiber works by absorbing many times its own weight in water.

3. **Eat wholegrain breads,** or fiber-enriched breads. They have over double the fiber of regular white bread.

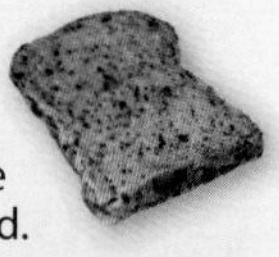

4. **Enjoy fruit as fresh fruit** with skin rather than as fruit juice. Enjoy wholegrain pasta, barley, brown rice, nuts and seeds.

5. **Eat more vegetables,** salads and legumes – especially cooked beans, lentils, potatoes with skins, avocado, broccoli, brussels sprouts, cabbage, carrots, celery, and peas.

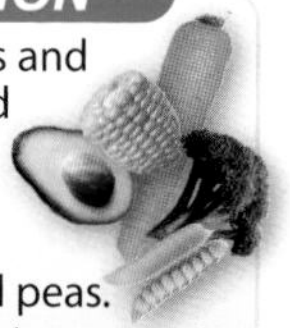

6. **Add bran** (barley/rice/wheat) or soy grits to soups, casseroles, yogurt, desserts, cookies, cakes. Also use whole-meal flour or soy flour in place of white flour. Use nuts, seeds, and ground linseed.

7. **Snack** on fresh or dried fruits, carrot or celery sticks, popcorn, nuts or seeds, wholegrain crackers, high-fiber bars (low-fat). Limit amounts if overweight.

8. **Exercise regularly** to strengthen abdominal muscles and stimulate the gut. Keep up water intake, especially in warm weather.

9. **Avoid** indiscriminate and regular use of harsh laxatives. They can overstimulate the intestinal muscles and may make normal bowel activity impossible. It may take several weeks to restore normal bowel function.

FOODS WITH ZERO FIBER

- **Dairy Products (Milk, Cheese, etc.)**
- **Meats, Poultry, Fish, Eggs**
- **Fats/Oils, Sugar/Syrups**

(Only foods of plant origin contain fiber.)

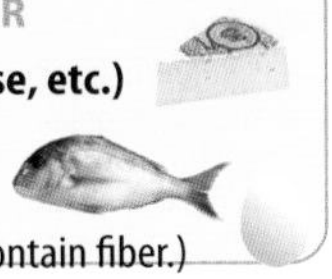

Breakfast Cereals

General Mills:	Fiber
Basic 4, 1 cup, 2 oz	3
Cheerios (Honey Nut; Multigrain), 1⅓ cups, 1 oz	4
Chex, Rice, cup	2
Cinnamon Toast Crunch, 1 cup, 1.4 oz	2
Fiber One, Original Bran, ⅔ cups, 1.4 oz	18
Kix, 1½ cups, 1.4 oz	3
Lucky Charms, 1 cup, 1.3 oz	2
Oatmeal Crisp Almond, 1 cup, 2 oz	6
Raisin Nut Bran, 3/4 cup, 1.7 oz	6
Total, Whole Grain, 0.875 oz	2
Trix, 1¼ cups, 1.4 oz	1
Wheat Chex, 1 cup, 2 oz	8
Wheaties, 1 cup, 1.26 oz	4
Kellogg's:	
All-Bran, Buds, ½ cup, 1.58 oz	17
Corn Flakes, 1½ cups, 1.4 oz	1
Frosted Flakes, 1 cuo, 1.4 oz	0.5
Frosted Mini Wheats, 2 oz	6
Krave, Chocolate, 1 pkg, 1.87 oz	3
Raisin Bran, 1 cup, 2 oz	7
Rice Krispies, 1½ cups, 1.4 oz	0
Special K, 1 cup, 1.4 oz	3
Kashi: Organic	
7 Whole Grain Puffs, 1½ cups, 1.4 oz	4
7 Whole Grain Flakes, 1¼ cups, 2.2 oz	7
Blueberry Clusters, 1 cup, 1.9 oz	3
GO: Rise, Original, 1¼ cuos, 2 oz	13
Go Defy, Crunch, ¾ cup, 1.9 oz	9
Honey Toasted Oat, 1 cup, 1.4 oz	5
Strawberry Fields, 1 cup, 1.95 oz	3
Warm Cinnamon Oat, 1 cup, 1.4 oz	5
Whole Wheat Biscuits, 31 pieces, 2.1 oz	7

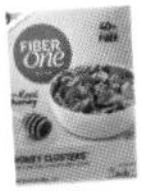

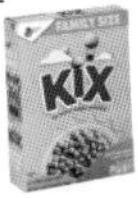

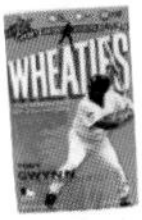

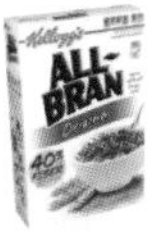

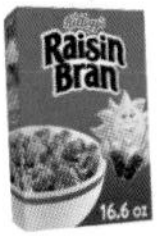

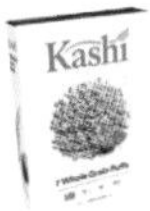

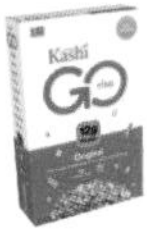

Fiber ~ Fiber (grams)

Breakfast Cereals (Cont)

Quaker:	Fiber
Corn Crunch, 1 cup, 1.3 oz	5
Life, Original, 1 cup, 1.45 oz	3
Oatmeal Squares, Cinnamon, 1 cup, 1.9 oz	5
Muesli, Raisin Date Almond, ½ cup, 1.8 oz	5
Multigrain Flakes, Honey Vanilla, ¾ cup, 2.2 oz	3
Quisp, 1¼ cups, 1.45 oz	0.5
Real Medleys, Multigrain, Cherry, ¾ cup, 1.9 oz	4
Simply Granola, Oats, Honey, Raisins & Alm., 2.4 oz	7
Post:	
Alpha Bits, 1 cup, 1 oz	2
Better Oats, Maple & Br. Sugar, 1 oz pouch	3
Bran Flakes, 1 cup, 1.34 oz	7
Dunkin', Mocha Latte, 1⅓ cups, 1.34 oz	0
Grape Nuts, Original, ½ cup, 2 oz	7
Great Grains, Blueberry Morning, 1 cup, 2 oz	4
Honey Bunches of Oats, Vanilla, 1 cup, 0.95 oz	4
Raisin Bran, 1¼ cups, 2.1 oz	9
Shredded Wheat, Original, Spoon, 1⅓ cups, 2 oz	8

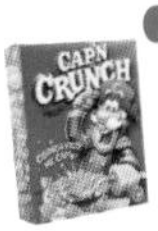

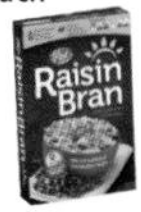

Brans & Supplements, Metamucil

Oat Bran: 1 Tbsp (level)	1
1/3 cup, (5 1/3 Tbsp), 1 oz	5
Rice Bran, raw. 1/3 cup, 1 oz	6
Wheat Bran, Unprocessed:	
Raw, 1 Tbsp	1.5
2 Tbsp (level), 1/4 oz	3
1/4 cup, (4 Tbsp), 1/2 oz	6
Wheat Germ, Raw, 1/4 cup, 1 oz	4
Psyllium Seed Husks, 2 Tbsp	8
Fibersure, 1 heaping tsp	5
Metamucil: Orange, 1 rnd Tbsp, 11g	3
Fiber Wafers (2)	6

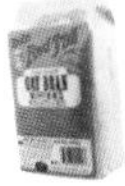
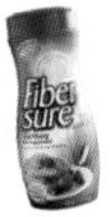

Hot Cereals, Oatmeal

Bulgur (Cracked Wheat), ckd, 1 cup	8
Corn/Hominy Grits, dry, 3 Tbsp, 1 oz	0.5
Cream of Wheat, cooked, 1 oz	1
Oatmeal, cooked 2/3 cup	3

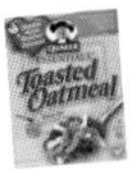

Fiber Counter

Breads & Crackers

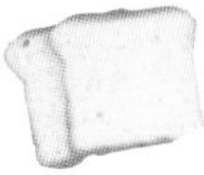

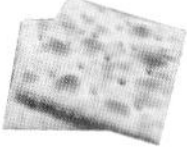

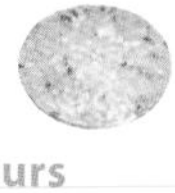

	Fiber
Bread: White, 1 slice, 1 oz	0.6
Whole-wheat, 1 slice, 1 oz	1.5
Wholegrain, 1 slice, 1 oz	2
Rye, Pumpernickel, 1 oz	1.5
Bagel/Roll/Bun, 1 medium, 2 oz	1.5
Pita, whole wheat, 6.5″ pocket	4.5
Crackers: Graham, average, 2	0.4
Saltine, 4 crackers	0.4
Crispbreads, average, 2	4
Matzo, 1 board, 1 oz	1
Rice Cakes, average, 1 cake	0.3
Tortilla: Regular, 6″	0.5
Whole-wheat, 6″	1.3

Barley, Pasta, Rice & Flours

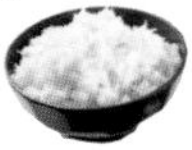

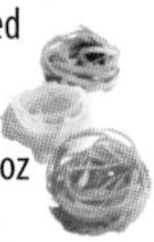

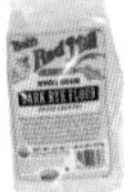

	Fiber
Barley, pearled, raw, 1/4 cup, 1.7 oz	8
Rice:	
White, cooked, 1 cup	0.6
Brown, cooked, 1 cup	3.5
Rice-A-Roni, average, 1 cup, prepared	1.5
Spaghetti/Noodles: Cooked, 1 cup	2
Whole-Wheat, cooked, 1 cup	4
Flour: Wheat, All-purpose, 1 cup, 4.5 oz	3.5
Whole-Wheat, 1 cup, 4.5 oz	15
Cornmeal, stone ground, 1 cup, 4.5 oz	13
Carob Flour, 1 cup, 3.5 oz	41
Hemp Wholemeal Flour, 1 cup, 3.5 oz	41
Rye Flour, 1 cup, 3.5 oz	15
Soy Flour: Defatted, 1 cup, 3.5 oz	17
Full-fat, raw, 1 cup, 3 oz	8
Soy Meal, defatted, 1 cup, 4.5 oz	14

Frozen Entrees & Dinners

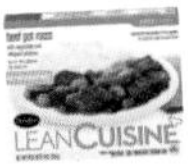

	Fiber
***Average All Brands**: Per Serving*	
Beans/Chili base, average	6-10
Potato/Pasta base, average	4-6
Vegetable base, average	3
Meat/Chicken base, average	2-3
Pizzas, 1/4 large, average	3
Vegetarian Soy Burgers, 1 pattie	4

Soups

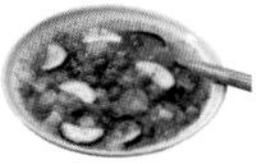

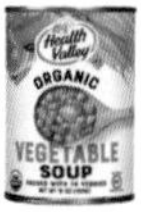

	Fiber
Chicken Noodle, 1 cup	0.5
Tomato Soup, average, 1 cup	0.5
Vegetable Soup, average, 1 cup	3
***Health Valley:** Per 1 Cup*	
Chicken & Rice	1
Minestrone	6
Split Pea	13
Tomato	5
Vegetable	4
Progresso, Tomato	6

Fast Foods & Restaurants

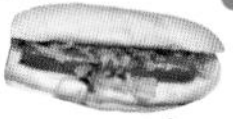

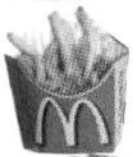

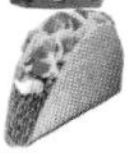

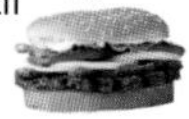

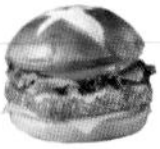

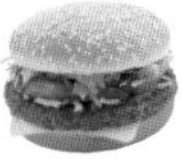

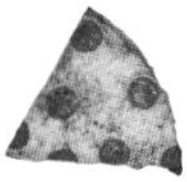

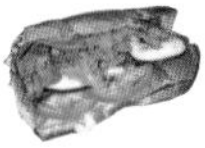

	Fiber
Hamburgers: Small, average	1.5
Large/Whopper, average	2.5
Hot Dog, Regular	1.5
French Fries: Small serving, 2.5 oz	2.5
Regular/Medium, 3.5 oz	3.5
Chicken Nuggets, 6 pack	0.5
Chicken Sandwich, average	2
Taco, average	4
Sundaes, Shakes, Soft Drinks	0
Arby's, Classic Roast Beef Sandwich	2
Burger King: Whopper	2
Impossible Whopper	4
Del Taco, Beyond 8 Layer Burrito	9
Denny's: House Salad, no dressing	3
Bacon Avocado Cheeseburger	5
Club Sandwich	8
Super Bird Sandwich	2
Domino's: 12″ Thin Crust, 1 slice	0.5
12″ Handmade Pan Crust, 1 slice	0.5
12″ Deluxe, Hand Tossed, 1 slice	1
McDonald's: Big Mac	3
Hamburger	1
Egg McMuffin	2
Quarter Pounder with Cheese	2
Pizza Hut: *Per 1 Slice, Medium*	
Original Pan Pizza: Cheese, Pepp.	2
Supreme	2
Thin 'n Crispy, Supreme	2
Hand-Tossed, average all varieties	2
Subway: 6″ 9 Grain Honey Oat Roll	4
6″ 9 Grain Wheat Roll	4
Habanero Wrap	2
Taco Bell: Bean Burrito, vegan	11
Power Menu Bowl, Veggie	10

Cakes, Cookies, Snack Bars

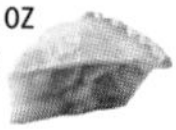

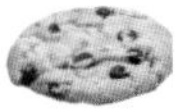

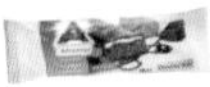

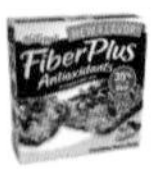

	Fiber
Apple/Fruit Pie, 1 serving, 4 oz	2
Cake: With plain flour, 1 serving, 3.4 oz	1.5
With whole-wheat flour, 1 serving	3
Carrot Cake, 4 oz	4
Cookies, oatmeal, (3 small/1 large)	1
Donuts, medium, 1.7 oz	0.7
Fruit Cake, 1 serving, 1.5 oz	2
Fig Bars, 1 cookie, 0.5 oz	0.7
Muffins, Oat Bran (2 small, 1 large), 4 oz	5
Granola Bars, average, 1 bar	2
Atkins Advantage Bars, av.	7
Clif Bars, 2.5 oz	4
Fiber One (Gen. Mills):	
Oats & Chocolate, 0.8 oz	9
Other Bars, 0.8oz	6
Fiber Plus, Chewy, 1.27 oz	9
Health Valley, Cereal Bars	0.5
Luna Bars, avg., 1.7 oz	3
Special K, Chocolate Protein Meal Bar, 1.6 oz	3

Chocolate, Chips, Popcorn

	Fiber
Cheese Balls/Curls/Twists	1
Chocolate, Hard Candy, 1 oz	0
Chocolate with nuts/fruit, 2 oz bar	1.5
Mars Bar, 1.8 oz	1
Potato Chips; corn chips, 1 oz	1
Popcorn, 3 cups	3
Pretzels, Twists (6)	1

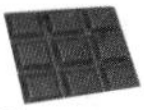
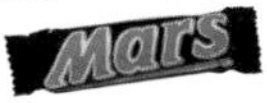

Nuts, Seeds

	Fiber
Almonds: Natural, 25 nuts, 1 oz	3.5
Blanched (skins removed), 1 oz	3
Cashews, Filberts, Pecans, 1 oz	1.7
Hepm Seeds, 3 Tbsp, 1 oz	9
Peanuts, Mixed Nuts, Coconut, 1 oz	2.5
Peanut Butter, 2 Tbsp, 1 oz	2
Pistachio Nuts, dried, shelled, 1 oz	3
Walnuts, Black/English, dried, 1 oz	2
Seeds: Amaranth, 2½ Tbsp, 1 oz	3.5
Flax Seeds, 3 Tbsp, 1 oz	7
Psyllium Seed Husks, 5 Tbsp, 1 oz	20
Quinoa Seeds, 3 Tbsp, 1 oz	1.7
Sesame Seeds, whole, 1 oz	3.4
Sesame Butter/Tahini, 2 Tbsp, 1.1 oz	1.4
Sunflower Kernels, ¼ cup, 1 oz	3.8

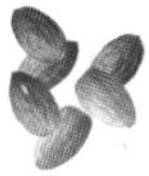
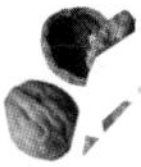
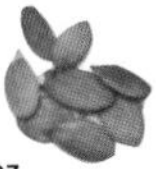

Fruit – Fresh

	Fiber
Apples: 1 medium, 5½ oz (whole)	
with skin + core	3.7
with skin, no core	3.2
without skin, no core	1.7
Apricots, 2 medium, 4 oz	1.5
Avocado, average, ½ medium	6
Banana, 1 medium, 6 oz (w. skin)	3
Blueberries, raw, ½ cup, 2.5 oz	1.7
Cherries, sweet, raw, 8 fruits, 1.6 oz	1
Grapefruit, average, ½ fruit, 10 oz	1.4
Grapes, 1 medium bunch, seedless, 7 oz	2
Kiwifruit, 1 medium, 2.7 oz	2.3
Mango, 1 medium, 11 oz (whole)	1.6
Melons, Cantaloupe, 4 oz (edible)	1
Nectarine, 1 medium, 4 oz	1.9
Olives, average all types, 7 jumbo, 2 oz	1.5
Oranges, 1 medium (7-8 oz w. skin)	
5½ oz (peeled)	3.8
Passionfruit, 2 medium, 2.5 oz	5
Peaches, 1 large, 6 oz	2
Pears, raw, 1 medium, 6 oz	4.5
Pineapple, 1 slice, 3 oz	1.2
Plums, 2 medium, 6 oz	1.8
Strawberries, 6 medium/3 large, 2 oz	1
Watermelon, 4 oz (edible)	0.5

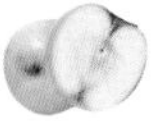
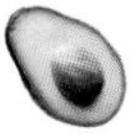
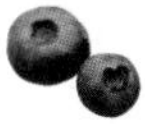
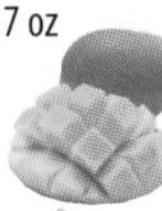
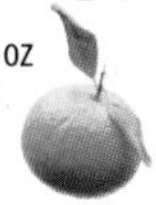
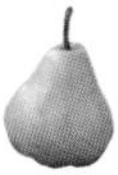
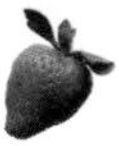

Fruit – Dried, Juice

	Fiber
Dried Fruit: Apricots, 8 halves, 1 oz	2.2
Dates (3 med); Raisins (2 Tbsp), 1 oz	1.5
Figs, 3 medium, 1½ oz	5
Prunes, 4 medium, 1 oz	2
Fruit Juice: Orange/Apple etc, 1 glass	<0.5
Prune Juice, 5 oz	1.4
Carrot Juice, 8 oz	1.8

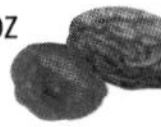
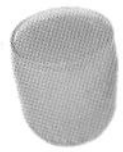

Vegetables

	Fiber
Asparagus, 4 medium spears	1.3
Bean Sprouts, ½ cup, 2 oz	1
Beans: Snap/Green, ½ cup, 2 oz	2
Baked Beans in Tom Sce, ½ c, 4.5 oz	5
Dried Beans, ckd, average, ½ cup	7
Beets, ckd, slices, ½ cup, 3 oz	1.7
Broccoli, cooked, ½ cup, 3 oz	2.4
Brussels Sprouts, ckd, ½ cup, 3 oz	3.5
Cabbage: White, ckd, ½ cup, 2.5 oz	1
Red, ckd, ½ cup, 2.5 oz	2
Carrots, 1 medium (7½"), ½ cup, 3 oz	2.5
Cauliflower, cooked, 3 flowerets, 2 oz	1.5
Celery, raw, diced, 1 cup, 3.5 oz	1.6
Chickpeas (Garbanzos), ckd, ½ c., 3 oz	6.5
Corn: Kernels, cooked, ½ cup, 2½ oz	2.5
Corn on the Cob, 1 ear, 5 oz	4
Cucumber/Lettuce/Mushrooms, 2 oz	0.5
Eggplant, raw, sliced, ½ cup, 1.5 oz	2
Lentils, cooked, ½ cup, 3.5 oz	8
Mixed Vegetables, frozen, cooked, ½ cup	3
Onions: Raw, 1 medium, 4 oz	1.5
Spring Onions, chop., ¼ cup, 1 oz	0.7
Peas: Green, raw, ½ cup, 2.5 oz	3.7
Cowpeas (Black-eyed), ckd, ½ cup	10
Split Peas, cooked, ½ cup, 3.5 oz	8
Peppers, sweet, raw, 1 large, 6 oz	3
Potatoes: 1 medium, with skin, 5 oz	4
1 medium, without skin	2.5
½ cup mashed, 3.5 oz	1.5
French Fries, small, 2.6 oz	3
Spinach, cooked, ½ cup, 3 oz	2.2
Squash: Summer, cooked, ½ cup, 3 oz	2.5
Winter, cooked, ½ cup, 3.5 oz	2.4
Tomatoes: 1 medium, 4.5 oz	1.5
Tomato Sauce, 1 cup	0.3
Soybean Products: Miso, ½ c., 5 oz	7.4
Tempeh, cooked, 1 piece, 3 oz	2
Tofu, ½ cup, 4.4 oz	0.4

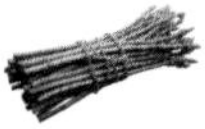
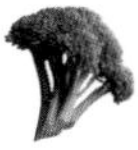
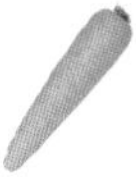
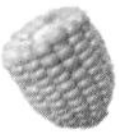
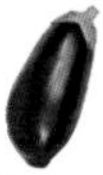
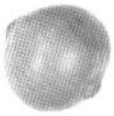
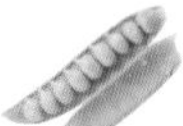
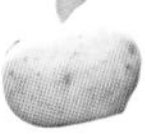
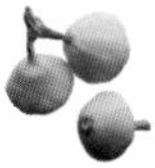
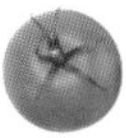

Salads:

	Fiber
Side Salad, average	1
Bean Salad, ½ cup	5
Coleslaw, ½ cup	1
Potato Salad, ½ cup	2

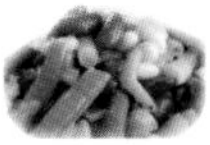

Protein Guide

General Notes

- **Protein has many important body functions.** It builds and repairs muscle, and is the basis of our body's organs, hormones, enzymes, and antibodies to fight infection.
- **Protein is also an emergency fuel** in the absence of sufficient carbohydrate and fats. For this reason, weight loss should be gradual so as to preserve protein levels in muscle, the heart and other body organs.
- **It is easy to obtain sufficient protein,** even if vegetarian. **Plant proteins are not inferior to animal proteins.** In fact, eating more soy and other plant proteins, and less animal protein, may help to build stronger bones and prevent osteoporosis, and may help to control blood cholesterol levels.
- **When changing to a vegetarian diet,** include legume beans (soy, chickpeas etc.), lentils, nuts, seeds, tofu, tempeh; as well as wholegrain cereals and flours. Also try nutritional yeast flakes, and plant-based meat substitutes (*Beyond Meat; Impossible* burgers). Dairy products (lower fat) and eggs can enhance nutrient intake.

Protein & Muscle

- Although muscles are built of protein, protein is not a special fuel for working muscle cells – carbohydrates and fats are.
- In fact, a diet high in protein (and fat) and low in carbohydrate can significantly reduce the performance of endurance sports athletes. **Carbohydrates** are the best fuel for muscles exercised for long periods.
- Any **extra protein** required by athletes and body-builders can easily be obtained from the extra food eaten to satisfy hunger and energy needs.
- Remember, **excessive protein** intake will not build bigger muscles. Any excess is converted and stored as fat. Excess protein can also strain the kidneys, which excrete the waste products of protein metabolism.

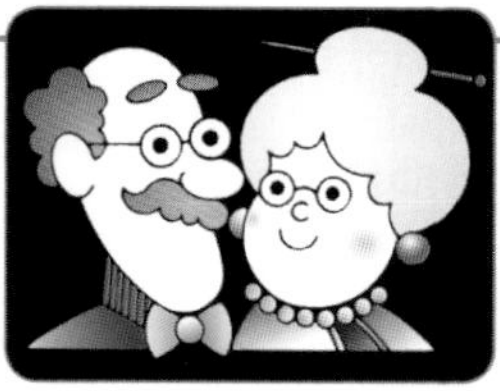

Elderly people (and dieters) must eat sufficient food to ensure adequate protein intake.

Inadequate protein leads to a drop in immune response with greater susceptibility to illness and infections. Muscle strength and muscle mass also drop.

Protein needs are easily met with sensible eating. Athletes who eat enough food for their energy needs can obtain sufficient protein.

RECOMMENDED DAILY PROTEIN INTAKE ~ HEALTHY RANGE ~

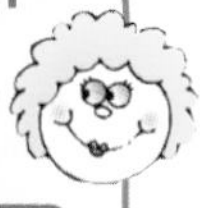

(Lower figure is RDA)

		PROTEIN
Children:	1-3 yrs	13g-26g
	4-8 yrs	19g-38g
	9-13 yrs	34g-64g
Males:	14-18 yrs	52g-120g
	19+	56g-120g
Females:	14+	46g-110g
Pregnancy:		71g-120g
Breastfeeding:		71g-120g

Note: On lower-calorie diets, aim for higher amounts of protein within the Healthy Range.

Pro ~ Protein (grams)

Meats, Sausages

	Pro
Bacon, 3 medium slices	6
Ground Beef Patty, lean, cooked, 3 oz	21
Ham: Luncheon, 2 slices, 1½ oz	7
Roasted, 2 pieces, 3 oz	18
Lamb chop, broiled, 3 oz	22
Liver, cooked, 3 oz	23
Pastrami, 3 slices, 1¾ oz	10
Pork, cooked, lean, 3 oz	24
Roast Beef, lean, 2 slices, 3 oz	24
Sausages: Bologna, 2 sl., 2 oz	7
Braunschweiger, 2 sl., 2 oz	8
Pork link, thick, 2 oz	6
Frankfurter, 1⅓ oz	5
Salami, hard, 3 slices, 1 oz	7
Steak: Average all cuts, lean (no fat)	
Small (4 oz raw/3 oz cooked)	23
Medium (6 oz raw/4¼ oz cooked)	34
Large (10 oz raw/7¼ oz cooked)	57

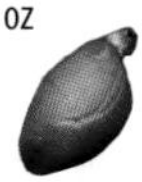
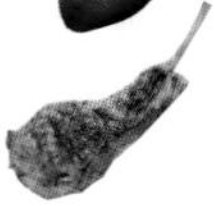
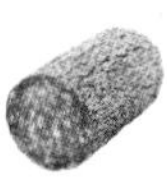
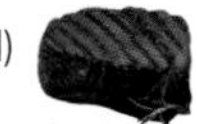

Meat Substitutes (Vegan)

	Pro
Beyond Meat: Beef/Burger, 4 oz	20
Sausages, 2 patties, 2 oz	11
Impossible, 4 oz Patty	19

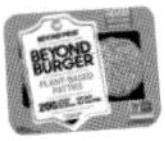

	Pro
Vegetarian Patties, av., 4 oz	13

Chicken/Turkey: *Without Skin*

	Pro
Chicken, cooked: Breast, Roasted, 4 oz	36
Leg/Thigh, Roasted, 2 oz	14
½ Whole Chicken	60
Drumstick, Rstd, 1 med., 3 oz	13
Turkey: Light meat, cooked, 3 oz	28
Dark meat, lean, 3 oz	24

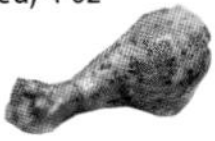

Fish

	Pro
Fresh Fish: *Per 4 oz, cooked*	
Cod, Flounder/Sole, Pollock	28
Catfish, Haddock, Halibut, M/Mahi	28
Ocean Perch, Swordfish, Orange Roughy	28
Canned Fish: Tuna, av., 3 oz	25
Salmon, pink, 3 oz	17
Salmon, red, 3 oz	17
Sardines, 3 whole (3"), 1¼ oz	9
Shellfish: Crabmeat, 3 oz	17.5
Clams, raw, 4 large/9 sml, 3 oz	11
Crayfish, cooked, 3 oz	20
Lobster, cooked, 3 oz	17
Oysters, raw, 6 medium, 3 oz	7
Scallops, 2 lge/5 small, 1 oz	5
Shrimp, raw, 6 large, 1½ oz	8.5
Fish Products: Fish Sticks, 4 sticks	10
Fish Portions, in batter, 4 oz	13
Gefilte Fish, 1 medium ball, 2 oz	8

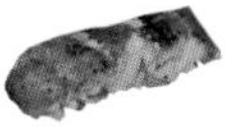
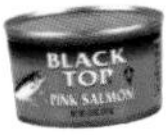

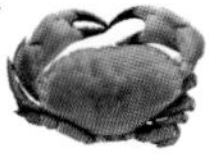
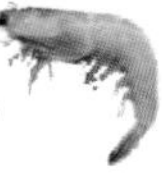

Eggs

	Pro
1 Large Egg, whole	6
Egg Yolk	3
Egg White	3
Omelet: Plain, 2 eggs	13
Ham & cheese	17
Egg Substitutes, (liquid):	
Egg Beaters, ¼ cup, 2 oz	4.5
Better 'n Eggs/Scramblers, ¼ cup, 2 oz	6

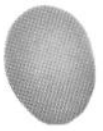
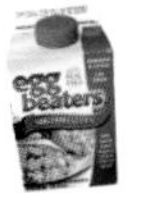

Milk, Yogurt, Ice Cream

	Pro
Milk: Whole: 2%, 1 cup	8
Low-Fat (1%); Fat-Free, 1 cup	8.5
Chocolate Milk, 1 cup	8
Thick Shake: Chocolate, 10 oz	9
Vanilla, 10 oz	11
Soymilk, (fortified), average, 1 cup	7
Soy Dream, Enriched, shelf-stable, 1 cup	7
Yogurt, average all brands:	
Plain, 6 oz	8
Fruit flavors, 6 oz	7
Chobani, Greek, Plain, 6 oz	14
Soy, fruit flavors, 6 oz	7
Ice Cream: Rich, ½ cup	2
Regular, Vanilla, ½ cup	2.5
Sherbet, ½ cup	1
Custard, baked, ½ cup	7

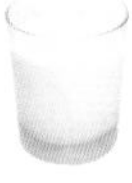
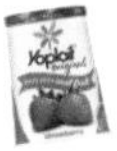

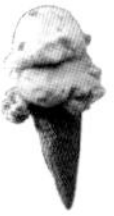

Cheese

	Pro
Hard Cheeses, average, 1 oz	7
Cottage Cheese, ½ cup	13
Cream Cheese, avg., 1 oz	2
Ricotta, part skim, ½ cup	14

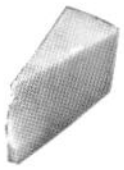

Bread, Bagels, Biscuits

	Pro
Bread: *With enriched flour*	
1 slice, 1 oz	2
4 thin slices, 4 oz	8
4 thick slices, 6 oz	12
Bagel, plain 2 oz	6
Biscuits, 1 oz	2
Pita Bread, 1 pita, 1½ oz	4
Pumpernickel, 1 slice, 1 oz	3

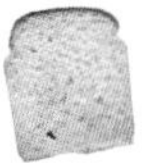
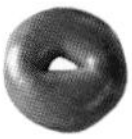

Infant/Baby Foods

	Pro
Infant Formula Milk:	
Enfamil/Gerber/Similac, Regular/Low Iron , 5 fl.oz	2.2
Isomil/Nursoy/ProSobee,	3
Baby Cereals: *Average all brands*	
Dry, 4 Tbsp, ½ oz	1
Jars, with fruit, 4½ oz	1

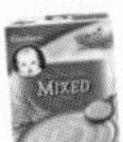

Protein Counter

Breakfast Cereals

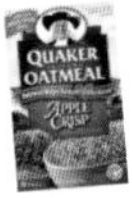

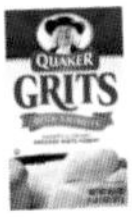

	Pro
Hot Cereals ~ *Cooked:*	
Bulgur, cooked, 1 cup, 5 oz	9
Oatmeal: Reg., non-fortified, 1 cup	6
Instant, fortified, avg., 1 pkt	4
Quaker, all flavors, 1/2 cup	5
Corn/Hominy Grits: 1 cup	3
Quaker: Reg., 3 Tbsp, 1 oz	3
Instant White, 1 packet	2
Cream of Wheat, 1 cup	4
Brands ~ *Ready-To-Eat*	
***General Mills*:**	
Cheerios, Original, 1¼ cups, 1.4 oz	5
Chex, Corn, 1¼ cups, 1.4 oz	3
Kix, Original,1½ cupss, 1.4 oz	3
Lucky Charms, Original, 3/4 cup, 1 oz	2
Total, Raisin Bran, 1¼ cups, 2.3 oz	4
Wheaties, 1 cup, 1.3 oz	3
Kashi:	
7 Whole Grain Flakes, 1¼ cups, 2.1 oz	7
GO: Love, Chocolate Crunch, ¾ cup, 1.83 oz	10
Rise, Original, 1¼ cups, 2 oz	12
Honey Toasted Oat, 1 cup, 1.41 oz	4
Super Loops, 1 cup, 1.35 oz	4
Warm Cinnamon Oat, 1 cup, 1.41 oz	4
Whole Wheat Biscuits, Autumn, 2 oz	7
Kellogg's:	
All-Bran, Original, 1.83 oz pkg	6
Apple Jacks, Original, 1⅓ cups, 1.4 oz	2
Corn Flakes, 1½ cups, 1.41 oz	3
Product 19, 1 cup, 1 oz	3
Rice Krispies, 1 1/4 cup, 1.2 oz	2
Special K: Original, 1.27 oz	7
Granola, Touch of Honey, ½ cup, 1.83 oz	6
Prottein, 1⅓ cups, 2 oz	15
***Post*:**	
Grape Nuts, Original, 1/2 cup, 2 oz	6
Raisin Bran, 1¼ cups, 2.1 oz	5
***Quaker*:**	
Corn Bran Crunch, 1 cup, 1.35 oz	2
Life, Vanilla, 1 cup, 1.45 oz	4
Multigrain Flakes, Honey Vanilla, ¾ cup, 2.2 oz	7
Simply Granola, Oats, Honey & Alm., ⅔ cup, 2.2 oz	7

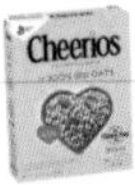

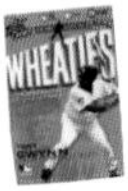

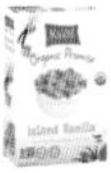

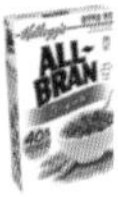

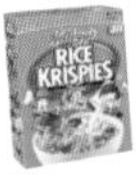

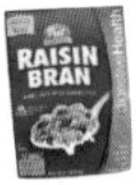

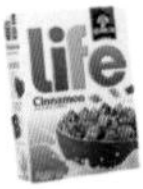

Brans & Wheatgerm

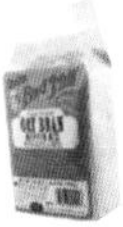

	Pro
Oat Bran, raw, 1 Tbsp	2
Rice Bran, raw, 2 Tbsp	1
Wheat Bran, unprocessed, 2 T.	1
Wheat Germ, 2 Tbsp, 1/2 oz	4

Grains & Flours, Yeast

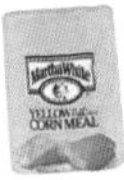

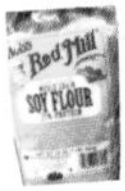

	Pro
Amaranth grain, cooked, 1/2 cup, 4.5 oz	5
Barley, 1/2 cup, 3.2 oz	12
Buckwheat Flour, Whole-groat, 1 cup	15
Carob Flour, 1 cup, 3.6 oz	5
Corn Flour, 1 cup, 4 oz	11
Corn Meal, 1 cup, 4 1/2 oz	8
Flour: White, 1 cup, 5.6 oz	9
Wholegrain, 1 cup, 4¼ oz	16
Hemp Wholemeal Flour, 1 cup, 3.5 oz	30
Millet, wholegrain, 1 cup, 3½ oz	12
Quinoa, raw, ⅓ cup, 1.5 oz	6
Rye Flour: Dark, 1 cup, 4 1/2 oz	18
Light, 1 cup, 3 1/2 oz	9
Soy Flour, full fat, 1 cup, 3 oz	29
Yeast: Brewers, 2 Tbsp, 1/2 oz	8
Nutritional Yeast Flakes *(Red Star),* 1 heaping Tbsp, 1/2 oz	8

Rice, Spaghetti, Macaroni

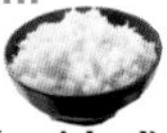

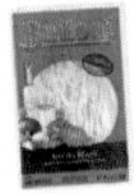

	Pro
Rice: Brown/White, average 1 cup cooked, 6 1/2 oz	5
Spaghetti/Macaroni/Noodles (enriched):	
Cooked, 1 cup, 4 1/2 oz	7
Canned: in Tomato Sce, 1/2 cup	2
with Meatballs, 1 cup, 8 oz	10
Macaroni & Cheese, 1 cup, 9 oz	8

Soups

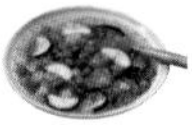

	Pro
With Noodles/Vegetables, 1 cup	3
With Meat/Beans/Peas, 1 cup	8

Fruit

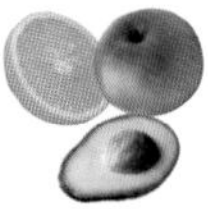

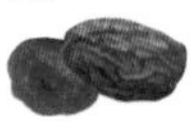

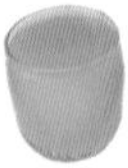

	Pro
Fresh/Canned:	
Average, all types, 1 medium/2 small fruit	1
Avocado, 1/2 medium	2
Dried Fruit: Apricots, 8 halves, 1 oz	1
Dates, 6 dates, 2 oz	1.5
Figs, 4 medium figs, 2 oz	2
Prunes, 5 medium, 1 1/2 oz	1
Raisins, 1 oz	1
Fruit Juice: Average, 1 cup	0.5
Prune Juice, 6 fl.oz	1
Tomato Juice, 1 cup, 8 fl.oz	1.5

Vegetables

Vegetables	Pro
Beans: Snap/green, 1/2 cup, 2 oz	1
Dried: Average all types, cooked, 1/2 cup	7
Baked Beans, 1/2 cup 4 1/2 oz	5
Bean Sprouts, mung, 1 c., 4 oz	3
Broccoli, raw, 1/2 cup, 1 1/2 oz	1.5
Cabbage; Cauliflower, raw, 1 c. 3 oz	1.5
Chickpeas, cooked, ½ cup, 3 oz	8
Corn: Raw, 1/2 cup kernels, 3 oz	2.5
1 ear trimmed to 3 1/2"	2
Lentils, cooked, 1/2 cup 3 1/2 oz	9
Mushrooms, raw, 1/2 c., sliced	1
Peas: Green, raw, 1/2 c., 2 1/2 oz	4
Split Peas, cooked, 1 cup, 7 oz	16
Potatoes: *Cooked:*	
1 medium, with skin, 5 oz	3.3
without skin, 4 oz	2.3
French Fries, small, 2.6 oz	2
Potato Salad, 1/2 cup, 4 oz	3.5
Pumpkin, 1/2 cup mashed, 4.3 oz	1
Seaweed, kelp, 1 oz	<1
Spinach, cooked, 1/2 cup, 3 oz	2.7
Squash, ckd, all types, 1/2 cup	1
Tomatoes, 1 medium, 4 1/2 oz	1
Vegetables, mixed, ckd, 1 cup	2.5
Soybeans, cooked, 1/2 cup, 3 oz	14

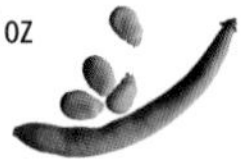
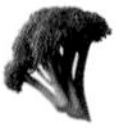
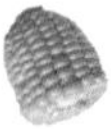
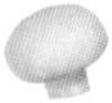
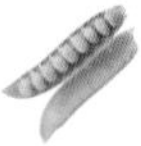
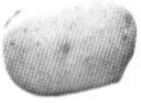
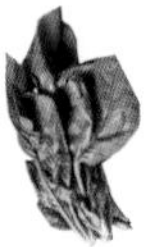

Tofu, Tempeh, Miso

Tofu, Tempeh, Miso	Pro
Tofu, raw, firm, 1/2 cup, 4 1/2 oz	10
Tempeh, 1/2 cup, 3 oz	16
Miso, 1/2 cup, 5 oz	16
Miso Soup, 1 cup	3
Soybean Protein *(TVP)*, 1 oz	18

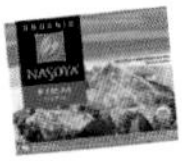

Cakes, Pastries, Pies

Cakes, Pastries, Pies	Pro
Banana Nut Bread, 4 oz	6
Carrot w. cream cheese frosting, 4 oz	4
Cheesecake, 1 piece, 4 oz	6
Chocolate, 1 piece, 2 oz	2
Fruitcake, 1 piece, 3 oz	4
Croissant, plain, small, 2 oz	5
Danish Pastry, 1 pastry, 2 1/4 oz	4
Donuts, average, 2 oz	4
Muffins, average, 1 med., 1 1/2 oz	3
Pancakes, 4" diam., two, 2 oz	4
Pies: Fruit, 1 piece, 5 1/2 oz	4
Pecan, 1 piece, 5 oz	7
Puddings, average, 1/2 cup, 4 1/2 oz	4
Waffles, 1 large, 2 1/2 oz	7

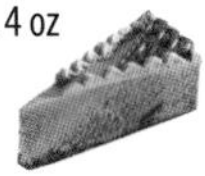
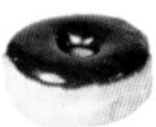
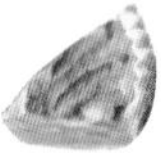

Peanut Butter

Peanut Butter	Pro
Regular: 2 Tbsp, 1.1 oz	8
Peter Pan Plus, 2 Tbsp, 1.1 oz	8

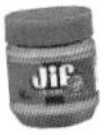

Sugar, Honey, Jam

Sugar, Honey, Jam	Pro
Sugar: White	0
Brown, 1 Tbsp	0
Molasses: Light/Med., 1 Tbsp	0
Blackstrap, 1 Tbsp, 3/4 oz	0
Corn Syrup, 1 Tbsp, 3/4 oz	0
Honey, Jams, Jelly	0

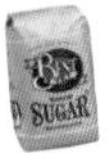

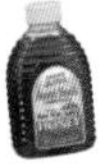

Candy, Chocolate, Carob

Candy, Chocolate, Carob	Pro
Candy, sugar-based	0
Chocolate: Plain, 2 oz bar	4
with nuts, 2 oz bar	6
Carob, plain, 2 oz	6

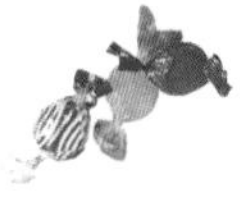

Cookies, Crackers, Chips

Cookies, Crackers, Chips	Pro
Cookies, average, 4 cookies	2
Crackers, Graham, 2 1/2" sq., (2)	1
Rice Cakes, average, one	1
Corn/Potato Chips, 1 oz	2

Nuts:

Nuts	Pro
Almonds, shelled, 20-25 nuts	6
Brazil Nuts, 7-8 medium nuts, 1 oz	4
Cashews, 12-16 nuts, 1 oz	5
Hemp Seeds, 3 tbsp, 1 oz	9
Macadamias, 1 oz	2
Peanuts, dry rsted, 40 nuts, 1 oz	6
Pecans, 24 halves, 1 oz	2
Walnuts, 15 halves, 1 oz	4

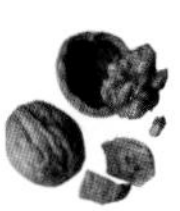

Seeds:

Seeds	Pro
Chia Seeds, raw, 2 Tbsp, 1.1 oz	5
Flax Seeds, 3 Tbsp, 1 oz	6
Sesame Seeds, dry, 1 Tbsp	2
Pumpkin Kernels, dry, hulled, 1 oz	7
Sunflower Seeds, dried, hulled, 1 oz	6

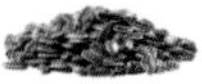

Granola & Food/Protein Bars

Granola & Food/Protein Bars	Pro
Granola Bars, average, 1 bar, 2 oz	2
Bariatrix, Proti-Bars (1), 1.4 oz	15
Cliff, Builder's Protein, av., 1 bar	20
GeniSoy, Protein Bars, 1.6 oz	15
Jenny Craig, Bars, av., 1 oz	10
Luna Protein, av., 1 bar	12
Met-Rx, "Big 100", av., 3.5 oz	31
Myoplex 30, all flavors, 3 oz	30
Optifast 800, all flavors, 1.72 oz	14
PowerBar, Protein Plus	20
Slim-Fast: Protein Meal Bars, 1.7 oz	10
Keto Meal Bar, 1.48 oz	7
***Special** K:* Keto Meal Bars, 2.2 oz	7
Protein Meal Bars, 1.5 oz	7

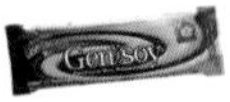

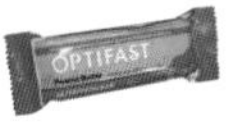

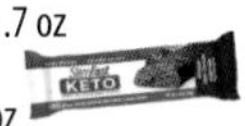

Protein Counter

High Protein Drinks & Powders

	Pro
Atkins, Shakes, 11 fl.oz	15
Bob's Red Mill, Protein Powders:	
Chia Protein, 1/3 cup, 1.45 oz	20
Pea Protein, ¼ cup, 1oz	21
Soy Protein, ¼ cup, 0.75 oz	17
Whey/Hemp Protein, ¼ cup, 0.75 oz	15
Boost, High Protein, 8 fl.oz bottle	20
Plus Protein Shake, 8 fl oz	14
Carnation, B'fast Essentials, 11 fl.oz	10
Ensure, Plus, 8 fl.oz bottle	13
Gatorade, Protein Recovery Shake, 11 oz	20
GNC, Lean Shake, 14 fl oz	25
Hemp Protein Powder, ¼ cup, 1 oz	14
Met-Rx Meal Replacement, RTD:	
High Protein; 51, 15 fl.oz	51
Myoplex, Original Nutrition Shake, 1 pkt	42
Optifast 800, prepared, 8 fl oz	16
Premier Protein, Chocolate, 11 fl.oz	20
Pure Protein Shake, 11 fl.oz	35
Slim-Fast Shakes: Keto, 11 fl.oz	8
Advanced Energy, 11 fl.oz	20
Special K, Protein Shakes, 10 fl.oz	15
Weider, Mass 1000, 4 scoops, 7 oz	34
Pumpkin Protein Powder, 2 Tbsp, ½ oz	9
Whey Protein Powder: 100%, plain, 1 oz	24
Choc Flavor, 1 scoop, 0.8 oz	18

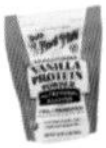
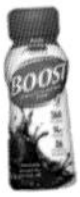

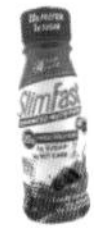

Coffee, Tea, Soda

	Pro
Coffee, Coffee Substitutes, 1 cup, 8 fl.oz	0
Coffee, with 2 oz milk, 1 cup, 8 fl.oz	2
Caffe latte, large, 16 fl.oz	12
Cappuccino, large, 16 fl.oz	8
Frappuccino, average, 16 fl.oz	6
Hot Chocolate, with milk, 1 cup, 8 fl.oz	8
Soft Drinks/Soda, Tea, all types	0

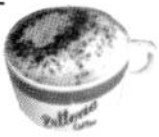
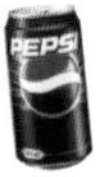

Beer, Wine, Spirits

	Pro
Beer, 12 fl.oz	1
Wines, red/white, 1 glass	0
Spirits/Liquor	0

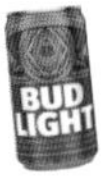

Fast-Foods/Burgers

	Pro
Pancakes, average all outlets, 3	8
Shakes, Chocolate, 16 fl.oz	12
Sundaes, Average all outlets	7
Arby's:	
Buffalo Chicken Slider	12
Buttermilk Crispy Chicken S'wich	24
Classic Roast Beef Sandwich	23
Fire-Roasted Philly	34
Burger King: Cheeseburger	15
Double Bacon Cheeseburger	24
Double Stacker King	61
Impossible Whopper	25
Whopper Sandwich	28

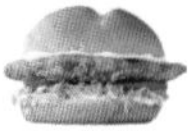
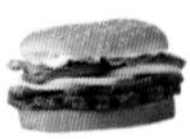

Fast Foods/Burgers (Cont)

	Pro
Carl's Jr: Beyond Famous Star with Cheese	33
Charbroiled Chicken Club Sandwich	44
Famous Star Burger with Cheese	28
Super Star Burger with Cheese	48
Del Taco: Beyond 8 Layer Burrito	27
Beyond Avocado Taco	12
Beyond Taco	19
Epic Beyond Original Mex	44
Domino's Pizza: *Hand Tossed (12")*	
Buffalo Chicken, 1 slice	12
Honolulu Hawaiian, 1 slice	10
Ultimate Pepperoni, 1 slice	11
KFC: Original Breast	39
Extra Crispy Chicken Tender	19
Kentucky Grilled, Breast	38
McDonald's: Big Mac	25
Buttermilk Crispy Chicken S'wch	27
Cheeseburger	15
Chicken McNuggets (4)	9
Filet-O-Fish	16
Hamburger	12
Quarter Pounder with Cheese	30
French Fries: Small, 2.5 oz	3
Large, 5.4 oz	7
Shakes, medium	14
Breakfast: Egg McMuffin	17
Bacon, Egg & Cheese McGriddles	18
Sausage Burrito	13
Sausage McMuffin with Egg	21
Pizza Hut: *Per Medium, 1 slice, 1/8 Pizza*	
Thin 'n Crispy, Supreme	10
Pan Pizzas, Hawaiian Chicken	11
Hand Tossed: Pepperoni Lover's	12
Ultimate Cheese Lover's	11
Red Robin, Veggie Burger	24
Subway : *6" Subs with standard toppings, no oil*	
Black Forest Ham	15
Meatball Marinara	20
Spicy Italian	20
Subway Club	20
Turkey Breast	15
Taco Bell: Bean Burrito, vegan	13
Burrito Supreme, Beef	16
Cheesy Gordita Crunch	21
Chicken Chalupa	16
Grilled Soft Beef Taco	9
Steak Chalupa	15
Wendy's:	
Grilled Asiago Ranch Chkn Club	42
Dave's Double Burger	49
Homestyle Chicken Sandwich	27
Jr Cheeseburger	19
White Castle, Impossible Burger w/o Chse Slider	9

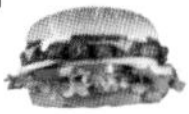
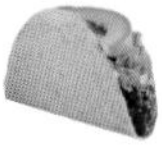
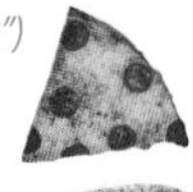
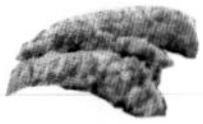
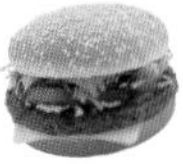
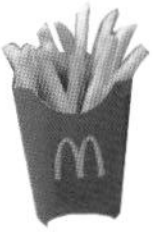
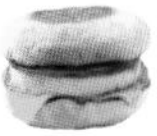
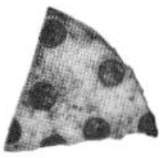
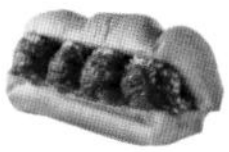
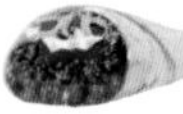
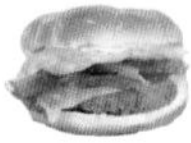

High Blood Pressure

Many American adults have hypertension (high blood pressure), and are unaware of it. It is generally symptomless, so **have your blood pressure checked annually** – particularly if it runs in the family.

Untreated hypertension overworks the heart, damages arteries and promotes atherosclerosis. This in turn greatly increases the risk of heart disease, stroke, blindness, kidney disease and impotence. The earlier hypertension is detected, the sooner it can be brought under control.

BLOOD PRESSURE CLASSIFICATION

For Adults Age 18 & Older ~ Not Acutely ill or on Medication (American Heart Association)

	DIASTOLIC		SYSTOLIC
Normal ➤	Below 80	and	Below 120
Prehypertension ➤	80-89	or	120-139
Hypertension:			
Stage 1 ➤	90-99	or	140-159
Stage 2 ➤	100 or more	or	160 or more

Treating Hypertension

Prehypertension (in the chart above) means you don't have high blood pressure now but are likely to develop it in the future.

You can take steps to lessen the risk by adopting healthy lifestyle habits such as:

- reducing sodium intake
- eating adequate fruit and vegetables
- losing weight if overweight
- limiting alcohol to 2 drinks or less daily
- quitting smoking
- exercising regularly, managing stress.

Stage 1 hypertension can often be treated with the above lifestyle changes.

Stage 2 hypertension usually requires drug therapy. However, salt restriction, abstaining from alcohol, and the above lifestyle changes will improve the success of drug therapy, and enable smaller drug doses to be prescribed.

HYPERTENSION DAMAGES ARTERIES & PROMOTES ATHEROSCLEROSIS

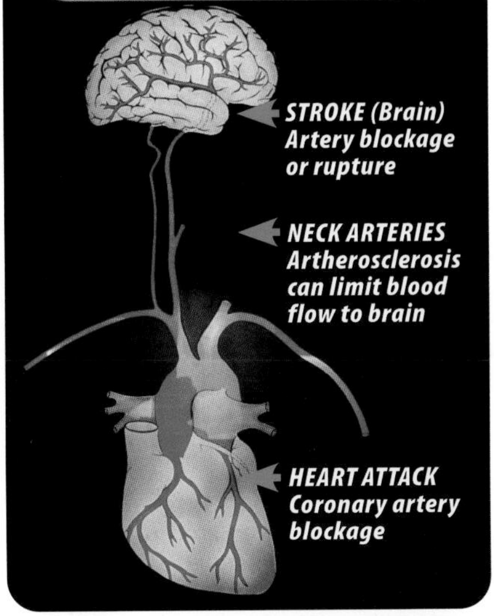

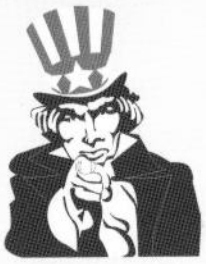

STROKE
KNOW THE WARNING SIGNS

Stroke is a medical emergency!
If you notice one or more of these signs, call 9-1-1 or your doctor immediately.

These signs may be signalling a possible stroke or transient ischemic attack:

- **Sudden weakness** or numbness in your face, arm, or leg on one side of your body.
- **Sudden confusion,** trouble speaking or understanding. Slurred speech.
- **Sudden trouble seeing,** in one or both eyes
- **Sudden trouble walking,** dizziness, loss of balance or coordination.
- **Sudden severe headache** - 'a bolt out of the blue' – with no apparent cause.

Extra Info: www.stroke.org

Salt & Sodium Guide

Salt & Sodium

- **Sodium is a mineral element** most commonly found in salt (sodium chloride). It also occurs naturally in much smaller amounts in animal and plant foods, and water – normally sufficient for our needs without having to add salt to our diet.
- **Sodium is required** for nerve and muscle function, as well as to balance the amount of fluid in our tissues and blood. Sodium acts like a sponge to attract and hold fluids in body tissues.
- **Excess sodium** can cause water retention, and increase the risk of developing hypertension. Very high salt intake may also increase the risk of stomach cancer.
- **Too little sodium** may cause low blood pressure (hypotension), and decrease blood flow to the heart, brain and kidneys – especially during exercise. (A certain blood volume is required to sustain the blood pressure needed for adequate blood flow in the capillaries).

Salt-Sensitive Persons

- **Normally, our kidneys** excrete excess dietary sodium. The thirst we feel after a salty meal is the body calling for water to dilute the sodium, and enable the kidneys to flush out excess sodium.
- **However, 'salt - sensitive'** persons (up to 70% of adults) tend to retain excess sodium (above approximately 3000mg daily) instead of excreting it. Such persons are more likely to develop hypertension and would benefit most from sodium restriction. Assume you are susceptible if there is a family history of hypertension.
- **Although not everyone will benefit, all Americans are being asked to moderate their salt and sodium intake** as a public health measure – particularly because so many do not know whether or not they have hypertension, and also because we do not know just who is salt-sensitive.

SAFE SODIUM LEVELS

The American Heart Association recommends a **maximum sodium intake of 1500mg per day** for adults with normal blood pressure.

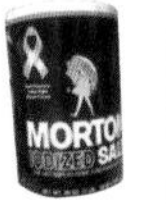

Persons with hypertension and kidney ailments are usually restricted to as little as **1000mg sodium per day**. Your doctor will discuss the correct sodium level for you.

FINDING HIDDEN SODIUM

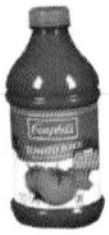

On average, **less than one third of our sodium intake comes from the salt shaker.** The rest is hidden in processed foods that have salt added during manufacture.

Sodium compounds added to food or medicinals can also contribute significant sodium.

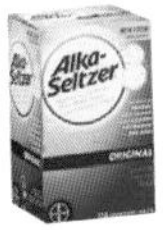

Sodium bicarbonate in particular is widely used in antacid tablets (such as *Alka Seltzer*) and powders. Sodium bicarbonate contains 27% sodium by weight. Each gram has 270mg of sodium. Large amounts of sodium can be unwittingly consumed – up to 600mg per tablet. (See Antacids ~ Page 280)

Example: 2 *Alka-Seltzer* Tablets = 1000mg sodium

Other sodium compounds include monosodium glutamate (MSG), sodium ascorbate, sodium nitrite, and sodium citrate.

POTASSIUM BALANCES SODIUM

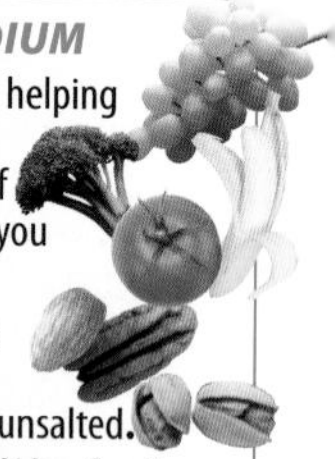

Potassium helps to balance sodium by helping the kidneys to excrete excess sodium. Fruit and vegetables are rich sources of potassium - another reason to ensure you have your 5-7 servings every day.

Nuts also provide potassium as well as magnesium and other heart-healthy nutrients and anti-oxidants. Eat them unsalted.

Note: This info is only for people with normal kidney function. Also not for persons on potassium-sparing diuretics.

ALCOHOL DANGER

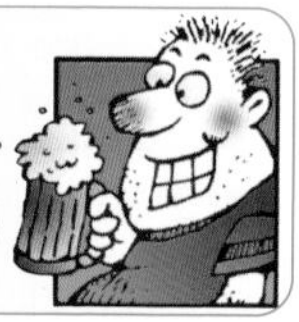

Excessive alcohol intake contributes to hypertension. Susceptible persons should avoid or limit alcohol intake to 1-2 drinks per day.

Salt Sodium Guide

Sodium accounts for only 40% of the weight of salt (sodium chloride). Examples:
1 gram (1000mg) Salt has 400mg Sodium
1 teaspoon (5g) Salt has 2000mg Sodium

HINTS TO REDUCE SODIUM

- **Cut down use of the salt shaker.** Start with an easy 50% cut in sodium by using Lite Salt (*Morton*) or *Cardia* Salt. Then gradually cut back until you can leave the salt shaker off the table. Sea salt is still high in sodium.
- **Use fresh herbs,** and salt-free seasonings to add flavor to food.
- **Choose low-sodium,** sodium-free, and reduced-sodium products in place of regular, salted products.
- **Check food labels for sodium levels.** FDA Guidelines for sodium descriptors are:
  - **Reduced Sodium:** At least 25% less sodium than the original product
  - **Low Sodium:** 140 mg or less/serving
  - **Very Low Sodium:** 35mg or less/serving
  - **Sodium Free:** Less than 5mg/serving
  - **No Salt Added:** Made without the salt normally added, but still contains the sodium that is a natural part of the food
- **Use reduced-sodium breads,** butter and margarine. Regular varieties are considered high in sodium in view of their significant contribution to our diet.
- **Go easy on salty condiments and sauces** such as ketchup, mustard, soy sauce, spaghetti sauces, and salad dressings. Use low-sodium varieties.
- **Limit pizzas and salty fast-foods.** Check the *CalorieKing.com* food database.
- **Avoid salty snack foods** such as potato chips, corn chips, salted nuts, pretzels and cheesy-flavored snacks. **Choose unsalted** popcorn, nuts or seeds. Eat more fruit.
- **Don't salt children's food** to your taste.
- **Avoid antacids with** sodium bicarbonate (such as *Alka-Seltzer*). They are high in sodium. Look for low-sodium alternatives.

FOODS HIGH IN SODIUM

- Bread (4 slices/day), Bagels, Biscuits
- Cheese, Butter, Margarine
- Pickles, Sauerkraut, Olives
- Condiments, Sauces
- Salad Dressings
- Canned vegetables/salads/beans
- Deli Salads (with dressing)
- Frozen/Packaged Meals/Entrees
- Soups: Canned/dry; bouillon cubes
- Meats: Ham, bacon, sausage, luncheon meats, smoked meats
- Canned Fish (in brine/salt)
- Sea Salt, Garlic/Celery Salt
- Snack Foods (potato chips, pretzels)
- Tomato Juice (Canned), V8 Vegetable Juice
- Fast Foods: Pizza, Burgers, Chicken
- *Alka-Seltzer* Antacid

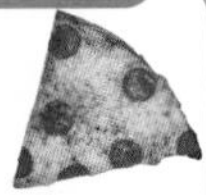
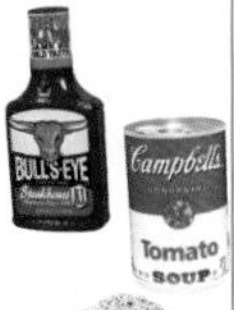

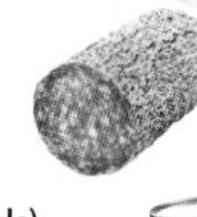
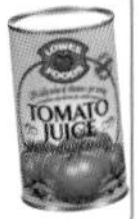

MODERATE SODIUM

- Meat, Fish, Poultry - Unprocessed
- Milk, Yogurt, Soy Drinks, Eggs
- Peanut Butter
- Breakfast Cereals (less than 200mg/serving)
- Chocolate Candy, Fruit/Nut Bars
- *Reduced Sodium & Low Sodium* Products

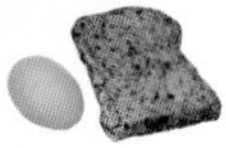
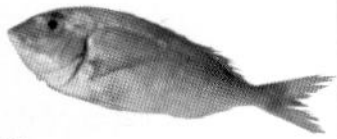

FOODS LOW IN SODIUM

- Products labelled *Very Low Sodium*, or *Sodium Free*
- Bread (No Salt Added)
- Fresh fruits and vegetables
- Canned and Dried Fruits
- Potatoes, Rice, Pasta
- Dried Beans & Lentils, Tofu
- Nuts & Seeds (unsalted)
- Corn & Popcorn (unsalted)
- Pepper, Spices, Herbs
- Jam, Honey, Syrup
- Candy, Gum
- Hard & Jelly Candy
- Coffee, Tea, Alcohol
- Fresh Fruit Juices, Water

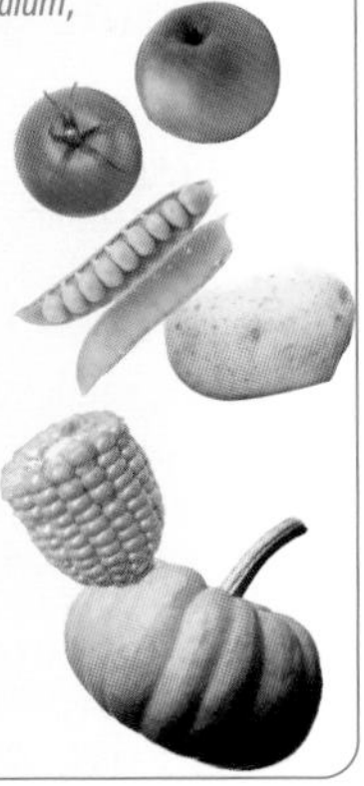

Sodium Counter

The American Heart Association recommends a sodium intake of less than 1500mg/day

Milk & Dairy Products

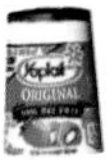
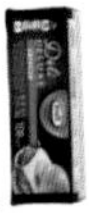

	Sodium
Milk: Whole/lowfat/skim, average	
1 glass, 8 fl.oz	120
Whole, low sodium, 1 cup	5
Choc Milk, 1 cup	130
Soy Milk, 8 fl.oz	30
Buttermilk, cultured, 8 fl.oz	250
Dry/Powder, skim, 1/4 cup, 1 oz	110
Yogurt, with fruit average, 8 oz	130
Cheese: Bleu, 1 oz	330
Cottage Cheese, Creamed, 1/2 cup, 4 oz	450
Kraft: American, Singles, 1 sl., 0.7 oz	240
American, Deli Deluxe, 2 slices, 0.9 oz	400
Philadelphia Cream Cheese, Tub, Orig.,1.1 oz	125
Parmesan, 1 oz	435
Ricotta Cheese, 1/2 cup, 4 oz	110
Swiss, Shredded Natural, 1oz	55
Triple Cheddar, 1 oz	170

Ice Cream, Frozen Yogurt

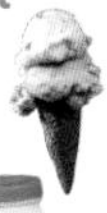

Ice Cream, average, 1/2 cup	50
Frozen Yogurt, 1/2 cup	50

Fats/Oils

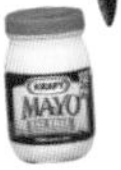
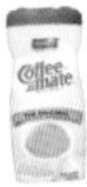

Butter/Margarine:	
Regular, 2 Tbsp, 1 oz	230
Unsalted, reg., 2 Tbsp, 1 oz	5
Mayonnaise, avg., 2 Tbsp, 1 oz	160
Oils/Lard/Drippings	0
Cream, average, 1 Tbsp	5
Coffee-Mate: Powdered, Original, 1 tsp	5
Liquid, all flavors	0-5

Eggs

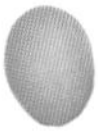
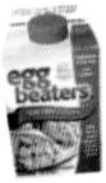

Whole, 1 large	70
Omelet: 2 egg, plain	220
With 1 oz Cheddar Cheese	400
Egg Beaters: Original, 3 Tbsp	90
Flavors, average, 3 Tbsp	140

Meats

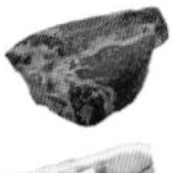
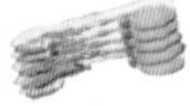

Meat, average all types, cooked	
Beef/Lamb/Veal/Pork, 4 oz	80
Corned Beef, cooked, 3 oz	800
Bacon, cooked, 2 slices, 0.5 oz	270
Ham, 3 oz	1100

Meat Substitutes (Vegan)

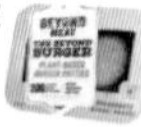

Beyond Meat: Beef/Burger, 4 oz	350
Sausage, cooked, 1 link	500

Sodium ~ Sodium (mg)

Sausages & Deli Meats

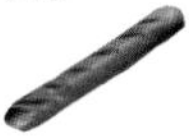
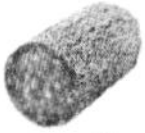
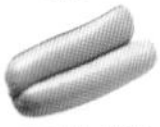
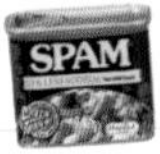

	Sodium
Bologna, 1 oz	280
Frankfurter, 2 oz	640
Ham, chopped, 0.8 oz slice	290
Liverwurst (Braunschweiger), 1 oz	320
Pepperoni, 5 slices, 1 oz	570
Salami: Cooked, 1 oz	350
dry/hard, 1 oz	600
Sausage, 1 oz link	220
Pork, 2 oz patty	260
Spam: Classic, 2 oz	790
25% Less Sodium, 2 oz	580
Turkey Roll, 1 oz	160

Chicken & Turkey

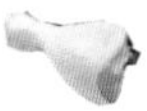

Chicken/Turkey, cooked, unsalted, 4 oz	80
Stuffing Mixes, average., ½ cup	500

Fish:

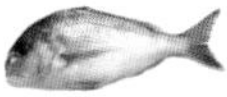
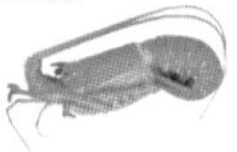
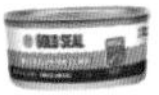
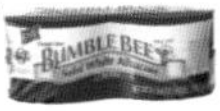

Fresh Fish: average, plain	
Cooked, 4 oz, without bone	60
Broiled w. butter, 4 oz	150
Breaded & fried, 4 oz	320
Fish fillets, batter-dipped 3 oz	350
Fish sticks, 1 oz stick	160
Gefilte Fish, with broth, 1 pce, 1.5 oz	220
Herring, pickled, 2 pces, 1 oz	260
Lobster, meat only, 4 oz	180
Oysters, fresh, 6 med., 3 oz	95
Salmon: Canned, 3 oz	460
No Salt Added, 3 oz	65
Smoked fish, average, 3 oz	650
Tuna: Canned, drained, 3 oz	160
Light, drained, 3 oz	200
No Added Salt, 3 oz	40
Spicy Flavored, 5 oz	260

Entrees & Meals

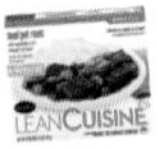
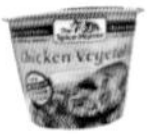

Frozen Meals, average	600-1300
Lean Cuisine, Favorites	500-800
Stouffer's, Meat Lovers Lasagna	750
Dinners, average	900-1200
Side Dishes, average	400-600
Pizza, frozen, 1/4 large, 6 oz	800-1200
Microwave, Cup Meals	900-1200
Cup Noodles, average	1050-1280

Soups

Item	Sodium
Condensed: Average, 1 cup, 8 oz	800-1000
Low Sodium, average	70
Chicken Noodle, average, 1 cup	900
Bouillon Cube, average	950
Top Ramen Noodle Soup, 3 oz pkg, av.	1600
Soup Cups, average	850
Soup Mixes, average, 1 cup	900

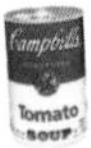

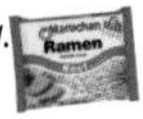

Condiments, Sauces, Dressings

Item	Sodium
A-1 Sauce, 1 Tbsp	280
Barbecue Sauce, 1 Tbsp	130
Bragg's Liquid Aminos, 1 tsp	350
Chili Sauce, 1 Tbsp	230
Ketchup: Tomato, 1 Tbsp	180
Low Sodium, 1 Tbsp	20
Mayonnaise, 1 Tbsp	80
Mustard, 1 tsp	70
Pizza Sauce, 1/2 cup	700
Salad Dressings, 2 Tbsp, 1 oz	160-400
Spaghetti Sauce, 1/2 cup	500
Soy Sauce: 1 Tbsp	900
Lite, 1 Tbsp	600
Sweet & Sour, 1/2 cup	250
Tabasco, 1 tsp	25
Vinegar, Lemon Juice	0
Worcestershire, 1 Tbsp	65
Tomato: Sauce, 1 cup	1200
Paste/Puree (salted), 1/2 cup	1000
No Salt Added, 1/2 cup	75

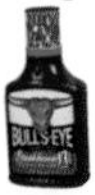

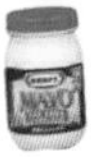

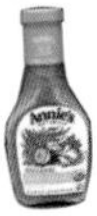
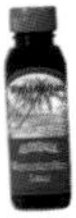
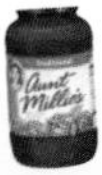

Salt & Salt Substitutes

Item	Sodium
Table Salt: 1 teaspoon, 6g	2400
Single Serve package, 1 g	400
Cardia Salt, 1 teaspoon	1080
Lite Salt, 1 teaspoon, 6g	1200
Morton, No Salt Substitute, 1 tsp	5
Garlic/Onion/Seasoned Salt, 1 tsp, 4g	1350
Garlic/Seasoned Salt 1 teaspoon, 4g	1300
Sea Salt, 1 teaspoon, 5g	2250

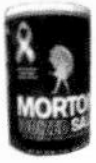

Seasonings, Herbs & Spices

Item	Sodium
Baking Powder, 1 tsp, 3g	340
Baking Soda (Sodium bicarb), 1 tsp, 3g	810
Accent, Flavor Enhancer, ¼ tsp	160
Chili Powder, 1 tsp, 3g	25
Curry Powder	0
Lemon Pepper 1 tsp	340
Meat Tenderizer, 1 tsp, 5g	1750
MSG (Monosodium Glutamate), 5g	500
Mrs Dash, Blends/Marinades	0
Old Bay: Seasoning, 1 tsp, 2.4 oz	560
Seasoning, Less Sodium, 1 tsp, 2.4 oz	360
Pepper, Mustard (dry), 1 tsp	1
Yeast, Nutritional, 1 Tbsp	10

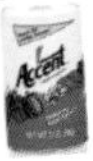

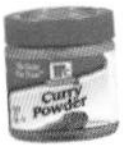

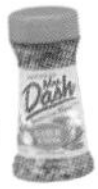

Breakfast Cereals

Item	Sodium
Kellogg's:	
All-Bran, Original, ⅔ cup, 1 oz	95
Special K, Original, 1¼ cups, 1.4 oz	270
Corn Flakes, 1½ cup,s 1 oz	300
Raisin Bran, 1 cup, 2 oz	200
Quaker:	
Corn Crunch, 1 cup, 1.3 oz	220
Multigrain Flakes, av., ¾ c., 2.2 oz	40
Real Medleys, ⅔ cup, 1.83 oz	15-45
Simply Granola, average, 1/2 cup	30-35
General Mills, Total, 1 cup, 1.4 oz	190
Oatmeal: Regular, 3/4 cup	1
Quaker, Instant Maple & Brown Sugar (1 pkt)	260

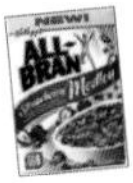

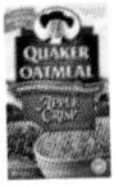

Breads, Bagels, Crackers

Item	Sodium
Bread: Thin Slice, average 1 oz	140
Thick Slice, 1.5 oz	210
Low Sodium, 1 oz	10
Bagels: Plain, medium, 2 oz	200
Large, take-out, average, 4 oz	550
Panera Bread, 3.8 oz	410
Biscuits, average, 1 oz	180
Bun/Roll: 1 medium, 1.5 oz	200
Large, 4 oz	560
Crackers: Saltine, 2 crackers	70
Low Salt, 2	25
Graham, 2 regular	50
Croissant, Plain, average, 2 oz	280
Rice Cakes, average	25
Ritz Crackers, Hint of Salt, 1 oz	60
RyVita, Original Crispbread, 2 slices	30

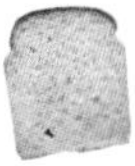
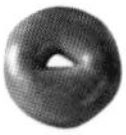
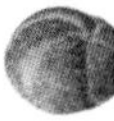
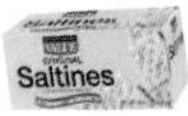

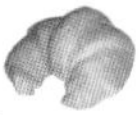

Cookies, Cakes, Desserts

Item	Sodium
Cookies: Average, 2-3 cookies, 1 oz	100
Average, 1 cookie, 2.5 oz	180
Baked Custard, 1/2 cup	100
Brownie, 1.5 oz	130
Carrot Cake, 8 oz	650
Cheesecake, 7 oz	350
Cinnamon Sweet Roll, 2 oz	250
Danish, Apple/Fruit	250
Donut, average	150
Muffins: 1 medium, 2 oz	150
1 extra large, 4 oz	300
Pancakes, (4"), x 3	360
Fruit Pies, average, 7 oz	600
Pudding: Average, 1/2 cup	160
Jell-O Instant Pudding Mix, 1/4 pkg	350
Waffles: Home-made, 7", 2.5 oz	350
Frozen: Average, 1.2 oz	260
Aunt Jemima, Homestyle, 3 pancakes	460

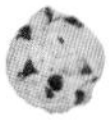
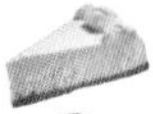
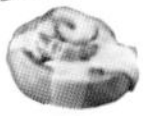
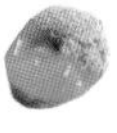
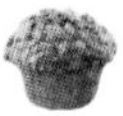
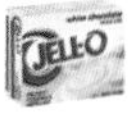

Sodium Counter

Fruit & Juices

	Sodium
Fresh Fruit, average all types, 1 serving	1
Dried/Canned Fruit, 1/2 cup	1
Fruit Juice: Fresh, squeezed, 6 fl.oz	1
Commercial, aver., 6 fl.oz	20
Tomato Juice *(Campbell's)*, 8 fl.oz	680
Low Sodium (No Salt Added), 8 fl.oz	140
V8 Vegetable *(Campbell's)*:	
11.5 fl.oz bottle	920
Low Sodium, 5.5 fl.oz can	95

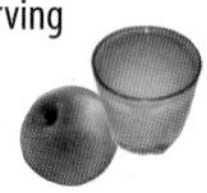
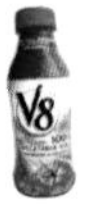

Vegetables

Fresh/Frozen (No Salt Added): Per 1/2 Cup	
Asparagus, Bean Sprouts, Corn	3
Beets, Carrots, Celery, 1/2 cup	40
Broccoli, Cabbage, Cauliflower	10
Cucumber, Green Beans, Mushroom, Okra	3
Onions, Peas, Potato, Pumpkin, Squash	3
Peppers, Hot Chili, raw, each	3
Spinach, Turnips, 1/2 cup, cooked	40
Tomato, 1 medium, 5 oz	10
Canned: Asparagus, 4 spears	300
Beans, baked in tomato sauce	450
Beets, 1/2 cup, 3 oz	240
Corn Kernels, 1/2 cup, 3 oz	190
Creamed, 1/2 cup, 4.5 oz	330
Mushrooms w. butter sce, 2oz	550
Peas, 1/2 cup, 3 oz	250
Sauerkraut, 1/2 cup, 4 oz	750

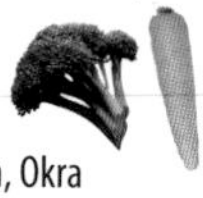
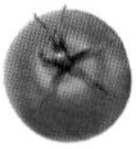
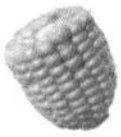
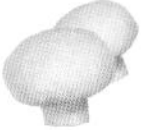

Pickles, Olives

Olives: pickled: Green, 1 large	90
Ripe/black, 1 large	40
Pickles: Bread & Butter, 4 slices, 1 oz	200
Dill, 1 pickle, 2.5oz	900
Sweet, 1 gherkin, 0.5 oz	130

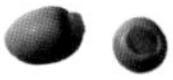
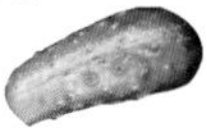

Soybean Products

Miso (Soy Paste), 1/4 c., 2.5 oz	2500
Soybean Protein Isolate, 1 oz	280
Tempeh, Natural, 1/2 cup, 3 oz	5
Tofu, average, 1/2 cup, 4 oz	5

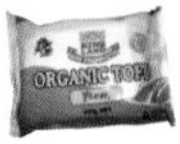

Jam, Honey, Syrups

Jam/Jelly, 1 Tbsp	2
Honey/Maple Syrup, 1 Tbsp	1
Log Cabin, Maple Syrup,2 Tbsp, 1 fl.oz	55
Syrup, Lite, 2 Tbsp, 1 fl.oz	95

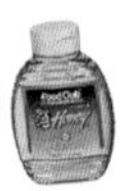

Peanut Butter

Peanut Butter: Regular, 2 Tbsp, 0.5 oz	190
Jif, Low Sodium, 2 Tbsp	65
Trader Joe's, Unsalted, 2 Tbsp	0

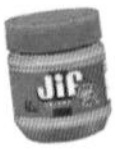

Snacks, Nuts

	Sodium
Cheese Balls/Curls, 1 oz	280
Cheetos, Cheddar Popcorn, 1 oz	260
Corn/Tortilla Chips: average, 1 oz	220
Fritos, Lightly Salted, 1 oz	80
Granola bars, average, 1 bar	80
Nuts: Plain, unsalted, 1 oz	1
Lightly salted, 1 oz	80
Salted or Honey Roasted, 1 oz	160
Popcorn: Plain (unsalted), 1 cup	1
Flavored, average, 1 cup	60
Salt added, 1 cup	180
Potato Chips: Plain, 1 oz	160
Lay's, Lightly Salted, 1 oz	65
Flavored, average, 1 oz	200
Pretzels: Regular, 3, 1 oz	450
Soft, salted, large	1000

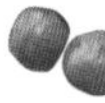
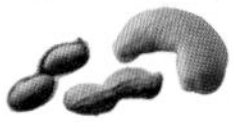
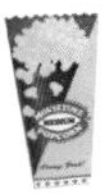
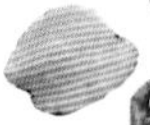
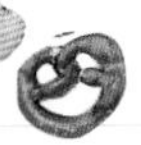
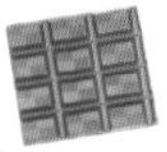

Candy, Chocolate

Chocolate, milk, 1 oz	30
Fudge, chocolate, 1 oz	55
Candy Bars, average, 1.5 oz	60
Hard Candy, 1 oz	10
Licorice, 1 oz	30

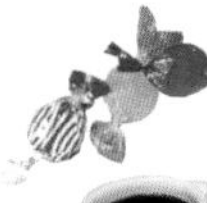

Beverages, Alcohol

Coffee or Tea, 1 cup	1
Cocoa: Dry, plain, 1 Tbsp	0
Mix, average, 1 envelope	120
Quik, 2 tsp	35
Soft Drinks, average, 8 fl.oz	20
Mineral Water: Perrier, 8 fl.oz	5
Gatorade, Thirst Quencher, 8 fl.oz	110
Red Bull: 8.4 fl.oz can	105
Sugar Free, 8.4 fl.oz	105
Water, Average, 1 cup, 8 fl.oz	5
Alcohol: Beer, average, 12 fl.oz	15
Wines, average, 4 fl.oz	10
Spirits (distilled), 1.5 fl.oz	1

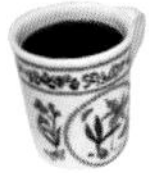
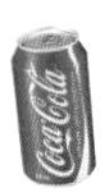

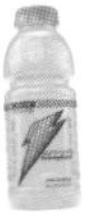

Antacids ~ Alka-Seltzer

	Sodium
Alka-Seltzer: *Per Tablet*	
Original; Heartburn	570
Extra Strength	590
Lemon Lime	500
Gold	310
Alka-Mints, chewable	0
Bromo Seltzer, 3/4 capful	760
Picot, 1 packet, 5g	670
Rolaids, All types	0
Tums, Regular/Extra Strength	0

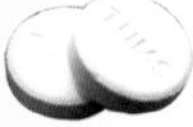

Cold & Flu ~ Alka-Seltzer Plus

Effervescents, average, 1 tablet	480
Fast Crystal Packs; Liquid Gels	0

Fast-Foods & Restaurants

Burger King:

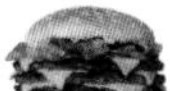
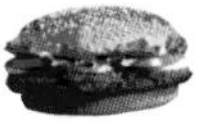

	Sodium
Bacon Double Cheeseburger	670
Cheeseburger	560
Double Stacker King	1871
Hamburger	385
Whoppers: Original	980
Triple with Cheesse	1475
Whopper Jr.	390
Impossible Whopper	1080
Chicken Sandwich, Original	1170
Sides: French Fries, medium, salted	570
Onion Rings, medium	1315
Breakfast, Ham, Egg & Cheese Croissan'wich	1000

Carl's Jr.:

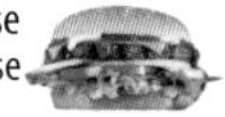

	Sodium
Burgers: Famous Star w/ Cheese	1270
Beyond Famous Star w/ Cheese	1600
The Big Carl	1380

Denny's:

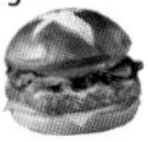
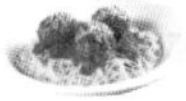
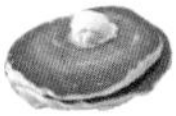

	Sodium
Burgers: Bacon Avocado Cheeseburger	1650
Slamburger	1780
Sandwiches: Club	2060
Mega Philly Cheese Melt	2120
Dinner: Brooklyn Spaghetti & Meatballs	2510
Premium Chicken Tenders	2360
Sides: Broccoli	110
Seasoned Fries	1110
Red-Skinned Potatoes	580
Breakfast: BlueberyPancakes (2)	1400
Moons Over My Hammy Omelette, w/ Hash	2200
Santa Fe Skillet	1700
Sides: Hash Browns, 1 serving	360
Sausages (2)	300

Jack In The Box:

	Sodium
Burgers: Bacon Ultimate Cheeseburger	1590
Jumbo Jack	580
Jumbo Jack Cheeseburger	990
Sandwiches: H'style Ranch Chicken Club	1869
Sourdough Grilled Chicken Club	1500

KFC:

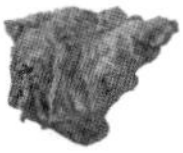
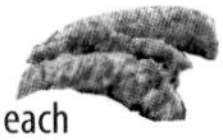
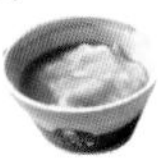

	Sodium
Chicken Breast: Original	1190
Extra Crispy	1150
Kentucky Grilled	710
Popcorn Nuggets, Large	1820
Sandwich, Crispy Twister	1260
Tenders, Extra Crispy Tenders, each	610
Wings, Nashville HotSpicy Crispy (1)	450
Sides: Macaroni & Cheese	590
Mashed Potatoes with Gravy	520
Potato Wedges	700

Fast-Foods & Restaurants

McDonalds:

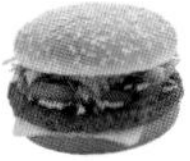
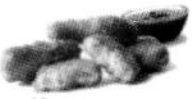
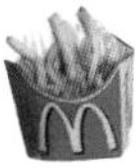
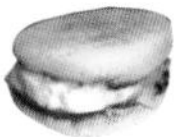

	Sodium
Burgers: Big Mac	1010
Cheeseburger	720
Double	1180
Hamburger	510
Quarter Pounder with Cheese	1150
Chicken McNuggets, 4 pieces	330
McChicken, Sandwich	560
French Fries: Small, 2.6 oz	180
Medium, 3.9 oz	260
Large, 5.9 oz	400
Ketchup, 1 package, 10g	90
Breakfast: Egg McMuffin	760
Big Breakfast	1490
Hash Browns, 2 oz	310
Hotcakes & Sausage	880
Sausage Burrito	800
Sausage McGriddles	990
Desserts/Shakes: Hot Fudge Sundae	180
Strawberry Banana Smoothie, medium	50

Pizza Hut:

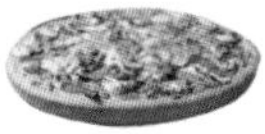

	Sodium
Original Pan Pizza: *Per Slice, Medium 12"*	
Meat Lovers	660
Cheese	450
Pepperoni Lover's	580
Supreme	500

Subway: *On 9 Grain Wheat Bread*

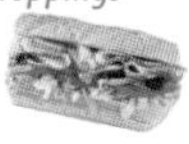
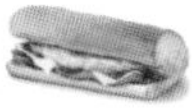

	Sodium
6" Sandwiches: *With Set Menu Toppings*	
Chicken Bacon Ranch Melt	1100
Meatball Marinara	1040
Spicy Italian	1240
6" Breakfast Flatbread S'wich: *With Set Menu Toppings*	
Bacon, Egg & Cheese	1200
Black Forest Ham, Egg & Chse	1180
Egg & Cheese	950
Steak, Egg & Cheese	1270

Taco Bell:

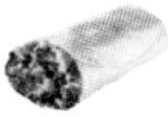
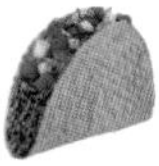

	Sodium
Burritos: Beefy 5-Layer	1250
Supreme, Chicken	1110
Chalupa Supreme, Chicken/Steak, av	545
Nachos: BellGrande, Chicken	1050
Steak	1030
Specialties, Cheese Quesadillas	990
Tacos: Soft Chicken	450
Crunchy Supreme	340

Index A - C

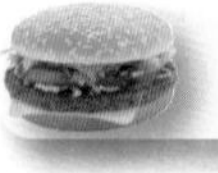

FAST-FOODS INDEX ~ PAGE 175 ~

D

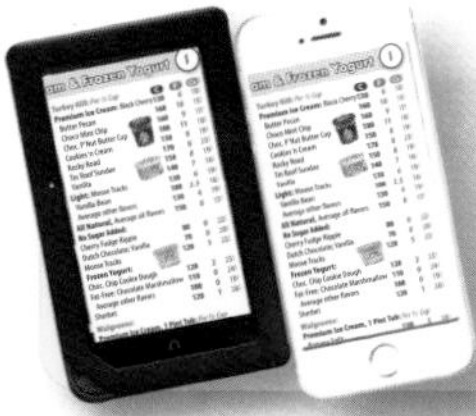

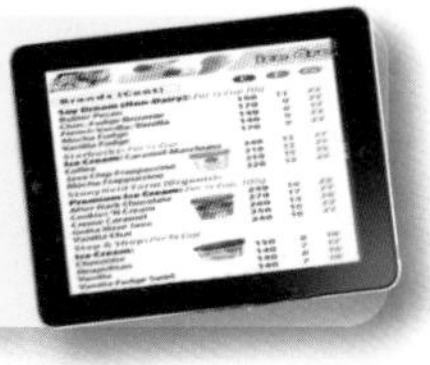

FAST-FOODS INDEX
~ PAGE 175 ~

Index P - S

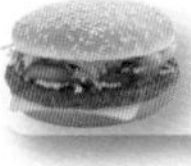

FAST-FOODS INDEX
~ PAGE 175 ~

Notes

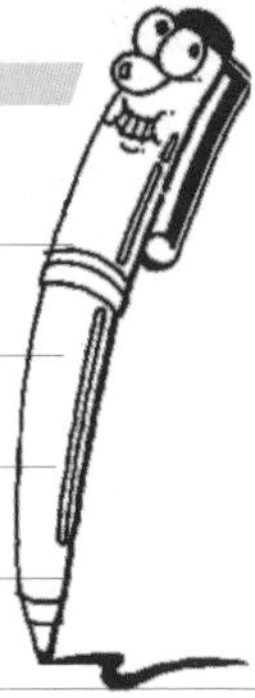